Glycerophospholipids in the

Akhlaq A. Farooqui and Lloyd A. Horrocks
Department of Molecular and Cellular Biochemistry,
The Ohio State University, Columbus, Ohio, U.S.A.

Glycerophospholipids in the Brain

Phospholipases A$_2$ in Neurological Disorders

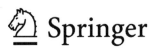 Springer

Akhlaq A. Farooqui
3120 Herrick Road
Columbus, OH 43221
USA

Lloyd A. Horrocks, Ph.D.
Department of Molecular and Cellular
   Biochemistry
The Ohio State University
Columbus, Ohio 43210-1218
USA
Horrocks.2@osu.edu

Library of Congress Control Number: 2006932152

ISBN-10: 0-387-36602-4
ISBN-13: 978-0387-36602-9

Printed on acid-free paper.

9 8 7 6 5 4 3 2 1

springer.com

Preface

Glycerophospholipids are amphipathic molecules that form the backbone of biological membranes, which are organized in bilayers and held together by hydrophobic, coulombic, and Van der Waal forces, and by hydrogen bonds. Biomembranes contain microdomains or lipid rafts that are rich in sphingolipids and cholesterol and serve as mobile platforms for signal transduction by clustering and organizing bilayer constituents including receptors, enzymes, and ion-channels. Thus, biomembranes are not simply inert physical barriers but are complex dynamic environments that regulate cellular function by modulating activities of membrane-bound enzymes, receptors, and ion channels.

Major advances in our understanding of signal transduction processes have occurred in last 20 years. A literature search on PubMed using the key word brain plus another key word illustrates the rapidly increasing interest in phospholipids and their metabolism in the brain (Table P-1). Although changes in the style of indexing at PubMed may skew these results, certainly the interest of researchers on phospholipids and phospholipases in the 5-year period increased at least 5-fold. The greatest increase was 14-fold for plasmalogen, indicating the realization of the very rapid turnover of these compounds and the role of choline plasmalogens (plasmenylcholine) as precursors of signaling molecules. We anticipate that this interest in research on brain phospholipids and phospholipases will continue at a rapid rate in coming years as more information on the composition of glycerophospholipid molecular species and the involvement of phospholipases in normal brain and the pathophysiology of neural trauma and neurodegenerative diseases becomes available.

Lipidomics and proteomics have emerged rapidly for the full characterization of the molecular species of phospholipids and for the enzymes associated with their metabolism. These techniques will be applied not only in whole brain, but also in neural membranes at cellular and subcellular levels as well as in biological fluids. These studies will help to understand the roles of phospholipid molecular species in gene expression, neural cell proliferation and differentiation, apoptosis, and maintenance of protein structure and function in normal brain, as well as in brain tissue from patients with neurological disorders. The phospholipases A_2 are a superfamily of enzymes that hydrolyze arachidonic acid and docosahexaenoic

TABLE P-1. PubMed search for papers with brain plus another keyword by year.

Other Keyword, Year	2000	2001	2002	2003	2004
Phospholipids	446	516	354	2871	5251
Phosphatidylcholine	136	141	79	714	1338
Plasmalogen	13	20	18	128	183
Phospholipase	268	293	236	763	2022
Phospholipases	186	211	171	594	1412
Phospholipase A$_2$	70	84	78	256	691
Phospholipase C	153	155	119	349	1092

This search was done on 31 March 2006.

acids from glycerophospholipids. These enzymes are involved in signal transduction, membrane homeostasis and remodeling, and neurodegeneration.

The main purpose of this book is to present readers with cutting edge information on glycerophospholipids and phospholipases A$_2$ and the generation of second messengers such as arachidonic and docosahexaenoic acids and their oxygenated metabolites (eicosanoids and docosanoids) in normal brain and brain from patients with neurological disorders. We attempt this in a form that is useful to students, teachers, and physicians, and to researchers in basic sciences, medicine, and the pharmaceutical industry. This book covers the involvement of phospholipases A$_2$ in neural trauma and neurodegenerative diseases and the therapeutic effects of phospholipase A$_2$ inhibitors in neurological disorders. These topics are of immense interest to neurochemists, neurologists, neuropharmacologists, and neurobiologists.

The book has 14 chapters. The first two chapters describe the metabolism of glycerophospholipids in brain, including those containing a vinyl ether group (plasmalogens). Chapters 3 and 4 cover innovative information on the properties and roles of phospholipases A$_2$ in the central nervous system. Chapters 5, 6, 7, 8, and 9 are devoted to the release of second messengers, such as arachidonic acid, docosahexaenoic acid, lyso glycerophospholipids, and lysophosphatidic acid, from neural membrane glycerophospholipids by phospholipases A$_2$ and their neurochemical effects on brain metabolism and function. Chapters 10 and 11 cover the involvement of phospholipases A$_2$ in neurological disorders, and the use of phospholipase A$_2$ inhibitors for the treatment of diseases associated with altered phospholipid metabolism. Chapter 12 describes the strengths and pitfalls of available methods for the assays of phospholipases A$_2$. Chapter 13 describes the association of phospholipases A$_2$ with neuropsychiatric disorders. Chapter 14 presents readers with future directions to follow to solve unresolved problems of brain phospholipid metabolism. Our choices of these topics are personal. They are based on our interests on phospholipid metabolism and phospholipases A$_2$ and on areas where major progress is being made. We hope that our attempt to consolidate the knowledge of glycerophospholipid metabolism and phospholipases A$_2$ in brain will provide the basis of more dramatic advances and developments on the roles of glycerophospholipid molecular species in the brain and on the consequences of altered glycerophospholipid metabolism in neurological disorders.

Akhlaq A Farooqui
Lloyd A Horrocks

Contents

Abbreviations

AA, arachidonic acid

DAG, diacylglycerol

Gpl, glycerophospholipid

Gro$P$Cho, *sn*-glycero-3-phosphocholine

Ins$P$, inositol monophosphate

InsP_2, inositol bisphosphate

InsP_3, inositol trisphosphate

Lyso-PtdCho, lysophosphatidylcholine

Lyso-PtdEtn, lysophosphatidylethanolamine

PtdGro, phosphatidylglycerol

PtdH, phosphatidic acid

PtdIns, phosphatidylinositol

PtdIns-4-P, phosphatidylinositol 4-phosphate

PtdIns-4,5-P_2, phosphatidylinositol 4,5-bisphosphate

PtdCho, phosphatidylcholine

PtdSer, phosphatidylserine

PlsEtn, ethanolamine plasmalogen, plasmenylethanolamine

PlsCho, choline plasmalogen, plasmenylcholine

Nomenclature of Glycerophospholipids

There is much confusion in the literature on phospholipids because shorthand abbreviations and the wrong nomenclature are used. The Nomenclature Commission of the International Union of Biochemistry and the International Union of Pure and Applied Chemistry issued rules for lipids in 1976 (IUPAC-IUB Commission on Biochemical Nomenclature, 1977; IUPAC-IUB Commission on Biochemical Nomenclature, 1978b; IUPAC-IUB Commission on Biochemical Nomenclature, 1978a; Fahy et al., 2005). The purpose of this section is to remind readers of these rules (Horrocks, 1989).

A phospholipid is a lipid containing phosphorus (P). A glycerophospholipid is a phospholipid containing glycerol (Gro). The term phosphoglycerides is not recommended. The stereospecific nomenclature of glycerophospholipids places the phosphate at the *sn*-3 position. Phosphatidyl, the radical of phosphatidic acid, is 1,2-diacyl-*sn*-glycero-3-phospho- (Ptd). Phosphatidylcholine is 1,2-diacyl-*sn*-glycero-3-phosphocholine (PtdCho). The majority of publications still use the ambiguous abbreviation PC for PtdCho. PC should be an impossible compound of carbon and phosphorus or it could be phosphocholine (*P*Cho). The *P* in italics is an approved abbreviation for the phosphate group. Table 1 gives some abbreviations.

Three classes of glycerophospholipids (Gpl) contain 2-acyl-*sn*-glycero-3-phosphocholine. In addition to 1,2-diacyl-*sn*-glycero-3-phosphocholine, there is 1-alk-1′-enyl-2-acyl-*sn*-glycero-3-phosphocholine (PlsCho, choline plasmalogen, plasmenylcholine) and 1-alkyl-2-acyl-*sn*-glycero-3-phosphocholine (PakCho), the precursor of platelet-activating factor, 1-alkyl-2-acetyl-*sn*-glycero-3-phosphocholine. The usual procedures of TLC or HPLC generally isolate these three classes together. It is not correct to designate the mixture of three classes as PtdCho or PC, because Ptd means two acyl groups in the molecule. The mixture should be named ChoGpl, choline glycerophospholipids. Plasmenyl is the radical 1-alk-1′-enyl-2-acyl-*sn*-glycero-3-phospho- (Pls). Plasmanyl is the official name for the radical 1-alkyl-2-acyl-*sn*-glycero-3-phospho-, which we abbreviate as Pak because there is no good three-letter abbreviation for plasmanyl.

TABLE 1. Abbreviations for constituents of phospholipids.

Cer	Ceramide
Cho	Choline
Etn	Ethanolamine
Gpl	Glycerophospholipid
Gro	Glycerol
Ins	Inositol
P	Phosphoric residue
Ser	Serine
Sph	Sphingosine

References

Fahy E., Subramaniam S., Brown H. A., Glass C. K., Merrill A. H. J., Murphy R. C., Raetz C. R. H., Russell D. W., Seyama Y., Shaw W., Shimizu T., Spener F., Van Meer G., VanNieuwenhze M. S., White S. H., Witztum J. L., and Dennis E. A. (2005). A comprehensive classification system for lipids. *J. Lipid Res.* 46:839–861.

Horrocks L. A. (1989). Nomenclature and structure of phosphatides. In: Szuhaj B. (ed.), *Lecithins: Sources, Manufacture and Uses*. Am. Oil Chemists' Soc., Champaign, IL, pp. 1–6.

IUPAC-IUB Commission on Biochemical Nomenclature (1977). The nomenclature of lipids. *Lipids* 12:455–468.

IUPAC-IUB Commission on Biochemical Nomenclature (1978a). Nomenclature of lipids. *J. Lipid Res.* 19:114–128.

IUPAC-IUB Commission on Biochemical Nomenclature (1978b). The nomenclature of lipids. *Biochem. J.* 171:21–35.

1
Phospholipid Metabolism in Brain

1.1 Introduction

Cellular membranes cannot exist without structural glycerophospholipids. They consist of a glycerol backbone, fatty acids, phosphoric acid, and a nitrogenous base. The membranes also contain cholesterol and sphingolipids. In glycerophospholipids, glycerol is esterified at carbon-3 (an α-carbon) with phosphoric acid and a nitrogenous base and at carbon atoms 1 and 2 with long chain fatty acids (Fig. 1.1). The phosphate at the α-carbon at the *sn*-3 position makes the glycerophospholipid molecule asymmetric.

Glycerophospholipids are amphipathic molecules with so-called polar and nonpolar ends. The polar end is the head group and the nonpolar end is the tail. The polar end is charged due to the ionization of the phosphate group and nitrogenous base and thus is hydrophilic. The polar ends face out toward the extracellular and intracellular spaces on either side of the hydrophobic inner area of the biomembrane. The nonpolar tail groups (fatty acyl, alkenyl, and alkyl chains) are hydrophobic and tend to aggregate in an aqueous environment. The degree of unsaturation in the long inward-pointing hydrocarbon tails of these molecules determines the membrane order, packing pattern, and fluidity. Thus, variations in the head group, length of the phospholipid acyl chains, and the degree of saturation produce changes in surface charge and physicochemical characteristics of neural membranes. Brain tissue contains relatively high amounts of glycerophospholipids. In adult brain, they account for 20 to 25% of the dry weight. In neural membranes, the glycerophospholipids, along with cholesterol and sphingolipids, represent approximately 50 to 60% of the total membrane mass with proteins accounting for most of the remainder.

Neural membranes contain two types of domains (Welti and Glaser, 1994; Wood et al., 2002; Lucero and Robbins, 2004). Synapses, gap junctions, and focal contacts represent the permanent membrane structural domains. Microdomains, also called lipid domains (lipid rafts), are less stable. In lipid domains, sphingolipids and cholesterol are segregated into glycerophospholipid-rich membrane areas (Brown and London, 1998a,b). Lipid domains play a crucial role in the expression and regulation of cellular membrane functions such as signaling,

1

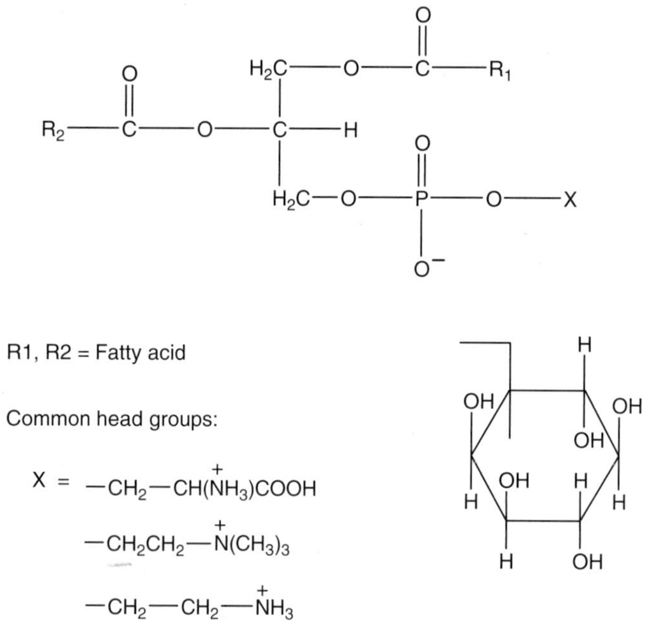

FIG. 1.1. Chemical structure of glycerophospholipids. R1 is mostly saturated fatty acid and R2 is mostly polyunsaturated fatty acid.

sorting, adhesion, and transport processes (Hooper, 1997; Wood et al., 2002; Pike, 2004). In addition, some lipid domains have the capacity to coalesce into larger domains called super-rafts or super-domains. These domains are involved in protein–protein interactions among proteins originally localized in different domains (Lucero and Robbins, 2004).

Caveolae are Ω-shaped membrane invaginations that are similar in composition to the lipid domains but contain a unique family of proteins, caveolins (Kurzchalia et al., 1992; Rothberg et al., 1992). They are involved in cell signaling, transcytosis, and in the regulation of cellular cholesterol homeostasis. The collective evidence suggests that lipid domains and caveolae are heterogeneous structures involved in modulation of membrane functions and cross talk between raft components (Lucero and Robbins, 2004; Pike, 2004).

Among the membranes of the brain, myelin contains the highest amount of glycerophospholipids. The major glycerophospholipids include ethanolamine plasmalogens and phosphatidylcholines. The phospholipid and molecular species compositions of myelin are very different from that of gray matter (Leray et al., 1994; Farooqui et al., 2000b).

Brain tissue has five major classes of glycerophospholipids. The first four classes, 1,2-diacyl glycerophospholipids, 1-alk-1′-enyl-2-acyl glycerophospholipids or plasmalogens, 1-alkyl-2-acyl glycerophospholipids, and phosphatidic acid, have a glycerol backbone with a fatty acid, usually unsaturated, at carbon-2 and a phosphobase (choline, ethanolamine, serine, or inositol) at carbon-3 of the glycerol moiety. The fifth class, of which the only representative is sphingomyelin, contains ceramide linked to phosphocholine through its primary hydroxyl group. These glycerophospholipids provide neural membranes with stability, fluidity, and permeability. They are also required for the proper function of integral membrane proteins, receptors, transporters, and ion-channels (Farooqui and Horrocks, 1985; Farooqui et al., 2000b).

1.2 Classes, Occurrence, and Distribution of Neural Glycerophospholipids

In biomembranes, glycerophospholipids are organized in bilayers that are held together by hydrophobic, coulombic, and van der Waal forces, and hydrogen bonds (Nagle and Tristram-Nagle, 2000). The most abundant glycerophospholipids in mammalian tissues are choline glycerophospholipids (ChoGpl), ethanolamine glycerophospholipids (EtnGpl), serine glycerophospholipids (SerGpl), and inositol glycerophospholipids (InsGpl). Each glycerophospholipid class may contain diacyl (PtdIns), alkylacyl (PakCho), or alkenylacyl types (PlsEtn), according to differences in the linkage of the hydrocarbon chain at the *sn*-1 position of the glycerol moiety, such as acyl, ether, and vinyl-ether bonds.

The number of unsaturated carbon–carbon bonds in the aliphatic groups at the *sn*-1 and *sn*-2 position of the glycerophospholipid is a key factor in determining the phase transition temperature and lateral diffusion velocity of membranes, thus playing important roles in events such as endo- and exocytosis, sorting of lipids, or membrane fusion.

Brain glycerophospholipids exhibit a high degree of heterogeneity with regard to molecular species, which results from the combination of the structures of the fatty chains at the *sn*-1 and *sn*-2 positions (Vecchini et al., 1997). Over 400 glycerophospholipid species with different structures can be identified in a single cell (Pearce and Komoroski, 2000; Farooqui et al., 2002; Isaac et al., 2003; Ivanova et al., 2004). In neural membranes each class of phospholipids exists as a heterogeneous mixture of molecular species (Isaac et al., 2003; Ivanova et al., 2004). The synthesis of different pools within a phospholipid subclass appears to be compartmentalized according to the fatty acid composition and the source of the head group (Farooqui et al., 2002). Each species contributes to the properties of the membrane. Presumably, the multiplicity of species is present for unique functional capabilities.

The distribution of phospholipids in neural membranes is normally asymmetric across the plane of the plasma membrane, with ethanolamine glycerophospholipids and phosphatidylserine (PtdSer) concentrated in the inner leaflet and choline glycerophospholipids and sphingomyelin concentrated in the outer leaflet (Freysz et al., 1982; Porcellati, 1983). This distribution of the membrane glycerophospholipids is quite stable. When the glycerophospholipids are redistributed so that PtdSer or PtdEtn is in the outer leaflet of the bilayer, an aminophospholipid translocase (flippase) restores the normal glycerophospholipid distribution (Daleke and Lyles, 2000; Pomorski et al., 2004). This maintenance of the normal composition of outer and inner leaflets requires 8% of the brain's consumption of ATP (Purdon and Rapoport, 1998).

In biomembranes, normal glycerophospholipid homeostasis is based on a balance between glycerophospholipid catabolism, resynthesis by reacylation, and de novo synthesis pathways (Porcellati, 1983). All of these processes of synthesis, reacylation, recycling of phosphoinositides, and maintenance of the inner and outer leaflets, requires up to 20% of the ATP consumed by brain (Purdon et al., 2002). Much of the remaining ATP maintains the distribution of ions.

As stated above, each class of phospholipid exists as a heterogeneous mixture of molecular species. The synthesis of different pools within a phospholipid subclass appears to be compartmentalized according to the fatty acid composition and the source of the head group (de novo synthesis versus modification and interconversion reactions) (Farooqui et al., 2000b). Thus, different pools of phospholipid molecular species may have different metabolic and physical properties depending upon their localization in different types of neural cells and membranes (Farooqui et al., 2000b, 2002). Neural membrane glycerophospholipids are rich in polyunsaturated fatty acids, which not only play a major role in determining many physical bilayer properties, such as phase transition temperature, bilayer thickness, area per molecule, acyl chain packing free volume, and lateral domains, but also serve other basic functions.

Receptors, enzymes, and ion-channels penetrate the glycerophospholipid bilayer in neural membranes to a varying degree. These protrude differentially through the membrane or are localized predominantly on the intracellular or extracellular membrane surface (Lee, 2003). Some membrane proteins connect with the intracellular cytoskeleton or extracellular matrix, restricting free diffusion of small molecules. Thus, proteins are dispersed like "icebergs in a sea of lipids" in the neural membranes (Pike, 2004). The interaction of an agonist with a receptor results in an enhancement of glycerophospholipid metabolism that results not only in the generation of second messengers, but also in the regulation of activities of membrane-bound enzymes, receptors, transporters, and ion-channels (Farooqui and Horrocks, 1985; Gagné et al., 1996; Farooqui et al., 2000b).

1.3 Biosynthesis of Neural Membrane Glycerophospholipids

Phosphatidic acid (PtdH) is an important intermediate, it being the main precursor of all neural membrane glycerophospholipids. It consists of glycerol-3-phosphate with long-chain fatty acids esterified at the *sn*-1 and *sn*-2 positions. The glycerophospholipid classes are defined based on the substituent at the *sn*-3 position of PtdH. PtdCho and PtdEtn are synthesized mainly via the CDP-choline or CDP-ethanolamine pathways (Kennedy cycle). This pathway involves three enzymic steps catalyzed by choline or ethanolamine kinases, phosphocholine or phosphoethanolamine cytidylyltransferases, and CDP-choline or CDP-ethanolamine:

1,2-diacylglycerol choline or ethanolamine phosphotransferases (Fig. 1.2). These enzymes are intracellular: choline and ethanolamine kinase are localized in cytosol, cytidylyltransferases are distributed between cytosol and membrane fractions, and phosphotransferases are integral membrane proteins that are predominantly present in endoplasmic reticulum (Vance, 1996; Ross et al., 1997; Mancini et al., 1999).

Among these reactions, the cytidylyltransferase reaction is the rate-limiting step for the CDP-choline and CDP-ethanolamine pathways. A novel mechanism that involves translocation of the enzyme between the cytosol and endoplasmic

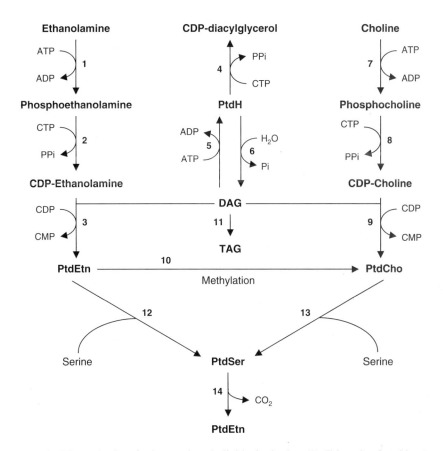

FIG. 1.2. Biosynthesis of glycerophospholipids in brain. (1) Ethanolamine kinase, (2) CTP: phosphoethanolamine cytidylyltransferase, (3) CDP-ethanolamine: 1,2-diacylglycerol phosphoethanolamine transferase, (4) Phosphatidate cytidylyltransferase, (5) Diacylglycerol kinase, (6) Phosphatidic acid phosphatase, (7) Choline kinase, (8) CTP: phosphocholine cytidylyltransferase, (9) CDP-choline: 1,2-diacylglycerol phosphocholine transferase, (10) Phosphatidylethanolamine N-methyltransferase, (11) Diacylglycerol acyltransferase, (12) and (13) Phosphatidylserine synthase, and (14) PtdSer-decarboxylase.

reticulum regulates non-neural cytidylyltransferase. The cytosolic cytidylyltransferase is inactive and the translocation of enzyme to endoplasmic reticulum results in its activation. The phosphorylation of cytidylyltransferase by cAMP-dependent kinase releases the enzyme from the membrane and renders it inactive (Kent, 1997). Subsequent dephosphorylation of the cytidylyltransferase renders it active by binding to endoplasmic reticulum membrane. To date, this type of regulation has not been observed with brain cytidylyltransferases (Araki and Wurtman, 1997). All these enzymes have been purified and characterized from several sources (Ishidate, 1997; Kent, 1997; McMaster and Bell, 1997a,b).

Cytidylyltransferases occur in multiple forms designated as CCT-α and CCT-β (Lykidis et al., 1998, 1999). Both isoforms have been purified. The CCT-α antibody does not cross react with CCT-β, indicating that these isoforms have different antigenic properties. Immunofluorescent microscopic studies indicate that CCT-α is localized in the nucleus, whereas CCT-β is located outside the cell nucleus. The CCT-α catalytic domain is a 50-amino acid amphipathic helix (domain M) with interfacial lysine residues that insert into membranes in response to activating lipids, such as fatty acids or diacylglycerols. These activating lipids increase membrane lateral packing stress or negative charge, resulting in domain M insertion into the bilayer (Attard et al., 2000). Among various tissues, brain has the highest level of CCT-β suggesting that this isoform may be actively involved in glycerophospholipid synthesis in brain.

Choline or ethanolamine phosphotransferases catalyze the final step of glycerophospholipid synthesis. These enzymes are mainly localized in the endoplasmic reticulum. They catalyze the transfer of phosphocholine or phosphoethanolamine to 1,2-diacylglycerol from CDP-choline or CDP-ethanolamine, with the release of CMP. Under physiological conditions, the synthesis of PtdCho or PtdEtn is favored because of the very rapid rephosphorylation of CMP to CTP that requires ATP.

The occurrence of choline phosphotransferase in the nuclear envelope suggests that the nucleus may be an important site for PtdCho synthesis during differentiation. Based on topographical studies, the choline phosphotransferase may be located on the outer leaflet with the ethanolamine phosphotransferase situated on the inner leaflet, or they have transmembrane localization in the brain microsomal vesicle (Freysz et al., 1982). When labeled CDP-choline and CDP-ethanolamine are used, isolated neuronal cells have a markedly higher activity (5- to 10-fold) of choline and ethanolamine glycerophospholipid synthesis compared to glial cells. This suggests that glial cells are less efficient than neurons in synthesizing these lipids (Binaglia et al., 1973).

The repeated methylation of PtdEtn with S-adenosylmethionine is another pathway for the synthesis of PtdCho. PtdEtn N-methyltransferase activity is associated with the endoplasmic reticulum and mitochondria. Purification and characterization of two methyltransferases has been reported from rat liver (Zachowski, 1993; Vance et al., 1997; Ilincheta de Boschero et al., 2000). PtdEtn methylation occurs in rat brain (Mozzi and Porcellati, 1979; Blusztajn et al., 1979; Dainous et al., 1982; Horrocks et al., 1986). It should be recognized here that brain is a very heterogeneous tissue and that PtdEtn methylation is higher in glial cells than in neurons (Tsvetnitsky et al., 1995). Myelin contains an intrinsic PtdEtn methyltransferase activity that plays an important role in the maintenance of the myelin structure. Decreased levels of S-adenosylmethionine are associated with demyelinating diseases (Bottiglieri and Hyland, 1994).

A minor pathway for the synthesis of PtdEtn involves the decarboxylation of serine glycerophospholipids. This enzyme has been purified, characterized, and cloned (Voelker, 1997).

PtdCho and PtdEtn contain more than one kind of fatty acid per molecule, so that a given class of these glycerophospholipids from any tissue actually represents a family of molecular species. In the PC12 cell cultures undergoing neurite outgrowth, the activity of CDP-choline: 1,2-diacylglycerol choline phosphotransferase, was increased by 50% after nerve growth factor treatment (Araki and Wurtman, 1997). In chicken brain, the specific activity of CDP-choline: 1,2-diacylglycerol choline phosphotransferase increases during embryonic development in parallel with the quantity of PtdCho (Freysz et al., 1972). Thus, PtdCho synthesis in brain tissue is dependent upon the availability of diacylglycerols. Based on various incorporation and enzymic studies, the composition of the diacylglycerols may be just as important as the specificity of biosynthetic enzymes for the synthesis of neural membrane glycerophospholipids (Porcellati, 1983).

In nervous tissue, PtdSer is synthesized exclusively by base-exchange (Mozzi et al., 2003; Buratta et al., 2004). The base-exchange reaction between PtdEtn and serine is initiated by an attack on the phosphodiester bond of PtdEtn or PtdCho by the hydroxyl group of serine. In the mitochondrial membrane, PtdCho is the major substrate for PtdSer synthesis. As there is no net change in the number or kind of bonds, this reaction is reversible and energy-independent. Phosphatidylserine synthases I and II catalyze the base-exchange reaction. Their activity is localized in endoplasmic reticulum and stimulated by Ca^{2+}. The base-exchange enzymes have been purified and cloned (Vance, 1996; Kuge and Nishijima, 1997; Ilincheta de Boschero et al., 2000; Vance and Vance, 2004).

The biosynthesis of PtdIns involves several enzymes. CDP-diacylglycerol synthase, an enzyme that catalyzes the biosynthesis of CDP-diacylglycerol, is localized in the endoplasmic reticulum for PtdIns synthesis and in mitochondria for synthesis of phosphatidylglycerol including cardiolipin (Heacock and Agranoff, 1997). PtdIns is synthesized by a reaction between CDP-diacylglycerol and inositol. Phosphatidylinositol synthase that is located in endoplasmic reticulum catalyzes this reaction. This enzyme has been purified, characterized, and cloned (Antonsson, 1997). In addition to de novo synthesis, an exchange reaction in which free *myo*-inositol is incorporated into phosphatidylinositol in the presence of manganese ions also synthesizes PtdIns.

Brain tissue contains several different phosphorylated forms of PtdIns (Table 1.1). They include PtdIns-4-P, PtdIns-4,5-P_2, PtdIns-3-P, PtdIns-3,4-P_2, and PtdIns-3,4,5-P_3 (Irvine, 1995; Tolias and Cantley, 1999). The most abundant of these are PtdIns-4-P and PtdIns-4,5-P_2. The kinases that catalyze the synthesis of PtdIns-4-P and PtdIns-4,5-P_2 (phosphatidylinositol kinase and phosphatidyl-4-phosphate kinase) have been purified and characterized from brain (Gehrmann

TABLE 1.1. PtdIns-kinases involved in the biosynthesis of phosphorylated phosphoinositides.

Substrate	Enzyme	Product	References
PtdIns	PtdIns-3-kinase	PtdIns-3-P	Fruman et al., 1998
PtdIns	PtdIns-4-kinase	PtdIns-4-P	Nakagawa et al., 1996
PtdIns	PtdIns-5-kinase	PtdIns-5-P	Tolias et al., 1998
PtdIns-3-P	PtdIns-5-kinase	PtdIns-3,5-P_2	Tolias et al., 1998
PtdIns-3-P	PtdIns-4-kinase	PtdIns-3,4-P_2	Tolias et al., 1998
PtdIns-5-P	PtdIns-3-kinase	PtdIns-3,5-P_2	Tolias et al., 1998
PtdIns-4-P	PtdIns-5-kinase	PtdIns-4,5-P_2	Rameh et al., 1997
PtdIns-5-P	PtdIns-4-kinase	PtdIns-4,5-P_2	Rameh et al., 1997
PtdIns-4-P	PtdIns-3-kinase	PtdIns-3,4-P_2	Carter et al., 1994
PtdIns-4,5-P_2	PtdIns-3-kinase	PtdIns-3,4,5-P_3	Carter et al., 1994
PtdIns-3,4-P_2	PtdIns-5-kinase	PtdIns-3,4,5-P_3	Stephens et al., 1991

et al., 1996; Nakagawa et al., 1996). Phosphatidylinositol-3-kinase is a multi-functional kinase that phosphorylates the D-3 position of PtdIns to produce PtdIns-3-P (Fukui et al., 1998). The addition of growth factors activates it and is responsible for the generation of second messengers involved in rearrangement of the cytoskeleton.

Interest in the phosphorylated forms of PtdIns rose immensely (Fig. 1.3) because they are substrates for hormone and growth factor-regulated phospholipase C. Their hydrolysis generates diacylglycerols and inositol polyphosphates that are well-known second messengers of neural cells (Bleasdale et al., 1985). In addition to its role as a second messenger-generating phospholipid, PtdIns-4,5-P_2 modulates the activity of several proteins, such as μ-calpain (Saido et al., 1992), ADP-ribosylation factor (Randazzo and Kahn, 1994), and Akt kinase/protein kinase B (Goswami et al., 2000). It also binds to actin regulatory proteins, such as profilin, cofilin, and gelsolin and inhibits their function (Takenawa et al., 1999). The collective evidence suggests that the interaction of PtdIns-4,5-P_2 with actin and regulatory proteins stimulates the development of stress fibers. A decreased level of PtdIns-4,5-P_2 leads to the depolymerization of actin. Therefore, changes in phosphorylated inositol glycerophospholipids not only influence second messenger generation, but also influence a variety of cellular processes including exocytosis, cytoskeletal reorganization, apoptosis, and membrane trafficking (Yin and Janmey, 2003).

1.4 Incorporation of Glycerophospholipids into Neural Membranes

Synthesis of glycerophospholipids occurs at the endoplasmic reticulum. Involvement of the endoplasmic reticulum in glycerophospholipid synthesis is dominant but not exclusive, because other subcellular organelles, such as the Golgi apparatus and mitochondria also synthesize glycerophospholipids with significant rates (Fang et al., 1998; Voelker, 2003; Vance and Vance, 2004). The

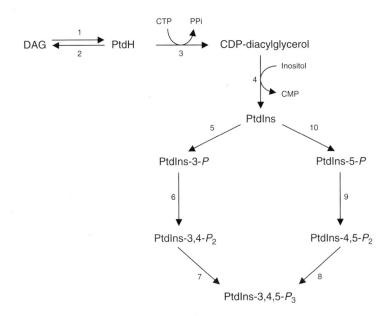

FIG. 1.3. Pathways showing phosphoinositide interconversion reactions. The continuous phosphorylation/dephosphorylation reactions allow a steady-state levels of PtdIns, PtdIns-4-P, PtdIns-4,5-P_2, and PtdIns-3,4,5-P_3. The cleavage of PtdIns-4,5-P_2 results in formation of Ins-1,4,5-P_3 and diacylglycerol (DAG). (1) DAG-kinase, (2) Phosphatidic acid phosphatase, (3) CDP-DAG synthase, (4) PtdIns synthase, (5) PtdIns-3-kinase, (6) PtdIns-3-P 4-kinase, (7) PtdIns-3,4-P_2 5-kinase, (8) PtdIns-4,5-P_2 3-kinase, (9) Type II PtdIns 4-kinase and (10) Type I PtdIns 5-kinase.

newly synthesized glycerophospholipids self-assemble into thermodynamically stable bimolecular layers. These layers form vesicles that detach from the endoplasmic reticulum and travel to other sites for donation of their glycerophospholipids to other membranous structures. This process involves spontaneous transfer of glycerophospholipid to other membranes and transport of glycerophospholipid molecules by phospholipid transfer proteins (Alb, Jr. et al., 1996; Voelker, 2003). Some glycerophospholipid transfer proteins are specific and others are not (Wirtz, 1997; Frayne et al., 1999; Komatsu et al., 2003). Multiple vesicular carriers exist with distinct mechanisms for the transfer of glycerophospholipids between subcellular compartments (Moreau and Cassagne, 1994; Voelker, 2004). Studies dealing with the transfer of glycerophospholipids from the endoplasmic reticulum to the mitochondria also indicate the importance of the spatial organization of the endoplasmic reticulum and the existence of specific proximity between various organelles (Pomorski et al., 2004).

Other important factors that affect the transfer of glycerophospholipids to other membranes are the occurrence of specific membrane domains and a sorting mechanism for glycerophospholipids (Sandra et al., 1993; Voelker, 2004). In general, glycerophospholipid sorting mechanisms are modulated by (a) microdomains,

(b) preferential partitioning of synthesized lipids into membrane regions of a certain curvature, and (c) preferential participation of synthesized lipids in specific protein–lipid or lipid–lipid interaction. An active transfer of glycerophospholipids between outer and inner leaflets occurs against concentration and electrical gradients by an enzymic mechanism (aminophospholipid transferase and flippases) (Pomorski et al., 2004). This process uses ATP to overcome the gradients. The nonenzymic transfer movement of glycerophospholipids from one side to the other (flip-flop movement) also occurs, but it is slow and measured in days or weeks. Thus, the distribution of glycerophospholipids in biomembranes is regulated not only by the activities of enzymes involved in their metabolism but also by the processes of transport and incorporation into the membrane (Pomorski et al., 2004).

1.5 Effect of Structural Variations of Glycerophospholipids on Neural Membrane Structure

Glycerophospholipids perform important functions in neural membranes. Certain sets of glycerophospholipids are selected for each membrane to give it unique characteristics suited to its role. These characteristics include membrane fluidity, permeability, local curvature, molecular packing or hydration, charge, and ability to regulate the activities of membrane-bound enzymes and ion-channels (Crews, 1982; Freysz et al., 1982). These characteristics are not the properties of individual glycerophospholipid classes but properties of an organized neural membrane as a whole. As all membranes possess a typical composition with more or less the same classes of glycerophospholipids, the ratios between these classes and their molecular species are unique and provide membranes from different organelles with specific characteristics (Van Meer, 1989; Farooqui et al., 2000b, 2002). In addition, most membranes from different organelles have some glycerophospholipid synthesizing activities (interconversion reactions).

Glycerophospholipids undergo a rapid deacylation–reacylation process involving phospholipase A_2 and acyltransferases (Sun and MacQuarrie, 1989; Farooqui et al., 2000a), resulting in continuous shuttling of fatty acids between different glycerophospholipid subclasses. The deacylation–reacylation cycle is responsible for the introduction of polyunsaturated fatty acids into glycerophospholipids. In this cycle, a glycerophospholipid is hydrolyzed by phospholipase A_2 generating a lysophospholipid that is rapidly re-esterified with another fatty acid. Thus in the unstimulated nerve cell, the availability of the lysophospholipid acceptor is a limiting factor for the acyl-CoA: lysophospholipid acyltransferase catalyzed reactions (Sun and MacQuarrie, 1989). The deacylation–reacylation cycle is an important mechanism for controlling the saturated and polyunsaturated glycerophospholipid acyl group composition in neural membranes (Yamashita et al., 1997).

Comparisons of molecular species in the choline, ethanolamine, and serine glycerophospholipids in synaptosomal plasma membranes (SPM) and myelin from the cerebral cortex of adult rats show important differences. SPM contain more polyunsaturated fatty acids than myelin, but comparisons of various glycerophospholipid classes show differences that are more interesting. Thus, ethanolamine and serine glycerophospholipids contain more of the docosahexaenoic acid, 22:6(n-3), in SPM than in myelin, and choline glycerophospholipids in SPM contain more saturated fatty acids. The 18:1 content of all three lipid classes is much higher in myelin than in SPM, whereas the 20:4(n-6) content is higher in ethanolamine glycerophospholipids and lower in serine glycerophospholipids (Porcellati, 1983). Studies on the composition of glycerophospholipids in various membranes are still in a developing state. To reconstruct a membrane composition found in vivo under physiological conditions, one has to determine the glycerophospholipid composition expressed in terms of mol/surface area for a specific membrane in a particular subcellular organelle of a specific tissue. Moreover, most studies to date are on membrane fractions that are frequently contaminated with membranes from other organelles.

Head group asymmetry determines the surface charge on glycerophospholipids. PtdSer and PtdIns are strongly anionic, PtdEtn is slightly anionic, and PtdCho and sphingomyelin are zwitterionic at neutral pH. The ratio of strongly anionic to zwitterionic glycerophospholipids varies widely between cell types, but is usually constant for a particular cell type among different species. Cations like Ca^{2+} and Mg^{2+} bind to anionic head groups at the inner half of the lipid bilayer. They can increase bilayer rigidity and induce lateral segregation of glycerophospholipids. Neural membranes therefore may act as a sink for those cations that can be released because of membrane perturbation. This process may be involved in many disease processes that are characterized by alterations in properties of neural membranes and levels of cations, such as Ca^{2+}, Mg^{2+}, and Fe^{3+} (Hall, 1992; Regan and Guo, 1998).

Neural membranes are also vulnerable to oxidative damage because membrane glycerophospholipids are rich in polyunsaturated fatty acids. Furthermore, the brain is rich in iron ions and surrounded by cerebrospinal fluid with little or no iron-binding capacity. Free radicals are formed in small amounts by normal cellular processes (Halliwell, 1994). The polyunsaturated fatty acid at the sn-2 position is most susceptible to free radical attack at the α-methylene carbon that is adjacent to the carbon–carbon double bond. The lipid hydroperoxides thus formed are not completely stable in vivo and, in the presence of iron, can further decompose to radicals that can propagate the chain reactions started by an initial free radical attack. Lipid hydroperoxides also generate aldehydes that can in turn cross-link enzymes and proteins making them inactive. The damage to neural membranes induced by lipid peroxidation has many potential consequences. These include: (a) changes in physicochemical properties of neural membranes (microviscosity) resulting in alterations in the orientation of optimal domains for the interaction of functional membrane proteins, such as receptors, enzymes, and ion-channels, (b) changes in the number of receptors and their affinity for neurotransmitters and drugs, and (c) inhibition of ion pump operation resulting in changes in ion homeostasis. The presence of peroxidized glycerophospholipids in neural membranes may also produce a membrane-packing defect, making the *sn*-2 ester bond more accessible to the action of PLA$_2$. In fact, glycerophospholipid hydroperoxides are better substrates for PLA$_2$ than are the native glycerophospholipids (McLean et al., 1993). The hydrolysis of peroxidized glycerophospholipids results in removal of peroxidized fatty acyl chains, which are reduced and re-esterified. Thus, the action of PLA$_2$ repairs and restores the physiological physicochemical state of neural membranes.

1.6 Catabolism of Neural Membrane Glycerophospholipids

Brain tissue actively catabolizes glycerophospholipids. Each portion of the glycerophospholipid molecule turns over at a different rate. Turnover rates of the phosphate group are different from those of the nitrogenous base and acyl groups at the *sn*-1 and *sn*-2 positions (Farooqui and Horrocks, 1985; Farooqui et al., 2000b). A group of enzymes called phospholipases hydrolyzes glycerophospholipids. Phospholipase A$_1$ (PLA$_1$) catalyzes the hydrolysis of the ester bond at the *sn*-1 position forming free fatty acids and a 2-acyl lysophospholipid. Phospholipase A$_2$ (PLA$_2$) acts on the fatty acid ester bond at the *sn*-2 position liberating free fatty acids and a 1-acyl lysophospholipid, which in turn can be acylated by acyl-CoA in the presence of acyltransferase. Alternatively, a lysophospholipase can hydrolyze a 1-acyl lysoglycerophospholipid forming fatty acids and a glycerophosphobase. Phospholipase C (PLC) hydrolyzes the phosphodiester bond at the *sn*-3 position forming 1,2-diacylglycerol and a phosphobase. Finally, phospholipase D (PLD) cleaves a glycerophospholipid into phosphatidic acid and a free base (Fig. 1.4). Phospholipases A$_1$, A$_2$, C, and D have been purified and characterized from

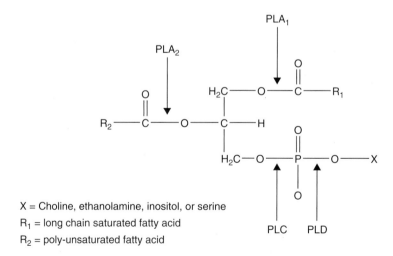

X = Choline, ethanolamine, inositol, or serine
R$_1$ = long chain saturated fatty acid
R$_2$ = poly-unsaturated fatty acid

Fɪɢ. 1.4. Site of action of phospholipases A$_1$, A$_2$, C and D on the glycerophospholipid molecule.

brain tissue (Hirashima et al., 1992; Rhee and Choi, 1992; Ross et al., 1995; Negre-Aminou et al., 1996; Pete and Exton, 1996; Exton, 1997, 1999; Yang et al., 1999; Farooqui et al., 2000c). All these enzymes occur in brain tissue in multiple forms. Many isoforms of PLC and PLD have been cloned from brain (Cheng et al., 1995; Park et al., 1997).

In neural membranes, PtdCho, PtdEtn, PtdSer, and PtdIns are hydrolyzed by specific PLA$_2$ activities (Farooqui et al., 1997b, 2000c). Lysophospholipids generated by the action of PLA$_1$ and PLA$_2$ are either hydrolyzed by a lysophospholipase, or used to regenerate phospholipids in the remodeling pathway (Farooqui et al., 2000a).

Mammalian brain phospholipases are part of a signal transduction network. *Cross-talk* between receptor-regulated effector systems through the generated second messengers (Fig. 1.5) is essential for maintaining normal neuronal and glial cell growth (Farooqui et al., 1992, 2004a). Suggestions on *cross-talk* between intracellular phospholipases A$_1$, A$_2$, C, and D are supported by the observation that all these enzymes can be stimulated by the same agonist and the products of one phospholipase can participate in the activation of others (Clark et al., 1995). Thus the stimulation of PLC generates diacylglycerol, which translocates and activates protein kinase C (PKC), leading to the activation of both PLA$_2$ and PLD. The other product of the PLC catalyzed reaction PtdIns(4,5)P_2, also stimulates PLA$_2$

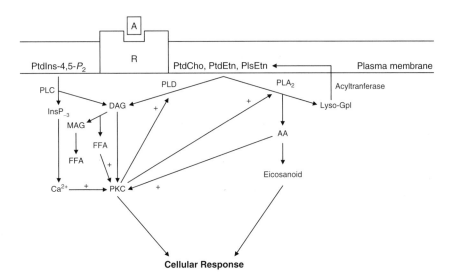

FIG. 1.5. Scheme showing the receptor-mediated degradation of neural membrane phospholipids by phospholipases A$_2$, C, and D. PtdIns 4,5-P_2, phosphatidylinositol 4,5-bisphosphate; PtdCho, phosphatidylcholine; PtdEtn, phosphatidylethanolamine; PlsEtn, ethanolamine plasmalogen; InsP_3, inositol 1,4,5-trisphosphate; DAG, diacylglycerol; FFA, free fatty acid, AA, arachidonic acid; Lyso-Gpl, lysoglycerophospholipids; MAG, monoacylglycerol; Ca^{2+}, intracellular calcium; PKC, protein kinase C.

(Hirabayashi et al., 2004) and inhibits PLD (Pasquare et al., 2004). Similarly, activation of PLA$_2$ generates arachidonic acid and eicosanoids. These second messengers activate PLD (Klein et al., 1995). Second messengers generated by PLA$_2$, PLC, and PLD are involved in modulation of neuronal plasticity through various pathways in different types of neural cells (Sun et al., 2004).

1.7 Phospholipid Metabolism in the Nucleus

Total phospholipid contents of nuclei are about 3% by weight, compared with 75% for protein and 22% for DNA. Nuclear phospholipids include phosphatidylinositol (PtdIns), phosphatidylcholine (PtdCho), and sphingomyelin (CerPCho) (Hunt et al., 2001; Irvine, 2003; Hammond et al., 2004). The nucleus also contains trace amounts of phosphatidylethanolamine (PtdEtn). This contrasts with the plasma membranes that contain considerable amounts of PtdCho, PtdEtn, PtdSer, and PtdIns (Hunt et al., 2001; Irvine, 2003). The phospholipid contents (per mg protein) of the nuclear membrane are approximately nine times that of whole nuclei. Although significant information is available on proportions of molecular species in plasma membranes (Farooqui et al., 2000b, 2002), very little is known about the phospholipid molecular species in the nucleus (Hunt et al., 2001).

Nuclear phospholipid metabolism is sensitive to differentiation and proliferation stimuli (Martelli et al., 2004b). During these processes, the quantitative ratios among phospholipids undergo significant changes depending upon the functional state of neurons, macroglia, and microglia and are modulated by interactions among them (Ledeen and Wu, 2004). Thus nuclear phospholipids have a composition and turnover different from those present in plasma membranes, microsomes, and mitochondria (Martelli et al., 1999, 2004b; Albi and Magni, 2004). Nuclear inositol polyphosphates serve as essential co-factors for several nuclear processes, including DNA repair, transcription regulation, and RNA dynamics (Hammond et al., 2004). Inositol polyphosphates in the nucleus represent high turnover activity switches for nuclear events.

Isolated nuclei contain several enzymes of phospholipid metabolism (Table 1.2). These include phosphatidylinositol synthetase (Baker and Chang, 1990b), acyl-*sn*-glycero-3-phosphate acyl transferase (Baker and Chang, 1990a), CTP: phosphocholine cytidylyltransferase (Morand and Kent, 1989), diacylglycerol acyltransferase (Baker and Chang, 1987), lysophosphatidic acid phosphohydrolase (Baker and Chang, 1990a,b), diacylglycerol kinase (Payrastre et al., 1992; Hozumi et al., 2003), sphingosine kinase (Kleuser et al., 2001), acetyltransferase (Baker and Chang, 1997), monoacylglycerol lipase (Baker and Chang, 1990a), phosphatidylinositol-specific phospholipase C (Payrastre et al., 1992; Albi et al., 2003), phospholipase A$_2$ (Antony et al., 2001, 2003), phospholipase D (Kanfer et al., 1996; Antony et al., 2001, 2003), phosphatidic acid phosphatase (Kanfer et al., 1996), and a magnesium-dependent neutral sphingomyelinase (Tamiya-Koizumi et al., 1989; Tamiya-Koizumi, 2002).

TABLE 1.2. Phospholipid metabolizing enzymes involved in generation and modulation of phospholipid metabolism in the nucleus.

Enzyme	References
Phosphatidylinositol synthetase	Baker and Chang, 1990b
Acyl-sn-glycero-3-phosphate acyltransferase	Baker and Chang, 1990a
CTP: phosphocholine cytidylyltransferase	Morand and Kent, 1989
Diacylglycerol acyltransferase	Baker and Chang, 1987
Lysophosphatidic acid phosphohydrolase	Baker and Chang, 1990a,b
Diacylglycerol kinase	Payrastre et al., 1992; Hozumi et al., 2003
Sphingosine kinase	Kleuser et al., 2001
Acetyltransferase	Baker and Chang, 1997
Diacylglycerol lipase	Farooqui and Horrocks, 2004
Monoacylglycerol lipase	Baker and Chang, 1990a,b; Farooqui and Horrocks, 2004
Phosphatidylinositol-specific phospholipase C	Martelli et al., 2004b
Phosphatidylcholine-specific phospholipase C	Albi and Viola, 1999; Antony et al., 2000
Isoforms of phospholipases A_2	Antony et al., 2001; Farooqui and Horrocks, 2004
Phospholipase D	Kanfer et al., 1996; Antony et al., 2003
Phosphatidic acid phosphatase	Kanfer et al., 1996
Mg^{2+}-dependent neutral sphingomyelinase	Tamiya-Koizumi et al., 1989; Tamiya-Koizumi, 2002
Phosphatidylinositol 4-kinase	Payrastre et al., 1992
CDP-choline: 1,2-diacylglycerol phosphocholine transferase	Fernández-Tome et al., 2004
PtdIns 3-, 4-, and 5-kinases	Martelli et al., 2004b; Payrastre et al., 1992

The second messengers generated by these enzymes modulate neural cell proliferation, differentiation, and apoptosis. These processes involve a coordinated expression of different genes along with alterations in activities of protein kinases, phospholipases, and protein phosphatases. During these processes the quantitative ratios among various phospholipids undergo significant changes depending upon the functional state of neurons, astrocytes, and oligodendrocytes, and are modulated by interaction among them (Lang et al., 1995; D'Santos et al., 1998; Farooqui et al., 2000b, 2002). Some extracellular stimuli (such as retinoic acid) produce bioactive lipid metabolites (such as diacylglycerol and arachidonic acid) only in the nucleus and not in the plasma membrane. Thus, in normal brain, agonist-mediated alterations in nuclear fraction are not a duplication of those changes that occur at the plasma membrane level (Martelli et al., 1999, 2002b, 2004b; Cocco et al., 2001). Furthermore, the enzymic properties of phospholipid metabolizing enzymes in the nuclear fraction are different from those found in plasma membrane, microsomes, and cytoplasm (Martelli et al., 2002b). For example, bombesin, a powerful mitogen, stimulates phosphoinositide metabolism at the plasma membrane level, but has no effect on phosphoinositide metabolism in the nucleus (Martelli et al., 2004a). Furthermore, insulin growth factor-1 (IGF-1) stimulates DAG-kinase activity in the nucleus, but not in whole homogenate (Martelli et al., 2004b).

1.8 Roles of Glycerophospholipids in Brain Metabolism

Besides being an integral component of neural membranes, glycerophospholipids have many other important functions (Fig. 1.6). They are dynamic molecules whose specific distribution and catabolism are the result of highly regulated processes that can lead to a host of important biological responses during signal transduction. Glycerophospholipids are involved in the following processes.

1.8.1 Glycerophospholipids as a Storage Depot for Second Messengers and Their Precursors

Glycerophospholipids are a reservoir for the generation of many bioactive mediators (Dennis et al., 1991; Exton, 1994; Farooqui et al., 1995, 1997b, 2000c). The activation of a single membrane receptor by an agonist (hormone, growth factor, or neurotransmitter) results in the stimulation of phospholipases and initiates a complex intracellular signaling cascade, as evidenced by the generation of various lipid second messengers (Fig. 1.3 and Table 1.3). This complexity is further enhanced by the fact that the synthesis of one messenger, depending on the time interval following receptor activation, involves different glycerophospholipid substrates and metabolic pathways (see below).

1.8.1a PLA$_2$-Generated Second Messengers

Arachidonic acid that is liberated by the action of PLA$_2$ on glycerophospholipids has been implicated both in physiological and pathological processes (Dennis

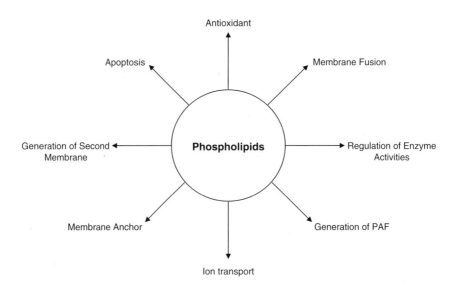

FIG. 1.6. Proposed roles of glycerophospholipids in neural membranes.

TABLE 1.3. Second messengers produced by the action of phospholipases on glycerophospholipids.

Phospholipids	Phospholipase	Second messengers	References
PtdCho, PtdEtn, PtdIns	A_2	Arachidonate, Eicosanoids, PAF	Dennis et al., 1991; Farooqui et al., 1997b; Farooqui and Horrocks, 2004
PtdIns	C	Diacylglycerol, Ins(1,4,5)P_3	Dennis et al., 1991; Exton, 1994
PlsEtn, PlsCho	A_2	Arachidonate, Eicosanoids, PAF	Farooqui et al., 1995
PtdCho	D	PtdH, Lyso-PtdH	Exton, 1997

Abbreviations used: Phosphatidylcholine (PtdCho), phosphatidylethanolamine (PtdEtn), phosphatidylserine (PtdSer), phosphatidylinositol (PtdIns), platelet-activating factor (PAF), choline plasmalogen (PlsCho), ethanolamine plasmalogen (PlsEtn), N-acylethanolamines (NAE), arachidonic acid (AA), cytidine monophosphate (CMP), cytidine triphosphate (CTP), adenosine triphosphate (ATP), phospholipase A_1 (PLA$_1$), phospholipase A_2 (PLA$_2$), phospholipase C (PLC), phospholipase D (PLD), protein kinase C (PKC), phosphatidylinositol 4,5-bisphosphate (PtdIns-4,5-P_2), inositol 1,4,5-trisphosphate (Ins-1,4,5-P_3), diacylglycerol (DAG), reactive oxygen species (ROS), low-density lipoprotein (LDL), synaptosomal plasma membrane (SPM).

et al., 1991; Farooqui et al., 1997a,b). For example, it modulates ion-channels and regulates the activity of protein kinases A and C, NADPH oxidase, DAG-kinase, and Na$^+$, K$^+$-ATPase (Farooqui et al., 1997a). Arachidonic acid also inhibits glutamate uptake that is mediated by excitatory amino acid transporters in intact cells, tissue slices, synaptosomes, and cultures of neurons and glia (Volterra et al., 1994). Arachidonic acid is metabolized to prostaglandins, leukotrienes, and thromboxanes. These metabolites are collectively called eicosanoids (Wolfe and Horrocks, 1994). They differ from other intracellular second messengers in one important way. Eicosanoids, because of their amphiphilic nature, can cross the cell membrane and leave the cell that generates them to act on neighboring cells. They have been implicated in the control of behavior (Chiu and Richardson, 1985), regulation of blood flow (Wolfe and Horrocks, 1994), and modulation of neural and immune functions (Katsuki and Okuda, 1995).

High concentrations of arachidonic acid produce a variety of detrimental effects on neural membrane structure, including a profound adverse effect on the capacity of brain mitochondria to produce ATP. Arachidonic acid uncouples oxidative phosphorylation and induces efflux of Ca^{2+} and K$^+$ from mitochondria (Katsuki and Okuda, 1995; Farooqui et al., 1997a).

Lysophospholipids, the other product of PLA$_2$-catalyzed reactions, have many effects on various systems. They can be precursors for PAF. Lysophosphatidylcholines (lyso-PtdCho) stimulate phenylalanine hydroxylase, alkaline phosphatase, cyclic 3,5-nucleotide phosphodiesterase, PKC, and glycosyl- and sialyltransferases (Weltzien, 1979). They also inhibit activities of acyl-CoA: lysophosphatidylcholine acyltransferase, lysophospholipase, guanylate cyclase, and adenylate cyclase (Weltzien, 1979).

1.8.1b PLC-Generated Second Messengers

The PLC family of enzymes hydrolyze phosphatidylinositol 4,5-bisphosphate (PtdIns-4,5-P_2) into inositol 1,4,5-trisphosphate (Ins-1,4,5-P_3) and diacylglycerol (DAG). Ins-1,4,5-P_3 stimulates the release of Ca^{2+}, mainly from the endoplasmic reticulum, and thereby activates Ca^{2+}/calmodulin-dependent kinases whereas DAG stimulates PKC (Farooqui et al., 1988). The formation of DAG often lasts for about 1 min and is limited to some extent by the availability of PtdIns-4,5-P_2. The activation of PLD catalyzes a second phase of DAG formation (see below). Either tyrosine kinase or PKC can activate PLD. Thus the initial breakdown of PtdIns-4,5-P_2 can then be coordinated with the activation of PLD and the generation of a second phase of DAG formation. This process is facilitated by the involvement of phosphatidic acid (PtdH) phosphohydrolase (phosphatidic acid phosphatase), which acts on the PtdH generated from PtdCho by PLD (Kanoh et al., 1999).

Phosphatidic acid phosphatase has a molecular mass of 35 kDa and occurs in multiple forms. The purified enzyme is N-glycosylated and possesses six transmembrane domains. The purified enzyme can dephosphorylate lysophosphatidate, ceramide-1-phosphate, and diacylglycerol pyrophosphate. The physiological significance of such broad substrate specificity remains unknown, but it is interesting to know that phosphatidic acid phosphatase metabolizes a wide range of lipid mediators derived from glycerophospholipid and sphingolipid metabolism (Kanoh et al., 1999). The availability of PtdCho, which is abundant in biomembranes, does not limit DAG formation by PLD. DAG formed from this process is involved in the activation of those PKC forms that do not require Ca^{2+} (Farooqui et al., 1988; Rhee and Choi, 1992).

1.8.1c PLD-Generated Second Messengers

PLD hydrolyzes PtdCho to PtdH and choline in response to various extracellular stimuli (Klein et al., 1995; Exton, 1997, 1999). PtdH stimulates the activities of kinases including PKCζ, monoacylglycerol acyltransferase, phosphatidylinositol 4-kinase, and PLCγ, and increases the GTP-bound form of Ras. PtdH can also serve as the precursor for lyso-phosphatidic acid (lyso-PtdH), which has paracrine or autocrine signal properties (Chun, 1999; Luquain et al., 2003; Kingsbury et al., 2004). It increases the activity of tyrosine kinases and Ras-Raf-MAP kinase, PLCγ, and PLD. Furthermore, both lyso-PtdH and PtdH inhibit the activity of adenylate cyclase through a pertussis-toxin sensitive mechanism thereby lowering cAMP levels. Lyso-PtdH also stimulates a heterotrimeric G-protein receptor linked to Gi that initiates tyrosine kinase activation and stimulates the Ras-Raf-MAP kinase.

Brain tissue contains the highest concentration of lyso-PtdH and the highest level of lyso-PtdH receptors and binding proteins (Das and Hajra, 1989). Lyso-PtdH decreases glutamate and glucose uptake in astrocytes and produces neuronal cell rounding and neurite retraction in neuroblastoma cells (Tokumura, 1995; Keller et al., 1996). Apoptotic cell death in embryonic brain during development is modulated by lyso-PtdH receptors (Chun et al., 1999). Lyso-PtdH is an important lipid mediator that is involved in many neuronal developmental processes including neurogenesis, neuronal migration, neuritogenesis, and myelination in embryonic and adult brain (Toman and Spiegel, 2002; Ye et al., 2002; Luquain et al., 2003; Saba, 2004; Fukushima, 2004).

In brain tissue, PtdH is converted to DAG that can stimulate PKC. In vitro, in the presence of a primary alcohol, PLD can also catalyze a transphosphatidylation reaction. This reaction exchanges the polar head group of the glycerophospholipid substrate with the given alcohol to form the corresponding phosphatidyl alcohol (Klein et al., 1995). This reaction does not occur in vivo. The collective evidence suggests that PLD is involved in membrane trafficking and various transport processes in which acidic glycerophospholipids may facilitate membrane budding and/or fusion (Jones et al., 1999).

1.8.2 Involvement of PtdSer and PtdEtn in Apoptosis

Morphologically, apoptosis is characterized by nuclear condensation, cell shrinkage, and bleb formation. In brain neuronal death as a result of apoptosis occurs not only during development, but also in neurodegenerative diseases, acute metabolic trauma (stroke), and mechanical trauma (head injury and spinal cord injury) (Farooqui et al., 2004b). During the execution of apoptosis, the cell changes the phospholipid asymmetry of the plasma membrane by rapidly translocating PtdSer to the outer leaflet where it functions as a tag on the dying cell for recognition and removal by phagocytes (Fadok et al., 1992; De Simone et al., 2003). A specific inside–outside PtdSer translocase may be involved in the loss of neural membrane asymmetry during apoptosis. This mechanism can explain the extremely rapid kinetics of PtdSer externalization on apoptotic cells (Martin, 1997). The removal of apoptotic bodies is of great functional importance for eliminating unwanted cells, thereby avoiding neural inflammation and risks of uncontrolled cell lysis. The detection of PtdSer on a cell surface can be made with a fluorescent conjugate of annexin V (Van den Eijnde et al., 1997; Zhang et al., 1997), a Ca^{2+}- and phospholipid-binding protein that inhibits PLA_2.

Ro09-0198, a peptide that specifically recognizes PtdEtn, is a useful probe for studying the transbilayer movement of PtdEtn in cell membranes. Ro09-0198 recognizes PtdEtn exposure on CTLL-2 cells undergoing apoptosis. The exposure of PtdEtn correlates well with PtdSer exposure on the outer leaflet. This suggests that a complete loss of asymmetric distribution of plasma membrane glycerophospholipids occurs during apoptosis (Emoto et al., 1997; Wang et al., 2004). This disruption of lipid asymmetry can lead to looser lipid packing that may allow PLA_2 to attack phospholipids in the outer leaflet. This hypothesis is supported by the observation that inhibitors of PLA_2 activity inhibit apoptosis (Farooqui et al., 1997b, 2004b). In CHO-K1 cells (a non-neural cell line) and GOTO cells (a human neuroblastoma cell line), the addition of exogenous PtdSer results in dose-dependent apoptotic cell death (Uchida et al., 1998). This cytotoxic effect is specific for PtdSer. PtdCho, PtdEtn, PtdIns, and PtdH have no effect on cell viability. PtdSer-induced apoptotic cell death is not due to the detergent action of lyso-PtdSer. A high concentration of lyso-PtdSer is required to induce the cytotoxic action of this metabolite. Cells incubated with lyso-PtdSer undergo extensive membrane fragmentation and swelling whereas cells treated with PtdSer become round and show a dramatic reduction in cellular volume while maintaining the membrane containment of cellular content.

The mechanism of PtdSer-induced apoptotic cell death may include peroxidation of PtdSer that precedes its externalization. The PtdSer content of apoptotic cells was three times higher than that of control cells. This suggests that the aberrant increase in cellular PtdSer content may be responsible for malregulation of cellular signaling pathways leading to apoptotic cell death (Uchida et al., 1998). A study on HN2-5 cells (a neuronal hippocampal cell line) also indicates that PtdSer externalization during apoptosis may be linked to the detachment of cells from the culture plates and rapid phagocytosis by microglia (Adayev et al., 1998).

Another important event is a significant increase (10–20%) in the proportion of saturated fatty acids in the acyl chains of PtdEtn, PtdSer, and PtdIns, but not in PtdCho, in HN2-5 cells (Singh et al., 1996). Such a change in fatty acid acyl group composition of neural membrane phospholipids may be associated with cell shrinkage, deformation, and porosity of membranes. These changes in membrane structures may allow the diffusion of deoxyribonucleases into cell nuclei inducing the fragmentation of chromosomal DNA that occurs in apoptosis.

Like glycerophospholipids, sphingolipids are important constituents of neural membranes. They also provide second messengers for signal transduction processes. Studies on sphingolipid metabolism in neural and non-neural cell lines show that the hydrolysis of sphingomyelin by sphingomyelinase (SMase) and the generation of ceramide are closely associated with apoptotic cell death (Hannun and Obeid, 1995). Polyunsaturated fatty acids, including arachidonic acid (AA), are also known to induce apoptosis (Vanags et al., 1997; Colquhoun, 1998). In addition, ceramide-induced cell death requires the release of AA and the stimulation of cPLA$_2$ activity (Hayakawa et al., 1993; MacEwan, 1996; Jayadev et al., 1997) (Fig. 1.7). A close interaction between the cPLA$_2$-generated second messenger, AA, and the SMase-generated second messenger, ceramide, occurs at several sites in signal transduction processes induced by the cytokines, tumor necrosis factor and interleukin-1β. These cytokines trigger apoptosis in neural and non-neural cell cultures. The mechanism is apparently by stimulation of both SMase and PLA$_2$ activities. These activities are stimulated in a dose- and concentration-dependent manner and this stimulation can be blocked with PLA$_2$ and SMase inhibitors (Vanags et al., 1997; Gomez-Muñoz, 1998). In non-neural cell cultures, a product of PLA$_2$ catalyzed reactions, AA, stimulates SMase (Robinson et al., 1997), and ceramide, the product of SMase, stimulates PLA$_2$ activity (Hayakawa et al., 1996; Sato et al., 1999; Farooqui et al., 2000b).

Melittin, an activator of PLA$_2$, mimics the effect of AA on sphingomyelin levels.

Ceramide is a potent inhibitor of PLD activation and can inhibit some isoforms of PKC (Gomez-Muñoz, 1998). Finally, sphingosine, a degradation product of ceramide, strongly inhibits phosphatidic acid phosphatase resulting in accumulation

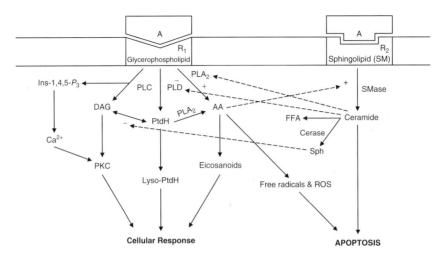

Fig. 1.7. Proposed schematic illustration of interactions between glycerophospholipid metabolites and sphingolipid metabolites in apoptosis. Note that arachidonic acid (AA) stimulates sphingomyelinase (SMase) and ceramide stimulates phospholipase A_2 activity. Free radicals and lipid peroxides may also play an important role in apoptosis. R1 and R2, receptors; A, agonist; DAG, diacylglycerol; Ins-1,4,5-P_3, inositol-1,4,5-trisphosphate; PtdH, phosphatidic acid; Lyso-PtdH, lyso-phosphatidic acid; PKC, protein kinase C; Sph, sphingosine; FFA, free fatty acid (hydroxy). The symbols (+, −) indicate stimulatory and inhibitory action of metabolites.

of PtdH and decreasing the formation of DAG. This results in the inhibition of PKC activity and induction of apoptosis (Gomez-Muñoz, 1998). Furthermore, sphingomyelin can be synthesized from ceramide through the transfer of phosphocholine derived from PtdCho. This reaction is catalyzed by phosphatidylcholine: ceramide cholinephosphotransferase (Gomez-Muñoz, 1998). Thus, the collective evidence from multiple studies supports the occurrence of cross talk between glycerophospholipid and sphingomyelin signaling pathways. This controlled and coordinated signaling may be involved in cell proliferation, differentiation, and apoptosis.

1.8.3 Phosphatidylinositol and Membrane Anchoring

Many proteins are attached to neural membranes by a glycosylphosphatidylinositol anchor which consist of phosphoethanolamine, glycans, and PtdIns (Low, 1989; Englund, 1993). Some of these proteins are enzymes such as acetylcholinesterase, alkaline phosphatase, aminopeptidase P, carboxypeptidase M, and 5′-nucleotidase (Hooper, 1997). These enzymes are all found in brain tissue and play important roles in various metabolic processes. Brain tissue also has the highest concentration of proteins covalently modified with lipids by acylation with myristic or palmitic acid or isoprenylation with farnesol and geraniol (Sinensky and Lutz, 1992).

On the neural surface, the glycosylphosphatidylinositol anchor may have many advantages over the transmembrane polypeptide anchor. The glycosylphosphatidylinositol anchor takes less space within the membrane than the transmembrane polypeptide anchor. Because of the lack of interaction with intracellular cytoskeletal proteins, glycosylphosphatidylinositol anchor-linked proteins, being outside, not only have more lateral mobility in neural membranes but can also help in directing the proteins and other molecules to the axonal membrane in hippocampal neurons (Sinensky and Lutz, 1992).

Glycosylphosphatidylinositol anchor-linked proteins, TAG-1, axonin-1, and the neural cell adhesion molecule, stimulate neurite outgrowth and axonal elongation in PC12 cells (Doherty and Walsh, 1993). Polyphosphoinositides are also involved in various membrane trafficking events such as secretory granule formation, fusion, and endocytosis (Martin, 1997).

1.8.4 Involvement of Glycerophospholipids in Regulation of Enzymic Activities

Many enzymes require glycerophospholipids for their activities. While this requirement can sometimes be met by any hydrophobic molecule, some enzymes are highly specific for a particular glycerophospholipid (Spector and Yorek, 1985; Yeagle, 1989). Thus PtdSer stimulates PKC, an enzyme involved in exocytosis, extracellular signal transduction, and cell division. An early process in the activation of PKC is the association of this enzyme with neural membranes through PtdSer in the presence of Ca^{2+}. This association of PKC to neural membrane induces an increase in surface pressure that can aid in the insertion of the protein domain of PKC into the membrane where this enzyme binds to diacylglycerol and becomes fully active.

PtdSer also induces changes in AMPA receptor binding by modulating PKC activity. The modulation of AMPA receptor function is reflected in a long lasting effect on synaptic plasticity (Gagné et al., 1996). The channel function of the acetylcholine receptor is also regulated by PtdSer (Sunshine and McNamee, 1992). PtdSer is also involved in the regulation of activities of Na^+, K^+-ATPase, diacylglycerol kinase, B-Raf protein kinase, and dynamin GTPase.

β-Hydroxybutyrate dehydrogenase, an enzyme found in the inner membrane of mitochondria, has an absolute requirement for PtdCho. PtdSer and PtdEtn cannot substitute for PtdCho in activating this enzyme. Other enzymes that require a specific phospholipid for their activity include Na^+, K^+-ATPase; Ca^{2+}, Mg^{2+}-ATPase; Ca^{2+}-ATPase; and adenylate cyclase (Farooqui and Horrocks, 1985; Spector and Yorek, 1985). These enzymes are involved in maintaining normal ion homeostasis in neurons and glial cells.

In the nucleus, glycerophospholipids (PtdIns) stimulate RNA synthesis, not only by modulating RNA polymerase activity, but also by affecting chromatin organization (Martelli et al., 1999). Metabolites of the phosphatidylinositol cycle bind to nucleoskeletal proteins (nuclear lamin B and DNA topoisomerase) and nuclear signaling proteins (phospholipase C) and affect gene expression (Martelli et al., 2002a,b; Ledeen and Wu, 2004). Nuclear inositol lipids may also be involved in mRNA transcription and/or processing and in DNA replication or repair potentially resulting in cell differentiation, proliferation, or apoptosis.

Furthermore, the interaction of glycerophospholipids with histones and non-histone chromosomal proteins suggests that the regulation of RNA polymerase with glycerophospholipids occurs at the level of template availability (D'Santos et al., 1998; Martelli et al., 2002a,b). The α isoform of CTP: choline phosphate cytidylyl-transferase, the rate-limiting enzyme of the Kennedy pathway, also occurs in the nucleus (Antony et al., 2000), and its activity is involved in temperature-sensitive mutation associated with cell survival. In the nucleus, glycerophospholipids and their second messengers play a major role in modulation of differentiation, apoptosis, and growth suppression (Ledeen and Wu, 2004; Hammond et al., 2004).

1.8.5 Other Roles of Glycerophospholipids

Glycerophospholipids are precursors for DAG, which activates protein kinase C when it is translocated to membranes (Farooqui et al., 1988). DAG also promotes the insertion of the regulatory domain of PKC into the hydrophobic core of membranes (Orr and Newton, 1992), probably through changes in membrane bilayer properties related to lipids with hexagonal-phase propensity (Senisterra and Epand, 1993). DAG favors membrane fusion (Nieva et al., 1989), a process that may be associated with neurotransmitter release. Glycerophospholipids also modulate activities of diacylglycerol kinase (Fanani et al., 2004) and 5-lipoxygenase (Pande et al., 2004).

PtdSer modulates binding properties of glutamate receptors involved in maintenance of long-term potentiation in neonatal and adult rat brain (Baudry et al., 1991; Gagné et al., 1996). PtdSer synthesis in cerebellar slices is inhibited by metabotropic glutamate receptor agonists (Buratta et al., 2004), indicating that metabotropic glutamate receptor stimulation decreases not only the incorporation of serine into PtdSer but also modulates the generation of excitatory post-synaptic currents in rat cerebellar slices. Collective evidence suggests that neural membrane PtdSer modulates long-lasting changes in learning and memory associated with neural membrane composition.

1.9 Conclusion

Glycerophospholipids are amphipathic molecules found in all cellular membranes, asymmetrically distributed between the two bilayers. They not only constitute the backbone of cellular membranes but also provide the membrane with a suitable environment, fluidity, and ion permeability. The degree of saturation and the length of phospholipid acyl chains are important determinants of neural membrane characteristics.

Glycerophospholipids are mainly synthesized at the endoplasmic reticulum and then transported to other membranous structures by phospholipid exchange and transfer proteins. Once glycerophospholipids are laid down in a biomembrane, they undergo the interconversion reactions, base-exchange, methylation, and decarboxylation. These reactions and activities of phospholipases may be responsible for the turnover, compositional maintenance, and rearrangements of glycerophospholipids in membranes. This process results in the modulation of membrane function.

Glycerophospholipids are multifunctional molecules. The functions include being a storage depot for second messengers and their precursors, involvement in membrane fusion and apoptosis, and regulation of the activities of membrane-bound enzymes and ion-channels. It is important to realize that the above discussion on metabolism, incorporation, and roles of glycerophospholipids does not describe the entire dynamics of glycerophospholipid metabolism in brain tissue, but rather provides an initial insight into the molecular complexity that is present in neural membranes.

References

Adayev T., Estephan R., Meserole S., Mazza B., Yurkow E. J., and Banerjee P. (1998). Externalization of phosphatidylserine may not be an early signal of apoptosis in neuronal cells, but only the phosphatidylserine-displaying apoptotic cells are phagocytosed by microglia. *J. Neurochem.* 71:1854–1864.

Alb J. G., Jr., Kearns M. A., and Bankaitis V. A. (1996). Phospholipid metabolism and membrane dynamics. *Curr. Opin. Cell Biol.* 8:534–541.

Albi E. and Magni M. P. V. (2004). The role of intranuclear lipids. *Biol. Cell* 96:657–667.

Albi E. and Viola M. M. (1999). Phosphatidylcholine-dependent phospholipase C in rat liver chromatin. *Biochem. Biophys. Res. Commun.* 265:640–643.

Albi E., Rossi G., Maraldi N. M., Magni M. V., Cataldi S., Solimando L., and Zini N. (2003). Involvement of nuclear phosphatidylinositol-dependent phospholipases C in cell cycle progression during rat liver regeneration. *J. Cell. Physiol.* 197:181–188.

Antonsson B. (1997). Phosphatidylinositol synthase from mammalian tissues. *Biochim. Biophys. Acta* 1348:179–186.

Antony P., Kanfer J. N., and Freysz L. (2000). Phosphatidylcholine metabolism in nuclei of phorbol ester activated LA-N-1 neuroblastoma cells. *Neurochem. Res.* 25:1073–1082.

Antony P., Freysz L., Horrocks L. A., and Farooqui A. A. (2001). Effect of retinoic acid on the Ca^{2+}-independent phospholipase A_2 in nuclei of LA-N-1 neuroblastoma cells. *Neurochem. Res.* 26:83–88.

Antony P., Freysz L., Horrocks L. A., and Farooqui A. A. (2003). Ca^{2+}-independent phospholipases A_2 and production of arachidonic acid in nuclei of LA-N-1 cell cultures: a specific receptor activation mediated with retinoic acid. *Mol. Brain Res.* 115:187–195.

Araki W. and Wurtman R. J. (1997). Control of membrane phosphatidylcholine biosynthesis by diacylglycerol levels in neuronal cells undergoing neurite outgrowth. *Proc. Natl Acad. Sci. USA* 94:11946–11950.

Attard G. S., Templer R. H., Smith W. S., Hunt A. N., and Jackowski S. (2000). Modulation of CTP:phosphocholine cytidylyltransferase by membrane curvature elastic stress. *Proc. Natl Acad. Sci. USA* 97:9032–9036.

Baker R. R. and Chang H. Y. (1987). The incorporation of fatty acids into triacylglycerols of isolated neuronal nuclear envelopes: the influence of thiol reducing reagents and chromatin. *Biochim. Biophys. Acta* 920:285–292.

Baker R. R. and Chang H. (1990a). Phosphatidylinositol synthetase activities in neuronal nuclei and microsomal fractions isolated from immature rabbit cerebral cortex. *Biochim. Biophys. Acta* 1042:55–61.

Baker R. R. and Chang H. Y. (1990b). The acylation of 1-acyl-*sn*-glycero-3-phosphate by neuronal nuclei and microsomal fractions of immature rabbit cerebral cortex. *Biochem. Cell Biol.* 68:641–647.

Baker R. R. and Chang H. Y. (1997). Neuronal nuclear acetyltransferases involved in the synthesis of platelet-activating factor are located in the nuclear envelope and show differential losses in activity. *Biochim. Biophys. Acta Lipids Lipid Metab.* 1345:197–206.

Baudry M., Massicotte G., and Hauge S. (1991). Phosphatidylserine increases the affinity of the AMPA/quisqualate receptor in rat brain membranes. *Behav. Neural Biol.* 55:137–140.

Binaglia L., Goracci G., Porcellati G., Roberti R., and Woelk H. (1973). The synthesis of choline and ethanolamine phosphoglycerides in neuronal and glial cells of rabbit in vitro. *J. Neurochem.* 21:1067–1082.

Bleasdale J. E., Eichberg J., and Hauser G. (1985). Inositol and phosphoinositides: metabolism and regulation, pp. 1–698. Humana Press, Clifton, NJ.

Blusztajn J. K., Zeisel S. H., and Wurtman R. J. (1979). Synthesis of lecithin (phosphatidylcholine) from phosphatidylethanolamine in bovine brain. *Brain Res.* 179:319–327.

Bottiglieri T. and Hyland K. (1994). S-adenosylmethionine levels in psychiatric and neurological disorders: a review. *Acta Neurol. Scand. Suppl.* 154:19–26.

Brown D. A. and London E. (1998a). Functions of lipid rafts in biological membranes. *Annu. Rev. Cell Dev. Biol.* 14:111–136.

Brown D. A. and London E. (1998b). Structure and origin of ordered lipid domains in biological membranes. *J. Membr. Biol.* 164:103–114.

Buratta S., Mambrini R., Miniaci M. C., Tempia F., and Mozzi R. (2004). Group I metabotropic glutamate receptors mediate the inhibition of phosphatidylserine synthesis in rat cerebellar slices: a possible role in physiology and pathology. *J. Neurochem.* 89:730–738.

Carter A. N., Huang R., Sorisky A., Downes C. P., and Rittenhouse S. E. (1994). Phosphatidylinositol 3,4,5-trisphosphate is formed from phosphatidylinositol 4,5-bisphosphate in thrombin-stimulated platelets. *Biochem. J.* 301:415–420.

Cheng H. F., Jiang M. J., Chen C. L., Liu S. M., Wong L. P., Lomasney J. W., and King K. (1995). Cloning and identification of amino acid residues of human phospholipase Cδ1 essential for catalysis. *J. Biol. Chem.* 270:5495–5505.

Chiu E. K. and Richardson J. S. (1985). Behavioral and neurochemical aspects of prostaglandins in brain function. *Gen. Pharmacol.* 16:163–175.

Chun J. (1999). Lysophospholipid receptors: implications for neural signaling. *Crit Rev. Neurobiol.* 13:151–168.

Chun J., Contos J. J. A., and Munroe D. (1999). A growing family of receptor genes for lysophosphatidic acid (LPA) and other lysophospholipids (LPs). *Cell Biochem. Biophys.* 30:213–242.

Clark J. D., Schievella A. R., Nalefski E. A., and Lin L.-L. (1995). Cytosolic phospholipase A$_2$. *J. Lipid Mediat. Cell Signal.* 12:83–117.

Cocco L., Martelli A. M., Gilmour R. S., Rhee S. G., and Manzoli F. A. (2001). Nuclear phospholipase C and signaling. *Biochim. Biophys. Acta Mol. Cell Biol. Lipids* 1530:1–14.

Colquhoun A. (1998). Induction of apoptosis by polyunsaturated fatty acids and its relationship to fatty acid inhibition of carnitine palmitoyltransferase I activity in Hep2 cells. *Biochem. Mol. Biol. Int.* 45:331–336.

Crews F. (1982). Rapid changes in phospholipid metabolism during secretion and receptor activation. *Int. Rev. Neurobiol.* 23:141–163.

D'Santos C. S., Clarke J. H., and Divecha N. (1998). Phospholipid signalling in the nucleus. *Biochim. Biophys. Acta Lipids Lipid Metab.* 1436:201–232.

Dainous F., Freysz L., Mozzi R., Dreyfus H., Louis J. C., Porcellati G., and Massarelli R. (1982). Synthesis of choline phospholipids in neuronal and glial cell cultures by the methylation pathway. *FEBS Lett.* 146:221–223.

Daleke D. L. and Lyles J. V. (2000). Identification and purification of aminophospholipid flippases. *Biochim. Biophys. Acta Mol. Cell Biol. Lipids* 1486:108–127.

Das A. K. and Hajra A. K. (1989). Quantification, characterization and fatty acid composition of lysophosphatidic acid in different rat tissues. *Lipids* 24:329–333.

De Simone R., Ajmone-Cat M. A., Tirassa P., and Minghetti L. (2003). Apoptotic PC12 cells exposing phosphatidylserine promote the production of anti-inflammatory and neuroprotective molecules by microglial cells. *J. Neuropathol. Exp. Neurol.* 62:208–216.

Dennis E. A., Rhee S. G., Billah M. M., and Hannun Y. A. (1991). Role of phospholipases in generating lipid second messengers in signal transduction. *FASEB J.* 5:2068–2077.

Doherty P. and Walsh F. S. (1993). Glycosylphosphatidylinositol anchored recognition molecules that mediate intracellular adhesion and promote neurite outgrowth. In: Massarelli R., Horrocks L. A., Kanfer J. N., and Löffelholz K. (eds.), *Phospholipids and Signal Transmission*. Springer-Verlag, Berlin, pp. 1–11.

Emoto K., Toyama-Sorimachi N., Karasuyama H., Inoue K., and Umeda M. (1997). Exposure of phosphatidylethanolamine on the surface of apoptotic cells. *Exp. Cell Res.* 232:430–434.

Englund P. T. (1993). The structure and biosynthesis of glycosyl phosphatidylinositol protein anchors. *Annu. Rev. Biochem.* 62:121–138.

Exton J. H. (1994). Phosphatidylcholine breakdown and signal transduction. Biochim. *Biophys. Acta Lipids Lipid Metab.* 1212:26–42.

Exton J. H. (1997). Phospholipase D: enzymology, mechanisms of regulation, and function. *Physiol. Rev.* 77:303–320.

Exton J. H. (1999). Regulation of phospholipase D. *Biochim. Biophys. Acta Mol. Cell Biol. Lipids* 1439:121–133.

Fadok V. A., Voelker D. R., Campbell P. A., Cohen J. J., Bratton D. L., and Henson P. M. (1992). Exposure of phosphatidylserine on the surface of apoptotic lymphocytes triggers specific recognition and removal by macrophages. *J. Immunol.* 148:2207–2216.

Fanani M. L., Topham M. K., Walsh J. P., and Epand R. M. (2004). Lipid modulation of the activity of diacylglycerol kinase α- and ζ-isoforms: Activation by phosphatidylethanolamine and cholesterol. *Biochemistry* 43:14767–14777.

Fang M., Rivas M. P., and Bankaitis V. A. (1998). The contribution of lipids and lipid metabolism to cellular functions of the Golgi complex. *Biochim. Biophys. Acta* 1404:85–100.

Farooqui A. A. and Horrocks L. A. (1985). Metabolic and functional aspects of neural membrane phospholipids. In: Horrocks L. A., Kanfer J. N., and Porcellati G. (eds.), *Phospholipids in the Nervous System, Vol. II: Physiological Role*. Raven Press, New York, pp. 341–348.

Farooqui A. A. and Horrocks L. A. (2004). Brain phospholipases A$_2$: a perspective on the history. *Prostaglandins Leukot. Essent. Fatty Acids* 71:161–169.

Farooqui A. A., Farooqui T., Yates A. J., and Horrocks L. A. (1988). Regulation of protein kinase C activity by various lipids. *Neurochem. Res.* 13:499–511.

Farooqui A. A., Hirashima Y., and Horrocks L. A. (1992). Brain phospholipases and their role in signal transduction. In: Bazan N. G., Toffano G., and Murphy M. (eds.), *Neurobiology of Essential Fatty Acids*. Plenum Press, New York, pp. 11–25.

Farooqui A. A., Yang H.-C., and Horrocks L. A. (1995). Plasmalogens, phospholipases A_2, and signal transduction. *Brain Res. Rev.* 21:152–161.

Farooqui A. A., Rosenberger T. A., and Horrocks L. A. (1997a). Arachidonic acid, neurotrauma, and neurodegenerative diseases. In: Yehuda S. and Mostofsky D. I. (eds.), *Handbook of Essential Fatty Acid Biology*. Humana Press, Totowa, NJ, pp. 277–295.

Farooqui A. A., Yang H. C., Rosenberger T. A., and Horrocks L. A. (1997b). Phospholipase A_2 and its role in brain tissue. *J. Neurochem.* 69:889–901.

Farooqui A. A., Horrocks L. A., and Farooqui T. (2000a). Deacylation and reacylation of neural membrane glycerophospholipids. *J. Mol. Neurosci.* 14:123–135.

Farooqui A. A., Horrocks L. A., and Farooqui T. (2000b). Glycerophospholipids in brain: their metabolism, incorporation into membranes, functions, and involvement in neurological disorders. *Chem. Phys. Lipids* 106:1–29.

Farooqui A. A., Ong W. Y., Horrocks L. A., and Farooqui T. (2000c). Brain cytosolic phospholipase A_2: localization, role, and involvement in neurological diseases. *Neuroscientist* 6:169–180.

Farooqui A. A., Farooqui T., and Horrocks L. A. (2002). Molecular species of phospholipids during brain development. Their occurrence, separation and roles. In: Skinner E. R. (ed.), *Brain Lipids and Disorders in Biological Psychiatry*. Elsevier Science B.V., Amsterdam, pp. 147–158.

Farooqui A. A., Antony P., Ong W. Y., Horrocks L. A., and Freysz L. (2004a). Retinoic acid-mediated phospholipase A_2 signaling in the nucleus. *Brain Res. Rev.* 45:179–195.

Farooqui A. A., Ong W. Y., and Horrocks L. A. (2004b). Biochemical aspects of neurodegeneration in human brain: Involvement of neural membrane phospholipids and phospholipases A_2. *Neurochem. Res.* 29:1961–1977.

Fernández-Tome M., Kraemer L., Federman S. C., Favale N., Speziale E., and Sterin-Speziale N. (2004). COX-2-mediated PGD_2 synthesis regulates phosphatidylcholine biosynthesis in rat renal papillary tissue. *Biochem. Pharmacol.* 67:245–254.

Frayne J., Ingram C., Love S., and Hall L. (1999). Localisation of phosphatidylethanolamine-binding protein in the brain and other tissues of the rat. *Cell Tissue Res.* 298:415–423.

Freysz L., Lastennet A., and Mandel P. (1972). Phosphocholine diglyceride transferase activity during development of the chicken brain. *J. Neurochem.* 19:2599–2605.

Freysz L., Dreyfus H., Vincendon G., Binaglia L., Roberti R., and Porcellati G. (1982). Asymmetry of brain microsomal membranes: correlation between the asymmetric distribution of phospholipids and the enzymes involved in their synthesis. In: Horrocks L. A., Ansell G. B., and Porcellati G. (eds.), *Phospholipids in the Nervous System*. Raven Press, New York, pp. 37–47.

Fruman D. A., Meyers R. E., and Cantley L. C. (1998). Phosphoinositide kinases. *Annu. Rev. Biochem.* 67:481–507.

Fukui Y., Ihara S., and Nagata S. (1998). Downstream of phosphatidylinositol-3 kinase, a multifunctional signaling molecule, and its regulation in cell responses. *J. Biochem.* (Tokyo) 124:1–7.

Fukushima N. (2004). LPA in neural cell development. *J. Cell. Biochem.* 92:993–1003.

Gagné J., Giguère C., Tocco G., Ohayon M., Thompson R. F., Baudry M., and Massicotte G. (1996). Effect of phosphatidylserine on the binding properties of glutamate receptors in brain sections from adult and neonatal rats. *Brain Res.* 740:337–345.

Gehrmann T., Vereb G., Schmidt M., Klix D., Meyer H. E., Varsanyi M., and Heilmeyer L. M., Jr. (1996). Identification of a 200 kDa polypeptide as type 3 phosphatidylinositol 4-kinase from bovine brain by partial protein and cDNA sequencing. *Biochim. Biophys. Acta* 1311:53–63.

Gomez-Muñoz A. (1998). Modulation of cell signalling by ceramides. *Biochim. Biophys. Acta Lipids Lipid Metab.* 1391:92–109.

Goswami R., Dawson S. A., and Dawson G. (2000). Multiple polyphosphoinositide pathways regulate apoptotic signalling in a dorsal root ganglion derived cell line. *J. Neurosci. Res.* 59:136–144.

Hall E. D. (1992). Novel inhibitors of iron-dependent lipid peroxidation for neurodegenerative disorders. *Ann. Neurol.* 32(Suppl.):S137–S142.

Halliwell B. (1994). Free radicals, antioxidants, and human disease: curiosity, cause, or consequence? *Lancet* 344:721–724.

Hammond G., Thomas C. L., and Schiavo G. (2004). Nuclear phosphoinositides and their functions. In: Stenmark H. (ed.), *Phosphoinositides in Subcellular Targeting and Enzyme Activation.* Springer-Verlag, Berlin, pp. 177–206.

Hannun Y. A. and Obeid L. M. (1995). Ceramide: an intracellular signal for apoptosis. *Trends Biochem. Sci.* 20:73–77.

Hayakawa M., Ishida N., Takeuchi K., Shibamoto S., Hori T., Oku N., Ito F., and Tsujimoto M. (1993). Arachidonic acid-selective cytosolic phospholipase A_2 is crucial in the cytotoxic action of tumor necrosis factor. *J. Biochem.* 268:11290–11295.

Hayakawa M., Jayadev S., Tsujimoto M., Hannun Y. A., and Ito F. (1996). Role of ceramide in stimulation of the transcription of cytosolic phospholipase A_2 and cyclooxygenase 2. *Biochem. Biophys. Res. Commun.* 220:681–686.

Heacock A. M. and Agranoff B. W. (1997). CDP-diacylglycerol synthase from mammalian tissues. *Biochim. Biophys. Acta* 1348:166–172.

Hirabayashi T., Murayama T., and Shimizu T. (2004). Regulatory mechanism and physiological role of cytosolic phospholipase A_2. *Biol. Pharm. Bull.* 27:1168–1173.

Hirashima Y., Farooqui A. A., Mills J. S., and Horrocks L. A. (1992). Identification and purification of calcium-independent phospholipase A_2 from bovine brain cytosol. *J. Neurochem.* 59:708–714.

Hooper N. M. (1997). Glycosyl-phosphatidylinositol anchored membrane enzymes. *Clin. Chim. Acta* 266:3–12.

Horrocks L. A., Yeo Y. K., Harder H. W., Mozzi R., and Goracci G. (1986). Choline plasmalogens, glycerophospholipid methylation, and receptor-mediated activation of adenylate cyclase. In: Greengard P. and Robison G. A. (eds.), *Advances in Cyclic Nucleotide and Protein Phosphorylation Research, Vol. 20.* Raven Press, New York, pp. 263–292.

Hozumi Y., Ito T., Nakano T., Nakagawa T., Aoyagi M., Kondo H., and Goto K. (2003). Nuclear localization of diacylglycerol kinase zeta in neurons. *Eur. J. Neurosci.* 18:1448–1457.

Hunt A. N., Clark G. T., Attard G. S., and Postle A. D. (2001). Highly saturated endonuclear phosphatidylcholine is synthesized in situ and colocated with CDP-choline pathway enzymes. *J. Biol. Chem.* 276:8492–8499.

Ilincheta de Boschero M. G., Roque M. E., Salvador G. A., and Giusto N. M. (2000). Alternative pathways for phospholipid synthesis in different brain areas during aging. *Exp. Gerontol.* 35:653–668.

Irvine R. F. (1995). Inositide evolution: what can it tell us about functions? *Biochem. Soc. Trans.* 23:27–35.

Irvine R. F. (2003). Nuclear lipid signalling. *Nature Rev. Mol. Cell Biol.* 4:349–360.

Isaac G., Bylund D., Mansson J. E., Markides K. E., and Bergquist J. (2003). Analysis of phosphatidylcholine and sphingomyelin molecular species from brain extracts using capillary liquid chromatography electrospray ionization mass spectrometry. *J. Neurosci. Meth.* 128:111–119.

Ishidate K. (1997). Choline/ethanolamine kinase from mammalian tissues. *Biochim. Biophys. Acta Lipids Lipid Metab.* 1348:70–78.

Ivanova P. T., Milne S. B., Forrester J. S., and Brown H. A. (2004). Lipid arrays: new tools in the understanding of membrane dynamics and lipid signaling. *Mol. Interv.* 4:86–96.

Jayadev S., Hayter H. L., Andrieu N., Gamard C. J., Liu B., Balu R., Hayakawa M., Ito F., and Hannun Y. A. (1997). Phospholipase A_2 is necessary for tumor necrosis factor α-induced ceramide generation in L929 cells. *J. Biol. Chem.* 272:17196–17203.

Jones D., Morgan C., and Cockcroft S. (1999). Phospholipase D and membrane traffic – Potential roles in regulated exocytosis, membrane delivery and vesicle budding. *Biochim. Biophys. Acta Mol. Cell Biol. Lipids* 1439:229–244.

Kanfer J. N., McCartney D., Singh I. N., and Freysz L. (1996). Phospholipase D activity of rat brain neuronal nuclei. *J. Neurochem.* 67:760–766.

Kanoh H., Kai M., and Wada I. (1999). Molecular characterization of the type 2 phosphatidic acid phosphatase. *Chem. Phys. Lipids* 98:119–126.

Katsuki H. and Okuda S. (1995). Arachidonic acid as a neurotoxic and neurotrophic substance. *Prog. Neurobiol.* 46:607–636.

Keller J. N., Steiner M. R., Mattson M. P., and Steiner S. M. (1996). Lysophosphatidic acid decreases glutamate and glucose uptake by astrocytes. *J. Neurochem.* 67:2300–2305.

Kent C. (1997). CTP:phosphocholine cytidylyltransferase. *Biochim. Biophys. Acta Lipids Lipid Metab.* 1348:79–90.

Kingsbury M. A., Rehen S. K., Ye X., and Chun J. (2004). Genetics and cell biology of lysophosphatidic acid receptor-mediated signaling during cortical neurogenesis. *J. Cell. Biochem.* 92:1004–1012.

Klein J., Chalifa V., Liscovitch M., and Löffelholz K. (1995). Role of phospholipase D activation in nervous system physiology and pathophysiology. *J. Neurochem.* 65:1445–1455.

Kleuser B., Maceyka M., Milstien S., and Spiegel S. (2001). Stimulation of nuclear sphingosine kinase activity by platelet-derived growth factor. *FEBS Lett.* 503:85–90.

Komatsu H., Westerman J., Snoek G. T., Taraschi T. F., and Janes N. (2003). L-α-Glycerylphosphorylcholine inhibits the transfer function of phosphatidylinositol transfer protein α. *Biochim. Biophys. Acta Mol. Cell Biol. Lipids* 1635:67–74.

Kuge O. and Nishijima M. (1997). Phosphatidylserine synthase I and II of mammalian cells. *Biochim. Biophys. Acta Lipids Lipid Metab.* 1348:151–156.

Kurzchalia T. V., Dupree P., Parton R. G., Kellner R., Virta H., Lehnert M., and Simons K. (1992). VIP21, a 21-kD membrane protein is an integral component of trans-Golgi-network-derived transport vesicles. *J. Cell Biol.* 118:1003–1014.

Lang D., Leray C., Mestre R., Massarelli R., Dreyfus H., and Freysz L. (1995). Molecular species analysis of 1,2-diglycerides on phorbol ester stimulation of LA-N-1 neuroblastoma cells during proliferation and differentiation. *J. Neurochem.* 65:810–817.

Ledeen R. W. and Wu G. S. (2004). Nuclear lipids: key signaling effectors in the nervous system and other tissues. *J. Lipid Res.* 45:1–8.

Lee A. G. (2003). Lipid–protein interactions in biological membranes: a structural perspective. *Biochim. Biophys. Acta* 1612:1–40.

Leray C., Sarliève L. L., Dreyfus H., Massarelli R., Binaglia L., and Freysz L. (1994). Molecular species of choline and ethanolamine glycerophospholipids in rat brain myelin during development. *Lipids* 29:77–81.

Low M. G. (1989). The glycosyl-phosphatidylinositol anchor of membrane proteins. *Biochim. Biophys. Acta* 988:427–454.

Lucero H. A. and Robbins P. W. (2004). Lipid rafts–protein association and the regulation of protein activity. *Arch. Biochem. Biophys.* 426:208–224.

Luquain C., Sciorra V. A., and Morris A. J. (2003). Lysophosphatidic acid signaling: how a small lipid does big things. *Trends Biochem. Sci.* 28:377–383.

Lykidis A., Murti K. G., and Jackowski S. (1998). Cloning and characterization of a second human CTP:phosphocholine cytidylyltransferase. *J. Biol. Chem.* 273:14022–14029.

Lykidis A., Baburina I., and Jackowski S. (1999). Distribution of CTP:phosphocholine cytidylyltransferase (CCT) isoforms. Identification of a new CCTβ splice variant. *J. Biol. Chem.* 274:26992–27001.

MacEwan D. J. (1996). Elevated $cPLA_2$ levels as a mechanism by which the p70 TNF and p75 NGF receptors enhance apoptosis. *FEBS Lett.* 379:77–81.

Mancini A., Del Rosso F., Roberti R., Orvietani P., Coletti L., and Binaglia L. (1999). Purification of ethanolaminephosphotransferase from bovine liver microsomes. Biochim. Biophys. *Acta Lipids Lipid Metab.* 1437:80–92.

Martelli A. M., Capitani S., and Neri L. M. (1999). The generation of lipid signaling molecules in the nucleus. *Prog. Lipid Res.* 38:273–308.

Martelli A. M., Bortul R., Tabellini G., Bareggi R., Manzoli L., Narducci P., and Cocco L. (2002a). Diacylglycerol kinases in nuclear lipid-dependent signal transduction pathways. *Cell. Mol. Life Sci.* 59:1129–1137.

Martelli A. M., Manzoli L., Faenza I., Bortul R., Billi A., and Cocco L. (2002b). Nuclear inositol lipid signaling and its potential involvement in malignant transformation. *Biochim. Biophys. Acta* 1603:11–17.

Martelli A. M., Fala F., Faenza I., Billi A. M., Cappellini A., Manzoli L., and Cocco L. (2004a). Metabolism and signaling activities of nuclear lipids. *Cell. Mol. Life Sci.* 61:1143–1156.

Martelli A. M., Manzoli L., and Cocco L. (2004b). Nuclear inositides: facts and perspectives. *Pharmacol. Ther.* 101:47–64.

Martin T. F. J. (1997). Phosphoinositides as spatial regulators of membrane traffic. *Curr. Opin. Neurobiol.* 7:331–338.

McLean L. R., Hagaman K. A., and Davidson W. S. (1993). Role of lipid structure in the activation of phospholipase A_2 by peroxidized phospholipids. *Lipids* 28:505–509.

McMaster C. R. and Bell R. M. (1997a). CDP-choline:1,2-diacylglycerol cholinephosphotransferase. *Biochim. Biophys. Acta Lipids Lipid Metab.* 1348:100–110.

McMaster C. R. and Bell R. M. (1997b). CDP-ethanolamine:1,2-diacylglycerol ethanolaminephosphotransferase. *Biochim. Biophys. Acta Lipids Lipid Metab.* 1348:117–123.

Morand J. N. and Kent C. (1989). Localization of the membrane-associated CTP:phosphocholine cytidylyltransferase in Chinese hamster ovary cells with an altered membrane composition. *J. Biol. Chem.* 264:13785–13792.

Moreau P. and Cassagne C. (1994). Phospholipid trafficking and membrane biogenesis. *Biochim. Biophys. Acta* Rev. Biomembr. 1197:257–290.

Mozzi R. and Porcellati G. (1979). Conversion of phosphatidylethanolamine to phosphatidylcholine in rat brain by the methylation pathway. *FEBS Lett.* 100:363–366.

Mozzi R., Buratta S., and Goracci G. (2003). Metabolism and functions of phosphatidylserine in mammalian brain. *Neurochem. Res.* 28:195–214.

Nagle J. F. and Tristram-Nagle S. (2000). Structure of lipid bilayers. *Biochim. Biophys. Acta* 1469:159–195.

Nakagawa T., Goto K., and Kondo H. (1996). Cloning, expression, and localization of 230-kDa phosphatidylinositol 4-kinase. *J. Biol. Chem.* 271:12088–12094.

Negre-Aminou P., Nemenoff R. A., Wood M. R., de la Houssaye B. A., and Pfenninger K. H. (1996). Characterization of phospholipase A_2 activity enriched in the nerve growth cone. *J. Neurochem.* 67:2599–2608.

Nieva J. L., Goñi F. M., and Alonso A. (1989). Liposome fusion catalytically induced by phospholipase C. *Biochemistry* 28:7364–7367.

Orr J. W. and Newton A. C. (1992). Interaction of protein kinase C with phosphatidylserine. 2. Specificity and regulation. *Biochemistry* 31:4667–4673.

Pande A. H., Moe D., Nemec K. N., Qin S., Tan S. H., and Tatulian S. A. (2004). Modulation of human 5-lipoxygenase activity by membrane lipids. *Biochemistry* 43:14653–14666.

Park S. K., Provost J. J., Bae C. D., Ho W. T., and Exton J. H. (1997). Cloning and characterization of phospholipase D from rat brain. *J. Biol. Chem.* 272:29263–29271.

Pasquare S. J., Salvador G. A., and Giusto N. M. (2004). Phospholipase D and phosphatidate phosphohydrolase activities in rat cerebellum during aging. *Lipids* 39:553–560.

Payrastre B., Nievers M., Boonstra J., Breton M., Verkleij A. J., and van Bergen en Henegouwen P. M. (1992). A differential location of phosphoinositide kinases, diacylglycerol kinase, and phospholipase C in the nuclear matrix. *J. Biol. Chem.* 267:5078–5084.

Pearce J. M. and Komoroski R. A. (2000). Analysis of phospholipid molecular species in brain by ^{31}P NMR spectroscopy. *Magn. Reson. Med.* 44:215–223.

Pete M. J. and Exton J. H. (1996). Purification of a lysophospholipase from bovine brain that selectively deacylates arachidonoyl-substituted lysophosphatidylcholine. *J. Biol. Chem.* 271:18114–18121.

Pike L. J. (2004). Lipid rafts: heterogeneity on the high seas. Biochem. J. 378:281–292.

Pomorski T., Holthuis J. C. M., Herrmann A., and Van Meer G. (2004). Tracking down lipid flippases and their biological functions. *J. Cell Sci.* 117:805–813.

Porcellati G. (1983). Phospholipid metabolism in neural membranes. In: Sun G. Y., Bazan N., Wu J. Y., Porcellati G., and Sun A. Y. (eds.), *Neural Membranes*. Humana Press, New York, pp. 3–35.

Purdon A. D. and Rapoport S. I. (1998). Energy requirements for two aspects of phospholipid metabolism in mammalian brain. *Biochem.* J. 335:313–318.

Purdon A. D., Rosenberger T. A., Shetty H. U., and Rapoport S. I. (2002). Energy consumption by phospholipid metabolism in mammalian brain. *Neurochem. Res.* 27:1641–1647.

Rameh L. E., Tolias K. F., Duckworth B. C., and Cantley L. C. (1997). A new pathway for synthesis of phosphatidylinositol-4,5-bisphosphate. *Nature* 390:192–196.

Randazzo P. A. and Kahn R. A. (1994). GTP hydrolysis by ADP-ribosylation factor is dependent on both an ADP-ribosylation factor GTPase-activating protein and acid phospholipids. *J. Biol. Chem.* 269:10758–10763.

Regan R. F. and Guo Y. P. (1998). Toxic effect of hemoglobin on spinal cord neurons in culture. *J. Neurotrauma* 15:645–653.

Rhee S. G. and Choi K. D. (1992). Regulation of inositol phospholipid-specific phospholipase C isozymes. *J. Biol. Chem.* 267:12393–12396.

Robinson B. S., Hii C. S. T., Poulos A., and Ferrante A. (1997). Activation of neutral sphingomyelinase in human neutrophils by polyunsaturated fatty acids. *Immunology* 91:274–280.

Ross B. M., Kim D. K., Bonventre J. V., and Kish S. J. (1995). Characterization of a novel phospholipase A$_2$ activity in human brain. *J. Neurochem.* 64:2213–2221.

Ross B. M., Moszczynska A., Blusztajn J. K., Sherwin A., Lozano A., and Kish S. J. (1997). Phospholipid biosynthetic enzymes in human brain. *Lipids* 32:351–358.

Rothberg K. G., Heuser J. E., Donzell W. C., Ying Y. S., Glenney J. R., and Anderson R. G. (1992). Caveolin, a protein component of caveolae membrane coats. *Cell* 68:673–682.

Saba J. D. (2004). Lysophospholipids in development: miles apart and edging in. *J. Cell. Biochem.* 92:967–992.

Saido T. C., Shibata M., Takenawa T., Murofushi H., and Suzuki K. (1992). Positive regulation of μ-calpain action by polyphosphoinositides. *J. Biol. Chem.* 267:24585–24590.

Sandra A., Van't Hof W., Van Genderen I., and Van Meer G. (1993). Lipid synthesis and targeting to the mammalian cell surface. In: Massarelli R., Horrocks L. A., Kanfer J. N., and Löffelholz K. (eds.), *Phospholipids and Signal Transmission*. Springer-Verlag, Berlin, pp. 13–37.

Sato T., Kageura T., Hashizume T., Hayama M., Kitatani K., and Akiba S. (1999). Stimulation by ceramide of phospholipase A_2 activation through a mechanism related to the phospholipase C-initiated signaling pathway in rabbit platelets. *J. Biochem.* (Tokyo) 125:96–102.

Senisterra G. and Epand R. M. (1993). Role of membrane defects in the regulation of the activity of protein kinase C. *Arch. Biochem. Biophys.* 300:378–383.

Sinensky M. and Lutz R. J. (1992). The prenylation of proteins. *BioEssays* 14:25–31.

Singh J. K., Dasgupta A., Adayev T., Shahmehdi S. A., Hammond D., and Banerjee P. (1996). Apoptosis is associated with an increase in saturated fatty acid containing phospholipids in the neuronal cell line, HN2-5. *Biochim. Biophys. Acta Lipids Lipid Metab.* 1304:171–178.

Spector A. A. and Yorek M. A. (1985). Membrane lipid composition and cellular function. *J. Lipid Res.* 26:1015–1035.

Stephens L. R., Hughes K. T., and Irvine R. F. (1991). Pathway of phosphatidylinositol(3,4,5)-trisphosphate synthesis in activated neutrophils. *Nature* 351:33–39.

Sun G. Y. and MacQuarrie R. A. (1989). Deacylation–reacylation of arachidonoyl groups in cerebral phospholipids. *Ann. NY Acad. Sci.* 559:37–55.

Sun G. Y., Xu J. F., Jensen M. D., and Simonyi A. (2004). Phospholipase A_2 in the central nervous system: implications for neurodegenerative diseases. *J. Lipid Res.* 45:205–213.

Sunshine C. and McNamee M. G. (1992). Lipid modulation of nicotinic acetylcholine receptor function: the role of neutral and negatively charged lipids. *Biochim. Biophys. Acta* 1108:240–246.

Takenawa T., Itoh T., and Fukami K. (1999). Regulation of phosphatidylinositol 4,5-bisphosphate levels and its roles in cytoskeletal re-organization and malignant transformation. *Chem. Phys. Lipids* 98:13–22.

Tamiya-Koizumi K. (2002). Nuclear lipid metabolism and signaling. *J. Biochem.* 132:13–22.

Tamiya-Koizumi K., Umekawa H., Yoshida S., Ishihara H., and Kojima K. (1989). A novel phospholipase A2 associated with nuclear matrix: stimulation of the activity and modulation of the Ca^{2+}-dependency by polyphosphoinositides. *Biochim. Biophys. Acta* 1002:182–188.

Tokumura A. (1995). A family of phospholipid autacoids: occurrence, metabolism and bioactions. *Prog. Lipid Res.* 34:151–184.

Tolias K. F. and Cantley L. C. (1999). Pathways for phosphoinositide synthesis. *Chem. Phys. Lipids* 98:69–77.

Tolias K. F., Rameh L. E., Ishihara H., Shibasaki Y., Chen J., Prestwich G. D., Cantley L. C., and Carpenter C. L. (1998). Type I phosphatidylinositol-4-phosphate 5-kinases synthesize the novel lipids phosphatidylinositol 3,5-bisphosphate and phosphatidylinositol 5-phosphate. *J. Biol. Chem.* 273:18040–18046.

Toman R. E. and Spiegel S. (2002). Lysophospholipid receptors in the nervous system. *Neurochem. Res.* 27:619–627.

Tsvetnitsky V., Auchi L., Nicolaou A., and Gibbons W. A. (1995). Characterization of phospholipid methylation in rat brain myelin. *Biochem. J.* 307:239–244.

Uchida K., Emoto K., Daleke D. L., Inoue K., and Umeda M. (1998). Induction of apoptosis by phosphatidylserine. *J. Biochem.* (Tokyo) 123:1073–1078.

Van den Eijnde S. M., Boshart L., Reutelingsperger C. P. M., De Zeeuw C. I., and Vermeij-Keers C. (1997). Phosphatidylserine plasma membrane asymmetry in vivo: a pancellular phenomenon which alters during apoptosis. *Cell Death Differ.* 4:311–316.

Van Meer G. (1989). Lipid traffic in animal cells. *Annu. Rev. Cell Biol.* 5:247–275.

Vanags D. M., Larsson P., Feltenmark S., Jakobsson P. J., Orrenius S., Claesson H. E., and Aguilar-Santelises M. (1997). Inhibitors of arachidonic acid metabolism reduce DNA and nuclear fragmentation induced by TNF plus cycloheximide in U937 cells. *Cell Death Differ.* 4:479–486.

Vance D. E. (1996). Glycerolipid biosynthesis in eukaryotes. In: Vance D. E. and Vance J. E. (eds.), *Biochemistry of Lipids, Lipoproteins, and Membranes*. Elsevier, New York, pp. 153–181.

Vance J. E. and Vance D. E. (2004). Phospholipid biosynthesis in mammalian cells. *Biochem. Cell Biol.* 82:113–128.

Vance D. E., Walkey C. J., and Cui Z. (1997). Phosphatidylethanolamine N-methyltransferase from liver. *Biochim. Biophys. Acta* 1348:142–150.

Vecchini A., Panagia V., and Binaglia L. (1997). Analysis of phospholipid molecular species. *Mol. Cell. Biochem.* 172:129–136.

Voelker D. R. (1997). Phosphatidylserine decarboxylase. *Biochim. Biophys. Acta Lipids Lipid Metab.* 1348:236–244.

Voelker D. R. (2003). New perspectives on the regulation of intermembrane glycerophospholipid traffic. *J. Lipid Res.* 44:441–449.

Voelker D. R. (2004). Genetic analysis of intracellular aminoglycerophospholipid traffic. *Biochem. Cell Biol.* 82:156–169.

Volterra A., Trotti D., and Racagni G. (1994). Glutamate uptake is inhibited by arachidonic acid and oxygen radicals via two distinct and additive mechanisms. *Mol. Pharmacol.* 46:986–992.

Wang X. J., Li N., Liu B., Sun H. Y., Chen T. Y., Li H. Z., Qiu J. M., Zhang L. H., Wan T., and Cao X. T. (2004). A novel human phosphatidylethanolamine-binding protein resists tumor necrosis factor alpha-induced apoptosis by inhibiting mitogen-activated protein kinase pathway activation and phosphatidylethanolamine externalization. *J. Biol. Chem.* 279:45855–45864.

Welti R. and Glaser M. (1994). Lipid domains in model and biological membranes. *Chem. Phys. Lipids* 73:121–137.

Weltzien H. U. (1979). Cytolytic and membrane-perturbing properties of lysophosphatidylcholine. *Biochim. Biophys. Acta* 559:259–287.

Wirtz K. W. A. (1997). Phospholipid transfer proteins revisited. *Biochem. J.* 324:353–360.

Wolfe L. S. and Horrocks L. A. (1994). Eicosanoids. In: Siegel G. J., Agranoff B. W., Albers R. W., and Molinoff P. B. (eds.), *Basic Neurochemistry*. Raven Press, New York, pp. 475–490.

Wood W. G., Schroeder F., Igbavboa U., Avdulov N. A., and Chochina V. V. (2002). Brain membrane cholesterol domains, aging and amyloid beta-peptides. *Neurobiol. Aging* 23:685–694.

Yamashita A., Sugiura T., and Waku K. (1997). Acyltransferases and transacylases involved in fatty acid remodeling of phospholipids and metabolism of bioactive lipids in mammalian cells. *J. Biochem.* (Tokyo) 122:1–16.

Yang H. C., Mosior M., Ni B., and Dennis E. A. (1999). Regional distribution, ontogeny, purification, and characterization of the Ca^{2+}-independent phospholipase A_2 from rat brain. *J. Neurochem.* 73:1278–1287.

Ye X. Q., Fukushima N., Kingsbury M. A., and Chun J. (2002). Lysophosphatidic acid in neural signaling. *NeuroReport* 13:2169–2175.

Yeagle P. (1989). Lipid regulation of cell membrane structure and function. *FASEB J.* 3:1833–1842.

Yin H. L. and Janmey P. A. (2003). Phosphoinositide regulation of the actin cytoskeleton. *Annu. Rev. Physiol.* 65:761–789.

Zachowski A. (1993). Phospholipids in animal eukaryotic membranes: transverse asymmetry and movement. *Biochem. J.* 294:1–14.

Zhang G., Gurtu V., Kain S. R., and Yan G. (1997). Early detection of apoptosis using a fluorescent conjugate of annexin V. *Biotechniques* 23:525–531.

2
Ether Lipids in Brain

2.1 General Considerations and Importance

Ether glycerophospholipids are major constituents of neural cell membranes. Depending on the substituents at carbon-1, most ether glycerophospholipids belong to one of two groups: (1) alkenyl–acyl glycerophospholipids and (2) alkyl–acyl glycerophospholipids. In mammalian tissues, alkenyl–acyl glycerophospholipids are represented by plasmalogens, whereas alkyl–acyl glycerophospholipids are represented by plasmalogen precursors, platelet-activating factors and its analogs and precursors. Plasmalogens contain a vinyl ether (enol ether) linkage at the *sn*-1 position with 16:0, 18:0, and 18:1 (n-7 and n-9) side chains (alk-1-enyl groups); an ester bond linking arachidonic acid, docosahexaenoic acid, or another unsaturated fatty acid at the *sn*-2 position; and a phosphoethanolamine or phosphocholine group at the *sn*-3 position of the glycerol moiety (Fig. 2.1). In contrast, platelet-activating factor (PAF) has an O-alkyl ether linkage at the *sn*-1 position (fatty alcohol side chain), a short acyl chain (acetyl moiety) at the *sn*-2 position, and a phosphocholine group at the *sn*-3 position of the glycerol moiety.

Plasmalogens are abundant in cholesterol-rich biological membranes such as myelin and the plasma membrane of red blood cells. Although considerable attention has been paid to the metabolism and role of platelet-activating factor in mammalian tissues (Honda et al., 2002), information on the role of plasmalogens in receptor-mediated metabolism is only now emerging (Farooqui and Horrocks, 2001). It is now evident that plasmalogens play important roles in neural cells, not only in signal transduction processes, but also in membrane fusion and antioxidant activity.

Abbreviations used: PlsEtn, plasmenylethanolamine (ethanolamine plasmalogen); PlsCho, plasmenylcholine (choline plasmalogen); PLA_2, phospholipase A_2; PLC, phospholipase C; PLD, phospholipase D; HDL, high-density lipoprotein; LDL, low-density lipoprotein; ROS, reactive oxygen species; LTP, long-term potentiation; HIV, human immunodeficiency virus; COX-2, cyclooxygenase-2; alkenyl-GP, 1-*O*-alk-1'-enyl-2-lyso-*sn*-glycero-3-phosphate; and mc-PAF, 1-*O*-hexadecyl-2-methylcarbamoyl-*sn*-glycerol-3-phosphocholine.

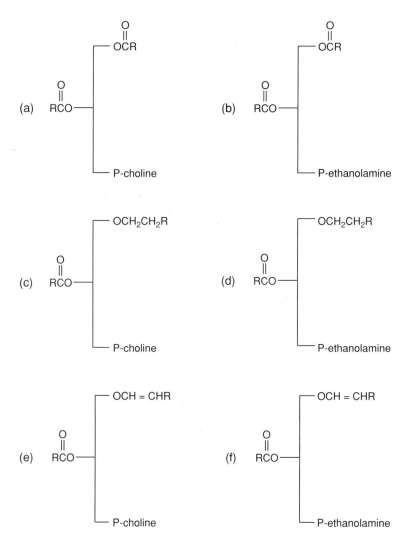

FIG. 2.1. Structures of glycerophospholipids containing choline and ethanolamine and ether glycerophospholipids. Phosphatidylcholine or 1, 2-diacyl-*sn*-glycero-3-phosphocholine (a); Phosphatidylethanolamine or 1, 2-diacyl-*sn*-glycero-3-phosphoethanolamine (b); Plasmanylcholine or 1-alkyl-2-acyl-*sn*-glycero-3-phosphocholine (c); Plasmanylethanolamine or 1-alkyl-2-acyl-*sn*-glycero-3-phosphoethanolamine (d); Plasmenylcholine (choline plasmalogen) or 1-alk-1′-enyl-2-acyl-*sn*-glycero-3-phosphocholine (e); and plasmenylethanolamine or 1-alk-1′-enyl-2-acyl-*sn*-glycero-3-phosphoethanolamine (f). Current nomenclature uses 1Z-alkenyl instead of alk-1′enyl (Fahy et al., 2005).

The overall physicochemical properties of ether glycerophospholipids are similar to those of ester-bonded glycerophospholipids except for differences in the phase transition temperature from gel to liquid crystalline and from lamellar to hexagonal phases. These differences may be responsible for determining physical properties of neural membranes such as bilayer thickness, area per molecule, side-chain packing, free volume, and lateral domains (Paltauf, 1994; Lohner, 1996). In artificial membrane systems, there are close similarities between the molecular arrangement of the ether glycerophospholipids and the corresponding ester-bonded analogs. The replacement of one or both acyl ester bonds with an alkenyl or alkyl ether bond produces changes in membrane properties (Lohner, 1996), such as a decrease in membrane dipole potential and alterations in thermotropic phase behavior, ion permeability, and side-chain mobility (Paltauf, 1994).

In comparison to the ester-bonded glycerophospholipids (Fig. 2.1), ether lipids have a greater propensity to facilitate membrane fusion. Proteins may interact differently with ether glycerophospholipids than with diacyl glycerophospholipids. For example, the selective binding of ethanolamine plasmalogen, which has predominantly unsaturated acyl groups, is essential for Ca^{2+} transport (Ford and Hale, 1996). Also, 1-O-hexadec-1′-enyl-2-arachidonyl-sn-glycero-3-phosphoethanolamine has a stimulatory effect on the Ca^{2+} pump (Duhm et al., 1993; Ford and Hale, 1996).

2.2 Plasmalogens

2.2.1 Biosynthesis

Enzymes for plasmalogen biosynthesis have not been purified and characterized from brain tissue. Several investigators have reviewed the biosynthesis of plasmalogens in non-neural tissues (Lee, 1998; Nagan and Zoeller, 2001; Murphy, 2001; Brites et al., 2004). Biosynthesis of plasmalogens is initiated in peroxisomes and completed in the endoplasmic reticulum. Thus, the first three enzymes of plasmalogen biosynthesis, dihydroxyacetone phosphate acyltransferase, alkyl dihydroxyacetone phosphate synthase, and acyl/alkyl dihydroxyacetone reductase, are located in peroxisomes. The endoplasmic reticulum contains the other enzymes, namely, 1-alkyl-sn-GroP acyltransferase, 1-alkyl-2-acyl-sn-GroP phosphohydrolase, and 1-alkyl-2-acyl-sn-Gro: CDP-choline (CDP-ethanolamine) choline (ethanolamine) phosphotransferase. Dihydroxyacetone phosphate acyltransferase catalyzes the acylation of dihydroxyacetone phosphate by acyl-CoA with formation of 1-acyl dihydroxyacetone phosphate (Fig. 2.2). The acyl group in this intermediate is then replaced by a long-chain alcohol that provides the oxygen for the ether linkage in the reaction catalyzed by alkyl dihydroxyacetone phosphate synthase. The carbonyl function in alkyl dihydroxyacetone phosphate is then reduced and acylated to give an alkyl analog of phosphatidic acid. This intermediate is dephosphorylated prior to introduction of the phosphocholine or phosphoethanolamine group (Lee, 1998; Nagan and Zoeller, 2001).

The conversion of 1-alkyl-2-acyl-sn-Gro$P$Etn to 1-alk-1′-enyl-2-acyl-sn-Gro$P$Etn (ethanolamine plasmalogen) is carried out by a cytochrome b5-dependent microsomal electron transport system. This system consists of cytochrome b5, NADH: cytochrome b5 reductase, and cyanide-sensitive 1-alkyl desaturase (Snyder et al., 1985). Choline plasmalogen is synthesized from ethanolamine

DHAP + Fatty acyl-CoA $\xrightarrow{1}$ Acyl-DHAP + CoA

Acyl-DHAP + ROH $\xrightarrow{2}$ 1-*O*-Alkyl-DHAP + RCOOH

1-*O*-Alkyl-DHAP + NADH + H⁺ $\xrightarrow{3}$ 1-*O*-Alkyl-glycerophosphate + NAD

1-*O*-Alkylglycerophosphate + Fatty acyl-CoA $\xrightarrow{4}$ 1-*O*-Alkyl-2-acyl-glycerophosphate + CoA

1-*O*-Alkyl-2-acyl-glycerophosphate $\xrightarrow{5}$ 1-*O*-Alkyl-2-acylglycerol + Pi

1-*O*-Alkyl-2-acylglycerol + CDP-Choline $\xrightarrow{6}$ 1-*O*-Alkyl-2-acyl-glycero-3-phosphoethanolamine + CDP

1-*O*-Alkyl-2-acyl-3-phosphoethanolamine $\xrightarrow{7}$ Ethanolamine plasmalogen

Ethanolamine plasmalogen $\xrightarrow{8}$ Choline plasmalogen

FIG. 2.2. Biosynthesis of plasmalogens in mammalian tissues. (1) dihydroxyacetone phosphate acyltransferase; (2) 1-acyl dihydroxyacetone phosphate synthase; (3) 1-alkyl dihydroxyacetone phosphate oxidoreductase; (4) 1-alkyl-*sn*-glycerophosphate acyltransferase; (5) 1-alkyl-2-acylglycerophosphate phosphohydrolase; (6) CDP-ethanolamine transferase; (7) 1-alkyl-2-acyl-*sn*-glycerophosphoethanolamine desaturase; and methyl transferases and base-exchange enzymes.

plasmalogen by polar-head group modifications by a base-exchange enzyme or N-methyltransferases (Paltauf, 1994; Horrocks et al., 1986; Lee, 1998). Plasmalogens are also synthesized from alkylglycerols, bypassing the first three steps through the action of a kinase, ATP: 1-alkyl-*sn*-glycerol phosphotransferase (alkylglycerol kinase). The product, 1-*O*-alkyl-2-lyso-*sn*-glycero-3-phosphate, enters the synthesizing cycle after the reductase step (Nagan and Zoeller, 2001). This pathway represents a salvage pathway for plasmalogen biosynthesis from partially degraded plasmalogen.

2.2.2 *Receptor-Mediated Degradation*

The release of arachidonic acid or docosahexaenoic acid from the *sn*-2 position of plasmalogens, catalyzed by the plasmalogen-selective PLA$_2$, is a receptor-mediated process related to signal transduction (Horrocks et al., 1986). This enzyme has been purified from several mammalian tissues, including brain, heart, and kidney (Hirashima et al., 1992; Hazen and Gross, 1993; Portilla and Dai, 1996). Brain plasmalogen-selective PLA$_2$ has a molecular mass of 39 kDa and does not require calcium (Hirashima et al., 1992; Farooqui et al., 1995). It is not affected by ATP and other nucleotides in the micromolar range, but is markedly inhibited by these nucleotides at 2 mM or above, the normal intracellular concentration of ATP. This differs from the heart plasmalogen-selective PLA$_2$, which is stimulated by the addition of ATP (Hazen et al., 1991) and is associated with phosphofructokinase as a complex with 400-kDa mol mass. Purified rabbit kidney plasmalogen-selective PLA$_2$ has a molecular mass of 28 kDa and a substrate preference for plasmenylcholine > phosphatidylcholine. The enzyme displays a fatty acid preference for arachidonic acid > palmitic acid. Nonionic detergents, Triton X-100 and Tween-20, stimulate the enzymic activity of brain plasmalogen-selective PLA$_2$. These detergents inhibit the activity of heart plasmalogen-selective PLA$_2$. Other detergents, such as octylglucoside, sodium deoxycholate, and sodium taurocholate, inhibit the plasmalogen-selective PLA$_2$ in a dose-dependent manner. The SH-group blocking agent, dithio-*bis*-2-nitrobenzoic acid, inhibits bovine brain plasmalogen-selective PLA$_2$. Other SH-group blocking agents, iodoacetate and N-ethylmaleimide, inhibit enzymic activity as well, but to a lesser degree. This PLA$_2$ is also inhibited by polyvalent anions (citrate > sulfate > phosphate) (Farooqui et al., 1995).

The turnover of arachidonic acid in ethanolamine and choline plasmalogens in brain is much greater than indicated by most labeling experiments because plasmalogens are not pulse labeled. The fractional turnover rate for arachidonic acid in choline plasmalogens is about 2% per hour. The corresponding rate for docosahexaenoic acid is more than 7%. The synthesis rates in adult rat brain microsomes give half-lives of 15 min for PlsCho and 2.9 h for PlsEtn (Rintala et al., 1999). The specific radioactivity of the arachidonic acid in choline plasmalogen molecular species at 24 hours is greater than that in any corresponding molecular species of PtdCho or PtdIns, the glycerophospholipids labeled initially with arachidonic acid (Horrocks, 1989). Although PlsCho fatty acids turn over very rapidly, the PlsCho and PlsEtn are not pulse labeled in the glycerol or alkenyl moieties; therefore in those portions of the molecules the turnover is slower.

Ether glycerophospholipids in rat brain are synthesized and turned over rapidly (Table 2.1) (Rosenberger et al., 2002). Because the ether side chains originate from fatty alcohols, hexadecanol labeled with tritium at the 1-position was used. Part of the hexadecanol is oxidized to palmitic acid, but in the process, the tritium is lost. All of the tritium in the glycerophospholipids should be in the ether side chains. Plasmalogen synthesis steps include desaturation of half of the hydrogen atoms at the 1-position of the alkyl group. The turnover rates and half-lives could

TABLE 2.1. Microsomal ether phospholipids in 3-month-old male rats (Rosenberger et al., 2002).

Phospholipid	Synthesis rate (nmol/g/min)	Turnover rate (%/min)	Half-life (min)
PakH		6.6	10.5
PakCho	1.2	1.9	36.5
PakEtn	9.3	2.6	26.7
PlsEtn	27.6	3.0	23.1
PlsCho	21.5	4.6	15.1

These values are for the awake unanesthetized rat. An intravenous infusion of [1,1-^{3}H]hexadecanol was administered for five minutes. The half-life of the PakH was too short to permit calculation of its synthesis rate. An indirect calculation gave the value of 10.5 nmol/g/min.

then be calculated from transfer coefficients and the rates of synthesis. PakH is the precursor for PakCho and PakEtn. PakEtn is the precursor for PlsEtn, which is the precursor for PlsCho.

The incorporation into myelin glycerophospholipids was very slow and always less than 10% of the total, at times up to two hours when it was 3% (Rosenberger et al., 2002). The incorporation was predominantly into gray matter, as shown with radioautographs. Much more radioactivity was in the synaptosomal fraction than in the microsomal fraction. The synaptosomal fraction contains plasma membranes and nerve endings with their mitochondria and synaptic vesicles. The microsomal fraction contains membranes from plasma membranes and endoplasmic reticulum. The results (Rosenberger et al., 2002) suggest the dynamic role of ether glycerophospholipids in plasticity and signaling in the brain.

Tritium-labeled glycerol was used with 18-day-old rats to determine the rate of PlsEtn synthesis in brain (Masuzawa et al., 1984). The rate was 32 nmol/g/min in excellent agreement with the rate found for older rats with hexadecanol. Turnover rates measured with the loss of radioactivity (Miller et al., 1977; Miller and Morell, 1978) are much longer than rates estimated from synthesis (Horrocks, 1969). The longer rates are due to recycling of radioactivity and sequestration into relatively stable pools of glycerophospholipids.

Receptor-mediated plasmalogen degradation by phospholipase A_2 may play an important role in signal transduction (Fig. 2.3). The stimulation of receptors on the cell surface by an agonist may cause the stimulation of Ca^{2+}-independent plasmalogen-selective PLA_2 and result in the generation of lysoplasmalogens (Horrocks et al., 1986) and arachidonic acid or docosahexaenoic acid. Under normal conditions, lysoplasmalogens are then either reacylated by CoA-independent transacylase or hydrolyzed by a lysoplasmalogenase (Jurkowitz et al., 1999).

Arachidonic acid is metabolized to bioactive molecules such as prostaglandins and leukotrienes (Farooqui et al., 2000c). These metabolites are known collectively as eicosanoids. Docosahexaenoic acid may be metabolized to 10, 17S-docosatrienes and 17S-resolvin (Hong et al., 2003; Marcheselli et al., 2003; Serhan et al., 2004; Serhan, 2005). The metabolites of docosahexaenoic acid metabolism are called docosanoids. Docosanoids have neuroprotective effects and not only antagonize the effects of eicosanoids, but also regulate both trafficking of leukocytes and downregulation of cytokines. The generation of eicosanoids may constitute the first wave of second messenger generation, the immediate phase of signal transduction, during receptor stimulation (Turini and Holub, 1994).

Lysoplasmalogens activate purified cyclic AMP-dependent protein kinase (Williams and Ford, 1997) independent of cAMP, indicating the involvement of plasmalogen-selective PLA_2 in nuclear signaling. Our recent studies support this. LA-N-1 cell nuclei contain plasmalogen-selective PLA_2 activity that is stimulated by retinoic acid in a dose- and time-dependent manner (Antony et al., 2001). A pan retinoic acid receptor antagonist, BMS943 (Antony et al., 2003; Farooqui et al., 2004a), blocks the stimulation of plasmalogen-selective PLA_2. Thus, the stimulation of plasmalogen-selective PLA_2 is a receptor-mediated process. The activation of a nuclear transcription factor, cAMP response element binding pro-

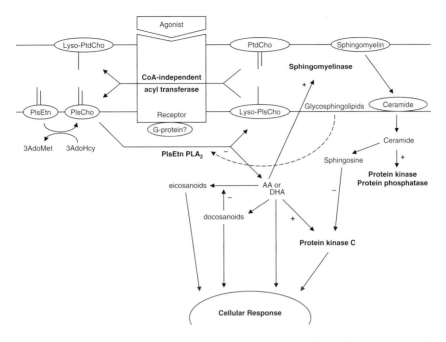

FIG. 2.3. A diagram showing the receptor-mediated degradation of plasmalogens by phospholipase A_2, cyclooxygenase, and lipoxygenase. Plasmenylethanolamine (PlsEtn); plasmenylcholine (PlsCho); lysoplasmenylcholine (lyso-PlsCho); lysophosphatidyl-choline (lyso-PtdCho); S-adenosyl-L-methionine (AdoMet); S-adenosyl-2-homocysteine (AdoHcy); plasmalogen-selective phospholipase A_2 (PlsEtn-PLA_2); glycerophospho-choline (GroPCho); and $-CH = O$ (aldehyde). 3 Mol of AdoMet is consumed during the methylation reaction. Note that docosanoids (10, 17S-docosatriene, 17S-resolvin, and neu-roprotectin), the metabolic products of docosahexaenoic acid, are anti-inflammatory and neuroprotective. They inhibit the generation of eicosanoids.

tein (CREB), also depends on the activity of plasmalogen-selective PLA_2. In addition, c-fos expression is also increased in response to perfusion with 500 nM lysoplasmenylcholine (Williams and Ford, 2001). All these studies indicate that metabolism of plasmalogens and lysoplasmalogens may be involved in signal transduction processes in the nucleus.

At the plasma membrane level, the generation of lysoplasmalogens can also induce changes in membrane permeability and fluidity and allow the influx of external Ca^{2+} via plasma membrane channels. Changes in the Ca^{2+} level result in the translocation of Ca^{2+}-dependent enzymes, including 85-kDa cytosolic PLA_2. This process induces the subsequent wave of second messenger generation, the late phase of signal transduction. Thus, plasmalogens provide second messengers that may be involved in early stages of signal transduction. In contrast, later stages of signal transduction utilize phosphatidylcholine.

Sphingomyelinase, an enzyme that generates ceramide, decreases the levels of plasmalogens in rat brain slices (Latorre et al., 1999). This effect can be mimicked by C2-ceramide (Latorre et al., 2003). The decrease in plasmalogens by sphingomyelinase or C2-ceramide is prevented by quinacrine, ganglioside, and bromoenol lactone, which are inhibitors of plasmalogen-selective PLA_2 activity (Farooqui and Horrocks, 2001). It is interesting to note that addition of the caspase-3 inhibitor, acetyl-L-aspartyl-L-glutamyl-L-valyl-L-aspartyl-chloromethylketone (Ac-DEVD-CMK), partially blocks the ceramide-induced stimulation of plasmalogen-selective PLA_2 without altering sphingomyelinase-elicited ceramide accumulation (Latorre et al., 2003). This suggests the involvement of plasmalogen hydrolysis in signal transduction related to apoptotic cell death at the nuclear level (Farooqui et al., 2004b). Arachidonic acid is known to stimulate sphingomyelinase and ceramide activates plasmalogen-selective PLA_2 activity (Farooqui et al., 2000b). Thus a close interaction between a plasmalogen-selective generated second messenger, arachidonic acid, and the sphingomyelinase-generated second messenger, ceramide, occurs in cytokine-induced apoptotic cell death. This type of cell death occurs in acute neural trauma and neurodegenerative diseases (Farooqui et al., 2000b).

2.2.3 Roles of Plasmalogens in Brain Tissue

Plasmalogens play important roles (Fig. 2.4) in mammalian brain (Lee, 1998; Nagan and Zoeller, 2001; Farooqui and Horrocks, 2001). Besides being the structural component of cellular membranes and a major reservoir for arachidonic and docosahexaenoic acids, plasmalogens are also involved in transport of ions across plasma membranes (Gross, 1985), membrane fusion (Lohner, 1996), protection of cellular membranes against oxidative stress (Zoeller et al., 1988; Engelmann et al., 1994), and the efflux of cholesterol from cells mediated by high-density

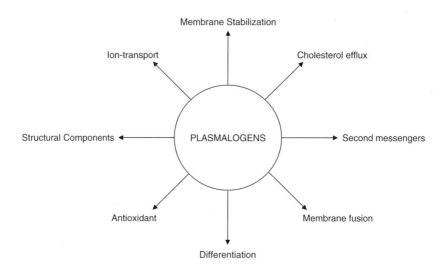

FIG. 2.4. Roles of plasmalogens in brain.

lipoprotein (HDL) (Mandel et al., 1998). Plasmalogens are also involved in cellular differentiation (Bichenkov and Ellingson, 1999).

2.2.3a Plasmalogens as Structural Components of Neural Membranes

Neural membranes contain considerable amounts of plasmalogens that impart different biophysical properties to membranes. The perpendicular orientation of the *sn*-2 acyl chain at the neural membrane surface and the lack of a carbonyl group at the *sn*-1 position in plasmalogens affect the hydrophilicity of the head group resulting in stronger intermolecular hydrogen bonding between the head groups (Lohner, 1996). These properties allow ethanolamine plasmalogens to adopt the inverse hexagonal phase and may be responsible for a different membrane potential compared to other glycerophospholipids (Horrocks and Sharma, 1982). This affects lipid packing, fluidity, and interactions with neural membrane receptors and ion channels.

Chronic *myo*-inositol administration increases PlsEtn by 10% and decreases brain PtdEtn by 5%, thus increasing the ratio between PlsEtn and PtdEtn by 15% (Pettegrew et al., 2001). The acute administration of *myo*-inositol plus ethanolamine also results in a positive correlation between the brain *myo*-inositol and the biosynthesis of ethanolamine glycerophospholipids with preferential synthesis of PlsEtn (Hoffman-Kuczynski and Reo, 2004). The molecular mechanism of the *myo*-inositol-induced increase in PlsEtn in rat brain remains unknown. *myo*-Inositol catabolism through the pentose phosphate cycle generates 2 mol of NADPH. This increase in NADPH level may be associated with increased PlsEtn synthesis in rat brain. An elevated PlsEtn/PtdEtn ratio can lead to tighter neural membrane packing. This may affect membrane dynamics and induce alterations in fluidity and permeability.

2.2.3b Plasmalogens as a Storage Depot for Second Messengers

Plasmalogens act as a reservoir for arachidonic and docosahexaenoic acids. These fatty acids are implicated in both physiological (synaptic plasticity) and pathophysiological (neurodegenerative) processes (Katsuki and Okuda, 1995). For example, arachidonic acid modulates ion channels and regulates the activity of many enzyme proteins such as protein kinase A, protein kinase C, NADPH oxidase, GTPase-activating protein, diacylglycerol kinase, and Na^+, K^+-ATPase (Farooqui et al., 1997). High concentrations of arachidonic acid have profound adverse effects on the ATP-producing capacity of mitochondria by uncoupling oxidative phosphorylation and inducing the efflux of Ca^{2+} and K^+ from mitochondria. In addition, arachidonic acid is also associated with regulation of gene expression (Jump et al., 1994). Arachidonic acid is metabolized to prostaglandins, leukotrienes, thromboxanes, and lipoxins. These metabolites are collectively called eicosanoids. These molecules are associated with various signal transduction processes.

Plasmalogens are also a reservoir for docosahexaenoic acid. Docosahexaenoic acid modulates dopaminergic, noradrenergic, glutamatergic, and serotonergic neurotransmission (Chalon et al., 1998; Zimmer et al., 2000; Hogyes et al., 2003);

and activates membrane-bound enzymes, ion channels, and receptors (Nishikawa et al., 1994; Haroutunian et al., 1986; Xiao and Li, 1999; Yehuda et al., 2002), memory processes (Fujimoto et al., 1989; Fujita et al., 2001), and gene expression (Nakanishi et al., 1994; Fernstrom, 1999; Farkas et al., 2000). The release of docosahexaenoic acid may be involved in vesicle formation during neurotransmitter release. This fatty acid is metabolized to docosanoids (Fig. 2.5). Docosahexaenoic acid and docosanoids may antagonize the effects of some eicosanoids (Serhan et al., 2004, 2005).

Under normal conditions, nearly all of the released arachidonic acid and docosahexaenoic acid is recycled back into neural membrane glycerophospholipids (Rapoport, 1999; Farooqui et al., 2000a). The action of plasmalogen-selective PLA$_2$ on 1-alkenyl-2-acyl-*sn*-GroPEtn results in generation of 1-alkenyl-2-lyso-*sn*-GroPEtn. This is an acceptor for the transfer of arachidonic acid from 1-alkyl-2-arachidonyl-*sn*-GroPCho. This reaction releases lysoplatelet-activating factor that can be acetylated to PAF (Uemura et al., 1991).

2.2.3c Plasmalogens and Generation of Long-Chain Aldehydes

Plasmalogens are highly sensitive to oxidative attack at the enol ether group at the *sn*-1 position (Yavin and Gatt, 1972). Arachidonic and docosahexaenoic acids at the *sn*-2 position of plasmalogens also undergo oxidation (Berry and Murphy, 2005), resulting in generation of ω-aldehyde and γ-hydroxy-α, β-unsaturated aldehydes, which are neurotoxic and deleterious for nerve cells. Plasmalogens also undergo epoxidation. These epoxides are hydrolyzed to long-chain α-hydroxy aldehydes (Felde and Spiteller, 1995). The levels of plasmalogen epoxide are enriched in heart after myocardial infarction (Dudda et al., 1996). Old bovine brain

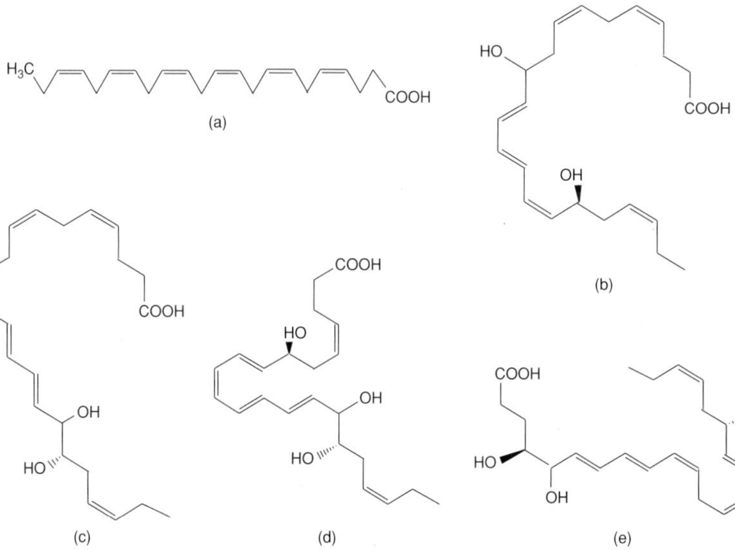

FIG. 2.5. Structures of docosahexaenoic acid and docosanoids.

contains a 30-fold higher amount of free α-hydroxy aldehyde and plasmalogen epoxide when compared with young bovine brain (Weisser et al., 1997). In human brain, the ratio of plasmalogen with respect to the long-chain α-hydroxy aldehyde remains constant during the lifetime.

The quotient of plasmalogen epoxide to plasmalogen increases with age, indicating that lipid peroxidation may be involved in decreasing the plasmalogen content in the aging brain (Weisser et al., 1997). Alterations in receptor function and ion channel activity in aged individuals may reflect this decrease. This may be caused by the reactivity of α-hydroxy aldehyde with membrane-bound proteins that are associated with optimal functioning of receptors and ion channels in neural membranes. At this stage, it is difficult to separate the consequences of lower plasmalogen levels that occur during normal aging from the decrease of plasmalogen level that occurs in certain neurological disorders (see below). However, both types of decrease in plasmalogen levels may compromise optimal membrane function by affecting fluidity, permeability, and other biophysical properties.

2.2.3d Plasmalogens and Membrane Fusion

Ethanolamine plasmalogens are major endogenous lipid constituents that facilitate membrane fusion of synaptic vesicles (Breckenridge et al., 1973). This is because of their high propensity to form inverse hexagonal phases. Plasmalogens influence biophysical properties of the neural membrane by stabilizing the hexagonal phase and altering critical temperature of the membrane (Ginsberg et al., 1998). In vitro, vesicles containing PlsEtn (PtdCho/PlsEtn/PtdSer, 45:45:10) undergo fusion 6-fold faster than those containing PtdEtn instead of PlsEtn (Lohner et al., 1991). The fusion rate also depends on the fatty acid composition. PlsEtn containing 20:4 at the *sn*-2 position fuses 5-fold faster than the corresponding PlsEtn with an 18:1 acyl chain.

This behavior of plasmalogens is related to phase transition temperature. It also depends on highly selective interaction and affinity of a fusion protein with vesicles containing PlsEtn (Glaser and Gross, 1995). The purified preparations of fusion protein have glyceraldehyde-3-phosphate dehydrogenase activity and are not affected by Ca^{2+} but have an obligatory requirement for PlsEtn and cholesterol. On an average, the fusion protein catalyzes one fusion event between two vesicles every millisecond. Whether this process occurs in vivo and plays a role in fusion of neurotransmitter vesicles is not established. However, the occurrence of high levels of plasmalogens in the synaptic plasma membrane and their interaction with a fusion protein suggests that plasmalogens may be involved in membrane fusion events such as endocytosis and exocytosis during neurotransmission, hormone release, and membrane vesicle trafficking (Glaser and Gross, 1995).

2.2.3e Plasmalogens and Ion Transport

The association of PlsEtn with Ca^{2+}-ATPase has been reported in skeletal muscle sarcoplasmic reticulum (Bick et al., 1991), which is actively involved in calcium transport (Gross, 1985). The sodium-calcium exchanger is predominantly found in the plasma membrane of excitatory cells and is an important component of excitation–secretion as well as excitation–contraction machinery (Ford and Hale, 1996). Based on reconstitution studies, and because of the acyl side-chain orientation, plasmalogens may provide a critical lipid environment in which anionic glycerophospholipids serve as boundary lipids for the regulation of the trans-sarcolemmal sodium–calcium exchanger (Ford and Hale, 1996).

The levels of PlsEtn in red blood cells are associated with maximal activity of the Na^+/K^+ pump (Duhm et al., 1993). The putative preferential lipid–protein interaction of PlsEtn with the membrane-embedded portion of the pump may induce a conformational change of the protein, thereby hindering the access of intracellular Na^+ to its binding site. Similarly, the presence of PlsCho in the vesicles may modulate the function of gramicidin ion channels. These observations on cardiac function are probably related to the effects of docosahexaenoic acid on arrhythmias (Kang and Leaf, 2000). DHA stimulates the synthesis of plasmalogens, as mentioned elsewhere in this discussion. DHA and plasmalogens may also be involved in the maintenance of ion pumps in neural membranes (Young et al., 2000).

2.2.4 Plasmalogen, Cholesterol Efflux, and Atherosclerosis

In mammalian tissues, cholesterol homeostasis is determined by de novo cholesterol synthesis, cellular uptake of cholesterol in low-density lipoproteins (LDL), and cholesterol efflux that is mediated by high-density lipoproteins. Studies on high-density lipoprotein (HDL)-mediated cholesterol efflux in the murine macrophage-like cell line RAW 264.7 and in a mutant RAW 108, derived from this cell line, indicate that the cellular plasmalogen content is related to HDL-mediated cholesterol efflux. Two observations support this suggestion. Cellular HDL-mediated cholesterol efflux is decreased in plasmalogen-deficient fibroblasts and macrophages. HDL-mediated cholesterol efflux is enhanced when cells are treated with 1-O-hexadecyl-sn-glycerol, a compound that restores the level of plasmalogens (Mandel et al., 1998).

A deficiency of ethanolamine plasmalogens also results in altered cholesterol transport in the CHO cell mutants, NRel-4 and NZel-1 (Munn et al., 2003). NRel-4 cells have a defect in dihydroxyacetone phosphate acyltransferase (DHAPAT) and NZel-1 cells have altered alkyl dihydroxyacetone phosphate synthase. In NRel-4 cells, ethanolamine plasmalogen is essential for specific cholesterol transport from the cell surface to acyl-CoA/cholesterol acyltransferase in the endoplasmic reticulum. Defective cholesterol transport can be restored when intermediates of ethanolamine plasmalogen biosynthesis are introduced into the system (Munn et al., 2003). The defect in cholesterol transport was also corrected when NRel-4 cells were transfected with a cDNA encoding the missing enzyme, DHAPAT. This suggests that plasmalogens play a very important role in HDL-mediated reverse cholesterol transport associated with atherosclerosis (Maeba and Ueta, 2003, 2004b).

HDL-mediated reverse cholesterol transport may be one of several important mechanisms by which this antiatherogenic lipoprotein slows the development of atherosclerosis. The reduction in the plasmalogen content of normal aortas with increasing donor age was more pronounced in arteriosclerotic aortas (Buddecke and Andresen, 1959). Based on their antioxidant properties, plasmalogens may play a crucial role in the pathogenesis of arteriosclerosis. Because plasmalogens are more susceptible to oxidation than phosphatidylcholine and sphingomyelin, HDL and plasmalogens may be preferred targets of lipid peroxidation before the bulk of polyunsaturated glycerophospholipids in LDL are attacked (Hofer et al., 1996). The importance of oxidized LDL in arteriosclerosis is supported by the finding of a higher oxidative susceptibility of LDL in patients with a higher degree of coronary arteriosclerosis. It is interesting to note that the PlsEtn content is lower by 20% in red cell membrane lipids in hyperlipidemic patients when compared with normolipidemic donors, suggesting that plasmalogens play an important role in cholesterol efflux (Engelmann et al., 1992).

2.2.5 Plasmalogens and Their Antioxidant Activity

Plasmalogens protect biological structures against free radical attack (Engelmann, 2004; Maeba and Ueta, 2004a). Thus plasmalogens not only protect cellular membranes of Chinese hamster ovary cells against oxidative stress (Zoeller et al., 1988), but also play an important role in defending low-density lipoprotein particles against oxidative stress (Engelmann et al., 1994). In neural membranes, transition metal ions (copper and iron) initiate lipid peroxidation by generating peroxyl and alkoxyl radicals from the decomposition of lipid hydroperoxides according to the following reactions.

$$LOOH + Cu^{2+}/Fe^{3+} \rightarrow LOO + H^+ + Cu^+/Fe^{2+} \tag{2.1}$$

$$LOOH + Cu^+/Fe^{2+} \rightarrow LO + OH^- + Cu^{2+}/Fe^{3+} \tag{2.2}$$

Plasmalogen-containing liposomes have a strong ability to chelate transition metal ions and thereby prevent the formation of peroxyl and alkoxyl radicals (Zommara et al., 1995; Sindelar et al., 1999). In biomembranes, the levels of plasmalogen are 25 to 100 times higher than vitamin E (Calzada et al., 1997; Hahnel et al., 1999). Both molecules are colocalized in lipoproteins and cellular membranes and are capable of scavenging peroxyl radicals. However, vitamin E scavenges peroxyl radicals with 20- to 25-fold higher efficiency than the plasmalogens (Hahnel et al., 1999), suggesting that vitamin E is the first line of cellular defense against oxidative stress. The other possibility is that neural cells contains a plasmalogen redox cycling system mediated by vitamin C (Yavin and Gatt, 1972; Engelmann, 2004), and this system plays an important role in defending neural cells from the oxidative stress.

The reactive brominating species generated by myeloperoxidase, as well as by activated neutrophils, also attack the vinyl ether bond of plasmalogens (Albert et al., 2002, 2003). This process results in the production of an α-chlorofatty aldehyde and lysophosphatidylcholine. They may have a profound effect on the host cell protein kinases and inhibit membrane transport proteins (Sasaki et al., 1993). Thus plasmalogens may serve as protective agents for the host cells by quenching ROS and hypohalous acids, and thus preventing them from interacting with other targets such as proteins and nucleic acids (Albert et al., 2002, 2003). Collective evidence suggests that plasmalogens represent the principal pool of antioxidant lipids in neural membranes and are targeted by oxidants. It is likely that an intramolecular competition occurs between the enol ether double bond and fatty acid double bond for reaction with oxidants (Berry and Murphy, 2005).

In contrast to the above view, studies based on the effect of menadione, an intracellular reactive oxygen species generator, on plasmalogen-deficient fibroblasts (Jansen and Wanders, 1997) and lactic acid on astrocytic cultures, suggest that plasmalogens do not play a major role in the protection of cells against superoxide anion radicals and lactic acid-induced oxidative stress (Fauconneau et al., 2001). The fatty aldehyde released from oxidized plasmalogens forms Schiff base adducts not only with malondialdehyde and 4-hydroxynonenals but also with PtdEtn (Stadelmann-Ingrand et al., 2004). Schiff base adducts may have a deleterious effect on neural cell membranes.

2.2.6 Plasmalogens in Differentiation

During development, the incorporation of [³H]ethanolamine into progenitor cells is in a ratio of 1.3 for [³H]PlsEtn to [³H]PtdEtn. When the progenitor cells are induced to differentiate with fetal calf serum, the ratio of [³H]PlsEtn to [³H]PtdEtn increased to 2.3 at 2 days of differentiation and remained at elevated levels of 2.3 to 2.7 through 6 days of differentiation. Although the ratio of [³H]PlsEtn to [³H]PtdEtn decreased after 6 days of differentiation, 1.8 times as much [³H]ethanolamine was still incorporated into [³H]PlsEtn than into [³H]PtdEtn at 9 days of differentiation (Bichenkov and Ellingson, 1999), suggesting that plasmalogens play an important role during differentiation. Plasmalogens and their metabolizing enzymes are present in the nucleus (Albi et al., 2004) and plasmalogen-selective PLA$_2$ is stimulated by retinoic acid (Antony et al., 2001). Retinoic acid treatment produces neuritic outgrowth in LA-N-1 cells. The pan retinoic acid receptor antagonist BMS493 not only inhibits PlsEtn-PLA2 activity but also blocks the formation of neuritic processes (Antony et al., 2003; Farooqui et al., 2004a).

2.3 Platelet-Activating Factor (PAF)

PAF (1-O-alkyl-2-acetyl-sn-glycerophosphocholine) (Fig. 2.6) is a potent biologically active ether lipid with diverse physiological and pathophysiological activities (Snyder, 1995; Bazan, 2003). Its production is tightly regulated both at the synthetic and degradative levels. PAF is released by a wide variety of cells, including macrophages, platelets, endothelial cells, mast cells, neutrophils, and neural cells. It exerts biological effects by activating the PAF receptors that con-

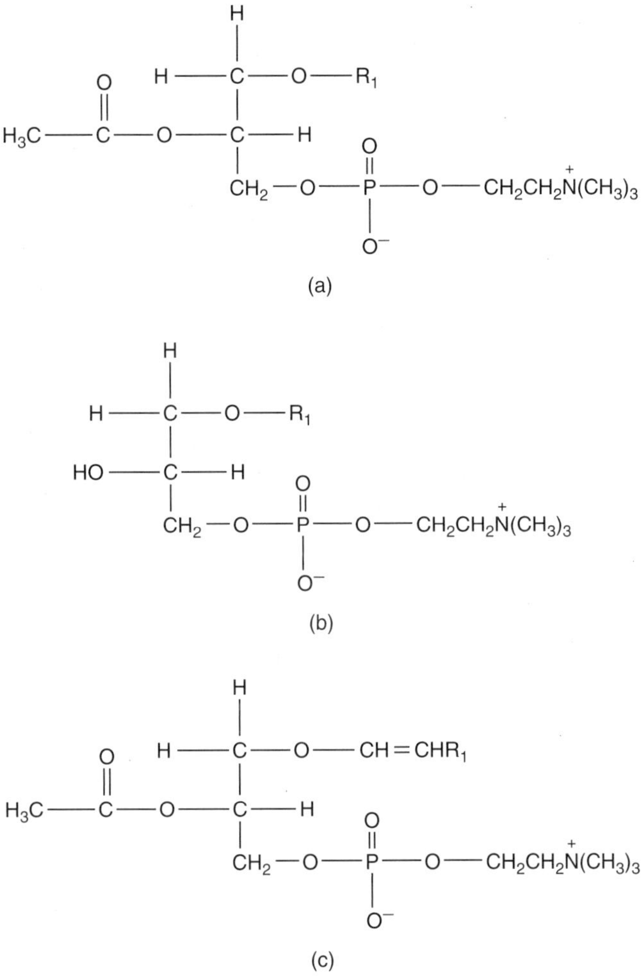

FIG. 2.6. Structures of platelet-activating factor and its analogs. Platelet-activating factor or 1-*O*-alkyl-2-acetyl-*sn*-glycero-3-phosphocholine (a); Lysoplatelet-activating factor or 2-lyso-1-*O*-alkyl-*sn*-glycero-3-phosphocholine (b); and the plasmalogen analog of platelet-activating factor or 1-alk-1′-enyl-2-acetyl-*sn*-glycero-3-phosphocholine (c).

sequently activate leukocytes, stimulate platelet aggregation, and induce the release of cytokines and expression of cell adhesion molecules (Maclennan et al., 1996; Honda et al., 2002; Blok et al., 2002). PAF receptors are linked to G-proteins and activate a variety of intracellular messenger systems such as calcium mobilization, arachidonic acid release, polyphosphoinositide turnover, generation of cAMP, and tyrosine phosphorylation (Chao and Olson, 1993; Ishii and Shimizu, 2000; Honda et al., 2002). PAF receptors have been cloned from a number of sources, including pig lungs and human leukocytes (Honda et al., 2002).

During inflammatory processes, PAF activates leukocytes tethered to the blood vessel wall via specific adhesion molecule expressed by endothelial cells. PAF activates a wide variety of cells, including neutrophils, eosinophils, monocytes, platelets, and endothelial cells.

Expression of PAF receptors in brain has been demonstrated by radioligand binding assay and Northern blotting and in situ hybridization in rats and mice (Marcheselli et al., 1990; Ishii et al., 1996). Although the synthesizing enzymes have not been purified and fully characterized from brain tissue, reports on the generation of PAF in mammalian brain are beginning to emerge (Francescangeli et al., 2000). In astrocytes, PAF upregulates nerve growth factor mRNA in a time- and concentration-dependent manner. This increase in nerve growth factor mRNA is suppressed by WEB 2086 and BN52021, potent PAF antagonists (Brodie, 1995; Yoshida et al., 2005). Astrocytic PAF may provide a neurotrophic signal to injured neurons; hence, interplay between PAF and the neurotrophic receptor may be involved in regenerative processes in brain tissue. The physiological activity of PAF is not limited to its proinflammatory function and neurotrophic effects. PAF is also involved in a variety of other settings, including reproduction; allergic reactions; brain functions; and circulatory system disturbances, such as atherosclerosis (Chao and Olson, 1993; Honda et al., 2002; Bazan, 2003).

2.3.1 PAF Biosynthesis

Three different pathways of PAF synthesis are known to occur in mammalian tissues (Snyder, 1995; Honda et al., 2002). They include a remodeling pathway, de novo synthesis, and an oxidative fragmentation pathway. The remodeling pathway occurs primarily in inflammatory cells (Fig. 2.7). In this pathway, the first step is the hydrolysis of arachidonate from 1-O-alkyl-2-arachidonyl-sn-glycero-3-phosphocholine by cytosolic phospholipase A$_2$ (cPLA$_2$). This results in the simultaneous generation of 1-O-alkyl-2-lyso-sn-glycero-3-phosphocholine (lyso-PAF) and arachidonic acid. This reaction is the basis of the interrelationship between the synthesis of PAF and eicosanoids. The second step of PAF production requires the conversion of lyso-PAF to PAF by the enzyme acetyl CoA: lyso-PAF acetyltransferase. Both these enzymes are activated by post-translational phosphorylation (Prescott et al., 1990).

Lyso-PAF formation can also be initiated by the selective transfer of arachidonate from 1-O-alkyl-2-arachidonyl-sn-glycero-3-phosphocholine to an acceptor lysophospholipid by a CoA-independent transferase activity (Prescott et al., 1990). It is interesting to note that the addition of exogenous lysoplasmalogens markedly stimulates the synthesis of PAF in the presence of acetyl-CoA (Blank et al., 1995). This suggests that plasmalogen-selective PLA$_2$, an enzyme that converts plasmalogens into lysoplasmalogens in the remodeling pathway, may modulate PAF synthesis.

The de novo synthesis of PAF requires three steps. In the first step, an acetyltransferase acetylates 1-O-alkyl-2-lyso-sn-glycerol 3-phosphate to form 1-O-alkyl-2-acetyl-sn-glycero-3-phosphate. The second step requires the action of a phosphohydrolase resulting in the generation of 1-O-alkyl-2-acetyl-sn-glycerol.

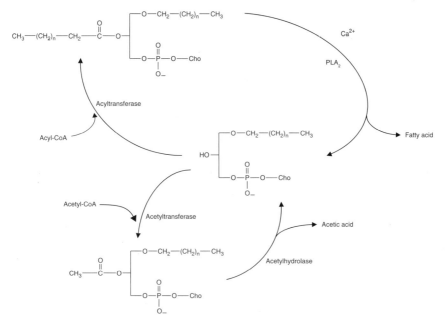

FIG. 2.7. Synthesis and degradation of platelet-activating factor by the remodeling pathway.

Finally the transfer of phosphocholine is catalyzed by dithiothreitol-insensitive choline phosphotransferase (Snyder, 1995).

The third pathway for the synthesis of PAF is the oxidative fragmentation of phosphatidylcholines. When exposed to oxidative conditions, 1-*O*-alkyl-2-arachidonyl-*sn*-glycerophosphocholine breaks down into a variety of species of 1-*O*-alkyl phospholipids containing different short-chain substituents at the *sn*-2 position. These 1-*O*-alkyl phospholipids interact with PAF receptors and induce a variety of biological effects (Stafforini et al., 1996). Analogs of PAF generated from ethanolamine plasmalogens (Fig. 2.6) are of considerable interest, because many cell types form significant amounts of this metabolite naturally. Although little is known about their physiological function, such analogs do exhibit biological activity at higher concentrations than PAF.

2.3.2 PAF Degradation

PAF is hydrolyzed by PAF acetylhydrolases (Fig. 2.7) found in all mammalian tissues (Snyder, 1995). Three isoforms of PAF acetylhydrolase occur in mammalian tissues. One isoform is extracellular and is found in plasma. The other two are intracellular and are found in brain and other visceral organs (Tjoelker and Stafforini, 2000; Arai, 2002). Although both these proteins are serine-dependent enzymes, their ability to hydrolyze PAF is quite different. Plasma PAF acetylhydrolase is a single 44-kDa polypeptide containing a lipase consensus motif (GXSXG). It is also expressed in macrophages and in tissues containing a high content of inflammatory cells (Derewenda and Derewenda, 1998; Arai, 2002). In addition to PAF acetylhydrolase activity, plasma LDL-PLA$_2$ also has a high level of PLA$_2$ activity toward phosphatidylcholine with either oxidized or short-chain fatty acids at the *sn*-2 position. The plasma PAF acetylhydrolase has a dual role in metabolism. It not only inactivates PAF released from inflammatory cells, but is also involved in the elimination of oxidized fatty acid residues in plasma lipoproteins (Tjoelker and Stafforini, 2000; Arai, 2002).

Bovine brain PAF acetylhydrolase is an α, β, γ heterotrimer (mol masses 26, 30, 45 kDa, respectively) with a catalytic serine residue in both the β and γ subunits. Two other PAF acetylhydrolases occur in mammalian tissues. An enzyme from erythrocytes is a 25-kDa homomer and that from mammalian kidney and liver is a 44-kDa polypeptide (Rice et al., 1998). The latter enzyme protects biomembrane phospholipids from oxidative damage.

2.3.3 Roles of PAF

The binding of PAF to PAF receptors activates diverse intracellular signal transduction pathways and processes (Table 2.2) that ultimately activate transcription factors, gene expression, and produce stimulation of phospholipases A$_2$, C, and D activities. The stimulation of these enzymes results in the generation of arachidonic acid, diacylglycerols, and inositol 1,4,5-trisphosphate. Arachidonic acid is metabolized to eicosanoids, diacylglycerols activate protein kinase C, and inositol 1,4,5-trisphosphate mobilizes calcium from intracellular stores (Izumi and Shimizu, 1995, 2000). PAF receptor antagonists block all these processes. PAF also stimulates phosphatidylinositol 3-kinase and mitogen-activated kinase (MAP) kinase and inhibits adenylate cyclase. Moreover, PAF also acts as an intracellular mediator (Marcheselli and Bazan, 1994). The binding of PAF to intracellular sites elicits gene expression in neuronal and glial cell lines (Bazan et al., 1994). Furthermore, PAF receptors are also involved in the release of prostaglandin E$_2$ from astrocytes. This release of prostaglandin E$_2$ is closely associated with pathological pain processing (Watkins et al., 2001).

PAF also stimulates the inducible isoform of prostaglandin synthase or cyclooxygenase (COX-2). This enzyme catalyzes the rate-limiting step in the oxidation of arachidonic acid to prostaglandins. An immediate early gene encodes

TABLE 2.2. Roles of platelet-activating factor in mammalian tissues.

Role	Reference
Modulation of signal transduction processes	Chao and Olson, 1993; Maclennan et al., 1996
Modulation of calcium mobilization	Yue et al., 1991
Modulation of gene transcription	Marcheselli and Bazan, 1994; Bazan et al., 1997
Modulation of long-term potentiation	del Cerro et al., 1990; Kato et al., 1994
Modulation of cerebrovascular system	Kochanek et al., 1988, 1990
Modulation of neuropeptide levels ·	Rougeot et al., 1990; Hashimoto et al., 1993
Modulation of immune response	Müller et al., 1993
Modulation of blood pressure	Wu et al., 1999

COX-2, which is responsible for prostaglandin synthesis in neuropathological processes. Preincubation of cells with the PAF antagonist BN 50730 blocks the stimulation of the immediate early gene responsible for COX-2 (Bazan et al., 1997). Thus, PAF is associated with short- and long-term responses of cells to stimulation or neural trauma.

Neuronal migration is a critical event in brain development. Migration of cerebellar granule cells is modulated by PAF through receptor-dependent and receptor-independent pathways (Tokuoka et al., 2003). L1S-1, a gene that may be mutated in developmental human brain, is a pivotal molecule that links PAF action and neuronal cell migration in studies both in vivo and in vitro. PAF binding sites are present in the nucleus. The addition of PAF to nuclear preparations enhances phosphoinositide hydrolysis (Miguel et al., 2001). Interplay among PAF, oxidative stress, and group-1 metabotropic glutamate receptors modulates neuronal survival in neuronal cultures (Zhu et al., 2004). This once again suggests that PAF antagonists could be used as neuroprotective agents in neural trauma.

Long-term potentiation (LTP) is a long-lasting enhancement of synaptic efficacy due to repeated stimulation of postsynaptic NMDA receptors. The influx of Ca^{2+}, stimulation of $cPLA_2$, and the release of arachidonic acid accompany LTP. It depends on gene expression, protein synthesis, and the establishment of new neuronal connections. PAF antagonists block the development of LTP (del Cerro et al., 1990; Kato et al., 1994; Kato and Zorumski, 1996), indicating that PAF modulates LTP. Thus, in rats, PAF antagonists impair spatial learning and inhibitory avoidance, whereas treatment with a synthetic nonhydrolyzable analog of PAF (mc-PAF, 1-O-hexadecyl-2-methylcarbamoyl-sn-glycerol-3-phosphocholine) enhances memory (Packard et al., 1996). In cultured cells of neuronal and glial origin, high concentrations of PAF are neurotoxic (Kornecki and Ehrlich, 1988; Nogami et al., 1997). Collective evidence suggests that PAF modulates excitatory synaptic transmission, neuronal plasticity, gene expression, and memory.

Intracarotid infusion of PAF decreases cerebral blood flow with a concomitant increase in the global cerebral metabolic rate for oxygen (Kochanek et al., 1988, 1990). PAF administration causes a dose-dependent decrease in spinal cord blood flow. This decrease in blood flow can be blocked by a PAF receptor antagonist (Faden and Halt, 1992). Although PAF does not cross the blood–brain barrier itself, it induces changes in blood–brain barrier permeability (Catalán et al., 1993). PAF is also an essential component of the intricate mechanism by which immune cells such as leukocytes are recruited to their targets (Zimmerman et al., 1996).

2.4 Antitumor Ether Lipids

Antitumor ether lipids are structural analogs of PAF, but lack the readily hydrolyzable ester substituent at the sn-2 position of glycerol moiety (Fig. 2.8). They contain a long carbon chain at sn-1 and a short chain at the sn-2 position. At the sn-3 position, phosphocholine is the head group. Examples of antitumor

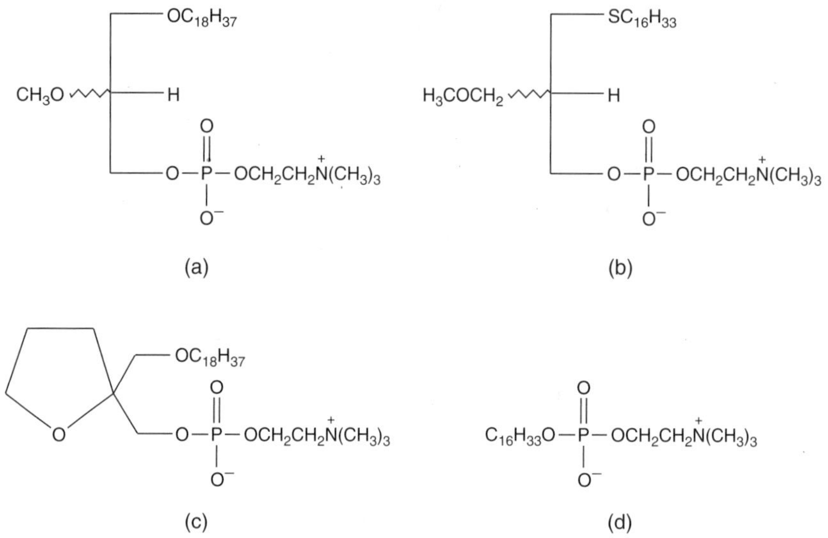

FIG. 2.8. Structures of the antitumor ether lipids. Edelfosine (ET 18-OCH$_3$) (a); ilmofosine (BM 41.440) (b); SR1 62–834 (c), and Miltefosine (HePC) (d).

ether lipids are edelfosine (1-O-octadecyl-2-O-methyl-rac-glycero-3-phosphocholine, Et-18-OCH$_3$), ilmofosine, and miltefosine (hexadecyl phosphocholine, HePC). They are unnatural compounds that are metabolized slowly by mammalian tissues.

They are useful as antitumor drugs because tumor and leukemic cells are more sensitive to the cytotoxic and cytostatic actions of these compounds than normal cells (Berkovic, 1998). The antitumor properties of these compounds include activation of macrophages, reduction of tumor cell invasion in vitro, inhibition of tumor metastases, inhibition of tumor development and shrinkage of tumors, differentiation of tumor cells, and selective inhibition of tumor cell proliferation (Berkovic et al., 1997; Arthur and Bittman, 1998). Whereas the majority of conventional anticancer drugs cause severe side effects due to bone marrow suppression, antitumor ether lipids exert minimal hematologic toxicity. Biochemically, antitumor ether lipids block de novo phosphatidylcholine synthesis by inhibiting CTP: phosphocholine cytidylyltransferase and promoting its translocation to membranes (van der Luit et al., 2002). Antitumor ether lipids also induce the expression of c-fos and c-jun in human leukemic cells and c-fos and zif/268 in astroglial cells by affecting transcription machinery (Mollinedo et al., 1994).

Antitumor ether lipids block various cell signaling pathways (Arthur and Bittman, 1998). They inhibit phosphoinositide-specific phospholipase C (Powis et al., 1992) and phosphatidylinositol-3-kinase (Berggren et al., 1993), and activate protein kinase C and phospholipase D depending on the state of maturation of human tumor cell line U937. Antitumor ether lipids differentially regulate PLA$_2$ activity in human leukemia cell line U937 (Berkovic et al., 1997). In immature cells, these antitumor ether lipids enhance PLA$_2$ activity, whereas in mature differentiated U937 cells PLA$_2$ activity is inhibited. These lipids also modulate intracellular calcium levels affecting activities of many enzymes involved in signal transduction processes. All these studies suggest that the antitumor action of ether lipids is not based on nonspecific membrane alterations, but involves downstream signaling pathways associated with the specific activation of receptors involved in tumor formation (such as CD95) at the plasma membrane of target tumor cells. These lipids are active against HIV (Carballeira, 2002). They can be used along with azidothymidine (AZT) to inhibit the replication of HIV. Antitumor ether lipids also possess antileishmanial activity (Unger et al., 1998) with a cure rate of 88 to 100%.

2.5 Other Ether Lipids

Arachidonoylglycerol (2-AG) is an endogenous cannabinoid receptor ligand that exerts its effects by binding to central and peripheral cannabinoid receptors (Sugiura et al., 1995; Mechoulam et al., 1995). An ether-linked analog of 2-AG, noladin ether (Fig. 2.9), has been isolated from pig brain (Hanuš et al., 2001). Noladin ether is also found in rat brain (Fezza et al., 2002). In contrast, recent mass spectrographic studies indicate that noladin ether is not found in brain tissue of rat, mouse, hamster, guinea pig, and pig (Oka et al., 2003). The reason for this discrepancy is not fully understood. The role of noladin ether in mammalian brain is not known. However, noladin ether may be another endogenous cannabinoid receptor ligand involved in the modulation of several cannabimimetic activities

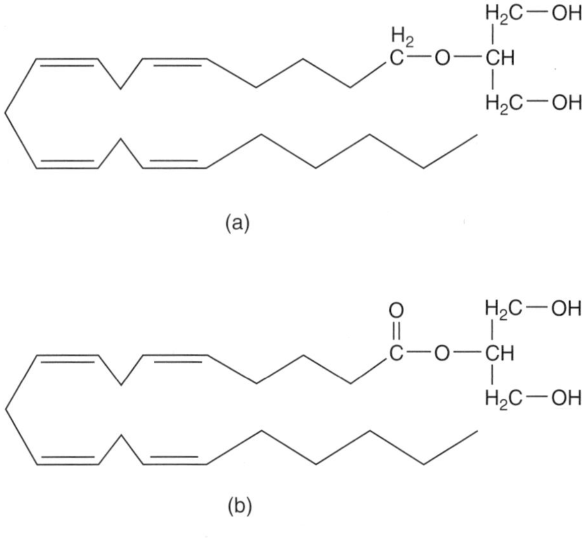

(a)

(b)

FIG. 2.9. Structures of noladin ether lipid (2-eicosa-5′,8′,11′,14′-tetraenylglycerol) (a) and 2-arachidonylglycerol (2-AG) (b).

TABLE 2.3. Roles of minor ether glycerophospholipids in mammalian tissues.

Ether glycerophospholipid	Role	Reference
1-O-Alkyl-2-acyl-sn-glycerophosphoinositol	Attachment with membrane	Cross, 1990
1-O-Alk-1'-enyl-2-lyso-sn-glycero-3-phosphate	Modulation of receptor function	Lu et al., 2002
1-O-Alk-1'-enyl-2-lyso-sn-glycero-3-phosphate	Modulation of receptor function	Liliom et al., 1998a
1-O-Alk-1'-enyl-2-acyl-sn-glycerol	Signal transduction	Hoffman et al., 1986

such as inhibition of lymphocyte proliferation, hypothermia, reduced locomotor activity, and analgesia (Hanuš et al., 2001; Fezza et al., 2002). Synthesis of phosphatidylinositol ether lipid analogs has also been reported (Gills and Dennis, 2004). These compounds inhibit serine/threonine kinase and Akt translocation.

1-O-Alkyl-2-acyl-sn-glycero-3-phosphoinositol is a component of glycosylphosphatidylinositol anchors (GPI anchors) that are involved in the attachment of several proteins to the cell surface (Paltauf, 1994). For example, the presence of alkyl ether lipids in GPI anchors has been reported in human and bovine acetylcholinesterase (Roberts et al., 1988). 1-O-Alkyl-1'-enyl-2-acyl-sn-glycerols and 1-O-alkyl-2-acyl-sn-glycerols are naturally occurring constituents of rabbit myocardium. The levels of these ether-linked diacylglycerols are markedly increased in rabbit heart tissue following ischemia (Ford and Gross, 1988, 1989). Similar to 1, 2-diacyl-sn-glycerols, 1-O-alkyl-1'-enyl-2-acyl-sn-glycerols and 1-O-alkyl-2-acyl-sn-glycerols stimulate protein kinase C and contribute to signal transduction processes during cell stimulation and trauma (Ford et al., 1989) (Table 2.3).

Ether glycerophospholipid species with a saturated ether linkage have been reported to modulate the activity of glucocorticoid receptors (Schulman et al., 1992). 1-O-alk-1'-enyl-2-lyso-sn-glycero-3-phosphate (alkenyl-GP or lyso PlsH) occurs in some commercially available sphingolipid preparations. Alkenyl-GP markedly stimulates mitogen-activated protein kinases and elicits mitogenic responses in 3T3 fibroblasts. This ether lipid may function as a component of a growth factor (Liliom et al., 1998a). This suggests that minor ether phospholipids not only facilitate the attachment of proteins with biomembranes, but also stabilize and modulate receptors localized in biomembranes. Alkenyl-GP has been recently detected in the fluid bathing the cornea. Corneal injury in rabbits produces a marked increase in the levels of this ether lipid along with lysophosphatidic acid (Liliom et al., 1998b). These lipids may be involved not only in maintaining the integrity of the normal cornea, but also in promoting the cellular regeneration of the injured cornea (Liliom et al., 1998b).

2.6 Conclusion

Ether glycerophospholipids are an integral component of neural membranes in which they exist in a dynamic flux, with continuous biosynthesis countered by continuous degradation. In biomembranes, plasmalogens, platelet-activating factor, and other minor ether lipids represent the ether glycerophospholipids. In mammalian tissues, plasmalogen-synthesizing enzymes are localized in peroxisomes and endoplasmic reticulum. Receptor-mediated degradation of plasmalogens is catalyzed by plasmalogen-selective calcium-independent PLA_2. In addition to being antioxidants and the reservoir for second messengers, plasmalogens may be involved in ion transport, membrane fusion, and efflux of cholesterol.

In mammalian tissues, PAF is mainly generated by the action of cytosolic calcium-dependent PLA_2 that releases lyso-PAF and arachidonic acid. Lyso-PAF is then acetylated to form PAF. PAF acetylhydrolases hydrolyze PAF. PAF and its analogs are involved in modulation of gene transcription and long-term potentiation and synaptic plasticity. Although considerable progress has been made on ether glycerophospholipid composition, synthesis, and degradation in biomembranes, only a few enzymes of ether glycerophospholipid metabolism have been purified, characterized, and cloned.

References

Albert C. J., Crowley J. R., Hsu F. F., Thukkani A. K., and Ford D. A. (2002). Reactive brominating species produced by myeloperoxidase target the vinyl ether bond of plasmalogens – Disparate utilization of sodium halides in the production of alpha-halo fatty aldehydes. *J. Biol. Chem.* 277:4694–4703.

Albert C. J., Thukkani A. K., Heuertz R. M., Slungaard A., Hazen S. L., and Ford D. A. (2003). Eosinophil peroxidase-derived reactive brominating species target the vinyl ether bond of plasmalogens generating a novel chemoattractant, alpha-bromo fatty aldehyde. *J. Biol. Chem.* 278:8942–8950.

Albi E., Cataldi S., Magni M. V., and Sartori C. (2004). Plasmalogens in rat liver chromatin: new molecules involved in cell proliferation. *J. Cell. Physiol.* 201:439–446.

Antony P., Freysz L., Horrocks L. A., and Farooqui A. A. (2001). Effect of retinoic acid on the Ca^{2+}-independent phospholipase A_2 in nuclei of LA-N-1 neuroblastoma cells. *Neurochem. Res.* 26:83–88.

Antony P., Freysz L., Horrocks L. A., and Farooqui A. A. (2003). Ca^{2+}-independent phospholipases A_2 and production of arachidonic acid in nuclei of LA-N-1 cell cultures: a specific receptor activation mediated with retinoic acid. *Mol. Brain Res.* 115:187–195.

Arai H. (2002). Platelet-activating factor acetylhydrolase. *Prostaglandins Other Lipid Mediat.* 68–69:83–94.

Arthur G. and Bittman R. (1998). The inhibition of cell signaling pathways by antitumor ether lipids. *Biochim. Biophys. Acta Lipids Lipid Metab.* 1390:85–102.

Bazan N. G. (2003). Synaptic lipid signaling: significance of polyunsaturated fatty acids and platelet-activating factor. *J. Lipid Res.* 44:2221–2233.

Bazan N. G., Fletcher B. S., Herschman H. R., and Mukherjee P. K. (1994). Platelet-activating factor and retinoic acid synergistically activate the inducible prostaglandin synthase gene. *Proc. Natl Acad. Sci.* USA 91:5252–5256.

Bazan N. G., Packard M. G., Teather L., and Allan G. (1997). Bioactive lipids in excitatory neurotransmission and neuronal plasticity. *Neurochem. Int.* 30:225–231.

Berggren M. I., Gallegos A., Dressler L. A., Modest E. J., and Powis G. (1993). Inhibition of the signalling enzyme phosphatidylinositol-3-kinase by antitumor ether lipid analogues. *Cancer Res.* 53:4297–4302.

Berkovic D. (1998). Cytotoxic etherphospholipid analogues. *Gen. Pharmacol.* 31:511–517.

Berkovic D., Luders S., Goeckenjan M., Hiddemann W., and Fleer E. A. (1997). Differential regulation of phospholipase A$_2$ in human leukemia cells by the etherphospholipid analogue hexadecylphosphocholine. *Biochem. Pharmacol.* 53:1725–1733.

Berry K. A. Z. and Murphy R. C. (2005). Free radical oxidation of plasmalogen glycerophosphocholine containing esterified docosahexaenoic acid: structure determination by mass spectrometry. *Antioxidants Redox Signal.* 7:157–169.

Bichenkov E. and Ellingson J. S. (1999). Temporal and quantitative expression of the myelin-associated lipids, ethanolamine plasmalogen, galactocerebroside, and sulfatide, in the differentiating CG-4 glial cell line. *Neurochem. Res.* 24:1549–1556.

Bick R. J., Youker K. A., Pownall H. J., Van Winkle W. B., and Entman M. L. (1991). Unsaturated aminophospholipids are preferentially retained by the fast skeletal muscle CaATPase during detergent solubilization. Evidence for a specific association between aminophospholipids and the calcium pump protein. *Arch. Biochem. Biophys.* 286:346–352.

Blank M. L., Smith Z. L., Fitzgerald V., and Snyder F. (1995). The CoA-independent transacylase in PAF biosynthesis: tissue distribution and molecular species selectivity. *Biochim. Biophys. Acta Lipids Lipid Metab.* 1254:295–301.

Blok W. L., Rabinovitch M., Zilberfarb V., Netea M. G., Buurman W. A., and Van der Meer J. W. M. (2002). The influence of dietary fish-oil supplementation on cutaneous *Leishmania amazonensis* infection in mice. *Cytokine* 19:213–217.

Breckenridge W. C., Morgan I. G., Zanetta J. P., and Vincendon G. (1973). Adult rat brain synaptic vesicles. II. Lipid composition. *Biochim. Biophys. Acta* 320:681–686.

Brites P., Waterham H. R., and Wanders R. J. A. (2004). Functions and biosynthesis of plasmalogens in health and disease. *Biochim. Biophys. Acta Mol. Cell Biol. Lipids* 1636:219–231.

Brodie C. (1995). Platelet activating factor induces nerve growth factor production by rat astrocytes. *Neurosci. Lett.* 186:5–8.

Buddecke E. and Andresen G. (1959). Quantitative Bestimmung der Acetalphosphatide (Plasmalogene) in der Aorta des Menschen unter Berucksichtigung der Arteriosklerose. Hoppe-Seyler's *Z. Physiol. Chem.* 314:38–45.

Calzada C., Bruckdorfer K. R., and Rice-Evans C. A. (1997). The influence of antioxidant nutrients on platelet function in healthy volunteers. *Atherosclerosis* 128:97–105.

Carballeira N. M. (2002). New advances in the chemistry of methoxylated lipids. *Prog. Lipid Res.* 41:437–456.

Catalán R. E., Martínez A. M., Aragonés M. D., Garde E., and Díaz G. (1993). Platelet-activating factor stimulates protein kinase C translocation in cerebral microvessels. *Biochem. Biophys. Res. Commun.* 192:446–451.

Chalon S., Delion-Vancassel S., Belzung C., Guilloteau D., Leguisquet A. M., Besnard J. C., and Durand G. (1998). Dietary fish oil affects monoaminergic neurotransmission and behavior in rats. *J. Nutr.* 128:2512–2519.

Chao W. and Olson M. S. (1993). Platelet-activating factor: receptors and signal transduction. *Biochem. J.* 292:617–629.

Cross G. A. M. (1990). Glycolipid anchoring of plasma membrane proteins. *Annu. Rev. Cell Biol.* 6:1–39.

del Cerro S., Arai A., and Lynch G. (1990). Inhibition of long-term potentiation by an antagonist of platelet-activating factor receptors. *Behav. Neural Biol.* 54:213–217.

Derewenda Z. S. and Derewenda U. (1998). The structure and function of platelet-activating factor acetylhydrolases. *Cell Mol. Life Sci.* 54:446–455.

Dudda A., Spiteller G., and Kobelt F. (1996). Lipid oxidation products in ischemic porcine heart tissue. *Chem. Phys. Lipids* 82:39–51.

Duhm J., Engelmann B., Schönthier U. M., and Streich S. (1993). Accelerated maximal velocity of the red blood cell Na+/K+ pump in hyperlipidemia is related to increase in 1-palmitoyl-2-arachidonoyl-plasmalogen phosphatidylethanolamine. *Biochim. Biophys. Acta Biomembr.* 1149:185–188.

Engelmann B. (2004). Plasmalogens: targets for oxidants and major lipophilic antioxidants. *Biochem. Soc. Trans.* 32:147–150.

Engelmann B., Streich S., Schönthier U. M., Richter W. O., and Duhm J. (1992). Changes of membrane phospholipid composition of human erythrocytes in hyperlipidemias. I. Increased phosphatidylcholine and reduced sphingomyelin in patients with elevated levels of triacylglycerol-rich lipoproteins. *Biochim. Biophys. Acta Lipids Lipid Metab.* 1165:32–37.

Engelmann B., Bräutigam C., and Thiery J. (1994). Plasmalogen phospholipids as potential protectors against lipid peroxidation of low density lipoproteins. *Biochem. Biophys. Res. Commun.* 204:1235–1242.

Faden A. I. and Halt P. (1992). Platelet-activating factor reduces spinal cord blood flow and causes behavioral deficits after intrathecal administration in rats through a specific receptor mechanism. *J. Pharmacol. Exp. Ther.* 261:1064–1070.

Fahy E., Subramaniam S., Brown H. A., Glass C. K., Merrill A. H. J., Murphy R. C., Raetz C. R. H., Russell D. W., Seyama Y., Shaw W., Shimizu T., Spener F., Van Meer G., VanNieuwenhze M. S., White S. H., Witztum J. L., and Dennis E. A. (2005). A comprehensive classification system for lipids. *J. Lipid Res.* 46:839–861.

Farkas T., Kitajka K., Fodor E., Csengeri I., Lahdes E., Yeo Y. K., Krasznai Z., and Halver J. E. (2000). Docosahexaenoic acid-containing phospholipid molecular species in brains of vertebrates. *Proc. Natl Acad. Sci. USA* 97:6362–6366.

Farooqui A. A. and Horrocks L. A. (2001). Plasmalogens: workhorse lipids of membranes in normal and injured neurons and glia. *Neuroscientist* 7:232–245.

Farooqui A. A., Yang H.-C., and Horrocks L. A. (1995). Plasmalogens, phospholipases A$_2$, and signal transduction. *Brain Res. Rev.* 21:152–161.

Farooqui A. A., Rosenberger T. A., and Horrocks L. A. (1997). Arachidonic acid, neurotrauma, and neurodegenerative diseases. In: Yehuda S. and Mostofsky D. I. (eds.), *Handbook of Essential Fatty Acid Biology.* Humana Press, Totowa, NJ, pp. 277–295.

Farooqui A. A., Horrocks L. A., and Farooqui T. (2000a). Deacylation and reacylation of neural membrane glycerophospholipids. *J. Mol. Neurosci.* 14:123–135.

Farooqui A. A., Horrocks L. A., and Farooqui T. (2000b). Glycerophospholipids in brain: their metabolism, incorporation into membranes, functions, and involvement in neurological disorders. *Chem. Phys. Lipids* 106:1–29.

Farooqui A. A., Ong W. Y., Horrocks L. A., and Farooqui T. (2000c). Brain cytosolic phospholipase A$_2$: localization, role, and involvement in neurological diseases. *Neuroscientist* 6:169–180.

Farooqui A. A., Antony P., Ong W. Y., Horrocks L. A., and Freysz L. (2004a). Retinoic acid-mediated phospholipase A$_2$ signaling in the nucleus. Brain Res. Rev. 45:179–195.

Farooqui A. A., Ong W. Y., and Horrocks L. A. (2004b). Biochemical aspects of neurodegeneration in human brain: involvement of neural membrane phospholipids and phospholipases A$_2$. *Neurochem. Res.* 29:1961–1977.

Fauconneau B., Stadelmann-Ingrand S., Favrelière S., Baudouin J., Renaud L., Piriou A., and Tallineau C. (2001). Evidence against a major role of plasmalogens in the resistance of astrocytes in lactic acid-induced oxidative stress in vitro. *Arch. Toxicol.* 74:695–701.

Felde R. and Spiteller G. (1995). Plasmalogen oxidation in human serum lipoproteins. *Chem. Phys. Lipids* 76:259–267.

Fernstrom J. D. (1999). Effects of dietary polyunsaturated fatty acids on neuronal function. *Lipids* 34:161–169.

Fezza F., Bisogno T., Minassi A., Appendino G., Mechoulam R., and Di Marzo V. (2002). Noladin ether, a putative novel endocannabinoid: inactivation mechanisms and a sensitive method for its quantification in rat tissues. *FEBS Lett.* 513:294–298.

Ford D. A. and Gross R. W. (1988). Identification of endogenous 1-O-alk-1'-enyl-2-acyl-*sn*-glycerol in myocardium and its effective utilization by choline phosphotransferase. *J. Biol. Chem.* 263:2644–2650.

Ford D. A. and Gross R. W. (1989). Differential accumulation of diacyl and plasmalogenic diglycerides during myocardial ischemia. *Circ. Res.* 64:173–177.

Ford D. A. and Hale C. C. (1996). Plasmalogen and anionic phospholipid dependence of the cardiac sarcolemmal sodium–calcium exchanger. *FEBS Lett.* 394:99–102.

Ford D. A., Miyake R., Glaser P. E., and Gross R. W. (1989). Activation of protein kinase C by naturally occurring ether-linked diglycerides. *J. Biol. Chem.* 264:13818–13824.

Francescangeli E., Boila A., and Goracci G. (2000). Properties and regulation of microsomal PAF-synthesizing enzymes in rat brain cortex. *Neurochem. Res.* 25:705–713.

Fujimoto K., Yao K., Miyazaki T., Hirano H., Nishikawa M., Kimura S., Murayama K., and Nonaka M. (1989). The effect of dietary docosahexaenoate on the learning ability of rats. In: Chandra R. K. (ed.), *Health Effects of Fish and Fish Oils*. ARTS Biomedical, The Netherlands, pp. 275–284.

Fujita S., Ikegaya Y., Nishikawa M., Nishiyama N., and Matsuki N. (2001). Docosahexaenoic acid improves long-term potentiation attenuated by phospholipase A_2 inhibitor in rat hippocampal slices. *Br. J. Pharmacol.* 132:1417–1422.

Gills J. J. and Dennis P. A. (2004). The development of phosphatidylinositol ether lipid analogues as inhibitors of the serine/threonine kinase, *Akt. Expert Opin. Invest. Drugs* 13:787–797.

Ginsberg L., Xuereb J. H., and Gershfeld N. L. (1998). Membrane instability, plasmalogen content, and Alzheimer's disease. *J. Neurochem.* 70:2533–2538.

Glaser P. E. and Gross R. W. (1995). Rapid plasmenylethanolamine-selective fusion of membrane bilayers catalyzed by an isoform of glyceraldehyde-3-phosphate dehydrogenase: discrimination between glycolytic and fusogenic roles of individual isoforms. *Biochemistry* 34:12193–12203.

Gross R. W. (1985). Identification of plasmalogen as the major phospholipid constituent of cardiac sarcoplasmic reticulum. *Biochemistry* 24:1662–1668.

Hahnel D., Beyer K., and Engelmann B. (1999). Inhibition of peroxyl radical-mediated lipid oxidation by plasmalogen phospholipids and α-tocopherol. *Free Radic. Biol. Med.* 27:1087–1094.

Hanuš L., Abu-Lafi S., Fride E., Breuer A., Vogel Z., Shalev D. E., Kustanovich I., and Mechoulam R. (2001). 2-Arachidonyl glyceryl ether, an endogenous agonist of the cannabinoid CB1 receptor. *Proc. Natl Acad. Sci. USA* 98:3662–3665.

Haroutunian V., Kanof P. D., Tsuboyama G. K., Campbell G. A., and Davis K. L. (1986). Animal models of Alzheimer's disease: behavior, pharmacology, transplants. *Can. J. Neurol. Sci.* 13:385–393.

Hashimoto K., Hirasawa R., and Makino S. (1993). Comparison of the effects of intra-third ventricular administration of interleukin-1 or platelet activating factor on ACTH secretion and the sympathetic-adrenomedullary system in conscious rats. *Acta Med. Okayama* 47:1–6.

Hazen S. L., Ford D. A., and Gross R. W. (1991). Activation of a membrane-associated phospholipase A$_2$ during rabbit myocardial ischemia which is highly selective for plasmalogen substrate. *J. Biol. Chem.* 266:5629–5633.

Hazen S. L. and Gross R. W. (1993). The specific association of a phosphofructokinase isoform with myocardial calcium-independent phospholipase A$_2$. Implications for the coordinated regulation of phospholipolysis and glycolysis. *J. Biol. Chem.* 268:9892–9900.

Hirashima Y., Farooqui A. A., Mills J. S., and Horrocks L. A. (1992). Identification and purification of calcium-independent phospholipase A$_2$ from bovine brain cytosol. *J. Neurochem.* 59:708–714.

Hofer G., Lichtenberg D., Kostner G. M., and Hermetter A. (1996). Oxidation of fluorescent glycero- and sphingophospholipids in human plasma lipoproteins: alkenylacyl subclasses are preferred targets. *Clin. Biochem.* 29:445–450.

Hoffman D. R., Truong C. T., and Johnston J. M. (1986). The role of platelet-activating factor in human fetal lung maturation [published erratum appears in Am. J. Obstet. Gynecol. 1987;157(1):179]. *Am. J. Obstet. Gynecol.* 155:70–75.

Hoffman-Kuczynski B. and Reo N. V. (2004). Studies of myo-inositol and plasmalogen metabolism in rat brain. *Neurochem. Res.* 29:843–855.

Hogyes E., Nyakas C., Kiliaan A., Farkas T., Penke B., and Luiten P. G. (2003). Neuroprotective effect of developmental docosahexaenoic acid supplement against excitotoxic brain damage in infant rats. *Neuroscience* 119:999–1012.

Honda Z., Ishii S., and Shimizu T. (2002). Platelet-activating factor receptor. *J. Biochem.* 131:773–779.

Hong S., Gronert K., Devchand P. R., Moussignac R. L., and Serhan C. N. (2003). Novel docosatrienes and 17S-resolvins generated from docosahexaenoic acid in murine brain, human blood, and glial cells — Autacoids in anti-inflammation. *J. Biol. Chem.* 278:14677–14687.

Horrocks L. A. (1969). Metabolism of the ethanolamine phosphoglycerides of mouse brain myelin and microsomes. *J. Neurochem.* 16:13–18.

Horrocks L. A. (1989). Sources of brain arachidonic acid uptake and turnover in glycerophospholipids. *Ann. NY Acad.* Sci. 559:17–24.

Horrocks L. A. and Sharma M. (1982). Plasmalogens and O-alkyl glycerophospholipids. In: Hawthorne J. N. and Ansell G. B. (eds.), *Phospholipids, New Comprehensive Biochemistry, Vol. 4.* Elsevier Biomedical Press, Amsterdam, pp. 51–93.

Horrocks L. A., Yeo Y. K., Harder H. W., Mozzi R., and Goracci G. (1986). Choline plasmalogens, glycerophospholipid methylation, and receptor-mediated activation of adenylate cyclase. In: Greengard P. and Robison G. A. (eds.), *Advances in Cyclic Nucleotide and Protein Phosphorylation Research, Vol. 20.* Raven Press, New York, pp. 263–292.

Ishii S. and Shimizu T. (2000). Platelet-activating factor (PAF) receptor and genetically engineered PAF receptor mutant mice. *Prog. Lipid Res.* 39:41–82.

Ishii S., Matsuda Y., Nakamura M., Waga I., Kume K., Izumi T., and Shimizu T. (1996). A murine platelet-activating factor receptor gene: cloning, chromosomal localization and up-regulation of expression by lipopolysaccharide in peritoneal resident macrophages. *Biochem. J.* 314 (Pt 2):671–678.

Izumi T. and Shimizu T. (1995). Platelet-activating factor receptor: gene expression and signal transduction. *Biochim. Biophys. Acta Lipids Lipid Metab.* 1259:317–333.

Jansen G. A. and Wanders R. J. A. (1997). Plasmalogens and oxidative stress: evidence against a major role of plasmalogens in protection against the superoxide anion radical. *J. Inherit. Metab. Dis.* 20:85–94.

Jump D. B., Clarke S. D., Thelen A., and Liimatta M. (1994). Coordinate regulation of glycolytic and lipogenic gene expression by polyunsaturated fatty acids. *J. Lipid Res.* 35:1076–1084.

Jurkowitz M. S., Horrocks L. A., and Litsky M. L. (1999). Identification and characterization of alkenyl hydrolase (lysoplasmalogenase) in microsomes and identification of a plasmalogen-active phospholipase A_2 in cytosol of small intestinal epithelium. *Biochim. Biophys. Acta Lipids Lipid Metab.* 1437:142–156.

Kang J. X. and Leaf A. (2000). Prevention of fatal cardiac arrhythmias by polyunsaturated fatty acids. *Am. J. Clin. Nutr.* 71:202S–207S.

Kato K. and Zorumski C. F. (1996). Platelet-activating factor as a potential retrograde messenger. *J. Lipid Mediat. Cell Signal.* 14:341–348.

Kato K., Clark G. D., Bazan N. G., and Zorumski C. F. (1994). Platelet-activating factor as a potential retrograde messenger in CA1 hippocampal long-term potentiation. *Nature* 367:175–179.

Katsuki H. and Okuda S. (1995). Arachidonic acid as a neurotoxic and neurotrophic substance. *Prog. Neurobiol.* 46:607–636.

Kochanek P. M., Nemoto E. M., Melick J. A., Evans R. W., and Burke D. F. (1988). Cerebrovascular and cerebrometabolic effects of intracarotid infused platelet-activating factor in rats. *J. Cereb. Blood Flow Metab.* 8:546–551.

Kochanek P. M., Melick J. A., Schoettle R. J., Magargee M. J., Evans R. W., and Nemoto E. M. (1990). Endogenous platelet activating factor does not modulate blood flow and metabolism in normal rat brain. *Stroke* 21:459–462.

Kornecki E. and Ehrlich Y. H. (1988). Neuroregulatory and neuropathological actions of the ether-phospholipid platelet-activating factor. *Science* 240:1792–1794.

Latorre E., Aragonés M. D., Fernández I., and Catalán R. E. (1999). Platelet-activating factor modulates brain sphingomyelin metabolism. *Eur. J. Biochem.* 262:308–314.

Latorre E., Collado M. P., Fernández I., Aragonés M. D., and Catalán R. E. (2003). Signaling events mediating activation of brain ethanolamine plasmalogen hydrolysis by ceramide. *Eur. J. Biochem.* 270:36–46.

Lee T. C. (1998). Biosynthesis and possible biological functions of plasmalogens. *Biochim. Biophys. Acta Lipids Lipid Metab.* 1394:129–145.

Liliom K., Fischer D. J., Virág T., Sun G., Miller D. D., Tseng J. L., Desiderio D. M., Seidel M. C., Erickson J. R., and Tigyi G. (1998a). Identification of a novel growth factor-like lipid, 1-*O*-*cis*-alk-1′-enyl-2-lyso-*sn*-glycero-3-phosphate (alkenyl-GP) that is present in commercial sphingolipid preparations. *J. Biol. Chem.* 273:13461–13468.

Liliom K., Guan Z., Tseng J. L., Desiderio D. M., Tigyi G., and Watsky M. A. (1998b). Growth factor-like phospholipids generated after corneal injury. *Am. J. Physiol.* 274:C1065–C1074.

Lohner K. (1996). Is the high propensity of ethanolamine plasmalogens to form non-lamellar lipid structures manifested in the properties of biomembranes? *Chem. Phys. Lipids* 81:167–184.

Lohner K., Balgavy P., Hermetter A., Paltauf F., and Laggner P. (1991). Stabilization of non-bilayer structures by the etherlipid ethanolamine plasmalogen. *Biochim. Biophys. Acta* 1061:132–140.

Lu J., Xiao Y. J., Baudhuin L. M., Hong G. Y., and Xu Y. (2002). Role of ether-linked lysophosphatidic acids in ovarian cancer cells. *J. Lipid Res.* 43:463–476.

Maclennan K. M., Smith P. F., and Darlington C. L. (1996). Platelet-activating factor in the CNS. *Prog. Neurobiol.* 50:585–596.

Maeba R. and Ueta N. (2003). Ethanolamine plasmalogens prevent the oxidation of cholesterol by reducing the oxidizability of cholesterol in phospholipid bilayers. *J. Lipid Res.* 44:164–171.

Maeba R. and Ueta N. (2004a). A novel antioxidant action of ethanolamine plasmalogens in lowering the oxidizability of membranes. *Biochem. Soc. Trans.* 32:141–143.

Maeba R. and Ueta N. (2004b). Determination of choline and ethanolamine plasmalogens in human plasma by HPLC using radioactive triiodide (1−) ion ($^{125}I_3^-$). *Anal. Biochem.* 331:169–176.

Mandel H., Sharf R., Berant M., Wanders R. J. A., Vreken P., and Aviram M. (1998). Plasmalogen phospholipids are involved in HDL-mediated cholesterol efflux: insights from investigations with plasmalogen-deficient cells. *Biochem. Biophys. Res. Commun.* 250:369–373.

Marcheselli V. L. and Bazan N. G. (1994). Platelet-activating factor is a messenger in the electroconvulsive shock-induced transcriptional activation of c-*fos* and *zif*-268 in hippocampus. *J. Neurosci. Res.* 37:54–61.

Marcheselli V. L., Rossowska M. J., Domingo M. T., Braquet P., and Bazan N. G. (1990). Distinct platelet-activating factor binding sites in synaptic endings and in intracellular membranes of rat cerebral cortex. *J. Biol. Chem.* 265:9140–9145.

Marcheselli V. L., Hong S., Lukiw W. J., Tian X. H., Gronert K., Musto A., Hardy M., Gimenez J. M., Chiang N., Serhan C. N., and Bazan N. G. (2003). Novel docosanoids inhibit brain ischemia-reperfusion-mediated leukocyte infiltration and pro-inflammatory gene expression. *J. Biol. Chem.* 278:43807–43817.

Masuzawa Y., Sugiura T., Ishima Y., and Waku K. (1984). Turnover rates of the molecular species of ethanolamine plasmalogen of rat brain. *J. Neurochem.* 42:961–968.

Mechoulam R., Ben Shabat S., Hanuš L., Ligumsky M., Kaminski N. E., Schatz A. R., Gopher A., Almog S., Martin B. R., and Compton D. R. (1995). Identification of an endogenous 2-monoglyceride, present in canine gut, that binds to cannabinoid receptors. *Biochem. Pharmacol.* 50:83–90.

Miguel B. G., Calcerrada M. C., Martin L., Catalán R. E., and Martínez A. M. (2001). Increase of phosphoinositide hydrolysis and diacylglycerol production by PAF in isolated rat liver nuclei. *Prostaglandins Other Lipid Mediat.* 65:159–166.

Miller S. L., Benjamin J. A., and Morell P. (1977). Metabolism of glycerophospholipids of myelin and microsomes in rat brain. Reutilization of precursors. *J. Biol. Chem.* 252:4025–4037.

Miller S. L. and Morell P. (1978). Turnover of phosphatidylcholine in microsomes and myelin in brains of young and adult rats. *J. Neurochem.* 31:771–777.

Mollinedo F., Gajate C., and Modolell M. (1994). The ether lipid 1-octadecyl-2-methyl-*rac*-glycero-3-phosphocholine induces expression of *fos* and *jun* proto-oncogenes and activates AP-1 transcription factor in human leukaemic cells. *Biochem. J.* 302:325–329.

Müller E., Dagenais P., Alami N., and Rola-Pleszczynski M. (1993). Identification and functional characterization of platelet-activating factor receptors in human leukocyte populations using polyclonal anti-peptide antibody. *Proc. Natl Acad. Sci. USA* 90:5818–5822.

Munn N. J., Arnio E., Liu D., Zoeller R. A., and Liscum L. (2003). Deficiency in ethanolamine plasmalogen leads to altered cholesterol transport. *J. Lipid Res.* 44:182–192.

Murphy R. C. (2001). Free-radical-induced oxidation of arachidonoyl plasmalogen phospholipids: Antioxidant mechanism and precursor pathway for bioactive eicosanoids. *Chem. Res. Toxicol.* 14:463–472.

Nagan N. and Zoeller R. A. (2001). Plasmalogens: biosynthesis and functions. *Prog. Lipid Res.* 40:199–229.

Nakanishi K., Yasugi E., Morita H., Dohi T., and Oshima M. (1994). Plasmenylethanolamine in human intestinal mucosa detected by an improved method for analysis of phospholipid. *Biochem. Mol. Biol. Int.* 33:457–462.

Nishikawa M., Kimura S., and Akaike N. (1994). Facilitatory effect of docosahexaenoic acid on N-methyl-D-aspartate response in pyramidal neurones of rat cerebral cortex. *J. Physiol.* (London) 475:83–93.

Nogami K., Hirashima Y., Endo S., and Takaku A. (1997). Involvement of platelet-activating factor (PAF) in glutamate neurotoxicity in rat neuronal cultures. *Brain Res.* 754:72–78.

Oka S., Tsuchie A., Tokumura A., Muramatsu M., Suhara Y., Takayama H., Waku K., and Sugiura T. (2003). Ether-linked analogue of 2-arachidonoylglycerol (noladin ether) was not detected in the brains of various mammalian species. *J. Neurochem.* 85:1374–1381.

Packard M. G., Teather L. A., and Bazan N. G. (1996). Effects of intrastriatal injections of platelet-activating factor and the PAF antagonist BN 52021 on memory. *Neurobiol. Learn. Mem.* 66:176–182.

Paltauf F. (1994). Ether lipids in biomembranes. *Chem. Phys. Lipids* 74:101–139.

Pettegrew J. W., Panchalingam K., Hamilton R. L., and McClure R. J. (2001). Brain membrane phospholipid alterations in Alzheimer's disease. *Neurochem. Res.* 26:771–782.

Portilla D. and Dai G. (1996). Purification of a novel calcium-independent phospholipase A_2 from rabbit kidney. *J. Biol. Chem.* 271:15451–15457.

Powis G., Seewald M. J., Gratas C., Melder D., Riebow J., and Modest E. J. (1992). Selective inhibition of phosphatidylinositol phospholipase C by cytotoxic ether lipid analogues. *Cancer Res.* 52:2835–2840.

Prescott S. M., Zimmerman G. A., and McIntyre T. M. (1990). Platelet-activating factor. *J. Biol. Chem.* 265:17381–17384.

Rapoport S. I. (1999). In vivo fatty acid incorporation into brain phospholipids in relation to signal transduction and membrane remodeling. *Neurochem. Res.* 24:1403–1415.

Rice S. Q. J., Southan C., Boyd H. F., Terrett J. A., Macphee C. H., Moores K., Gloger I. S., and Tew D. G. (1998). Expression, purification and characterization of a human serine-dependent phospholipase A_2 with high specificity for oxidized phospholipids and platelet activating factor. *Biochem. J.* 330:1309–1315.

Rintala J., Seemann R., Chandrasekaran K., Rosenberger T. A., Chang L., Contreras M. A., Rapoport S. I., and Chang M. C. J. (1999). 85 kDa cytosolic phospholipase A_2 is a target for chronic lithium in rat brain. *NeuroReport* 10:3887–3890.

Roberts W. L., Myher J. J., Kuksis A., and Rosenberry T. L. (1988). Alkylacylglycerol molecular species in the glycosylinositol phospholipid membrane anchor of bovine erythrocyte acetylcholinesterase. *Biochem. Biophys. Res. Commun.* 150:271–277.

Rosenberger T. A., Oki J., Purdon A. D., Rapoport S. I., and Murphy E. J. (2002). Rapid synthesis and turnover of brain microsomal ether phospholipids in the adult rat. *J. Lipid Res.* 43:59–68.

Rougeot C., Junier M. P., Minary P., Weidenfeld J., Braquet P., and Dray F. (1990). Intracerebroventricular injection of platelet-activating factor induces secretion of adrenocorticotropin, beta-endorphin and corticosterone in conscious rats: a possible link between the immune and nervous systems. *Neuroendocrinology* 51:267–275.

Sasaki Y., Asaoka Y., and Nishizuka Y. (1993). Potentiation of diacylglycerol-induced activation of protein kinase C by lysophospholipids. *FEBS Lett.* 320:47–51.

Schulman G., Bodine P. V., and Litwack G. (1992). Modulators of the glucocorticoid receptor also regulate mineralocorticoid receptor function. *Biochemistry* 31:1734–1741.

Serhan C. N. (2005). Novel ω-3-derived local mediators in anti-inflammation and resolution. *Pharmacol. Ther.* 105:7–21.

Serhan C. N., Arita M., Hong S., and Gotlinger K. (2004). Resolvins, docosatrienes, and neuroprotectins, novel omega-3-derived mediators, and their endogenous aspirin-triggered epimers. *Lipids* 39:1125–1132.

Sindelar P. J., Guan Z. Z., Dallner G., and Ernster L. (1999). The protective role of plasmalogens in iron-induced lipid peroxidation. *Free Radic. Biol. Med.* 26:318–324.

Snyder F. (1995). Platelet-activating factor: the biosynthetic and catabolic enzymes. *Biochem. J.* 305:689–705.

Snyder F., Lee T.-C., and Wykle R. L. (1985). Ether-linked glycerolipids and their bioactive species: enzymes and metabolic regulation. In: Martonosi A. N. (ed.), *The enzymes of biological membranes*. Plenum Publishing Corporation, New York, pp. 1–58.

Stadelmann-Ingrand S., Pontcharraud R., and Fauconneau B. (2004). Evidence for the reactivity of fatty aldehydes released from oxidized plasmalogens with phosphatidylethanolamine to form Schiff base adducts in rat brain homogenates. *Chem. Phys. Lipids* 131:93–105.

Stafforini D. M., Prescott S. M., Zimmerman G. A., and McIntyre T. M. (1996). Mammalian platelet-activating factor acetylhydrolases. *Biochim. Biophys. Acta* 1301:161–173.

Sugiura T., Kondo S., Sukagawa A., Nakane S., Shinoda A., Itoh K., Yamashita A., and Waku K. (1995). 2-Arachidonoylglycerol: a possible endogenous cannabinoid receptor ligand in brain. *Biochem. Biophys. Res. Commun.* 215:89–97.

Tjoelker L. W. and Stafforini D. M. (2000). Platelet-activating factor acetylhydrolases in health and disease. *Biochim. Biophys. Acta* 1488:102–123.

Tokuoka S. M., Ishii S., Kawamura N., Satoh M., Shimada A., Sasaki S., Hirotsune S., Wynshaw-Boris A., and Shimizu T. (2003). Involvement of platelet-activating factor and LIS1 in neuronal migration. *Eur. J. Neurosci.* 18:563–570.

Turini M. E. and Holub B. J. (1994). The cleavage of plasmenylethanolamine by phospholipase A_2 appears to be mediated by the low affinity binding site of the TxA_2/PGH_2 receptor in U46619-stimulated human platelets. *Biochim. Biophys. Acta Lipids Lipid Metab.* 1213:21–26.

Uemura Y., Lee T. C., and Snyder F. (1991). A coenzyme A-independent transacylase is linked to the formation of platelet-activating factor (PAF) by generating the lyso-PAF intermediate in the remodeling pathway. *J. Biol. Chem.* 266:8268–8272.

Unger C., Maniera T., Kaufmann-Kolle P., and Eibl H. (1998). In vivo antileishmanial activity of hexadecylphosphocholine and other alkylphosphocholines. *Drugs Today* 34(Suppl. F):133–140.

van der Luit A. H., Budde M., Ruurs P., Verheij M., and Van Blitterswijk W. J. (2002). Alkyl-lysophospholipid accumulates in lipid rafts and induces apoptosis via raft-dependent endocytosis and inhibition of phosphatidylcholine synthesis. *J. Biol. Chem.* 277:39541–39547.

Watkins L. R., Milligan E. D., and Maier S. F. (2001). Glial activation: a driving force for pathological pain. *Trends Neurosci.* 24:450–455.

Weisser M., Vieth M., Stolte M., Riederer P., Pfeuffer R., Leblhuber F., and Spiteller G. (1997). Dramatic increase of alpha-hydroxyaldehydes derived from plasmalogens in the aged human brain. *Chem. Phys. Lipids* 90:135–142.

Williams S. D. and Ford D. A. (1997). Activation of myocardial cAMP-dependent protein kinase by lysoplasmenylcholine. *FEBS Lett.* 420:33–38.

Williams S. D. and Ford D. A. (2001). Calcium-independent phospholipase A_2 mediates CREB phosphorylation and c-fos expression during ischemia. *Am. J. Physiol. Heart Circ. Physiol.* 281:H168–H176.

Wu R., Lemne C., De Faire U., and Frostegard J. (1999). Antibodies to platelet-activating factor are associated with borderline hypertension, early atherosclerosis and the metabolic syndrome. *J. Intern. Med.* 246:389–397.

Xiao Y. F. and Li X. Y. (1999). Polyunsaturated fatty acids modify mouse hippocampal neuronal excitability during excitotoxic or convulsant stimulation. *Brain Res.* 846:112–121.

Yavin E. and Gatt S. (1972). Oxygen-dependent cleavage of the vinyl ether linkage of plasmalogens. 2. Identification of the low molecular weight active component and the reaction mechanism. *Eur. J. Biochem.* 25:437–446.

Yehuda S., Rabinovitz S., Carasso R. L., and Mostofsky D. I. (2002). The role of polyunsaturated fatty acids in restoring the aging neuronal membrane. *Neurobiol. Aging* 23:843–853.

Yoshida H., Imaizumi T., Tanji K., Sakaki H., Metoki N., Hatakeyama M., Yamashita K., Ishikawa A., Taima K., Sato Y., Kimura H., and Satoh K. (2005). Platelet-activating factor enhances the expression of nerve growth factor in normal human astrocytes under hypoxia. *Mol. Brain Res.* 133:95–101.

Young C., Gean P. W., Chiou L. C., and Shen Y. Z. (2000). Docosahexaenoic acid inhibits synaptic transmission and epileptiform activity in the rat hippocampus. *Synapse* 37:90–94.

Yue T. L., Gleason M. M., Gu J. L., Lysko P. G., Hallenbeck J., and Feuerstein G. (1991). Platelet-activating factor (PAF) receptor-mediated calcium mobilization and phosphoinositide turnover in neurohybrid NG108-15 cells: studies with BN50739, a new PAF antagonist. *J. Pharmacol. Exp. Ther.* 257:374–381.

Zhu P. M., DeCoster M. A., and Bazan N. G. (2004). Interplay among platelet-activating factor, oxidative stress, and group I metabotropic glutamate receptors modulates neuronal survival. *J. Neurosci. Res.* 77:525–531.

Zimmer L., Delion-Vancassel S., Durand G., Guilloteau D., Bodard S., Besnard J. C., and Chalon S. (2000). Modification of dopamine neurotransmission in the nucleus accumbens of rats deficient in n-3 polyunsaturated fatty acids. *J. Lipid Res.* 41:32–40.

Zimmerman G. A., Elstad M. R., Lorant D. E., McIntyre T. M., Prescott S. M., Topham M. K., Weyrich A. S., and Whatley R. E. (1996). Platelet-activating factor (PAF): signalling and adhesion in cell–cell interactions. *Adv. Exp. Med. Biol.* 416:297–304.

Zoeller R. A., Morand O. H., and Raetz C. R. H. (1988). A possible role for plasmalogens in protecting animal cells against photosensitized killing. *J. Biol. Chem.* 263:11590–11596.

Zommara M., Tachibana N., Mitsui K., Nakatani N., Sakono M., Ikeda I., and Imaizumi K. (1995). Inhibitory effect of ethanolamine plasmalogen on iron- and copper-dependent lipid peroxidation. *Free Radical Biol. Med.* 18:599–602.

3
Phospholipases A$_2$ in Brain

3.1 Introduction

The phospholipases A$_2$ (PLA$_2$, EC 3.1.1.4) form an expanding superfamily of esterases that specifically hydrolyze the acyl ester bond at the *sn*-2 position of glycerol in membrane glycerophospholipids to produce free fatty acids and lysoglycerophospholipids. Under normal conditions, a small portion of the released arachidonic acid, 20:4 n-6, is converted to inflammatory mediators (prostaglandins, leukotrienes, and thromboxanes), but the majority of this fatty acid is reincorporated into the brain glycerophospholipids (Leslie, 2004). AA acts via conversion to inflammatory metabolites and directly modulates neural cell function by various mechanisms, such as altering the fluidity and polarization state of membranes, activating protein kinase C, stimulating Ca^{2+} release, modulating the activity of several important enzymes, and regulating gene transcription (Molloy et al., 1998). The other product of PLA$_2$-catalyzed reactions, lysoglycerophospholipids, can include the immediate precursor of platelet-activating factor, another potent inflammatory mediator (Farooqui et al., 2000a). Lysoglycerophospholipids may also change membrane fluidity and permeability. The accumulation of lysoglycerophospholipids is controlled by either reacylation to native glycerophospholipids (Farooqui et al., 2000b) or by hydrolysis to water-soluble glycerophosphodiesters, such as glycerophosphocholine by lysophospholipases (Farooqui et al., 1985). A tight regulation of PLA$_2$ activity is necessary for maintaining basal levels of arachidonic acid, lysoglycerophospholipids, and PAF for normal brain function.

The existence of PLA$_2$ enzymes has been known for over 100 years, but it is only within the last 15 years that their metabolic importance in neurochemical processes has been recognized. The first report on PLA$_2$ activity in brain tissue appeared in 1962 when Gallai-Hatchard observed the formation of lysoglycerophospholipids from diacyl glycerophospholipids in human brain preparations (Balboa et al., 2002). Subsequently, Webster and Cooper (1968) reported the presence of PLA$_1$ and PLA$_2$ activities in rat brain slices and homogenates. Woelk (1978) detected PLA$_2$ activity in neurons. Among the subcellular fractions, mitochondrial and synaptosomal fractions contain most of the PLA$_2$ activity (Webster and Cooper, 1968; Kim et al., 1995). PLA$_2$ from human cerebral cortex and rat brain mitochondria display greater activity with 1,2-diacyl-*sn*-glycero-3-phosphocholine than with the 1-alk-1′enyl-2-acyl and 1-alkyl-2-acyl analogs (Woelk et al., 1974). The enzyme requires Ca^{2+} ions for optimal activity. Synaptic membranes of bovine brain contain a Ca^{2+}/calmodulin-dependent PLA$_2$ (Moskowitz et al., 1982, 1983). This enzyme is inhibited by ATP and cAMP and may be involved in neurotransmitter release. Under normal conditions, PLA$_2$ activity is involved in the generation of lipid mediators that are closely associated with glycerophospholipid turnover, neurotransmitter release, long-term potentiation, memory processes, and membrane repair. Normally, the released fatty acids are recycled into neural glycerophospholipids by a deacylation/reacylation pathway to maintain their normal composition (Farooqui et al., 2000a).

However, under pathological conditions, increased PLA$_2$ activity causes the loss of essential neural membrane glycerophospholipids, resulting in altered neural membrane fluidity and permeability, ion homeostasis, increased free fatty acid release, and accumulation of lipid peroxides. High levels of free radicals and lipid peroxides in brain produce oxidative stress. These processes along with compromised energy metabolism may result in neurodegeneration in acute neuronal trauma and neurodegenerative diseases (Farooqui and Horrocks, 1994).

3.2 Multiplicity and Properties of Phospholipase A$_2$ in Brain Tissue

With recent advances in the molecular and cellular biology of PLA$_2$, more than 20 isoforms with PLA$_2$ activity have been identified. PLA$_2$ enzymes are subdivided into several groups depending upon their structure, enzymic properties, subcellular localization, and cellular function (Table 3.1) (Dennis, 1997; Farooqui et al., 1997a; Chakraborti, 2003; Sun et al., 2004; Phillis and O'Regan, 2004). These groups include secretory phospholipase A$_2$ (sPLA$_2$), cytosolic phospholipase A$_2$ (cPLA$_2$), plasmalogen-selective phospholipase A$_2$ (PlsEtn-selective PLA$_2$), and calcium-independent phospholipase A$_2$ (iPLA$_2$). Each class of PLA$_2$ is further subdivided into isozymes for which there are 14 for sPLA$_2$, at least four for cPLA$_2$, and two for iPLA$_2$. Gene coding for sPLA$_2$, cPLA$_2$, and iPLA$_2$ occurs in different regions of brain, in neurons, microglia, and astrocytes (Zanassi et al., 1998; Molloy et al., 1998; Balboa et al., 2002). PLA$_2$ isoforms have been partially purified and characterized from brain tissue (Hirashima et al., 1992; Ross et al., 1995; Yang et al., 1999), but none have been cloned and fully characterized.

3.2.1 sPLA$_2$

sPLA$_2$ is synthesized intracellularly. Then it is secreted and acts in extracellular compartments. sPLA$_2$ has a molecular mass of 14 kDa and is mainly associated with synaptosomes and synaptic vesicle fractions (Kim et al., 1995; Matsuzawa

TABLE 3.1. Physicochemical and kinetic properties of various isoforms of brain PLA$_2$ activities.

Property	sPLA$_2$	cPLA$_2$-α	cPLA$_2$-β	cPLA$_2$-γ	PlsEtn-selective PLA$_2$	iPLA$_2$
Localization	Extracellular	Cytosol	Cytosol	Cytosol	Cytosol	Cytosol
Mol. Mass	14–18 kDa	85 kDa	114 kDa	61 kDa	39 kDa	80 kDa
Effect of Ca^{2+}	Stimulated (mM)	Translocation	Translocation	Translocation	No effect	No effect
Substrate	PtdCho	PtdCho	PtdCho	PtdCho	PlsEtn	PtdCho
Fatty acid specificity	None	AA	AA	AA	AA DHA	Lino
Chromosome	–	1	15	19	–	7
CalB domain	Absent	Present	Present	Absent	Not known	Absent
Effect of AACOCF$_3$	No effect	Inhibited	Inhibited	Inhibited	Inhibited	Inhibited
Effect of BEL	No effect	Inhibited	Inhibited	Inhibited	Inhibited	Inhibited

Data are summarized from Farooqui et al. (2000b), Hirashima et al. (1992), Yang et al. (1999), and Matsuzawa et al. (1996).

PtdCho, phosphatidylcholine; PlsEtn, ethanolamine plasmalogen; AA, arachidonic acid; Lino, Linoleic acid; AACOCF$_3$, arachidonyltrifluoromethyl ketone; BEL, bromoenol lactone.

et al., 1996). At least 14 different subfamilies of sPLA$_2$ occur in mammalian tissues. sPLA$_2$ binds to two types of cell surface receptors (Fig. 3.1), namely the N type, identified in neurons; and the M type, identified in skeletal muscles, of sPLA$_2$ receptors (Hanasaki and Arita, 2002; Murakami and Kudo, 2004; Hanasaki, 2004). Brain sPLA$_2$ contains a secretion peptide and requires mM Ca^{2+} for enzymic activity. It shows no selectivity for particular fatty acyl chains in the glycerophospholipids. This enzyme is present in all regions of mammalian brain. The highest activity of sPLA$_2$ is found in medulla oblongata, pons, and hippocampus, with moderate activity in the hypothalamus, thalamus, and cerebral cortex, and low activity in the cerebellum and olfactory bulb (Thwin et al., 2003). At the cellular level, the sPLA$_2$ transcript is found in astrocytes (Zanassi et al., 1998; Mosior et al., 1998). mRNAs encoding multiple forms of sPLA$_2$ (sPLA$_2$-X, -1B, -X, and -V) occur in rat retina (Kolko et al., 2004). The multiple forms of sPLA$_2$ may be involved in retinal degeneration.

sPLA$_2$ is present in differentiated PC12 cells and in rat brain synaptic vesicles, indicating that neurons also express sPLA$_2$ activity (Matsuzawa et al., 1996). Rat brain synaptosomes or differentiated PC12 cells release sPLA$_2$ upon stimulation via acetylcholine and glutamate receptors or via voltage-dependent Ca^{2+} channels through depolarization. Thus, sPLA$_2$ may play an important role in neuronal metabolism (Kim et al., 1995; Matsuzawa et al., 1996). Based on pharmacological studies, the sPLA$_2$ released from neuronal cells may modulate the degranulation process leading to the release of neurotransmitters. Inhibitors of sPLA$_2$ activity block this release. For the expression of neurotoxicity, the released

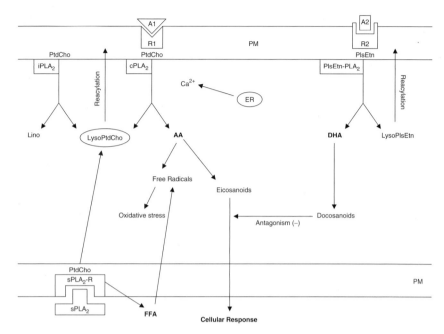

Fig. 3.1. A hypothetical diagram showing interactions among metabolites generated by sPLA$_2$, cPLA$_2$, iPLA$_2$, and PlsEtn-selective PLA$_2$. PM, plasma membrane; A1, agonist; R1, receptor; A2, agonist; R2, receptor; PtdCho, phosphatidylcholine; PlsEtn, ethanolamine plasmalogen; Lyso-PtdCho, lysophosphatidylcholine, Lyso-PlsEtn, lysoethanolamine plasmalogen; ER, endoplasmic reticulum; Lino, linoleic acid; AA, arachidonic acid; DHA, docosahexaenoic acid; FFA, free fatty acid; sPLA$_2$, secretory phospholipase A$_2$; cPLA$_2$, cytosolic phospholipase A$_2$; iPLA$_2$, calcium-independent phospholipase A$_2$; PlsEtn-PLA$_2$, plasmalogen-selective phospholipase A$_2$.

sPLA$_2$ binds to the presynaptic membrane, enters the lumen of the synaptic vesicle during the retrieval of the vesicle from the plasma membrane, and then hydrolyzes glycerophospholipids in the inner leaflet of synaptic vesicles, changing the glycerophospholipid composition and thus impairing its endocytosis. The stimulation of sPLA$_2$ in synaptic vesicles correlates with the induction of vesicle–vesicle aggregation, and this process plays a central role in presynaptic neurotransmission (Moskowitz et al., 1983; Matsuzawa et al., 1996; Wei et al., 2003). In brain sPLA$_2$ is expressed in astrocytes and can be induced in response to proinflammatory cytokines, such as tumor necrosis factor-α and interleukin-1β (Lin et al., 2004).

Mitochondrial fractions from rat brain, PC12 cells, and U251 astrocytoma cell cultures contain significant sPLA$_2$ and iPLA$_2$ activities (Macchioni et al., 2004). It is rather strange that a secretory protein, sPLA$_2$, is found in an intracellular organelle, the mitochondria. Heparan sulfate, a glycosaminoglycan, may play an important role in internalization and attachment of PLA$_2$ isoforms to intracellular organelles (Farooqui et al., 1994; Boilard et al., 2003). A reduction in the mito-chondrial membrane potential causes the release of sPLA$_2$. This sPLA$_2$, along with other PLA$_2$ isoforms, may be involved in neural cell injury (Farooqui et al., 1997b; Macchioni et al., 2004).

Glutamate and its analogs stimulate sPLA$_2$ activity in a dose- and time-dependent manner (Kim et al., 1995; Xu et al., 2003). The addition of sPLA$_2$ to cortical cultures synergistically increases the neurotoxicity of glutamate. Glutamatergic synaptic activity may be modulated by sPLA$_2$ and its receptors on neuronal surface (DeCoster et al., 2002; Kolko et al., 2002). In PC12 cells, sPLA$_2$ induces neurite outgrowth. Mutants with a reduced sPLA$_2$ activity exhibit a comparable reduction in neurite-inducing activity (Nakashima et al., 2003), indicating that sPLA$_2$ performs a neurotrophin-like role in the central nervous system.

3.2.2 cPLA$_2$

Although brain tissue contains cPLA$_2$ activity, it has never been purified to homo-geneity and characterized from brain. Studies with rat brain have indicated that the cytosolic fraction contains two forms of PLA$_2$ activity, PLA$_2$-H and PLA$_2$-L. PLA$_2$-H has an apparent molecular mass of 200 to 500 kDa. Ca^{2+} partially inhibits its activity. In contrast, PLA$_2$-L has a molecular mass of 100 kDa and requires Ca^{2+} (Yoshihara and Watanabe, 1990). Based on several enzymic properties, such as Ca^{2+} sensitivity, molecular mass, and Ca^{2+}-mediated translocation, PLA$_2$-L appears to be identical to cPLA$_2$ (Yoshihara et al., 1992). cPLA$_2$ prefers arachi-donic acid over other fatty acids and does not use Ca^{2+} for catalysis, although sub-micromolar Ca^{2+} concentrations are needed for membrane binding (Clark et al., 1987; Farooqui et al., 2000b). Owing to the presence of a Ca^{2+}-dependent glyc-erophospholipid-binding domain at the N-terminal region, cPLA$_2$ is translocated in a Ca^{2+}-dependent manner from cytosol to the nuclear or other cellular mem-branes (Clark et al., 1987; Hirabayashi et al., 2004), where other downstream enzymes, including the cyclooxygenases and lipoxygenases responsible for the metabolism of arachidonic acid to eicosanoids, are located. This gives cPLA$_2$ access to its membrane-associated glycerophospholipid substrate (Fig. 3.1). However, we do not know the manner in which cPLA$_2$ is activated by extracellu-lar stimuli and whether this activation occurs at specific sites (Hirabayashi et al., 2004). The C-terminal region of cPLA$_2$ contains the phosphorylation site and cat-alytic site. These sites may be involved in regulation of the enzymic activity. The activation of cPLA$_2$ can be through serine residues, notably Ser 505 and Ser 727, by mitogen-activated protein kinase (MAPK) and protein kinase C (PKC) (Hirabayashi and Shimizu, 2000; Hirabayashi et al., 2004). cPLA$_2$ also contains putative pleckstrin homology domains responsible for the ability of this enzyme to interact and bind with anionic glycerophospholipids. Thus cPLA$_2$ activity is also modulated through a cooperative binding mechanism with glycerophospho-lipids containing arachidonic acid (Burke et al., 1995) or through binding of anionic glycerophospholipids, such as phosphatidylinositol 4,5-bisphosphate

(PIP$_2$), phosphatidylinositol 3,4,5-trisphosphate (PIP$_3$), or ceramide 1-phosphate (Mosior et al., 1998; Pettus et al., 2004; Hirabayashi et al., 2004). The N-terminal C2 domain of non-neural cPLA$_2$ contains an antiparallel β-sandwich composed of two four-stranded sheets. Folding of the C2 domain of cPLA$_2$ is similar to those of protein kinase C, synaptotagmin, and phospholipase C and is necessary for the translocation of cPLA$_2$ from cytosol to plasma, endoplasmic reticulum, Golgi, and nuclear membranes (Evans et al., 2004).

This cPLA$_2$-α activity is present in the cytosolic fraction of brains from various animal species. It can be separated from other PLA$_2$ activities by Sephadex G-75 column chromatography (Yang et al., 1997). cPLA$_2$ activity is present in the cytosolic fraction of forebrain, midbrain, hindbrain, and spinal cord from the rat. Hindbrain displays the highest specific activity (19.5 pmol/min/mg), followed by spinal cord (15.2 pmol/min/mg), midbrain (6.3 pmol/min/mg), and forebrain (4.5 pmol/min/mg) (Ong et al., 1999b).

The basal expression of cPLA$_2$-α mRNA under normal conditions is very low in neuronal and glial cells of brain tissue (Owada et al., 1994). In human cerebral cortex, cPLA$_2$ is present in astrocytes of gray matter (Stephenson et al., 1994). Colocalization with glial fibrillary acidic protein (GFAP) suggests that cPLA$_2$-α is predominantly associated with protoplasmic astrocytes from gray matter. Astrocytes of the white matter are not immunoreactive, suggesting that the functional role of gray matter may be different from white matter astrocytes (Stephenson et al., 1999). In cortical cultures, cPLA$_2$-α is expressed by both astrocytes and neurons (Luo et al., 1998). In the rat, forebrain and midbrain are very lightly stained with cPLA$_2$-α antibody, except for the arcuate nucleus and mammillary nuclei (Fig. 3.2A–C). The hindbrain, in contrast, contained many densely labeled nuclei (Fig. 3.2D). Apart from the facial motor nucleus (Fig. 3.2D), dense staining is observed in the initial portions of the ascending auditory pathway, including the dorsal and ventral cochlear nuclei (Fig. 3.3A), and the superior olivary nucleus (Fig. 3.3B), which receives afferents from the dorsal cochlear nucleus (Beyerl, 1978). In addition, dense staining is also observed in some of the nuclei projecting to the cerebellar cortex, including the external cuneate nucleus (Fig. 3.3C) and the inferior olivary nucleus (Desclin, 1974). Purkinje neurons of the cerebellar cortex itself are labeled (Fig. 3.3D), and deep cerebellar nuclei, which receive afferents from the Purkinje neurons are also labeled (Fig. 3.3D). Electron microscopic studies indicate that most of the cPLA$_2$-α is present in dendrites postsynaptic to unlabeled axon terminals, and in a small number of myelinated axons (Ong et al., 1999b). Recent immunolabeling and in situ hybridization studies indicate that cPLA$_2$-α is localized in somata and dendrites of Purkinje cells, whereas cPLA$_2$-β is present in granule cells of rat brain (Shirai and Ito, 2004). cPLA$_2$-α is predominately found in astrocytes of gray matter (Farooqui et al., 2000b; Pardue et al., 2003), as well as in hippocampal neurons (Sandhya et al., 1998; Kishimoto et al., 1999; Strokin et al., 2003b), where under physiological conditions, cPLA$_2$-α may be involved in second messenger generation and long-term potentiation (LTP), a mechanism involved in memory storage.

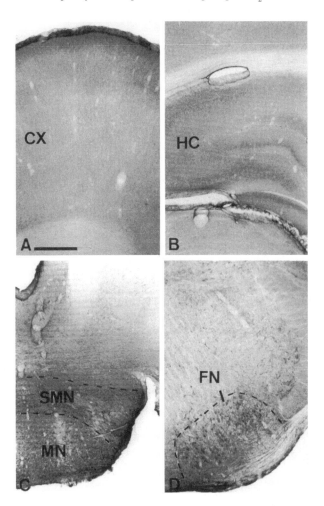

FIG. 3.2. A, B: sections through the rat frontal cortex (CX) and hippocampus (HC), show-ing light staining to cPLA₂. C: section through the hypothalamus, showing dense staining of the mamillary nucleus (MN) and supramamillary nucleus (SMN). D: section through the pons, showing dense staining of the facial nucleus (FN). The approximate boundaries of nuclei are indicated by dashed lines. Scale = 630 μm. This figure is reproduced from Farooqui et al. (2000b) with permission from Sage Science Press.

In rat and monkey spinal cord (Ong et al., 1999a), dense staining of cPLA₂-α can be observed in cell bodies and the neuropil in the dorsal horn (Fig. 3.4A), and in motor neurons of the ventral horn (Fig. 3.4B). As in brain regions, cPLA₂-α immunoreactivity is located in dendrites (Fig. 3.4C) and a small number of myeli-nated axons. The widespread distribution of cPLA₂ activity in cervical, thoracic, lumbar, and sacral motor neurons in spinal cord and in various regions of brain

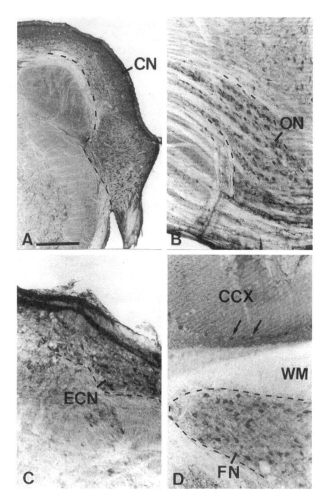

FIG. 3.3. A: section through the pons, showing dense staining of the dorsal and ventral cochlear nuclei (CN). B: section through the pons, showing dense staining of the superior olivary nucleus (ON). C: section through the medulla oblongata, showing dense staining of the external cuneate nucleus (ECN). D: section through the cerebellum, showing dense staining of Purkinje neurons (arrows) in the cerebellar cortex (CCX), and the fastigial nucleus (FN). The cerebellar white matter (WM) is not labeled. The approximate boundaries of nuclei are indicated by dashed lines. Scale: A = 630 µm, B–D = 250 µm. This figure is reproduced from Farooqui et al. (2000b) with permission from Sage Science Press.

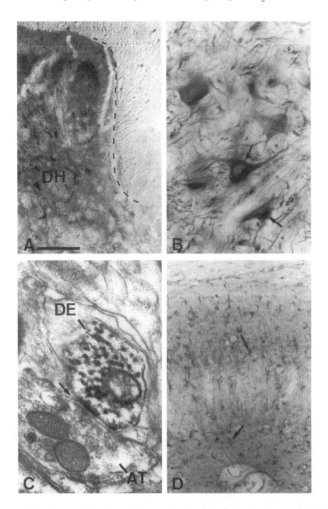

F$_{IG}$. 3.4. A: section through the dorsal horn of a lumbar spinal segment (DH, demarcated by dashed line), showing dense staining of cell bodies and the neuropil. B: section through the ventral horn of a lumbar spinal segment, showing dense staining of motor neurons (arrows). C: electron micrograph of the ventral horn of a sacral spinal segment, showing a synapse (arrow) between an unlabeled axon terminal (AT) and a labeled dendrite (DE). D: field CA1 of the hippocampus, from a rat that was injected with kainate 2 weeks earlier. In contrast to normal hippocampus (Fig. 3.1B), large numbers of cPLA$_2$-positive, reactive astrocytes (arrows) are present in the degenerating CA field. Scale: A,B = 50 μm; C = 0.3 μm, D = 160 μm. This figure is reproduced from Farooqui et al. (2000b) with permission from Sage Science Press.

suggests that cPLA$_2$ activity may play an important role in regulating the levels of arachidonic acid, eicosanoids, and PAF.

Three paralogs of cPLA$_2$ occur in brain and other non-neural tissues (Diaz-Arrastia and Scott, 1999; Farooqui et al., 2000b; Hirabayashi et al., 2004). They are cPLA$_2$-α (mol. mass: 85 kDa), cPLA$_2$-β (mol. mass: 114 kDa), and cPLA$_2$-γ (mol. mass: 61 kDa). These three paralogs contain two catalytic domains inter-spaced with paralog specific sequences. The lipase motif, GXSGS, is located in the catalytic domain. cPLA$_2$-β is found mainly in the cerebellum and shares more similarities with cPLA$_2$-α than with cPLA$_2$-γ. cPLA$_2$-γ lacks the C2 domain, but contains a prenyl-group-binding motif that behaves as a lipid anchor and allows binding of the enzyme to the membrane. Recombinantly expressed cPLA$_2$-γ liberates arachidonic acid from phosphatidylcholine. Unlike cPLA$_2$-α, cPLA$_2$-γ also acts on other fatty acid residues at the sn-2 and sn-1 positions of glycerophospholipids. cPLA$_2$-α has a remarkable specificity for arachidonic acid at the sn-2 position. It also has sn-1 lysophospholipase activity and a weak translocase activity associated with it. cPLA$_2$-β prefers to cleave fatty acids at the sn-1 position, and cPLA$_2$-γ efficiently hydrolyzes fatty acid at sn-1 as well as sn-2 positions of glycerol moiety (Song et al., 1999). The overexpression of cPLA$_2$-γ increases the proportions of polyunsaturated fatty acids in phosphatidylethanolamine, indicating that this paralog can modulate glycerophospholipid compositions (Asai et al., 2003). cPLA$_2$-γ is constitutively expressed in the endoplasmic reticulum where it is involved in remodeling and maintaining the glycerophospholipid composition under oxidative stress. cPLA$_2$-β displays much lower activity with [2-arachidonoyl]PtdCho than do the other two paralogs.

The genes for human cPLA$_2$-α, -β, -γ map to chromosomes 1, 15, and 19, respectively. Phosphorylation sites for mitogen-activated protein kinase are present only in cPLA$_2$-α and are not conserved in cPLA$_2$-β and cPLA$_2$-γ. cPLA$_2$-α activity is uniformly distributed in various regions of rat brain (Farooqui et al., 2000b). A new paralog of cPLA$_2$ is mainly found in skin and was named cPLA$_2$-δ (mol. mass 109 kDa) (Chiba et al., 2004). In contrast to other cPLA$_2$ paralogs, cPLA$_2$-δ prefers to release linoleic acid instead of arachidonic acid. Considerable information is available on cPLA$_2$-α (Farooqui et al., 2000b). Recently, the mRNA for cPLA$_2$-β and cPLA$_2$-δ has been identified by reverse transcription-polymerase chain reaction analysis in human brain tissue (Pickard et al., 1999; Song et al., 1999; Hirabayashi et al., 2004), but the role of these paralogs of cPLA$_2$ in brain tissue remains speculative. Since cPLA$_2$-δ mainly occurs in skin, it is proposed that this paralog plays a critical role in inflammation in psoriatic lesions (Chiba et al., 2004).

3.2.3 PlsEtn-Selective PLA$_2$

This enzyme hydrolyzes arachidonic acid and docosahexaenoic acid from the sn-2 position of plasmalogens, a special type of glycerophospholipid with a vinyl ether linkage at the sn-1 position of the glycerol backbone (Farooqui and Horrocks, 2001). This enzyme was purified and characterized from bovine brain cytosol

(Hirashima et al., 1992), rabbit kidney (Portilla and Dai, 1996), and rabbit heart (Hazen and Gross, 1993). Bovine brain PlsEtn-selective PLA$_2$ has an apparent molecular mass of 39 kDa. Nonionic detergents, Triton X-100 and Tween-20, stimulate the enzymic activity. Bromoenol lactone, an inhibitor that markedly inhibits iPLA$_2$, does not inhibit PlsEtn-selective PLA$_2$. Low μM ATP concentrations have no effect on PlsEtn-selective PLA$_2$ activity, but 2-mM ATP markedly inhibits its activity. DTNB, iodoacetate, and N-ethylmaleimide inhibit bovine brain PlsEtn-selective PLA$_2$ in a dose-dependent manner (Farooqui et al., 1995). Various polyvalent anions, citrate > sulfate > phosphate, and metal ions, Ag$^+$, Hg^{2+} and Fe^{3+}, also inhibit this enzyme in a dose-dependent manner. Glycosaminoglycans markedly inhibit bovine brain PlsEtn-selective PLA$_2$ with an inhibition pattern of heparan sulfate > hyaluronic acid > chondroitin sulfate > heparin. N-acetylneuraminic acid, gangliosides, and sialoglycoproteins also inhibit this PLA$_2$ (Yang et al., 1994b). Other glycosphingolipids, such as cerebrosides and sulfatides, have no effect. However, ceramide markedly stimulates PlsEtn-selective PLA$_2$ activity in a time- and dose-dependent manner (Latorre et al., 2003). Treatment of rat brain slices with *Staphylococcus aureus* sphingomyelinase or C2-ceramide produces a marked decrease in PlsEtn levels suggesting the stimulation of PlsEtn-selective PLA$_2$ activity. Bromoenol lactone, a potent inhibitor of iPLA$_2$, does not affect this stimulation, but quinacrine and gangliosides, nonspecific inhibitors of PlsEtn-selective PLA$_2$, completely block it (Yang et al., 1994a,b; Latorre et al., 2003). These studies have led to the suggestion that the degradation of plasmalogen by PlsEtn-selective PLA$_2$ is a receptor-mediated process (Farooqui and Horrocks, 2001; Latorre et al., 2003; Farooqui et al., 2003) and may involve an interaction between plasmalogen metabolism and sphingolipid metabolism.

PlsEtn-selective PLA$_2$ was localized immunochemically in neurons and astrocytes (Farooqui and Horrocks, 2001). The co-localization of PlsEtn-selective PLA$_2$ with glial fibrillary acidic protein suggests that this PLA$_2$ is predominantly associated with astrocytes (Fig. 3.5). This is in contrast to cPLA$_2$-α, which is present in neurons as well as astrocytes (Sandhya et al., 1998; Kishimoto et al., 1999). PlsEtn-selective PLA$_2$ releases arachidonic acid and docosahexaenoic acid in rat brain astrocytes and cyclic AMP and Ca^{2+} regulate these enzymes differentially (Strokin et al., 2003a). Since plasmalogens are major glycerophospholipids of neural membranes, PlsEtn-selective PLA$_2$ may be involved mainly in generating docosahexaenoic acid (DHA), a 22-carbon essential fatty acid with six double bonds. This fatty acid is highly enriched in synaptosomal membranes, synaptic vesicles, and growth cones, and accounts for more than 17% by weight of the total fatty acids in the brain of adult rats (Hamano et al., 1996).

3.2.4 iPLA$_2$

The cytosolic fraction from brain contains an 80-kDa Ca^{2+}-independent phospholipase A$_2$ (iPLA$_2$) activity. This enzyme was purified from rat brain to homogeneity using multiple column chromatographic procedures with a very low

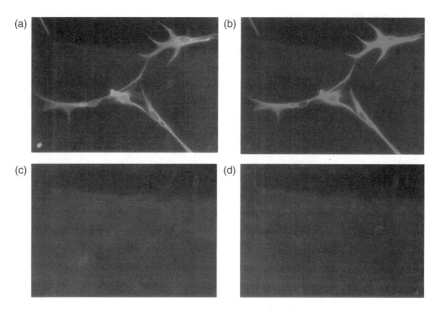

FIG. 3.5. Colocalization of plasmalogen-selective PLA$_2$ and glial fibrillary acidic protein (GFAP) in astrocytic cortical cultures. Dual labeling was performed with antiplasmalogen-selective PLA$_2$ (a) and anti-GFAP (b) and visualized with a fluorescein filter for PLA$_2$ and rhodamine filter for GFAP. Negative controls for PLA$_2$ (*See Colour Plate*) (c) and GFAP (d). Magnification (x40).

yield. The purified enzyme had a specific activity of 4.3 µmol/min/mg. The peptide sequence of this enzyme has considerable homology to sequences of the iPLA$_2$ from P388D1 macrophages, CHO cells, and human B lymphocytes (Yang et al., 1999). This iPLA$_2$ hydrolyzes the *sn*-2 fatty acid from PtdCho with its preferences linoleoyl > palmitoyl > oleoyl > arachidonoyl group. iPLA$_2$ has a unique amino acid sequence containing a lipase consensus sequence and eight ankyrin repeats. Bromoenol lactone strongly inhibits this enzyme and ATP augments its activity.

iPLA$_2$ is present in all brain regions with the highest activity in striatum, hypothalamus, and hippocampus. The gene encoding iPLA$_2$ was identified (Molloy et al., 1998). Alternative splicing can generate multiple iPLA$_2$ isoforms with distinct tissue distribution and localization (Larsson et al., 1998). Also, iPLA$_2$ is negatively regulated by truncated splice variant proteins that prevent the formation of active iPLA$_2$ tetramers (Luscher et al., 1992; Larsson et al., 1998; Seashols et al., 2004). Native iPLA$_2$ is a homotetramer that is potentially formed through interactions between N-terminal ankyrin repeats (Ackermann and Dennis, 1995). Five splice variants of iPLA$_2$ have been reported to occur in various tissues (Larsson et al., 1998; Shirai and Ito, 2004). One splice variant, iPLA$_2$-1, lacks exon 9 (165 base pairs), whereas four other variants, iPLA$_2$-2, iPLA$_2$-3, iPLA$_2$-ankyrin-1, and iPLA$_2$-ankyrin-2, contain exon 9. The presence of this exon makes these splice variants membrane bound because exon 9 encodes hydrophobic amino acids (Larsson et al., 1998; Shirai and Ito, 2004). Rat cerebellum contains iPLA$_2$-1, iPLA$_2$-2, or iPLA$_2$-3 but not iPLA$_2$-ankyrin-1 or iPLA$_2$-ankyrin-2.

In the normal monkey brain, iPLA$_2$ immunoreactivity is observed in structures derived from the telencephalon, including the cerebral cortex, septum, amygdala, and striatum (Fig. 3.6), whereas structures derived from the diencephalon, including the thalamus, hypothalamus, and subthalamic nucleus are lightly labeled. The brainstem is also generally lightly labeled, with the exception of the central gray and the locus ceruleus. The neuropil of the cerebellar cortex is moderately densely stained. Immunoreactivity is observed in neuronal nuclei and axon terminals at electron microscopy. Glial cells and mural cells in the walls of blood vessels do not show iPLA$_2$ immunoreactivity (Ong et al., 2006). In rat brain,

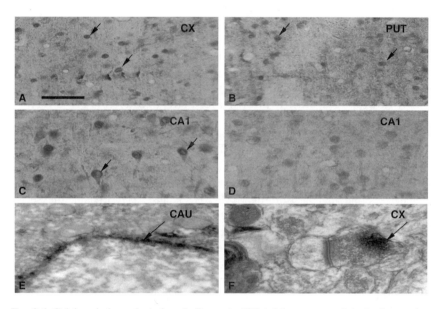

FIG. 3.6. Calcium-independent phospholipase A$_2$ (iPLA$_2$) immunoreactivity in the monkey brain (*Macacca fascicularis*). Regions derived from the telencephalon, including the cortex, striatum, and hippocampus, are densely labeled. A–C: Sections through the temporal cortex (A), putamen (B), and field CA1 of the hippocampus (C), immunolabeled with affinity purified goat antibody to iPLA$_2$ (Santa Cruz Biotechnology, sc-14466; diluted 1:500 from the 200 µg/ml supplied solution). Label is observed in nuclei and on the nuclear envelope of neurons (arrows) and fine processes in the neuropil. The latter were found to be dendrites and axon terminals with electron microscopy. D: section through the hippocampus incubated with antigen-absorbed antibody, showing only background labeling. E: electron micrograph of a neuron in the caudate nucleus, showing dense labeling of the nuclear envelope (arrow). F: electron micrograph of a labeled axon terminal (arrow) in the frontal cortex. Abbreviations: CX: cortex; PUT: putamen; CAU: caudate nucleus. Scale: A–D: 50 µm; E: 1 µm; and F: 0.4 µm. Details of this work are published in Ong et al. (2006).

iPLA$_2$ is present in granule cells, stellate cells, and the nuclei of Purkinje cells (Shirai and Ito, 2004). The olfactory bulb, hippocampus CA1-3, dentate gyrus, and brain stem have strong signals of iPLA$_2$ immunoreactivity.

In non-neural cells, the cleavage of iPLA$_2$ by caspase-3 is associated with the execution of apoptosis (Atsumi et al., 1998, 2000). The proposed role of iPLA$_2$ in glycerophospholipid remodeling and apoptosis is based on the use of bromoenol lactone, a specific inhibitor, but this compound actually inhibits other enzymes, such as diacylglycerol lipase and phosphatidate phosphohydrolase (Moriyama et al., 1999; Winstead et al., 2000; Fuentes et al., 2003). This makes it difficult to define the role of iPLA$_2$ in glycerophospholipid metabolism (Farooqui et al., 2000a; Akiba and Sato, 2004; Pérez et al., 2004). iPLA$_2$ plays an important role in long-term potentiation and long-term depression. Activity-dependent changes in synaptic strength are believed to underlie certain forms of learning and memory in the hippocampus (Fitzpatrick and Baudry, 1994; Wolf et al., 1995; Fujita et al., 2001). iPLA$_2$ is also important in neural cell proliferation, apoptosis, and differentiation (Farooqui et al., 2004; Akiba and Sato, 2004).

3.3 Platelet-Activating Factor Acetylhydrolases (PAF-AH)

Brain tissue contains PAF acetylhydrolase, a unique PLA$_2$ that hydrolyzes the acetyl group from the sn-2 position of the glycerol moiety of PAF and thus abolishes the diverse and potent actions of PAF. Unlike other secreted PLA$_2$ activities, PAF acetylhydrolase does not require Ca^{2+} for activity. The PAF-AH family includes two intracellular isoforms (PAF-AH Ib and PAF-AH II) and one secretory isoform (PAF-AH) (Snyder, 1995; Derewenda and Derewenda, 1998; Tjoelker and Stafforini, 2000; Karasawa et al., 2003).

Bovine brain PAF-AH 1b has a molecular mass of approximately 100 kDa. SDS gel electrophoresis revealed three distinct subunits with molecular mass of 26, 30, and 45 kDa. The 45-kDa α-subunit is not essential for the catalytic activity. The 26- and 30-kDa subunits have catalytic activity (Higuchi et al., 1996; McMullen et al., 2000). The 45-kDa β-subunit of PAF-AH1b has received considerable attention because it has striking homology (99%) with a protein encoded by the causal gene LIS-1 for Miller-Dieker lissencephaly, a human disease characterized by a smooth cerebral surface and abnormal neuronal migration (Hattori et al., 1994). This strongly suggests that the modulation of PAF concentration is crucial for brain development (Adachi et al., 1995; Manya et al., 1998; McMullen et al., 2000).

Besides the 45-kDa subunit, the bovine brain PAF-AH Ib complex consists of two 26-kDa catalytic subunits, $\alpha 1$ and $\alpha 2$, which share 63% sequence identity with each other. The amino acid sequences of these subunits have poor homology with plasma PAF-AH and PAF-AHI I (Karasawa et al., 2003). Collective evidence suggests that brain PAF-AH is a unique PLA$_2$ in which dimerization is essential for both stability and catalytic activity. In addition to

Colour Plate

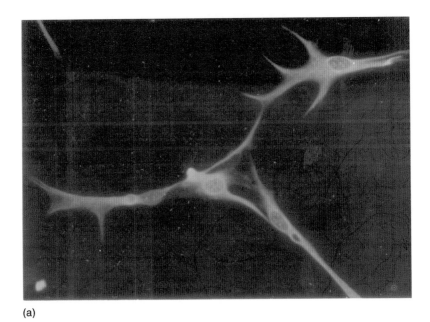

(a)

FIG. 3.5. Colocalization of plasmalogen-selective PLA_2 and glial fibrillary acidic protein (GFAP) in astrocytic cortical cultures. Dual labeling was performed with antiplasmalogen-selective PLA_2 (a) and anti-GFAP.

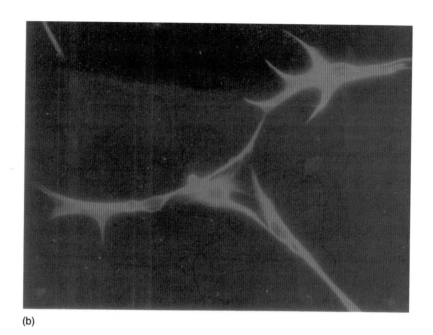

(b)

FIG. 3.5. *Continued* (b) and visualized with a fluorescein filter for PLA$_2$ and rhodamine filter for GFAP. Negative controls for PLA$_2$.

PAF acetylhydrolase activity, this enzyme also contains high PLA$_2$ activity toward phosphatidylcholine with either oxidized or short chain fatty acids at the *sn*-2 position (Gilbert et al., 1996).

3.4 Other Brain Phospholipases A$_2$

Other brain PLA$_2$ activities are incompletely characterized and have not been classified. Bovine brain microsomes contain an 18.5-kDa PtdIns-specific Ca^{2+}-dependent PLA$_2$ (Gray and Strickland, 1982). It has very little activity with PtdEtn, PtdSer, and PtdH. It prefers *sn*-2 fatty acids, with an activity pattern of 20:4 > 18:1 > 18:0 > 16:0. Divalent metal ions, Mg^{2+}, Mn^{2+}, and Zn^{2+}, activate it. Detergents, such as Triton-X-100 (0.02–0.03%) and n-octylglucoside (30 mM), stimulate the enzymic activity.

Two Ca^{2+}-independent PLA$_2$ activities were isolated from nerve growth cones. One enzyme selectively hydrolyzes phosphatidylinositol (mol. mass: 65 kDa) and the other acts on PtdEtn (mol. mass: 100 kDa) (Negre-Aminou et al., 1996). The PtdIns-selective enzyme is greatly enriched in the cytosolic fraction of fetal brain and is resistant to reducing agents. Attempts to establish an interaction or relationship between the PtdIns-PLA$_2$ and PtdEtn-selective PLA$_2$ remain inconclusive.

A calcium-sensitive 180-kDa PLA$_2$ was isolated from human brain cytosol. This enzyme does not require Ca^{2+} for its basal activity, but its activity is increased 2- to 3-fold by 2 mM Ca^{2+}. It hydrolyzes ethanolamine glycerophospholipids 8-fold faster than choline glycerophospholipids (Table 3.2). This human brain PLA$_2$ is heat sensitive and is activated by dithiothreitol (DTT).

Purification of a novel calcium-independent phospholipase from rat brain that releases various fatty acids from the *sn*-1 and *sn*-2 positions was reported (Ueda et al., 1993). This enzyme shows a high activity under alkaline conditions. The partially purified enzyme has a molecular mass of 300 kDa and hydrolyzes PtdCho, PtdEtn, PtdIns, and PtdH with equal efficiency, but PtdSer is not a good

TABLE 3.2. Properties of the incompletely characterized and unclassified brain phospholipases A$_2$.

Enzyme	Source (brain)	Localization	Mol. Mass (kDa)	Substrate specificity	Ca^{2+} requirement
PLA$_2$	Bovine	Microsomes	18.5	PtdIns	Dependent
PLA$_2$	Rat	Growth cones	65	PtdIns	Independent
PLA$_2$	Rat	Growth cones	100	PtdEtn	Independent
PLA$_2$	Rat	Cytosol	300	PtdCho, PtdEtn, PtdIns, PtdH	Independent
PLA$_2$	Human	Cytosol	180	PtdEtn	Dependent
PLA$_2$	Rat	Cytosol	58	PtdH	Independent

Data are summarized from Thomson and Clark (1995), Gray and Strickland (1982), Ross et al. (1995), Negre-Aminou et al. (1996), and Yoshida et al. (1998).

substrate. The purified enzyme is not selective for the arachidonyl group, but cleaves oleic and linoleic acids from PtdCho with equal efficiency. Based on kinetic properties, we conclude that this phospholipase is distinct from other phospholipases A_2, sPLA$_2$, cPLA$_2$, PlsEtn-selective PLA$_2$, and iPLA$_2$.

The occurrence of a calcium-independent PtdIns-specific PLA$_1$ in bovine brain has also been reported (Ueda et al., 1993). The relationship between rat brain 300-kDa PLA$_2$ and the above bovine PLA$_1$ remains unknown. A calcium-independent PtdH-specific PLA$_2$ activity was purified from rat brain (Thomson and Clark, 1995). At its optimum pH of 6.0, this enzyme shows little activity toward PtdCho, PtdEtn, and diacylglycerol. It has a molecular mass of 58 kDa.

3.5 Brain Nuclear PLA$_2$ Activities

In general, the function of signal transduction is to convey extracellular signals from the cell surface to the nucleus to induce a biological response at the gene level. Major proportions of the isoforms of PLA$_2$ activities occur mainly in the cytoplasm and in subcellular organelles found in the cytoplasmic compartment. In LA-N-1 cells, about 10% of the PLA$_2$ activity is localized in the nucleus (Antony et al., 2001, 2003; Ong et al., 2006). Low levels of PLA$_2$ isoforms must be viewed in the context that the isolated nuclei contain less than 3% of the total protein present in homogenates. Two calcium-independent PLA$_2$ activities are present in the nuclear preparation. One selectively hydrolyzes PtdEtn and the other acts on PlsEtn (Antony et al., 2001, 2003). It is well known that cytosolic cPLA$_2$ translocates from cytosol to plasma membranes, endoplasmic reticulum, and perinuclear membranes to act on glycerophospholipid substrates during signal transduction processes (Clark et al., 1987; Hirabayashi et al., 2004). At present, nothing is known about the relationship between the translocated cPLA$_2$ in plasma membrane, endoplasmic reticulum, or perinuclear membrane with the intrinsic nuclear PLA$_2$ isoforms.

Nuclear PtdEtn-selective and PlsEtn-selective PLA$_2$ have kinetic properties similar to those of the cytosolic enzymes. However, the nuclear enzymes respond differently to various PLA$_2$ inhibitors. The treatment of LA-N-1 cells with retinoic acid produces an increase in the specific activities of the PLA$_2$ hydrolyzing PtdEtn and PlsEtn only in the nuclear fraction. The pan-retinoic acid receptor antagonist, BMS493, blocks this stimulation, indicating a receptor-mediated process (Antony et al., 2003). The mechanism of the retinoic acid-mediated stimulation remains unknown. However, it seems possible that the interaction of retinoic acid with the retinoic acid receptor induces the synthesis of new PtdEtn-selective and PlsEtn-selective PLA$_2$ molecules. The pool sizes of nuclear PtdEtn-selective and PlsEtn-selective PLA$_2$ and the relatively small differences in specific activities of nuclear and cytosolic enzymes do not support that hypothesis. The other possibility is that the interaction of retinoic acid with its nuclear receptor induces the translocation of cytoplasmic PtdEtn-selective and PlsEtn-selective PLA$_2$ enzymes to the nucleus where phosphorylation activates them before they are transferred back to the cytoplasm. The treatment of LA-N-1 cells with cycloheximide partially prevents the stimulation in PLA$_2$ activity indicating some inhibition of protein synthesis in LA-N-1 cell nuclei (Antony et al., 2003). Unlike nuclear enzymes, retinoic acid does not affect cytosolic PtdEtn-selective and PlsEtn-selective PLA$_2$ activities. Some extracellular stimuli, such as neurotransmitters, growth factors, and neuromodulators, generate bioactive lipid metabolites at the neural cell surface through signal transduction networks associated with the plasma membrane. Other extracellular stimuli, such as retinoic acid, enter the plasma membrane through diffusion and are carried to the nucleus where they produce bioactive lipid metabolites, such as diacylglycerol, arachidonic acid and its metabolites, only in the nucleus. Thus, agonist-mediated alterations of second messengers in the nucleus may not be a duplication of those changes that occur at the plasma membrane and endoplasmic reticulum (Martelli et al., 2002, 2003).

3.6 Regulation of Isoforms of PLA$_2$ in Brain Tissue

The multiplicity of phospholipases A$_2$ in brain tissue provides for diversity in function and specificity for the regulation of enzymic activity in response to a wide range of extracellular signals. However, at the same time it complicates the analysis of their function. The complexity of this problem becomes obvious when one considers the coupling of various isoforms of PLA$_2$ with different receptors in a single neural cell and tries to associate PLA$_2$ activity with neuronal function and disease processes. The isoforms of PLA$_2$ do not function interchangeably but act in parallel to transduce signals (Farooqui et al., 1997a). Various isoforms of PLA$_2$ likely act on different pools of glycerophospholipids located in different types of neural cells. Different coupling mechanisms involving common second messengers may regulate these isoforms. This process may provide neural cells and brain tissue with great versatility in ensuring that neural cells efficiently utilize arachidonic acid and its metabolites. In brain tissue, the activity of PLA$_2$ isoforms may depend not only on the structural, physicochemical, and dynamic properties of neural membranes, but also on the interaction of extracellular signals with neural cell receptors. The activation of PLA$_2$ isoforms in neural cells is the rate-limiting step for the production of inflammatory lipid mediators, including eicosanoids and platelet-activating factor and anti-inflammatory mediators from docosahexaenoic acid (Serhan, 2004, 2005; Serhan et al., 2004). Therefore, a tight regulation of PLA$_2$ isozymes is very important for normal brain function. The regulation of PLA$_2$ activity is quite complex and is mediated by several factors and mechanisms, such as the microenvironment, gene expression, and secretion. Table 3.3 lists some of these factors and processes.

The level of the intracellular calcium ions and phosphorylation regulates cPLA$_2$ activity. Ca^{2+} mediates the binding of the enzyme to the glycerophospholipid substrate without being involved in the catalytic mechanism itself. An increase in the intracellular calcium ion concentration causes translocation of

TABLE 3.3. Factors and mechanism regulating activities of isozymes of brain PLA$_2$.

Enzyme	Regulatory factor and mechanism
sPLA$_2$	Ca^{2+}, cytokines, and annexins (Gerke and Moss, 1997; Murakami et al., 1997)
cPLA$_2$	Ca^{2+}, phosphorylation, cytokines, growth factors, and annexins (Gerke and Moss, 1997; Murakami et al., 1997; Hernández et al., 1999, 2000)
iPLA$_2$	Oligomerization (Larsson et al., 1998)
PlsEtn-selective PLA$_2$	Glycosaminoglycans, gangliosides (Yang et al., 1994a,b)

cPLA$_2$ to nuclear and other cellular membranes through a calcium-dependent lipid-binding motif (Clark et al., 1995). The translocation of cPLA$_2$ allows the interaction between the enzymic protein and its glycerophospholipid substrate and brings cPLA$_2$ into close proximity with other downstream enzymes responsible for the conversion of arachidonic acid into eicosanoids. This enzyme also contains a consensus sequence for mitogen-activated protein kinase (Pro-Leu-Ser-505-Pro). In astrocytes, Ser-505 is phosphorylated by both p38-MAP kinase and c-Jun N-terminal kinase (Hernández et al., 1999). Phosphorylation of cPLA$_2$ increases its intrinsic activity by 2- to 4-fold as measured in vitro. Thus, this enzyme is regulated both by docking to the cell membrane for accessing its glycerophospholipid substrate and by phosphorylation (Clark et al., 1995).

In non-neural systems, cPLA$_2$ inhibitory proteins (annexins) modulate cPLA$_2$ activity. Two models for cPLA$_2$ modulation have been proposed. One model requires the binding of annexin to glycerophospholipid in the presence of Ca^{2+}, resulting in the inhibition of cPLA$_2$ activity due to substrate depletion. In the other model, an annexin produces inhibition of enzyme activity by binding with cPLA$_2$ (Kim et al., 2001a,b). In these experiments, the specific binding of annexin to cPLA$_2$ was verified by immunoprecipitation studies. Studies on the regulation of cPLA$_2$ activity in non-neural cells are complicated by the presence of several annexins, at least five, and also by the occurrence of several paralogs of cPLA$_2$ activity. Thus detailed investigations are required on the type of cPLA$_2$, binding parameters, and the type of annexin involved in cPLA$_2$-mediated signaling in non-neural cells. cPLA$_2$ inhibitory proteins occur in brain but they have not been tested with purified brain cPLA$_2$.

PLA$_2$-activating proteins are found in non-neural cells, such as monocytes and endothelial cells (Clark et al., 1987). Aplysia neurons and rat cerebral cortex also contain PLA$_2$-activating proteins (Calignano et al., 1991). Protein kinase C phosphorylates the partially purified PLA$_2$ stimulatory protein. This phosphorylation may regulate isoforms of PLA$_2$ in neurons (Calignano et al., 1991).

High concentrations of Ca^{2+} stimulate brain sPLA$_2$ activity in brain tissue and astrocytic cultures. The other mechanism involved in regulation of sPLA$_2$ activity is expression of its gene. IL-6, tumor necrosis factor-α (TNF-α), and growth factors with tyrosine kinase receptors upregulate cPLA$_2$ and sPLA$_2$ expression, whereas glucocorticoids downregulate cPLA$_2$ and sPLA$_2$ activities in astrocytic cultures (Hernández et al., 2000). This sensitivity to glucocorticoids is consistent with the presence of a putative glucocorticoid response element in the promoter region of the $cPLA_2$ gene (Tay et al., 1994). The presence of $sPLA_2$, $iPLA_2$, and $cPLA_2$ transcripts (Zanassi et al., 1998; Yang et al., 1999; Balboa et al., 2002) in astrocytes is in agreement with the notion that these cells are capable of responding to cytokines with the induction of PLA_2 isozyme activities.

At present, nothing is known about the regulation of PlsEtn-selective PLA_2. However, since glycosaminoglycans and gangliosides are inhibitors, they may be involved in regulation of this enzyme (Yang et al., 1994a,b). The relationship among isoforms of PLA_2 may be quite complex. However, it is increasingly evident that in brain tissue isozymes of PLA_2 are parts of a complex signal transduction network. Cross-talk among various receptors through the generation of second messengers is essential for maintaining normal neural cell function (Farooqui et al., 2000b).

3.7 Conclusions

Good progress has been made on the isolation and characterization of brain PLA_2 during the past 15 years. These enzymes constitute a large family of structurally and mechanistically distinct proteins involved in hydrolysis of neural membrane glycerophospholipids. The PLA_2 family includes $sPLA_2$, $cPLA_2$, $iPLA_2$, PlsEtn-selective PLA_2, and many other enzymes with PLA_2 activities that have not been classified. Their reaction products act as intracellular second messengers, which can be converted to inflammatory and anti-inflammatory lipid mediators. These include the proinflammatory eicosanoids from arachidonic acid and the anti-inflammatory docosanoids (10,17S-docosatriene and neuroprotectin) from docosahexaenoic acid. Beside these metabolites, proinflammatory platelet-activating factor is also generated through the action of PLA_2 on neural membrane glycerophospholipids.

The relationship between isozymes of PLA_2 and cellular processes in which their diverse lipid messenger products are involved is coming into better perspective in recent years. Thus, $sPLA_2$ degrades glycerophospholipid substrates without fatty acid selectivity and have biological functions that reflect their catalytic activities with different types of $sPLA_2$ receptors. In contrast, $cPLA_2$ isoforms specifically liberate arachidonic acid from neural membrane glycerophospholipids through receptor-mediated mechanisms. This fatty acid is metabolized to eicosanoids. PlsEtn-selective PLA_2 catalyzes the release of docosahexaenoic acid from plasmalogens. This fatty acid is metabolized to docosanoids, which are known to oppose the effects of eicosanoids. A tight regulation of phospholipase A_2 isozymes is necessary for maintaining physiological levels of free fatty acids, including arachidonic acid and its metabolites in the various types of neural cells. Thus, under normal conditions, PLA_2 isozymes control low levels of second messengers in neural cells and modulate neurochemical processes for normal brain function. Under pathological situations, high levels of these metabolites initiate neurochemical processes associated with inflammation, cell injury, and cell death.

References

Ackermann E. J. and Dennis E. A. (1995). Mammalian calcium-independent phospholipase A_2. *Biochim. Biophys. Acta Lipids Lipid Metab.* 1259:125–136.

Adachi H., Tsujimoto M., Hattori M., Arai H., and Inoue K. (1995). cDNA cloning of human cytosolic platelet-activating factor acetylhydrolase gamma-subunit and its mRNA expression in human tissue. *Biochem. Biophys. Res. Commun.* 214:180–187.

Akiba S. and Sato T. (2004). Cellular function of calcium-independent phospholipase A_2. *Biol. Pharm. Bull.* 27:1174–1178.

Antony P., Freysz L., Horrocks L. A., and Farooqui A. A. (2001). Effect of retinoic acid on the Ca^{2+}-independent phospholipase A_2 in nuclei of LA-N-1 neuroblastoma cells. *Neurochem. Res.* 26:83–88.

Antony P., Freysz L., Horrocks L. A., and Farooqui A. A. (2003). Ca^{2+}-independent phospholipases A_2 and production of arachidonic acid in nuclei of LA-N-1 cell cultures: a specific receptor activation mediated with retinoic acid. *Mol. Brain Res.* 115:187–195.

Asai K., Hirabayashi T., Houjou T., Uozumi N., Taguchi R., and Shimizu T. (2003). Human group IVC phospholipase A_2 (cPLA$_2$γ) — Roles in the membrane remodeling and activation induced by oxidative stress. *J. Biol. Chem.* 278:8809–8814.

Atsumi G., Tajima M., Hadano A., Nakatani Y., Murakami M., and Kudo I. (1998). Fas-induced arachidonic acid release is mediated by Ca^{2+}-independent phospholipase A_2 but not cytosolic phospholipase A_2 which undergoes proteolytic inactivation. *J. Biol. Chem.* 273:13870–13877.

Atsumi G., Murakami M., Kojima K., Hadano A., Tajima M., and Kudo I. (2000). Distinct roles of two intracellular phospholipase A_2s in fatty acid release in the cell death pathway. Proteolytic fragment of type IVA cytosolic phospholipase $A_{2\alpha}$ inhibits stimulus-induced arachidonate release, whereas that of type VI Ca^{2+}-independent phospholipase A_2 augments spontaneous fatty acid release. *J. Biol. Chem.* 275:18248–18258.

Balboa M. A., Varela-Nieto I., Lucas K. K., and Dennis E. A. (2002). Expression and function of phospholipase A_2 in brain. *FEBS Lett.* 531:12–17.

Beyerl B. D. (1978). Afferent projections to the central nucleus of the inferior colliculus in the rat. *Brain Res.* 145:209–223.

Boilard E., Bourgoin S. G., Bernatchez C., Poubelle P. E., and Surette M. E. (2003). Interaction of low molecular weight group IIA phospholipase A_2 with apoptotic human T cells: role of heparan sulfate proteoglycans. *FASEB J.* 17:1068–1080.

Burke J. R., Witmer M. R., Tredup J., Micanovic R., Gregor K. R., Lahiri J., Tramposch K. M., and Villafranca J. J. (1995). Cooperativity and binding in the mechanism of cytosolic phospholipase A_2. *Biochemistry* 34:15165–15174.

Calignano A., Piomelli D., Sacktor T. C., and Schwartz J. H. (1991). A phospholipase A_2-stimulating protein regulated by protein kinase C in Aplysia neurons. *Mol. Brain Res.* 9:347–351.

Chakraborti S. (2003). Phospholipase A_2 isoforms: a perspective. *Cell. Signal.* 15:637–665.

Chiba H., Michibata H., Wakimoto K., Seishima M., Kawasaki S., Okubo K., Mitsui H., Torii H., and Imai Y. (2004). Cloning of a gene for a novel epithelium-specific cytosolic phospholipase A_2, cPLA$_2$δ, induced in psoriatic skin. *J. Biol. Chem.* 279:12890–12897.

Clark M. A., Conway T. M., Shorr R. G. L., and Crooke S. T. (1987). Identification and isolation of a mammalian protein which is antigenically and functionally related to the phospholipase A_2 stimulatory peptide melittin. *J. Biol. Chem.* 262:4402–4406.

Clark J. D., Schievella A. R., Nalefski E. A., and Lin L.-L. (1995). Cytosolic phospholipase A$_2$. *J. Lipid Mediat. Cell Signal.* 12:83–117.

DeCoster M. A., Lambeau G., Lazdunski M., and Bazan N. G. (2002). Secreted phospholipase A$_2$ potentiates glutamate-induced calcium increase and cell death in primary neuronal cultures. *J. Neurosci. Res.* 67:634–645.

Dennis E. A. (1997). The growing phospholipase A$_2$ superfamily of signal transduction enzymes. *Trends Biochem. Sci.* 22:1–2.

Derewenda Z. S. and Derewenda U. (1998). The structure and function of platelet-activating factor acetylhydrolases. *Cell Mol. Life Sci.* 54:446–455.

Desclin J. C. (1974). Histological evidence supporting the inferior olive as the major source of cerebellar climbing fibers in the rat. *Brain Res.* 77:365–384.

Diaz-Arrastia R. and Scott K. S. (1999). Expression of cPLA2-β and cPLA2-γ, novel paralogs of group IV cytosolic phospholipase A2 in mammalian brain. *Soc. Neurosci. Abstr.* 25:2206.

Evans J. H., Gerber S. H., Murray D., and Leslie C. C. (2004). The calcium binding loops of the cytosolic phospholipase A$_2$ C2 domain specify targeting to Golgi and ER in live cells. *Mol. Biol. Cell* 15:371–383.

Farooqui A. A. and Horrocks L. A. (1994). Excitotoxicity and neurological disorders: involvement of membrane phospholipids. *Int. Rev. Neurobiol.* 36:267–323.

Farooqui A. A. and Horrocks L. A. (2001). Plasmalogens: workhorse lipids of membranes in normal and injured neurons and glia. *Neuroscientist* 7:232–245.

Farooqui A. A., Pendley C. E., II, Taylor W. A., and Horrocks L. A. (1985). Studies on diacylglycerol lipases and lysophospholipases of bovine brain. In: Horrocks L. A., Kanfer J. N., and Porcellati G. (eds.), *Phospholipids in the Nervous System, Vol. II: Physiological Role.* Raven Press, New York, pp. 179–192.

Farooqui A. A., Yang H.-C., and Horrocks L. A. (1994). Purification of lipases, phospholipases and kinases by heparin-Sepharose chromatography. *J. Chromatogr.* 673:149–158.

Farooqui A. A., Yang H.-C., and Horrocks L. A. (1995). Plasmalogens, phospholipases A$_2$, and signal transduction. *Brain Res. Rev.* 21:152–161.

Farooqui A. A., Yang H. C., Rosenberger T. A., and Horrocks L. A. (1997a). Phospholipase A$_2$ and its role in brain tissue. *J. Neurochem.* 69:889–901.

Farooqui A. A., Yang H.-C., and Horrocks L. A. (1997b). Involvement of phospholipase A$_2$ in neurodegeneration. *Neurochem. Int.* 30:517–522.

Farooqui A. A., Horrocks L. A., and Farooqui T. (2000a). Deacylation and reacylation of neural membrane glycerophospholipids. *J. Mol. Neurosci.* 14:123–135.

Farooqui A. A., Ong W. Y., Horrocks L. A., and Farooqui T. (2000b). Brain cytosolic phospholipase A$_2$: localization, role, and involvement in neurological diseases. *Neuroscientist* 6:169–180.

Farooqui A. A., Ong W. Y., and Horrocks L. A. (2003). Plasmalogens, docosahexaenoic acid, and neurological disorders. In: Roels F., Baes M., and de Bies S. (eds.), *Peroxisomal Disorders and Regulation of Genes.* Kluwer Academic/Plenum Publishers, London, pp. 335–354.

Farooqui A. A., Antony P., Ong W. Y., Horrocks L. A., and Freysz L. (2004). Retinoic acid-mediated phospholipase A$_2$ signaling in the nucleus. *Brain Res. Rev.* 45:179–195.

Fitzpatrick J. S. and Baudry M. (1994). Blockade of long-term depression in neonatal hippocampal slices by a phospholipase A$_2$ inhibitor. *Dev. Brain Res.* 78:81–86.

Fuentes L., Pérez R., Nieto M. L., Balsinde J., and Balboa M. A. (2003). Bromoenol lactone promotes cell death by a mechanism involving phosphatidate phosphohydrolase-1 rather than calcium-independent phospholipase A$_2$. *J. Biol. Chem.* 278:44683–44690.

Fujita S., Ikegaya Y., Nishikawa M., Nishiyama N., and Matsuki N. (2001). Docosahexaenoic acid improves long-term potentiation attenuated by phospholipase A$_2$ inhibitor in rat hippocampal slices. *Br. J. Pharmacol.* 132:1417–1422.

Gerke V. and Moss S. E. (1997). Annexins and membrane dynamics. *Biochim. Biophys. Acta Mol. Cell Res.* 1357:129–154.

Gilbert J. J., Stewart A., Courtney C. A., Fleming M. C., Reid P., Jackson C. G., Wise A., Wakelam M. J., and Harnett M. M. (1996). Antigen receptors on immature, but not mature, B and T cells are coupled to cytosolic phospholipase A2 activation: expression and activation of cytosolic phospholipase A2 correlate with lymphocyte maturation. *J. Immunol.* 156:2054–2061.

Gray N. C. C. and Strickland K. P. (1982). The purification and characterization of a phospholipase A$_2$ activity from the 106000×g pellet (microsomal fraction) of bovine brain acting on phosphatidylinositol. *Can. J. Biochem.* 60:108–117.

Hamano H., Nabekura J., Nishikawa M., and Ogawa T. (1996). Docosahexaenoic acid reduces GABA response in substantia nigra neuron of rat. *J. Neurophysiol.* 75:1264–1270.

Hanasaki K. (2004). Mammalian phospholipase A$_2$: phospholipase A$_2$ receptor. *Biol. Pharm. Bull.* 27:1165–1167.

Hanasaki K. and Arita H. (2002). Phospholipase A$_2$ receptor: a regulator of biological functions of secretory phospholipase A$_2$. *Prostaglandins Other Lipid Mediat.* 68–69:71–82.

Hattori M., Adachi H., Tsujimoto M., Arai H., and Inoue K. (1994). Miller-Dieker lissencephaly gene encodes a subunit of brain platelet-activating factor acetylhydrolase. *Nature* 370:216–218.

Hazen S. L. and Gross R. W. (1993). The specific association of a phosphofructokinase isoform with myocardial calcium-independent phospholipase A$_2$. Implications for the coordinated regulation of phospholipolysis and glycolysis. *J. Biol. Chem.* 268:9892–9900.

Hernández M., Bayón Y., Sánchez Crespo M., and Nieto M. L. (1999). Signaling mechanisms involved in the activation of arachidonic acid metabolism in human astrocytoma cells by tumor necrosis factor-α: phosphorylation of cytosolic phospholipase A$_2$ and transactivation of cyclooxygenase-2. *J. Neurochem.* 73:1641–1649.

Hernández M., Nieto M. L., and Sánchez Crespo M. (2000). Cytosolic phospholipase A$_2$ and the distinct transcriptional programs of astrocytoma cells. *Trends Neurosci.* 23:259–264.

Higuchi Y., Hattori H., Hattori R., and Furusho K. (1996). Increased neurons containing neuronal nitric oxide synthase in the brain of a hypoxic–ischemic neonatal rat model. *Brain Dev.* 18:369–375.

Hirabayashi T. and Shimizu T. (2000). Localization and regulation of cytosolic phospholipase A$_2$. *Biochim. Biophys. Acta* 1488:124–138.

Hirabayashi T., Murayama T., and Shimizu T. (2004). Regulatory mechanism and physiological role of cytosolic phospholipase A$_2$. *Biol. Pharm. Bull.* 27:1168–1173.

Hirashima Y., Farooqui A. A., Mills J. S., and Horrocks L. A. (1992). Identification and purification of calcium-independent phospholipase A$_2$ from bovine brain cytosol. *J. Neurochem.* 59:708–714.

Karasawa K., Harada A., Satoh N., Inoue K., and Setaka M. (2003). Plasma platelet activating factor-acetylhydrolase (PAF-AH). *Prog. Lipid Res.* 42:93–114.

Kim D. K., Rordorf G., Nemenoff R. A., Koroshetz W. J., and Bonventre J. V. (1995). Glutamate stably enhances the activity of two cytosolic forms of phospholipase A_2 in brain cortical cultures. *Biochem. J.* 310:83–90.

Kim S. W., Ko J., Kim J. H., Choi E. C., and Na D. S. (2001a). Differential effects of annexins I, II, III, and V on cytosolic phospholipase A_2 activity: specific interaction model. *FEBS Lett.* 489:243–248.

Kim S. W., Rhee H. J., Ko J. S., Kim Y. J., Kim H. G., Yang J. M., Choi E. C., and Na D. S. (2001b). Inhibition of cytosolic phospholipase A_2 by annexin I — specific interaction model and mapping of the interaction site. *J. Biol. Chem.* 276:15712–15719.

Kishimoto K., Matsumura K., Kataoka Y., Morii H., and Watanabe Y. (1999). Localization of cytosolic phospholipase A_2 messenger RNA mainly in neurons in the rat brain. *Neuroscience* 92:1061–1077.

Kolko M., Rodriguez de Turco E. B., Diemer N. H., and Bazan N. G. (2002). Secretory phospholipase A_2-mediated neuronal cell death involves glutamate ionotropic receptors. *NeuroReport* 13:1963–1966.

Kolko M., Christoffersen N. R., Barreiro S. G., and Bazan N. G. (2004). Expression and location of mRNAs encoding multiple forms of secretory phospholipase A_2 in the rat retina. *J. Neurosci. Res.* 77:517–524.

Larsson P. K. A., Claesson H. E., and Kennedy B. P. (1998). Multiple splice variants of the human calcium-independent phospholipase A_2 and their effect on enzyme activity. *J. Biol. Chem.* 273:207–214.

Latorre E., Collado M. P., Fernández I., Aragonés M. D., and Catalán R. E. (2003). Signaling events mediating activation of brain ethanolamine plasmalogen hydrolysis by ceramide. *Eur. J. Biochem.* 270:36–46.

Leslie C. C. (2004). Regulation of arachidonic acid availability for eicosanoid production. *Biochem. Cell Biol.* 82:1–17.

Lin T. N., Wang Q., Simonyi A., Chen J. J., Cheung W. M., He Y. Y., Xu J., Sun A. Y., Hsu C. Y., and Sun G. Y. (2004). Induction of secretory phospholipase A_2 in reactive astrocytes in response to transient focal cerebral ischemia in the rat brain. *J. Neurochem.* 90:637–645.

Luo J., Lang J. A., and Miller M. W. (1998). Transforming growth factor $\beta 1$ regulates the expression of cyclooxygenase in cultured cortical astrocytes and neurons. *J. Neurochem.* 71:526–534.

Luscher T. F., Tanner F. C., and Dohi Y. (1992). Age, hypertension and hypercholesterolaemia alter endothelium-dependent vascular regulation. *Pharmacol. Toxicol.* 70:S32–S39.

Macchioni L., Corazzi L., Nardicchi V., Mannucci R., Arcuri C., Porcellati S., Sposini T., Donato R., and Goracci G. (2004). Rat brain cortex mitochondria release group II secretory phospholipase A_2 under reduced membrane potential. *J. Biol. Chem.* 279: 37860–37869.

Manya H., Aoki J., Watanabe M., Adachi T., Asou H., Inoue Y., Arai H., and Inoue K. (1998). Switching of platelet-activating factor acetylhydrolase catalytic subunits in developing rat brain. *J. Biol. Chem.* 273:18567–18572.

Martelli A. M., Manzoli L., Faenza I., Bortul R., Billi A., and Cocco L. (2002). Nuclear inositol lipid signaling and its potential involvement in malignant transformation. *Biochim. Biophys. Acta* 1603:11–17.

Martelli A. M., Tabellini G., Borgatti P., Bortul R., Capitani S., and Neri L. M. (2003). Nuclear lipids: new functions for old molecules? *J. Cell Biochem.* 88:455–461.

Matsuzawa A., Murakami M., Atsumi G., Imai K., Prados P., Inoue K., and Kudo I. (1996). Release of secretory phospholipase A_2 from rat neuronal cells and its possible function in the regulation of catecholamine secretion. *Biochem. J.* 318:701–709.

McMullen, T. W. P., Li, J., Sheffield, P. J., Aoki, J., Martin, T. W., Arai, H., Inoue, K., and Derewenda, Z. S. (2000). The functional implications of the dimerization of the catalytic subunits of the mammalian brain platelet-activating factor acetylhydrolase (Ib). *Protein Eng.* 13(12):865–871.

Molloy G. Y., Rattray M., and Williams R. J. (1998). Genes encoding multiple forms of phospholipase A$_2$ are expressed in rat brain. *Neurosci. Lett.* 258:139–142.

Moriyama T., Urade R., and Kito M. (1999). Purification and characterization of diacylglycerol lipase from human platelets. *J. Biochem.* (Tokyo) 125:1077–1085.

Mosior M., Six D. A., and Dennis E. A. (1998). Group IV cytosolic phospholipase A$_2$ binds with high affinity and specificity to phosphatidylinositol 4,5-bisphosphate resulting in dramatic increases in activity. *J. Biol. Chem.* 273:2184–2191.

Moskowitz N., Schook W., and Puszkin S. (1982). Interaction of brain synaptic vesicles induced by endogenous Ca^{2+}-dependent phospholipase A$_2$. *Science* 216:305–307.

Moskowitz N., Puszkin S., and Schook W. (1983). Characterization of brain synaptic vesicle phospholipase A$_2$ activity and its modulation by calmodulin, prostaglandin E$_2$, prostaglandin F$_{2\alpha}$, cyclic AMP and ATP. *J. Neurochem.* 41:1576–1586.

Murakami M. and Kudo I. (2004). Secretory phospholipase A$_2$. *Biol. Pharm. Bull.* 27:1158–1164.

Murakami M., Nakatani Y., Atsumi G., Inoue K., and Kudo I. (1997). Regulatory functions of phospholipase A$_2$. *Crit. Rev. Immunol.* 17:225–283.

Nakashima S., Ikeno Y., Yokoyama T., Kuwana M., Bolchi A., Ottonello S., Kitamoto K., and Arioka M. (2003). Secretory phospholipases A$_2$ induce neurite outgrowth in PC12 cells. *Biochem. J.* 376:655–666.

Negre-Aminou P., Nemenoff R. A., Wood M. R., de la Houssaye B. A., and Pfenninger K. H. (1996). Characterization of phospholipase A$_2$ activity enriched in the nerve growth cone. *J. Neurochem.* 67:2599–2608.

Ong W. Y., Horrocks L. A., and Farooqui A. A. (1999a). Immunocytochemical localization of cPLA$_2$ in rat and monkey spinal cord. *J. Mol. Neurosci.* 12:123–130.

Ong W. Y., Sandhya T. L., Horrocks L. A., and Farooqui A. A. (1999b). Distribution of cytoplasmic phospholipase A$_2$ in the normal rat brain. *J. Hirnforsch.* 39:391–400.

Ong W. Y., Yeo J. F., Ling S. F., and Farooqui A. A. (2005). Immunocytochemical localization of calcium-independent phospholipase A$_2$ (iPLA$_2$) in rat and monkey spinal cord. *J. Neurocytol.* 34:447–458.

Owada Y., Tominaga T., Yoshimoto T., and Kondo H. (1994). Molecular cloning of rat cDNA for cytosolic phospholipase A$_2$ and the increased gene expression in the dentate gyrus following transient forebrain ischemia. *Mol. Brain Res.* 25:364–368.

Pardue S., Rapoport S. I., and Bosetti F. (2003). Co-localization of cytosolic phospholipase A$_2$ and cyclooxygenase-2 in Rhesus monkey cerebellum. *Mol. Brain Res.* 116:106–114.

Pérez R., Melero R., Balboa M. A., and Balsinde J. (2004). Role of group VIA calcium-independent phospholipase A$_2$ in arachidonic acid release, phospholipid fatty acid incorporation, and apoptosis in U937 cells responding to hydrogen peroxide. *J. Biol. Chem.* 279:40385–40391.

Pettus B. J., Bielawska A., Subramanian P., Wijesinghe D. S., Maceyka M., Leslie C. C., Evans J. H., Freiberg J., Roddy P., Hannun Y. A., and Chalfant C. E. (2004). Ceramide 1-phosphate is a direct activator of cytosolic phospholipase A$_2$. *J. Biol. Chem.* 279:11320–11326.

Phillis J. W. and O'Regan M. H. (2004). A potentially critical role of phospholipases in central nervous system ischemic, traumatic, and neurodegenerative disorders. *Brain Res. Rev.* 44:13–47.

Pickard R. T., Strifler B. A., Kramer R. M., and Sharp J. D. (1999). Molecular cloning of two new human paralogs of 85-kDa cytosolic phospholipase A_2. *J. Biol. Chem.* 274:8823–8831.

Portilla D. and Dai G. (1996). Purification of a novel calcium-independent phospholipase A_2 from rabbit kidney. *J. Biol. Chem.* 271:15451–15457.

Ross B. M., Kim D. K., Bonventre J. V., and Kish S. J. (1995). Characterization of a novel phospholipase A_2 activity in human brain. *J. Neurochem.* 64:2213–2221.

Sandhya T. L., Ong W. Y., Horrocks L. A., and Farooqui A. A. (1998). A light and electron microscopic study of cytoplasmic phospholipase A_2 and cyclooxygenase-2 in the hippocampus after kainate lesions. *Brain Res.* 788:223–231.

Seashols S. J., del Castillo Olivares A., Gil G., and Barbour S. E. (2004). Regulation of group VIA phospholipase A_2 expression by sterol availability. *Biochim. Biophys. Acta Mol. Cell Biol. Lipids* 1684:29–37.

Serhan C. N. (2004). A search for endogenous mechanisms of anti-inflammation uncovers novel chemical mediators: missing links to resolution. *Histochem. Cell Biol.* 122:305–321.

Serhan C. N. (2005). Novel ω-3-derived local mediators in anti-inflammation and resolution. *Pharmacol. Ther.* 105:7–21.

Serhan C. N., Arita M., Hong S., and Gotlinger K. (2004). Resolvins, docosatrienes, and neuroprotectins, novel omega-3-derived mediators, and their endogenous aspirin-triggered epimers. *Lipids* 39:1125–1132.

Shirai Y. and Ito M. (2004). Specific differential expression of phospholipase A_2 subtypes in rat cerebellum. *J. Neurocytol.* 33:297–307.

Snyder F. (1995). Platelet-activating factor: the biosynthetic and catabolic enzymes. *Biochem. J.* 305:689–705.

Song C., Chang X. J., Bean K. M., Proia M. S., Knopf J. L., and Kriz R. W. (1999). Molecular characterization of cytosolic phospholipase $A_{2-\beta}$. *J. Biol. Chem.* 274:17063–17067.

Stephenson D. T., Manetta J. V., White D. L., Chiou X. G., Cox L., Gitter B., May P. C., Sharp J. D., Kramer R. M., and Clemens J. A. (1994). Calcium-sensitive cytosolic phospholipase A_2 (cPLA$_2$) is expressed in human brain astrocytes. *Brain Res.* 637:97–105.

Stephenson D., Rash K., Smalstig B., Roberts E., Johnstone E., Sharp J., Panetta J., Little S., Kramer R., and Clemens J. (1999). Cytosolic phospholipase A_2 is induced in reactive glia following different forms of neurodegeneration. *Glia* 27:110–128.

Strokin M., Sergeeva M., and Reiser G. (2003a). Docosahexaenoic acid and arachidonic acid release in rat brain astrocytes is mediated by two separate isoforms of phospholipase A_2 and is differently regulated by cyclic AMP and Ca^{2+}. *Br. J. Pharmacol.* 139:1014–1022.

Strokin M., Sergeeva M., and Reiser G. (2003b). Docosahexaenoic acid and arachidonic acid release in rat brain astrocytes is mediated by two separate isoforms of phospholipase A_2 and is differently regulated by cyclic AMP and Ca^{2+}. *Br. J. Pharmacol.* 139:1014–1022.

Sun G. Y., Xu J. F., Jensen M. D., and Simonyi A. (2004). Phospholipase A_2 in the central nervous system: implications for neurodegenerative diseases. *J. Lipid Res.* 45:205–213.

Tay A., Maxwell P., Li Z., Goldberg H., and Skorecki K. (1994). Isolation of promoter for cytosolic phospholipase A_2 (cPLA$_2$). *Biochim. Biophys. Acta* 1217:345–347.

Thomson F. J. and Clark M. A. (1995). Purification of a phosphatidic-acid-hydrolysing phospholipase A_2 from rat brain. *Biochem. J.* 306:305–309.

Thwin M. M., Ong W. Y., Fong C. W., Sato K., Kodama K., Farooqui A. A., and Gopalakrishnakone P. (2003). Secretory phospholipase A_2 activity in the normal and kainate injected rat brain, and inhibition by a peptide derived from python serum. *Exp. Brain Res.* 150:427–433.

Tjoelker L. W. and Stafforini D. M. (2000). Platelet-activating factor acetylhydrolases in health and disease. *Biochim. Biophys. Acta* 1488:102–123.

Ueda H., Kobayashi T., Kishimoto M., Tsutsumi T., Watanabe S., and Okuyama H. (1993). The presence of Ca^{2+}-independent phospholipase A$_1$ highly specific for phosphatidylinositol in bovine brain. *Biochem. Biophys. Res. Commun.* 195:1272–1279.

Webster G. R. and Cooper M. (1968). On the site of action of phosphatide acyl-hydrolase activity of rat brain homogenates on lecithin. *J. Neurochem.* 15:795–802.

Wei S., Ong W. Y., Thwin M. M., Fong C. W., Farooqui A. A., Gopalakrishnakone P., and Hong W. J. (2003). Differential activities of secretory phospholipase A$_2$ (sPLA$_2$) in rat brain and effects of sPLA$_2$ on neurotransmitter release. *Neuroscience* 121:891–898.

Winstead M. V., Balsinde J., and Dennis E. A. (2000). Calcium-independent phospholipase A$_2$: structure and function. *Biochim. Biophys. Acta* 1488:28–39.

Woelk H., Goracci G., and Porcellati G. (1974). The action of brain phospholipases A2 on purified, specifically labelled 1,2-diacyl-, 2-acyl-1-alk-1'-enyl- and 2-acyl-1-alkyl-sn-glycero-3-phosphorylcholine. Hoppe-Seyler's Z. *Physiol. Chem.* 335:75–81.

Woelk H., Goracci G., Arienti G., and Porcellati G. (1978). On the activity of phospholipases A$_1$ and A$_2$ in glial and neuronal cells. *Adv. Prostaglandin Thromboxane Res.* 3:77–83.

Wolf M. J., Izumi Y., Zorumski C. F., and Gross R. W. (1995). Long-term potentiation requires activation of calcium-independent phospholipase A$_2$. *FEBS Lett.* 377:358–362.

Xu J. F., Yu S., Sun A. Y., and Sun G. Y. (2003). Oxidant-mediated AA release from astrocytes involves cPLA$_2$ and iPLA$_2$. *Free Radic. Biol. Med.* 34:1531–1543.

Yang H.-C., Farooqui A. A., and Horrocks L. A. (1994a). Effects of glycosaminoglycans and glycosphingolipids on cytosolic phospholipases A$_2$ from bovine brain. *Biochem. J.* 299:91–95.

Yang H.-C., Farooqui A. A., and Horrocks L. A. (1994b). Effects of sialic acid and sialoglycoconjugates on cytosolic phospholipases A$_2$ from bovine brain. *Biochem. Biophys. Res. Commun.* 199:1158–1166.

Yang H.-C., Farooqui A. A., Rammohan K. W., Haun S. E., and Horrocks L. A. (1997). Occurrence and characterization of plasmalogen-selective phospholipase A$_2$ in brain of various animal species. *J. Neurochem.* 69:S205C.

Yang H. C., Mosior M., Ni B., and Dennis E. A. (1999). Regional distribution, ontogeny, purification, and characterization of the Ca^{2+}-independent phospholipase A$_2$ from rat brain. *J. Neurochem.* 73:1278–1287.

Yoshida H., Tsujishita Y., Hullin F., Yoshida K., Nakamura S., Kikkawa U., and Asaoka Y. (1998). Isolation and properties of a novel phospholipase A from rat brain that hydrolyses fatty acids at *sn*-1 and *sn*-2 positions. *Ann. Clin. Biochem.* 35:295–301.

Yoshihara Y. and Watanabe Y. (1990). Translocation of phospholipase A$_2$ from cytosol to membranes in rat brain induced by calcium ions. *Biochem. Biophys. Res. Commun.* 170:484–490.

Yoshihara Y., Yamaji M., Kawasaki M., and Watanabe Y. (1992). Ontogeny of cytosolic phospholipase A$_2$ activity in rat brain. *Biochem. Biophys. Res. Commun.* 185:350–355.

Zanassi P., Paolillo M., and Schinelli S. (1998). Coexpression of phospholipase A$_2$ isoforms in rat striatal astrocytes. *Neurosci. Lett.* 247:83–86.

4
Roles of Phospholipases A_2 in Brain

Most of our knowledge about the role of PLA_2 isoforms in brain comes from in vitro cell biology, neuropharmacology, and neuropathology studies. In brain tissue, PLA_2 isoforms perform housekeeping as well as signaling functions. Housekeeping functions of PLA_2 isoforms include phospholipid turnover, neural membrane remodeling, and removal of peroxidized fatty acids from phospholipid hydroperoxides. Under normal conditions, changes in PLA_2 activity induce alterations in the level of essential phospholipids affecting membrane fluidity, permeability, and ion homeostasis transiently. The reacylation of lysoglycerophospholipids through a series of energy-dependent reactions results in the restoration of the normal glycerophospholipid content of neural membranes.

Under pathological conditions (ischemia), in contrast, PLA_2-mediated hydrolysis of neural membrane glycerophospholipids produces free fatty acids and lysoglycerophospholipids at rates greater than that of membrane repair (reacylation), resulting in an accumulation of free fatty acids (Sun and MacQuarrie, 1989). This process produces irreversible changes in membrane integrity, loss of ion homeostasis, and abnormalities in cellular function (Farooqui and Horrocks, 1991).

The PLA_2 signaling functions in neural membranes are modulated by the generation of various second messengers. These messengers include eicosanoids (prostaglandins, leukotrienes, and lipoxins), docosanoids (resolvins and neuroprotectins), lysoglycerophospholipids, and platelet-activating factor (PAF). They modulate cellular function by acting through extracellular as well as intracellular receptors (Farooqui et al., 2000b,c). Besides modulating the generation of second messengers, PLA_2 isoforms are also involved in maintaining neural cell membrane homeostasis through the recycling of fatty acid moieties in glycerophospholipid molecular species of brain tissues. Although the relative contributions of PLA_2 isoforms in the release of various second messengers and maintenance of phospholipid molecular mass in neural membrane are still unknown, it is evident that PLA_2 isoforms play important roles in the efficient control of the acylation–deacylation cycle and in the regulation of the production of eicosanoids, platelet-activating factor, and docosanoids. These second messengers are involved in the modulation of neurotransmitter release, long-term potentiation, membrane repair, cell cycle, regeneration, and neurodegeneration.

4.1 PLA$_2$ Isoforms and Neurotransmitter Release

Under normal conditions in the brain tissue, most neuron-to-neuron and neuron-to-muscle cell communication occurs through the release of neurotransmitters from the synaptic vesicle at the synapse via exocytosis (Ghijsen et al., 2003; Li and Chin, 2003; Rohrbough and Broadie, 2005). Before exocytosis, neurotransmitter-filled synaptic vesicles are docked at a specialized area of the presynaptic membrane called the active zone. The docked vesicles then go through a maturation process called priming to become fusion competent. In response to the calcium ion influx induced by the action potential, primed vesicles undergo rapid exocytotic fusion with the neuronal plasma membrane and release their contents into the synaptic cleft (Li and Chin, 2003). The released neurotransmitter diffuses across the synaptic cleft and activates neurotransmitter receptors in the postsynaptic membrane. Exocytosis can also occur in the absence of calcium ion (Burgoyne and Morgan, 1995; Nishio et al., 1996; Abu-Raya et al., 1998). After exocytosis, synaptic vesicles quickly undergo endocytosis and recycle close to the site of exocytosis in the backfield of the synaptic nerve terminal. Synaptic vesicles take 60 sec to go through the whole synaptic cycle (Ghijsen et al., 2003). Although the molecular mechanism of neurotransmitter release remains unknown, calcium ion entry may be through voltage-sensitive channels and the activation of calcium-dependent PLA$_2$ may be an important part of the neurotransmitter-releasing mechanism (Moskowitz et al., 1982; Bloch-Shilderman et al., 2002). This suggestion is based on the observation that activation of both calcium-dependent PLA$_2$ and calcium-independent PLA$_2$ in synaptic vesicles correlates with the induction of vesicle formation. Inhibitors of PLA$_2$ activity suppress exocytosis and block neurotransmitter release in rat brain and PC12 cell preparations (Matsuzawa et al., 1996; Abu-Raya et al., 1998; Bloch-Shilderman et al., 2002; Wei et al., 2003). Furthermore, arachidonic acid, a product of reactions catalyzed by PLA$_2$, facilitates the insertion and translocation of protein kinase C in neural membranes. Protein kinase C is also involved in neurotransmitter release in cultured cells of neuronal and glial origin (Bramham et al., 1994). Collective evidence thus suggests that both calcium-dependent PLA$_2$ and calcium-independent PLA$_2$ modulate neurotransmitter release by direct and indirect mechanisms in various brain preparations (Fig. 4.1) (Bramham et al., 1994; Bloch-Shilderman et al., 2002; Ghijsen et al., 2003).

In pathological situations, such as ischemia, neurotransmitter release occurs by depolarization-induced reversal of the sodium-dependent high-affinity amino acid plasma membrane transporter (Ghijsen et al., 2003). Thus, an ischemic insult in the four-vessel occlusion model of cerebral ischemia and reperfusion is accompanied by a marked increase in levels of glutamate and GABA neurotransmitter release. This increase in neurotransmitter release can be blocked by quinacrine, a nonspecific PLA$_2$ inhibitor, suggesting the involvement of PLA$_2$ neurotransmitter release (O'Regan et al., 1995b). Based on biophysical and neuropharmacological studies, it is proposed that PLA$_2$ disrupts the integrity of the synaptic vesicle in a calcium-dependent manner (O'Regan et al., 1996). This loss of membrane

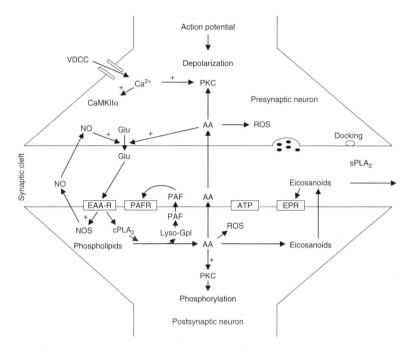

FIG. 4.1. Hypothetical model showing neurotransmitter (glutamate) release and interactions between second messengers of phospholipid metabolism. Glutamate, Glu; excitatory amino acid receptors, EAA-R; cytosolic phospholipase A$_2$, cPLA$_2$; secretory phospholipase A$_2$, sPLA$_2$; platelet-activating factor, PAF; platelet-activating factor receptor, PAF-R, lysoglycerophospholipid, lyso-Gpl; arachidonic acid, AA; reactive oxygen species, ROS; protein kinase C, PKC; eicosanoid receptor, EPR; calcium-/calmodulin-dependent protein kinase, CaMKIIα; nitric oxide, NO; voltage-dependent calcium channel, VDCC.

integrity allows the neurotransmitter to diffuse from intracellular compartment into the synaptic cleft. A PLA$_2$ inhibitor also can block this efflux of neurotransmitters, suggesting that PLA$_2$ activity is involved in neurotransmitter release under pathological conditions (O'Regan et al., 1995a,b).

4.2 PLA$_2$ Isoforms in Long-Term Potentiation (LTP)

Two forms of synaptic plasticity, long-term potentiation (LTP) and long-term depression (LTD), are major cellular mechanisms involved in learning and memory (Bliss and Collingridge, 1993; Chen and Tonegawa, 1997). These mechanisms involve depolarization of the postsynaptic membranes and calcium entry mediated by N-methyl-D-aspartate (NMDA) receptors. LTP is defined as a persistent increase in synaptic efficacy following brief high frequency stimulation of a monosynaptic pathway in the hippocampus. This phenomenon serves as a good electrophysiological model of memory formation (Williams et al., 1989). The induction of LTP is triggered by the postsynaptic entry of calcium through the NMDA receptor channel, whereas the maintenance is regulated by presynaptic mechanisms. The induction of LTP in dentate gyrus results in the activation of calcium-dependent PLA$_2$ and liberation of arachidonic acid from neural membrane glycerophospholipids. Phosphatidylcholine contents are significantly reduced following the induction of LTP. This suggests that phosphatidylcholine is the major glycerophospholipid that is metabolized by cPLA$_2$ during LTP (Clements et al., 1991). Released arachidonic acid crosses the synaptic cleft to act presynaptically as a retrograde messenger through activation of the γ-isoform of protein kinase C (Linden and Routtenberg, 1989; Izquierdo and Medina, 1995). This isoform of protein kinase C together with cPLA$_2$ plays an important role in the induction and maintenance of LTP (Bernard et al., 1994; Murakami and Routtenberg, 2003). In addition, protein kinase C activity mediated by arachidonic acid is involved in the phosphorylation of a 43-kDa growth associated protein (GAP-43). This protein is highly expressed in growth cones during neuronal development and synaptic remodeling. The phosphorylation of GAP-43 is associated with persistence of LTP in the dentate gyrus and CA1 area of hippocampus (Hulo et al., 2002). Lysophosphatidylcholine, the other product of the cPLA$_2$-catalyzed reaction, also facilitates hippocampal neurotransmission (Nomura et al., 2001). Thus, both products generated by PLA$_2$ are involved in the induction and maintenance of LTP. Injections of the cPLA$_2$ inhibitor, palmitoyl trifluoromethylketone, into rat hippocampus impair memory formation, indicating further that cPLA$_2$ activity and its metabolites are closely involved in LTP and memory formation (Schaeffer et al., 2005; Schaeffer and Gattaz, 2005).

Calcium-independent PLA$_2$ (iPLA$_2$) also participates in LTP induction (Wolf et al., 1995). The treatment of hippocampal slices with bromoenol lactone (BEL), a specific and potent inhibitor of iPLA$_2$, prior to tetanic stimulation prevents the induction of LTP. Importantly, the addition of arachidonic acid and docosahexaenoic acid during the tetanic stimulation induces LTP suggesting that iPLA$_2$ mediates the induction and maintenance of LTP (Wolf et al., 1995; Fujita et al., 2001). Intracerebroventricular injections of BEL in mice markedly affect spatial performance (Fujita et al., 2000), supporting the view that iPLA$_2$ is involved in spatial memory formation. Both the NMDA and AMPA types of glutamate receptors are coupled to isoforms of PLA$_2$ in neural membranes (Lazarewicz et al., 1990; Farooqui et al., 1994) and therefore participate in the modulation of LTP.

Kinases phosphorylate AMPA receptors. This can directly modulate AMPA receptor function and surface expression at synapses (Song and Huganir, 2002). Incubation of rat brain slices with BEL enhances phosphorylation of serine residue 831 on the AMPA receptor GluR1 subunit in a synaptosomal P2 fraction. In contrast, a cPLA$_2$ inhibitor, AACOCF$_3$, increases phosphorylation on serine residues 880/891 on the AMPA receptor GluR2/3 subunit. These effects are restricted to the AMPA receptor and no changes are observed in phosphorylation of the NMDA receptor NR1 subunit (Ménard et al., 2005a). The blockade of protein phosphatases by okadaic acid does not occlude the effects of BEL and AACOCF$_3$, indicating that the increase in AMPA receptor phosphorylation induced by a PLA$_2$ inhibitor does not rely on a decrease in dephosphorylation reactions. However, pretreatment of rat brain slices with a cell permeable inhibitor of protein kinase C prevents the phosphorylation induced by BEL and AACOCF$_3$ on the Ser 831 and Ser 880/891 sites of GluR1 and GluR2/3 subunits, respectively. This suggests that the cPLA$_2$ and iPLA$_2$ systems differentially influence the AMPA receptor properties and function in rat brain through mechanisms involving protein kinase C activity (Ménard et al., 2005b). The ability of iPLA$_2$ inhibitors to increase GluR1 phosphorylation can be mimicked by MK-886, a 5-lipoxygenase inhibitor, but not by blockers of 12-lipoxygenase or cyclooxygenase.

Altogether, these studies suggest that iPLA$_2$ activity through the generation of 5-lipoxygenase metabolites regulates AMPA receptor phosphorylation of GluR1 subunits in the CA1 area of the hippocampus and that AMPA receptors are involved in LTP. Collective evidence suggests that both iPLA$_2$ and cPLA$_2$ participate in the induction and maintenance of LTP. It is proposed that NMDA receptors trigger modification of AMPA receptor phosphorylation by transiently increasing postsynaptic calcium levels, producing a long-term stimulation of protein kinases (Baudry and Lynch, 2001) associated with long-lasting modification of synaptic function.

Low, 1 to 2 Hz, but more prolonged stimulation, 3 to 15 min, of a synapse and NMDA receptor-mediated calcium ion influx leads to LTD. Preincubation of hippocampal slices with iPLA$_2$ inhibitor blocks LTD formation (Okada et al., 1989), indicating that iPLA$_2$ is also involved in LTD. Treatment of hippocampal slices with arachidonate also mimics the LTD formation (Massicotte, 2000). Based on several studies, protein phosphorylation of GluR2 at Ser880 mediated by protein kinase A may modulate synaptic transmission by inducing receptor internalization, an event that may contribute to LTD formation in hippocampus as well as cerebellum (Chung et al., 2003; Seidenman et al., 2003). Collective evidence suggests that NMDA receptor-dependent LTD is associated with protein phosphatase activity and dephosphorylation of GluR1 and GluR2 AMPA receptor subunits is a key step in its expression mechanism (St-Gelais et al., 2004; Ménard et al., 2005b).

4.3 Involvement of PLA$_2$ Isoforms in Membrane Repair

Polyunsaturated fatty acids in neural membrane glycerophospholipids are susceptible to attack by reactive oxygen species. This results in generation of lipid hydroperoxides, peroxidized glycerophospholipids, and their degraded products (Farooqui et al., 2000b). The presence of peroxidized glycerophospholipids in neural membranes produces a packing defect making the *sn*-2 ester bond more accessible to the action of PLA$_2$ isoforms. In fact, glycerophospholipid hydroperoxides are better substrates for PLA$_2$ isozymes than the native nonperoxidized glycerophospholipids (McLean et al., 1993). The hydrolysis of peroxidized glycerophospholipids results in the removal of peroxidized fatty acyl chains, which are reduced and re-esterified (Farooqui et al., 2000a). Thus, the action of PLA$_2$ isoforms repairs and restores the appropriate physicochemical state of the membrane and prevents peroxidative cross-linking reactions. Without such repair, peroxidized glycerophospholipids would accumulate and produce alterations in neural membrane permeability and ion homeostasis.

Some peroxidized lipids exhibit specific biological activities, such as the activation of Ras, NFκB, MAP-kinase, and c-Jun kinase. Increasing evidence points to a role of oxidized glycerophospholipids as modulators of inflammatory reactions. These lipids accumulate at sites of inflammation such as atherosclerotic lesions. They influence a variety of cellular functions such as chemokine production and expression of adhesion molecules (Furnkranz and Leitinger, 2004). Oxidized glycerophospholipids also act as ligands for pattern-recognition receptors. These receptors detect conserved pathogen-associated molecular patterns during innate immune defense. Peroxidized glycerophospholipids may create a polar environment and decreased glycerophospholipid packing, markedly affecting signal transduction processes (Furnkranz and Leitinger, 2004). Furthermore, the polar nature of oxidized free fatty acids facilitates their expulsion to the aqueous phase. This process prolongs the catalytic activities of enzymes that are usually subjected to product inhibition (Reynolds et al., 1993). The significance of these studies in vivo remains unknown. However, it is worth noting that membrane structural organization markedly influences activities on many enzymes, including PLA$_2$ isoforms.

4.4 PLA$_2$ Isoforms in Modulation of Neurite Outgrowth and Regeneration

Increases in PLA$_2$ activities with release of arachidonic acid and its metabolites have an important but yet undefined role in neurite outgrowth, regeneration, and growth-dependent signal transduction processes (Suburo and Cei de Job, 1986; Katsuki and Okuda, 1995; Obermeier et al., 1995; Hornfelt et al., 1999). Treatment of NG 108-15 cells with PLA$_2$ inhibitors impairs neurite outgrowth formation (Smalheiser et al., 1996), whereas activators of PLA$_2$ activity, such as melittin, activate neurite outgrowth indicating the involvement of PLA$_2$-generated metabolites in neurite outgrowth formation. The molecular mechanism of the neurite outgrowth induced by arachidonic acid remains unknown. However, the activation of protein kinase C isozymes by arachidonic acid may play an important role in neurite formation (Katsuki and Okuda, 1995).

The role of cPLA$_2$ isoforms in axonal outgrowth has also been investigated in dorsal root ganglia (DRG) neurons. Methyl arachidonoyl fluorophosphonate (MAFP), a cPLA$_2$ inhibitor, reduces the axonal outgrowth length about 50%, and causes rapid collapse of the growth cone, an effect that is counteracted by the addition of arachidonic acid (AA), suggesting the involvement of PLA$_2$ activity. Other studies in DRG indicate that these PLA$_2$ inhibitors exert a biphasic effect on elongation of axons. They enhance outgrowth at low concentrations and inhibit outgrowth at higher concentration (Suburo and Cei de Job, 1986). Similarly, studies on initial stages of neural regeneration in the snail, *Helisoma trivolvis*, indicate that PLA$_2$ activity is necessary for the completion of neuronal regeneration (Geddis and Rehder, 2003). Collective evidence thus suggests the importance of PLA$_2$ activity for growth cone motility and axonal outgrowth in the adult central and peripheral nervous systems. In non-neural cells, arachidonic acid and its metabolites facilitate heterodimerization between peroxisome proliferator-activated receptor and retinoid X receptor. This process may also be involved in the expression of genes related to differentiation that are associated with neurite outgrowth formation. Lysoglycerophospholipids, the other product of PLA$_2$-catalyzed reaction, stimulate mitogen-activated protein kinase and protein kinase C. Both these enzymes are closely associated with neuronal cell proliferation and differentiation. These studies strongly link cPLA$_2$ activity to axonal outgrowth and growth cone function via mechanisms involving arachidonic acid, its metabolites, and lysoglycerophospholipids.

PlsEtn-PLA$_2$ releases docosahexaenoic acid (DHA) from plasmalogens (Farooqui and Horrocks, 2001; Strokin et al., 2003). Like arachidonic acid, treatment of hippocampal cultures with DHA also increases neurite length and the number of branches indicating that DHA promotes neuritic growth in vitro (Calderon and Kim, 2004). The action of DHA on hippocampal cultures seems to be very specific because supplementation with other fatty acids under identical conditions has no effect on neuritic growth. Interestingly, hippocampal neurons cultured from rats deficient in n-3 fatty acids show decreased neurite growth compared to neurons obtained from rats with adequate n-3 fatty acids. Subsequent DHA supplementation of neurons deficient in n-3 fatty acids promotes recovery of neuritic growth close to the level observed in neurons with adequate n-3 fatty acids (Calderon and Kim, 2004). The molecular mechanism involved in DHA-mediated neuritic outgrowth in not fully understood. However, there are several possibilities. DHA modulates signal transduction pathways by increasing the phosphatidylserine content in neuronal membranes, which in turn promotes the activation of Raf-1 and the PtdIns-3 kinase pathways (Kim et al., 2000; Akbar and Kim, 2002). Raf-1 and the PtdIns-3 kinase pathways play important roles in inducing neurite outgrowth in PC12 and H19-7 hippocampal cell lines (Kobayashi et al., 1997; Kita et al., 1998). DHA also stimulates glycerophospholipid synthesis in differentiated PC12 cells (Ikemoto et al., 1999). Since neurite outgrowth requires the synthesis of glycerophospholipids for incorporation into neural membrane, this mechanism may play an important role in neuritic outgrowth. Finally, both arachidonic acid and DHA can also act as endogenous ligands for nuclear retinoid receptor RXR. It modulates activities of transcription factors and gene expression in developing an adult brain (Antony et al., 2003; Lengqvist et al., 2004).

A newly discovered isoform of sPLA$_2$ (sPLA$_2$-X) also induces neurite outgrowth in PC12 cell cultures. This process correlates with the ability of sPLA$_2$-X to generate lysophosphatidylcholine (lyso-PtdCho) and induce G2A, a G-protein-coupled receptor involved in signaling mediated by lyso-PtdCho (Masuda et al., 2005; Ikeno et al., 2005). Neuritogenesis induced by lyso-PtdCho in PC12 cells may involve opening of L-type calcium ion channels and stimulation of protein kinase C and mitogen-activated protein kinases. Calcium ion influx through voltage-gated channels can also trigger a variety of cellular events leading to neuritogenesis via the concerted action of various calcium-binding proteins and cell adhesion molecules (Doherty et al., 1991; Kater and Mills, 1991). Other sPLA₂ isoforms such as sPLA₂-IIA have no effect on neurite outgrowth, but bee venom sPLA₂ and fungal sPLA₂ induce neurite outgrowth in a manner dependent on their catalytic activity. A combination of sPLA₂ and nerve growth factor induces more neurite outgrowth than sPLA₂ alone. The nerve growth factor–mediated neurite extension of PC12 cells can be significantly attenuated by both an anti-sPLA₂ antibody and an siRNA procedure (Masuda et al., 2005), indicating that sPLA₂ is an important player in neuritogenesis.

4.5 PLA₂ Isoforms in Inflammatory and Anti-Inflammatory Processes

Neuroinflammation is a complex defensive process designed to remove or inactivate noxious agents and inhibit their detrimental effects for the restoration of normal tissue structure and function. Although neuroinflammation is a neuroprotective mechanism, its persistence can initiate tissue damage and a disease process in the brain tissue (Correale and Villa, 2004). At the cellular level, neuroinflammation involves activation of astrocytes and microglia and their interactions with neurons, endothelial cells, and polymorphonuclear leukocytes. The activation of microglia contributes to neurodegeneration by the elaboration of proinflammatory cytokines such as interleukin-1 and tumor necrosis factor-α. The release of cytokines and growth factors modulates the generation of arachidonic acid by PLA₂ isozymes, the formation of proinflammatory eicosanoids by cyclooxygenases, and the synthesis of platelet-activating factor (PAF) by PLA₂ and an acetyltransferase (Bazan, 2003; Farooqui and Horrocks, 2004). The specific receptors for eicosanoids and platelet-activating factor occur in the brain tissue. Following PAF receptor occupancy, sPLA₂ is secreted from astrocytes and microglial cells and rapidly associates itself with its receptors on the outer neuronal membrane. Alterations in membrane lipid packing and asymmetry due to receptor occupancy result in the activation of sPLA₂ at the outer surface initiating the synthesis of prostaglandins. Prostaglandins not only initiate inflammatory responses, but also mediate resolution (Serhan, 2002). There are two phases in inflammatory responses: one at the onset for the generation of proinflammatory eicosanoids and the other at resolution for the synthesis of proresolving eicosanoids (Gilroy et al., 2004). The first phase of arachidonic acid formation involves the expression and stimulation of iPLA₂ with the generation of PGE₂, LTB₄, and PAF through cyclooxygenase-2, lipoxygenase, and acetyl-CoA acetyltransferase reactions, respectively. The second phase of arachidonic acid release utilizes sPLA$_2$ as well as cPLA$_2$ and is associated with the generation of PAF, lipoxin, and the proresolving prostaglandin, PGD$_2$ (Gilroy et al., 2004).

Prostaglandins serve as autocrine factors regulating platelet aggregation, vascular tone, and edema and are also involved in neuronal responses to pain (Yeo et al., 2004). Platelet-activating factor modulates the expression of COX-2 and also induces the release of cytokines and expression of cell adhesion molecules (Bazan, 2003). All these metabolites contribute to the induction and maintenance of the inflammatory process. Neuroinflammation can be both a cause, and a consequence, of chronic oxidative stress. Collective evidence suggests that modulation of PLA$_2$ isoforms by cytokines and the generation of arachidonic acid and its metabolites are central to inflammatory events that occur in the brain tissue after traumatic and metabolic injuries (Farooqui et al., 2000b, 2002). The most compelling evidence for the involvement of cPLA$_2$ isoforms in neuroinflammation comes from cPLA$_2$ knockout mice. These animals show reduced inflammation with decreased prostaglandin and leukotriene production and greater resistance to ischemic injury (Bonventre et al., 1997). Systemic administration of LPS in cPLA$_2$ knockout and wild-type mice indicates that cPLA$_2$-deficient mice have significantly less cyclooxygenase-2 (COX-2) mRNA with less expression of COX-2 in response to LPS than wild-type mice (Sapirstein et al., 2005), indicating that cPLA$_2$-α modulates COX-2 activity and PGE2 levels. Similarly, sPLA$_2$ knockout mice show a low incidence of atherosclerosis (Grass, 1999; Webb, 2005). These observations strongly implicate sPLA$_2$ in the progression of inflammation during atherogenesis.

Plasmalogen-selective phospholipase A$_2$ releases docosahexaenoic acid from neural membrane plasmalogens. This fatty acid attenuates prostaglandin synthesis by inhibiting cyclooxygenase and intracellular calcium signaling, which produces changes in the activity of cPLA$_2$ and hence lowers the amount of arachidonic acid available for prostaglandin synthesis (Hong et al., 2003; Marcheselli et al., 2003; Serhan et al., 2004a). These second messengers are collectively called docosanoids. They antagonize the effects of eicosanoids and modulate leukocyte trafficking as well as downregulate the expression of cytokines in glial cells (Hong et al., 2003; Marcheselli et al., 2003; Serhan et al., 2004a). Addition of neuroprotectin D1 to retinal epithelial cells counteracts the apoptotic DNA damage triggered by treatment with oxidative agents. Neuroprotectin D1 also upregulates the expression of the antiapoptotic proteins Bcl-2 and Bcl-xL, while downregulating the proapoptotic proteins Bax and Bad (Serhan et al., 2004b; Bazan, 2005a,b). The specific receptors for these bioactive lipid metabolites also occur in neural and non-neural tissues. These receptors include resolvin D receptors (resoDR1), resolvin E receptors (resoER1), and neuroprotectin D receptors (NPDR) Characterization of these receptors in brain tissue is in progress (Marcheselli et al., 2003; Serhan et al., 2004a,b). Microglial cells release cytokines in the brain. The D class resolvins block the transcription of interleukin (IL)-1β induced by tumor necrosis factor α and are potent regulators of PMN infiltration in brain (Serhan et al., 2004a). Collective evidence suggests that the generation of docosanoids may be an internal protective mechanism for preventing brain damage (Marcheselli et al., 2003; Mukherjee et al., 2004; Serhan, 2005a,b; Bazan, 2005b).

4.6 Involvement of PLA$_2$ Isoforms in the Cell Cycle

Very little is known about activities of PLA$_2$ isoforms and glycerophospholipid alterations during the development of the brain and the maturation of neuronal and glial cells (Ledeen and Wu, 2004; Farooqui et al., 2004a). However, alterations in the activities of cPLA$_2$ and iPLA$_2$ and glycerophospholipid contents occur during the cell cycle in non-neural cells. cPLA$_2$ activity is high during mitosis, decreases later, and increases again in the G1 and G1/S phases. During these phases, the elevation in cPLA$_2$ activity is due to increased phosphorylation rather than increased cPLA$_2$ protein expression. This suggestion is supported by studies in which phosphatase treatment of cPLA$_2$ reduces its activity (van Rossum et al., 2002). Inhibition of cPLA$_2$ activity with arachidonoyl trifluoromethyl ketone in early G1 phase markedly reduces DNA synthesis. Thus, cPLA$_2$ plays an important role in cell cycle progression. Cyclooxygenase inhibitors have no effect on cell cycle progression into S phase (van Rossum et al., 2002), indicating that the cPLA$_2$-dependent progression is not mediated by arachidonic acid metabolites generated by cyclooxygenase. However, the lipoxygenase inhibitors, caffeic acid and nordihydroguaiaretic acid, inhibit DNA synthesis when added in early G1 phase (van Rossum et al., 2002). In CHO-K1 and Jurkat T cells, the mass of PtdCho doubles during late G1 and early S phases when the rate of PtdCho catabolism is lowest (Manguikian and Barbour, 2004). iPLA$_2$ activity peaks during G2/M and late S phases and declines during G1 phase. It is lowest at the G1/S transition and during early S phase. Thus, the accumulation of PtdCho correlates with a decrease in iPLA$_2$ activity. These alterations in iPLA$_2$ activity during the cell cycle are not only involved in glycerophospholipid turnover, but are also responsible for the accumulation of PtdCho during late G1 and early S phases (Roshak et al., 2000; Ng et al., 2004; Manguikian and Barbour, 2004). The molecular mechanism involved in modulation of iPLA$_2$ is not fully understood. The decline in iPLA$_2$ activity during G1 phase is not caused by a loss in iPLA$_2$ protein mass, but may be due to decreased catalytic activity of the iPLA$_2$ protein.

4.7 PLA$_2$ Isoforms in Tubule Formation and Membrane Trafficking

After their synthesis on microsomes, newly synthesized secretory and membrane proteins undergo structural maturation, including folding, oligomeric assembly, glycosylation, and formation of disulfide bonds, in the endoplasmic reticulum. Most proteins leave the endoplasmic reticulum for the Golgi complex. In the Golgi complex they are modified, sorted, and directed to their diverse destinations by virtue of specific targeting sequences (Jamora, 1999). The Golgi complex contains several isoforms of PLA$_2$, including cPLA$_2$, iPLA$_2$, and sPLA$_2$-X (Grewal et al., 2005; Masuda et al., 2005; Shirai et al., 2005). These isoforms are implicated in maintaining normal Golgi structure and function during Golgi formation (Choukroun et al., 2000), tubulation (de Figueiredo et al., 1999), and membrane remodeling (Schmidt et al., 1999). In addition, several studies using PLA$_2$ inhibitors highlight the importance of PLA$_2$ activity in trafficking between the Golgi complex and the endoplasmic reticulum (de Figueiredo et al., 1998, 1999; Polizotto et al., 1999; Drecktrah and Brown, 1999), endocytosis (Mayorga et al., 1993), exocytosis (Slomiany et al., 1998), and the intracellular trafficking of secretory proteins (Tagaya et al., 1993; Choukroun et al., 2000). Since these inhibitors have a broad range of specificity, the association to a specific PLA$_2$ isoform is not clear. Nevertheless, in non-neural cells, the cPLA$_2$-α isoform seems to be predominantly located at the trans-Golgi stack and trans-Golgi network following elevation of cytosolic calcium ion or treatment with ceramide-1-phosphate (Subramanian et al., 2005), where it may be involved in trafficking events and maintenance of Golgi complex structure and function (Slomiany et al., 1992; Choukroun et al., 2000; Brown et al., 2003; Grewal et al., 2003; Herbert et al., 2005). Brefeldin A (BFA), a fungal metabolite, causes the redistribution of cPLA$_2$-α in Golgi-derived membranes in epithelial cells. It was used to develop in vivo and in vitro models for the formation of tubules from the Golgi complex to endoplasmic reticulum and from the trans-Golgi network to endosomes in hepatocytes. The PLA$_2$ inhibitors ONO-RS-082, arachidonoyl trifluoromethylketone, and bromoenol lactone prevent, and the PLA$_2$ activators melittin and PLA$_2$-activating protein peptide stimulate, BFA-mediated Golgi tubulation and retrograde trafficking in vivo and in vitro (de Figueiredo et al., 1998, 1999; Kuroiwa et al., 2001). These observations implicate PLA$_2$ isoforms in membrane tubule formation from the Golgi complex (Polizotto et al., 1999). The molecular mechanism of tubule formation remains elusive. However, PLA$_2$ isoforms may act on Golgi membranes to generate lysoglycerophospholipids in the outer leaflet of the lipid bilayer. The conversion of cylindrical and cone-shaped native glycerophospholipids to inverted cone-shaped lysoglycerophospholipids may allow an outward bending of the membrane resulting in the formation of tubules (Brown et al., 2003; Grewal et al., 2003; Chambers et al., 2005). Arachidonic acid, the other product of PLA$_2$-catalyzed reactions, promotes membrane bilayer to form the HII phase (Burger and Verkleij, 1990). The formation of the HII phase is imperative during membrane fusion events. Thus, the activation of PLA$_2$ isoforms initiates the formation of tubules and induces membrane curvature and bending, whereas activation of lysoglycerophospholipid acyltransferase has the opposite effect on membrane curvature and tubule formation. An elevated level of lysoglycerophospholipids in Golgi membranes may induce tubule formation due to increased membrane curvature. This process may have a direct effect on membrane structure and trafficking events (Chambers et al., 2005). Interestingly, the lysoglycerophospholipid acyltransferase inhibitor, Cl-976, also causes the accumulation of lysoglycerophospholipids and induces tubule formation and retrograde trafficking (Drecktrah et al., 2003; Chambers et al., 2005). Based on the effect of PLA$_2$ inhibitors and the lysoglycerophospholipid acyltransferase inhibitor, glycerophospholipid to lysoglycerophospholipid ratios may play an important role in controlling Golgi membrane shape and function (Brown et al., 2003).

Collective evidence suggests that cPLA$_2$-α plays an important role in membrane trafficking events (de Figueiredo et al., 1998, 1999; Kuroiwa et al., 2001). cPLA$_2$ not only inhibits the delivery of aquaporin-2 to the plasma membrane, but also disrupts the cisternal morphology of the Golgi complex (Brown et al., 2003). This suggests that cPLA$_2$ has a direct effect on the structure and function of the Golgi membrane complex. Furthermore, the overexpression of sPLA$_2$ in RBL mast cells induces an increased release of histamine. This enhancement may be due to the generation of lysoglycerophospholipids that influence the fusogenic properties of RBL mast cell plasma membranes (Chambers et al., 2005).

4.8 PLA$_2$ Isoforms in Neurodegeneration

Neurodegeneration is defined as a process that results in death of neurons, astrocytes, and oligodendrocytes in the brain and spinal cord. Apoptosis and necrosis are the two basic mechanisms of cell death that occur in the brain and spinal cord. Necrosis is characterized by passive cell swelling, intense mitochondrial damage with rapid loss of ATP, alterations in membrane permeability, high calcium ion influx, and disruption of ion homeostasis. This type of cell death leads to membrane lysis and release of intracellular components that induce an inflammatory reaction (Majno and Joris, 1995). In contrast, apoptosis is an active process in which caspases are stimulated. Caspases are a family of cysteine-dependent endoproteases with specificity for aspartate residues in proteins. Different caspases play distinct roles in apoptotic cell death during neurodegeneration. They may act either as an upstream initiator of a proteolytic cascade, such as caspase-8 and caspase-9, or as a downstream effector such as caspase-3 that hydrolyzes intracellular proteins related to signal transduction. These proteins include protein kinase C, cPLA$_2$, iPLA$_2$, PLC, and cytoskeletal proteins such as α-spectrin, β-spectrin, actin, vimentin, presenilins, Bcl-2 family of apoptosis-related proteins, and DNA-modulating enzymes (Sastry and Rao, 2000). Apoptotic cell death is accompanied by cell shrinkage, dynamic membrane blebbing, chromatin condensation, DNA laddering, loss of plasma membrane asymmetry, maintenance of ATP, mitochondrial oxyradical generation, and a mild calcium ion overload (Sastry and Rao, 2000). Inhibitors of gene transcription and translation can block apoptosis, indicating that this type of cell death requires ongoing protein synthesis. Although the molecular mechanisms underlying the execution phase, such as caspase involvement, are well described, those occurring during the early stage of the apoptotic process in neural cells are not well understood (Pittman et al., 1998; Ueda and Fujita, 2004).

4.8.1 Involvement of PLA$_2$ Isoforms in Apoptosis

During the execution phase of apoptosis, phosphatidylserine translocates to the outer leaflet of the phospholipid bilayer. This results in the loss of membrane asymmetry. Phosphatidylserine externalization functions as a tag on the dying neural cell for recognition and removal by phagocytosis and results in looser phospholipid packing in the outer leaflet allowing calcium ion entry. The mild alteration in calcium homeostasis and its short duration may lead to neuronal degeneration by the activation of caspases and PLA$_2$ resulting in apoptotic cell death. Inhibitors of caspases and PLA$_2$ block apoptotic cell death (Wissing et al., 1997; Atsumi et al., 1998, 2000; Pirianov et al., 1999). During apoptotic cell death, the released fatty acids are not free fatty acids, but are esterified fragments of lipids, indicating the shedding of membranes and the release of apoptotic bodies (Zhang et al., 1999). This suggests that the stimulation of caspases is followed by the activation of PLA$_2$ activity. Several isoforms, cPLA$_2$, iPLA$_2$, sPLA$_2$, and PlsEtn-PLA$_2$, may be involved in apoptotic cell death in the brain tissue.

The treatment of neural and non-neural cell cultures with tumor necrosis factor-α (TNF-α), a proinflammatory cytokine, results in caspase-mediated proteolytic cleavage and activation of cPLA$_2$ activity causing apoptotic cell death (Fig. 4.2). The tetrapeptide inhibitor of caspase activity, acetyl-Asp-Val-Asp-aldehyde, and the cPLA$_2$ inhibitor, arachidonoyl trifluoromethylketone, AACOCF$_3$, block TNF-α-mediated cell death. This suggests the involvement of cPLA$_2$ in apoptotic cell death (Wissing et al., 1997). Ceramide-mediated cell death also requires the release of arachidonic acid and the stimulation of cPLA$_2$ activity (Hayakawa et al., 1993, 1996; MacEwan, 1996; Pirianov et al., 1999). Cells resistant to TNF-α-mediated cytotoxicity have lower levels of cPLA$_2$ activity, whilst introduction of this enzyme into enzyme-deficient cells restores TNF-α-mediated cytotoxicity. The cPLA$_2$-generated second messenger, arachidonic acid, interacts closely with the sphingomyelinase-generated second messenger, ceramide, at several sites in the cytokine-induced signal transduction process (Fig. 4.3). In non-neural cells, cytokines stimulate both sphingomyelinase and cPLA$_2$ activities in a dose- and time-dependent manner. Inhibitors of cPLA$_2$ and sphingomyelinase block this stimulation (Vanags et al., 1997). The product of the cPLA$_2$-catalyzed reaction, arachidonic acid, stimulates sphingomyelinase (Robinson et al., 1997), and ceramide, the product from sphingomyelinase, stimulates cPLA$_2$ activity (Sato et al., 1999). Furthermore, ceramide-1-phosphate, a product of ceramide kinase, increases the membrane affinity of cPLA$_2$-α and allosterically stimulates this enzyme (Subramanian et al., 2005). Sphingosine-1 phosphate, a product of sphingosine kinase, activates cyclooxygenase during cytokine-mediated prostaglandin E$_2$ synthesis (Pettus et al., 2003, 2004, 2005). A combination of these sphingolipid metabolites produces a synergistic effect on prostaglandin E$_2$ synthesis, suggesting a coordinated regulation of glycerophospholipid metabolism with sphingolipid-generated metabolites. This suggests cross-talk between receptor-mediated glycerophospholipid and sphingomyelin

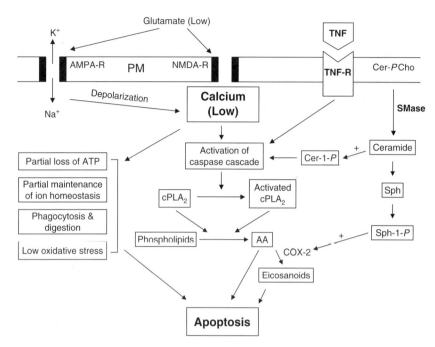

FIG. 4.2. Involvement and activation of cPLA$_2$ and iPLA$_2$ in apoptotic cell death mediated through tumor necrosis factor (TNF)-α or NMDA or AMPA receptors. Plasma membrane, PM; α-amino-3-hydroxy-5-methyl-4-isoxazole propionate receptor, AMPA-R; N-methyl-D-aspartate receptor, NMDA-R; cytosolic phospholipase A$_2$, cPLA$_2$; calcium-independent phospholipase A$_2$, iPLA$_2$; ceramide-1-phosphate, Cer-1-*P*; sphingosine, Sph; sphingomyelinase, SMase; sphingosine-1-phosphate, Sph-1-*P*; arachidonic acid, AA; and cyclooxygenase, COX-2.

signaling pathways. This type of cross-talk with controlled and coordinated signaling may be involved in apoptotic cell death under physiological conditions (Leist and Nicotera, 1998; Ueda and Fujita, 2004).

Fas-mediated apoptosis requires the participation of iPLA$_2$ (Fig. 4.4). During this process, iPLA$_2$ activity is stimulated and bromoenol lactone, BEL, an iPLA$_2$ inhibitor, prevents apoptotic cell death suggesting that iPLA$_2$ is involved in Fas-mediated cell death (Atsumi et al., 1998, 2000). Induction of apoptosis in non-neural cells produces an increased release of 16:0-lyso-PtdCho and 18:0-lyso-PtdCho, which act as chemotactic factors for macrophages. The inhibition of caspases or iPLA$_2$ blocks the enhanced release of lyso-PtdCho from apoptotic cells (Lauber et al., 2003).

The Bcl-2 protein family is also a key regulator of apoptotic cell death associated with diverse stimuli (Adams and Cory, 1998). Thus, Bcl-2 and Bcl-xl inhibit, whereas Bax and Bad promote apoptotic cell death. The exact mechanism by

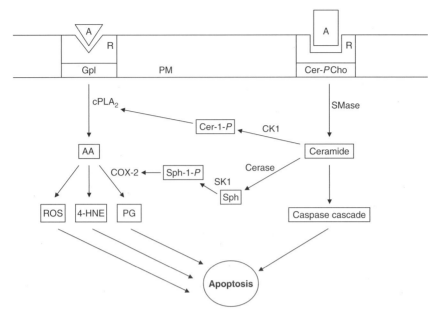

Fig. 4.3. Interactions between metabolites of glycerophospholipid metabolism and sphingolipid metabolism in apoptotic cell death. Agonist, A; receptor, R; glycerophospholipid, Gpl; cytosolic phospholipase A$_2$, cPLA$_2$; sphingomyelinase, SMase; arachidonic acid, AA; reactive oxygen species, ROS; 4-hydroxynonenal, 4-HNE; prostaglandin, PG; lysophosphatidylcholine, lyso-PtdCho; ceramide-1-phosphate, Cer-1-P; ceramide kinase, CKI; sphingomyelin, Cer-PCho; sphingosine-1 phosphate, Sph-1-P; sphingosine kinase, SKI; ceramidase, Cerase; and sphingomyelinase, SMase.

which Bcl-2 proteins control apoptotic cell death remains unknown. However, the ratio of antiapoptotic proteins to proapoptotic proteins plays a critical role in determining whether cells survive or die (Adams and Cory, 1998). During apoptosis, rat brain mitochondria release cytochrome c in the presence of truncated forms of BID (tBID) and BAX. This process is independent of the mitochondrial permeability transition, but depends on the generation of reactive oxygen species and the augmentation of iPLA$_2$ activity (Brustovetsky et al., 2005). Propanolol blocks all these processes, whereas 4-bromophenacyl bromide and bromoenol lactone suppress only iPLA$_2$ and the release of the apoptogenic factor, Cyt c. The treatment of brain mitochondria with a mixture of tBID and BAX not only inhibits cytochrome c release, but also suppresses iPLA$_2$ activity. This indicates a correlation between iPLA$_2$ activity and the release of cytochrome c from brain mitochondria. An increased degradation of glycerophospholipids by iPLA$_2$ in the outer mitochondrial membrane may lead to the release of cytochrome c. This release of cytochrome c may initiate apoptotic cell death (Brustovetsky et al., 2005).

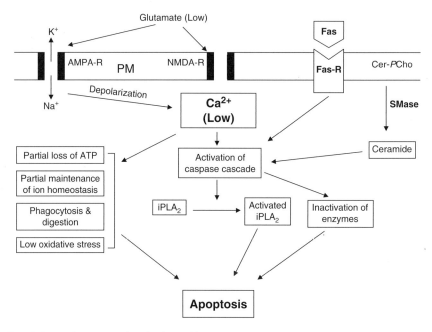

FIG. 4.4. Involvement and activation of iPLA$_2$ in apoptotic cell death mediated by tumor necrosis factor (TNF)-α or Fas. Plasma membrane, PM; α-amino-3-hydroxy-5-methyl-4-isoxazole propionate receptor, AMPA-R; N-methyl-D-aspartate receptor, NMDA-R; Fas receptor, Fas-R; sphingomyelin, Cer-PCho; calcium-independent phospholipase A$_2$, iPLA$_2$; and sphingomyelinase, SMase.

Stimulation of sPLA$_2$ in cytokine-mediated apoptosis in neuron-rich cultures also occurs (Yagami et al., 2005). sPLA$_2$ inhibitors can prevent apoptotic cell death in neuronal cultures (Zhao et al., 2002; Yagami et al., 2002b). An increase in cytokine levels leads to the secretion of sPLA$_2$-IIA from astrocytes (Oka and Arita, 1991). This sPLA$_2$ potentiates calcium influx through L-type voltage-sensitive calcium ion channels (Yagami et al., 2003), resulting in the stimulation of sPLA$_2$ and the liberation of arachidonic acid and prostaglandin D$_2$ (Yagami et al., 2002b). S2474, a cyclooxygenase-2 and 5-lipoxygenase inhibitor (Inagaki et al., 2000), prevents sPLA$_2$-IIA-induced prostaglandin D$_2$ generation and rescues neurons from apoptotic cell death. Collective evidence suggests that sPLA$_2$ participates in apoptotic cell death (Yagami et al., 2002a, 2003, 2005).

PlsEtn-PLA$_2$ is another target for ceramide-induced apoptosis (Latorre et al., 2003). Quinacrine, a nonspecific PLA$_2$ inhibitor, and 1-O-octadecyl-2-methyl-rac-glycero-3-phosphocholine, a CoA-independent transacylase inhibitor, block ceramide-mediated effects. Therefore, PlsEtn-PLA$_2$ and transacylase activities are tightly coupled. Based on various pharmacological experiments, caspase-3 may activate PlsEtn-PLA$_2$. This suggests an interaction between plasmalogen and sphingomyelin catabolism. Collective evidence suggests that all isoforms of

PLA$_2$ are involved in apoptotic cell death and that the level of free arachidonic acid is a critical signal for apoptotic cell death. Other fatty acids such as oleic and palmitic acids do not provide a signal for apoptosis.

4.8.2 Involvement of PLA$_2$ Isoforms in Necrosis

Necrosis occurs due to excessive physical or chemical injury. As stated earlier, swelling, organelle and cellular rupture, and inflammatory reactions due to activation of microglial cells characterize necrosis. A drastic decrease in ATP levels accompanies necrosis. Cellular ATP levels are determined by three parameters: glucose uptake, mitochondrial ATP production, and cellular ATP consumption (Ueda and Fujita, 2004). Although details of the mechanisms underlying decreased mitochondrial ATP synthesis remain unknown, the generation of reactive oxygen species (ROS) and damage to the mitochondrial membrane are likely candidates. During excitotoxic injury, abnormal mitochondrial metabolism is accompanied by sustained calcium ion overload, rapid decrease in ATP, and alterations in cellular redox due to the depletion of reduced glutathione (Farooqui and Horrocks, 1994; Weber, 1999; Wullner et al., 1999). A rise in intracellular calcium ion stimulates activities of a number of calcium-dependent enzymes, including isoforms of PLA$_2$, calpains, and nitric oxide synthase (Fig. 4.5)

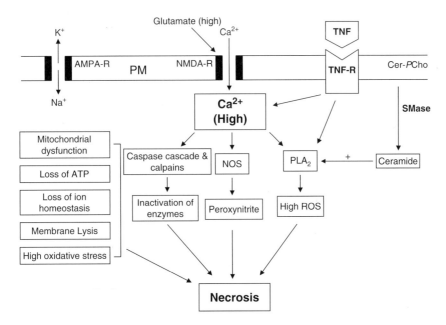

Fig. 4.5. Involvement of phospholipase A$_2$ stimulation mediated through receptors in necrotic cell death. Plasma membrane, PM; α-amino-3-hydroxy-5-methyl-4-isoxazole propionate receptor, AMPA-R; N-methyl-D-aspartate receptor, NMDA-R; sphingomyelin, Cer-PCho; phospholipase A$_2$, PLA$_2$; sphingomyelinase, SMase; and nitric oxide synthase, NOS.

(Farooqui and Horrocks, 1994). The activation of PLA$_2$ isoforms releases arachidonic acid from neural membrane glycerophospholipids and sets in motion an uncontrolled "arachidonic acid cascade." The latter includes the synthesis and accumulation of eicosanoids, isoprostanes, and 4-hydroxynonenal (4-HNE) (Farooqui et al., 2004b). The 4-HNE impairs the activities of key metabolic enzymes, including Na$^+$, K$^+$-ATPase, glucose 6-phosphate dehydrogenase, and several kinases (Farooqui and Horrocks, 2006). 4-HNE also disrupts transmembrane signaling, and the glucose and glutamate transporters in astrocytes (Mark et al., 1997; Camandola et al., 2000; Tamagno et al., 2003). The arachidonic acid cascade also potentiates the accumulation of lipid hydroperoxides. These lipid hydroperoxides inhibit reacylation of glycerophospholipids in neural membranes (Zaleska and Wilson, 1989). This inhibition constitutes another mechanism whereby oxidative processes contribute to necrotic cell death in neural cells. Furthermore, in rat glioma cells, arachidonic acid promotes cell death by changing from apoptosis to necrosis through lipid peroxidation initiated by lipid hydroperoxides produced by 12-lipoxygenase under glutathione depletion (Higuchi and Yoshimoto, 2002). Altogether, these studies suggest that PLA$_2$-generated metabolites play an important role in apoptotic and necrotic cell death.

References

Abu-Raya S., Bloch-Shilderman E., Shohami E., Trembovler V., Shai Y., Weidenfeld J., Yedgar S., Gutman Y., and Lazarovici P. (1998). Pardaxin, a new pharmacological tool to stimulate the arachidonic acid cascade in PC12 cells. *J. Pharmacol. Exp. Ther.* 287:889–896.

Adams J. M. and Cory S. (1998). The Bcl-2 protein family: arbiters of cell survival. *Science* 281:1322–1326.

Akbar M. and Kim H. Y. (2002). Protective effects of docosahexaenoic acid in staurosporine-induced apoptosis: involvement of phosphatidylinositol-3 kinase pathway. *J. Neurochem.* 82:655–665.

Antony P., Freysz L., Horrocks L. A., and Farooqui A. A. (2003). Ca^{2+}-independent phospholipases A$_2$ and production of arachidonic acid in nuclei of LA-N-1 cell cultures: a specific receptor activation mediated with retinoic acid. *Mol. Brain Res.* 115:187–195.

Atsumi G., Tajima M., Hadano A., Nakatani Y., Murakami M., and Kudo I. (1998). Fas-induced arachidonic acid release is mediated by Ca^{2+}-independent phospholipase A$_2$ but not cytosolic phospholipase A$_2$ which undergoes proteolytic inactivation. *J. Biol. Chem.* 273:13870–13877.

Atsumi G., Murakami M., Kojima K., Hadano A., Tajima M., and Kudo I. (2000). Distinct roles of two intracellular phospholipase A$_2$s in fatty acid release in the cell death pathway. Proteolytic fragment of type IVA cytosolic phospholipase A$_{2\alpha}$ inhibits stimulus-induced arachidonate release, whereas that of type VI Ca^{2+}-independent phospholipase A$_2$ augments spontaneous fatty acid release. *J. Biol. Chem.* 275:18248–18258.

Baudry M. and Lynch G. (2001). Remembrance of arguments past: how well is the glutamate receptor hypothesis of LTP holding up after 20 years? *Neurobiol. Learn. Mem.* 76:284–297.

Bazan N. G. (2003). Synaptic lipid signaling: significance of polyunsaturated fatty acids and platelet-activating factor. *J. Lipid Res.* 44:2221–2233.

Bazan N. G. (2005a). Neuroprotectin D1 (NPD1): A DHA-derived mediator that protects brain and retina against cell injury-induced oxidative stress. *Brain Pathol.* 15:159–166.

Bazan N. G. (2005b). Synaptic signaling by lipids in the life and death of neurons. *Mol. Neurobiol.* 31:219–230.

Bernard J., Lahsaini A., and Massicotte G. (1994). Potassium-induced long-term potentiation in area CA1 of the hippocampus involves phospholipase activation. *Hippocampus* 4:447–453.

Bliss T. V. P. and Collingridge G. L. (1993). A synaptic model of memory: long-term potentiation in the hippocampus. *Nature* 361:31–39.

Bloch-Shilderman E., Abu-Raya S., Trembovler V., Boschwitz H., Gruzman A., Linial M., and Lazarovici P. (2002). Pardaxin stimulation of phospholipases A$_2$ and their involvement in exocytosis in PC-12 cells. *J. Pharmacol. Exp. Ther.* 301:953–962.

Bonventre J. V., Huang Z. H., Taheri M. R., O'Leary E., Li E., Moskowitz M. A., and Sapirstein A. (1997). Reduced fertility and postischaemic brain injury in mice deficient in cytosolic phospholipase A$_2$. *Nature* 390:622–625.

Bramham C. R., Alkon D. L., and Lester D. S. (1994). Arachidonic acid and diacylglycerol act synergistically through protein kinase C to persistently enhance synaptic transmission in the hippocampus. *Neuroscience* 60:737–743.

Brown W. J., Chambers K., and Doody A. (2003). Phospholipase A$_2$ (PLA$_2$) enzymes in membrane trafficking: Mediators of membrane shape and function. *Traffic* 4:214–221.

Brustovetsky T., Antonsson B., Jemmerson R., Dubinsky J. M., and Brustovetsky N. (2005). Activation of calcium-independent phospholipase A$_2$ (iPLA$_2$) in brain mitochondria and release of apoptogenic factors by BAX and truncated BID. *J. Neurochem.* 94:980–994.

Burger K. N. and Verkleij A. J. (1990). Membrane fusion. *Experientia* 46:631–644.

Burgoyne R. D. and Morgan A. (1995). Ca^{2+} and secretory-vesicle dynamics. *Trends Neurosci.* 18:191–196.

Calderon F. and Kim H. Y. (2004). Docosahexaenoic acid promotes neurite growth in hippocampal neurons. *J. Neurochem.* 90:979–988.

Camandola S., Poli G., and Mattson M. P. (2000). The lipid peroxidation product 4-hydroxy-2,3-nonenal increases AP-1-binding activity through caspase activation in neurons. *J. Neurochem.* 74:159–168.

Chambers K., Judson B., and Brown W. J. (2005). A unique lysophospholipid acyltransferase (LPAT) antagonist, CI-976, affects secretory and endocytic membrane trafficking pathways. *J. Cell Sci.* 118:3061–3071.

Chen C. and Tonegawa S. (1997). Molecular genetic analysis of synaptic plasticity, activity-dependent neural development, learning, and memory in the mammalian brain. *Annu. Rev. Neurosci.* 20:157–184.

Choukroun G. J., Marshansky V., Gustafson C. E., McKee M., Hajjar R. J., Rosenzweig A., Brown D., and Bonventre J. V. (2000). Cytosolic phospholipase A$_2$ regulates Golgi structure and modulates intracellular trafficking of membrane proteins. *J. Clin. Invest.* 106:983–993.

Chung H. J., Steinberg J. P., Huganir R. L., and Linden D. J. (2003). Requirement of AMPA receptor GluR2 phosphorylation for cerebellar long-term depression. *Science* 300:1751–1755.

Clements M. P., Bliss T. V. P., and Lynch M. A. (1991). Increase in arachidonic acid concentration in a postsynaptic membrane fraction following the induction of long-term potentiation in the dentate gyrus. *Neuroscience* 45:379–389.

Correale J. and Villa A. (2004). The neuroprotective role of inflammation in nervous system injuries. *J. Neurol.* 251:1304–1316.

de Figueiredo P., Drecktrah D., Katzenellenbogen J. A., Strang M., and Brown W. J. (1998). Evidence that phospholipase A$_2$ activity is required for Golgi complex and trans Golgi network membrane tubulation. *Proc. Natl Acad. Sci. USA* 95:8642–8647.

de Figueiredo P., Polizotto R. S., Drecktrah D., and Brown W. J. (1999). Membrane tubule-mediated reassembly and maintenance of the Golgi complex is disrupted by phospholipase A$_2$ antagonists. *Mol. Biol. Cell* 10:1763–1782.

Doherty P., Ashton S. V., Moore S. E., and Walsh F. S. (1991). Morphoregulatory activities of NCAM and N-cadherin can be accounted for by G protein-dependent activation of L- and N-type neuronal Ca^{2+} channels. *Cell* 67:21–33.

Drecktrah D. and Brown W. J. (1999). Phospholipase A$_2$ antagonists inhibit nocodazole-induced Golgi ministack formation: evidence of an ER intermediate and constitutive cycling. *Mol. Biol. Cell* 10:4021–4032.

Drecktrah D., Chambers K., Racoosin E. L., Cluett E. B., Gucwa A., Jackson B., and Brown W. J. (2003). Inhibition of a Golgi complex lysophospholipid acyltransferase induces membrane tubule formation and retrograde trafficking. *Mol. Biol. Cell* 14:3459–3469.

Farooqui A. A. and Horrocks L. A. (1991). Excitatory amino acid receptors, neural membrane phospholipid metabolism and neurological disorders. *Brain Res. Rev.* 16:171–191.

Farooqui A. A. and Horrocks L. A. (1994). Excitotoxicity and neurological disorders: involvement of membrane phospholipids. *Int. Rev. Neurobiol.* 36:267–323.

Farooqui A. A. and Horrocks L. A. (2001). Plasmalogens: Workhorse lipids of membranes in normal and injured neurons and glia. *Neuroscientist* 7:232–245.

Farooqui A. A. and Horrocks L. A. (2004). Plasmalogens, platelet activating factor, and other ether lipids. In: Nicolaou A. and Kokotos G. (eds.), *Bioactive Lipids*. Oily Press, Bridgwater, England, pp. 107–134.

Farooqui A. A. and Horrocks L. A. (2006). Phospholipase A$_2$-generated lipid mediators in brain: the good, the bad, and the ugly. *Neuroscientist* 12:245.

Farooqui, A. A., Anderson, D. K., and Horrocks, L. A. (1994). Potentiation of diacylglycerol and monoacylglycerol lipase activities by glutamate and its analogs. *J. Neurochem.* 62:S74B.

Farooqui A. A., Horrocks L. A., and Farooqui T. (2000a). Deacylation and reacylation of neural membrane glycerophospholipids. *J. Mol. Neurosci.* 14:123–135.

Farooqui A. A., Horrocks L. A., and Farooqui T. (2000b). Glycerophospholipids in brain: their metabolism, incorporation into membranes, functions, and involvement in neurological disorders. *Chem. Phys. Lipids* 106:1–29.

Farooqui A. A., Ong W. Y., Horrocks L. A., and Farooqui T. (2000c). Brain cytosolic phospholipase A$_2$: localization, role, and involvement in neurological diseases. *Neuroscientist* 6:169–180.

Farooqui A. A., Ong W. Y., Lu X. R., and Horrocks L. A. (2002). Cytosolic phospholipase A$_2$ inhibitors as therapeutic agents for neural cell injury. *Curr. Med. Chem. — Anti-Inflammatory Anti-Allergy Agents* 1:193–204.

Farooqui A. A., Antony P., Ong W. Y., Horrocks L. A., and Freysz L. (2004a). Retinoic acid-mediated phospholipase A$_2$ signaling in the nucleus. *Brain Res. Rev.* 45:179–195.

Farooqui A. A., Ong W. Y., and Horrocks L. A. (2004b). Biochemical aspects of neurodegeneration in human brain: involvement of neural membrane phospholipids and phospholipases A$_2$. *Neurochem. Res.* 29:1961–1977.

Fujita S., Ikegaya Y., Nishiyama N., and Matsuki N. (2000). Ca²⁺-independent phospholipase A₂ inhibitor impairs spatial memory of mice. *Jpn. J. Pharmacol.* 83:277–278.

Fujita S., Ikegaya Y., Nishikawa M., Nishiyama N., and Matsuki N. (2001). Docosahexaenoic acid improves long-term potentiation attenuated by phospholipase A₂ inhibitor in rat hippocampal slices. *Br. J. Pharmacol.* 132:1417–1422.

Furnkranz A. and Leitinger N. (2004). Regulation of inflammatory responses by oxidized phospholipids structure–function relationships. *Curr. Pharm. Des.* 10:915–921.

Geddis M. S. and Rehder V. (2003). Initial stages of neural regeneration in *Helisoma trivolvis* are dependent upon PLA₂ activity. *J. Neurobiol.* 54:555–565.

Ghijsen W. E., Leenders A. G., and Lopes da Silva F. H. (2003). Regulation of vesicle traffic and neurotransmitter release in isolated nerve terminals. *Neurochem. Res.* 28:1443–1452.

Gilroy D. W., Newson J., Sawmynaden P. A., Willoughby D. A., and Croxtall J. D. (2004). A novel role for phospholipase A₂ isoforms in the checkpoint control of acute inflammation. *FASEB J.* 18:489–498.

Grass D. S. (1999). Transgenics in in vivo models of inflammation. In: Morgan D. W. and Marshall L. A. (eds.), *In Vivo Models of Inflammation*. Birkhauser Verlag, Berlin, pp. 291–305.

Grewal S., Ponnambalam S., and Walker J. H. (2003). Association of cPLA₂-α and COX-1 with the Golgi apparatus of A549 human lung epithelial cells. *J. Cell Sci.* 116:2303–2310.

Grewal S., Herbert S. P., Ponnambalam S., and Walker J. H. (2005). Cytosolic phospholipase A₂-α and cyclooxygenase-2 localize to intracellular membranes of EA.hy.926 endothelial cells that are distinct from the endoplasmic reticulum and the Golgi apparatus. *FEBS J.* 272:1278–1290.

Hayakawa M., Ishida N., Takeuchi K., Shibamoto S., Hori T., Oku N., Ito F., and Tsujimoto M. (1993). Arachidonic acid-selective cytosolic phospholipase A₂ is crucial in the cytotoxic action of tumor necrosis factor. *J. Biochem.* 268:11290–11295.

Hayakawa M., Jayadev S., Tsujimoto M., Hannun Y. A., and Ito F. (1996). Role of ceramide in stimulation of the transcription of cytosolic phospholipase A₂ and cyclooxygenase 2. *Biochem. Biophys. Res. Commun.* 220:681–686.

Herbert S. P., Ponnambalam S., and Walker J. H. (2005). Cytosolic phospholipase A₂₋α mediates endothelial cell proliferation and is inactivated by association with the Golgi apparatus. *Mol. Biol. Cell* 16:3800–3809.

Higuchi Y. and Yoshimoto T. (2002). Arachidonic acid converts the glutathione depletion-induced apoptosis to necrosis by promoting lipid peroxidation and reducing caspase-3 activity in rat glioma cells. *Arch. Biochem. Biophys.* 400:133–140.

Hong S., Gronert K., Devchand P. R., Moussignac R. L., and Serhan C. N. (2003). Novel docosatrienes and 17S-resolvins generated from docosahexaenoic acid in murine brain, human blood, and glial cells — Autacoids in anti-inflammation. *J. Biol. Chem.* 278:14677–14687.

Hornfelt M., Ekström P. A. R., and Edström A. (1999). Involvement of axonal phospholipase A₂ activity in the outgrowth of adult mouse sensory axons *in vitro*. *Neuroscience* 91:1539–1547.

Hulo S., Alberi S., Laux T., Muller D., and Caroni P. (2002). A point mutant of GAP-43 induces enhanced short-term and long-term hippocampal plasticity. *Eur. J. Neurosci.* 15:1976–1982.

Ikemoto A., Kobayashi T., Emoto K., Umeda M., Watanabe S., and Okuyama H. (1999). Effects of docosahexaenoic and arachidonic acids on the synthesis and distribution of aminophospholipids during neuronal differentiation of PC12 cells. *Arch. Biochem. Biophys.* 364:67–74.

Ikeno Y., Konno N., Cheon S. H., Bolchi A., Ottonello S., Kitamoto K., and Arioka M. (2005). Secretory phospholipases A$_2$ induce neurite outgrowth in PC12 cells through lysophosphatidylcholine generation and activation of G2A receptor. *J. Biol. Chem.* 280:28044–28052.

Inagaki M., Tsuri T., Jyoyama H., Ono T., Yamada K., Kobayashi M., Hori Y., Arimura A., Yasui K., Ohno K., Kakudo S., Koizumi K., Suzuki R., Kawai S., Kato M., and Matsumoto S. (2000). Novel antiarthritic agents with 1,2-isothiazolidine-1,1-dioxide (γ sultam) skeleton: cytokine suppressive dual inhibitors of cyclooxygenase-2 and 5-lipoxygenase. *J. Med. Chem.* 43:2040–2048.

Izquierdo I. and Medina J. H. (1995). Correlation between the pharmacology of long-term potentiation and the pharmacology of memory. *Neurobiol. Learn. Mem.* 63:19–32.

Jamora C. (1999). 100 years of Golgi complexities. *Trends Cell Biol.* 9:37–38.

Kater S. B. and Mills L. R. (1991). Regulation of growth cone behavior by calcium. *J. Neurosci.* 11:891–899.

Katsuki H. and Okuda S. (1995). Arachidonic acid as a neurotoxic and neurotrophic substance. *Prog. Neurobiol.* 46:607–636.

Kim H. Y., Akbar M., Lau A., and Edsall L. (2000). Inhibition of neuronal apoptosis by docosahexaenoic acid (22:6n-3). Role of phosphatidylserine in antiapoptotic effect. *J. Biol. Chem.* 275:35215–35223.

Kita Y., Kimura K. D., Kobayashi M., Ihara S., Kaibuchi K., Kuroda S., Ui M., Iba H., Konishi H., Kikkawa U., Nagata S., and Fukui Y. (1998). Microinjection of activated phosphatidylinositol-3 kinase induces process outgrowth in rat PC12 cells through the Rac-JNK signal transduction pathway. *J. Cell Sci.* 111(Pt 7):907–915.

Kobayashi M., Nagata S., Kita Y., Nakatsu N., Ihara S., Kaibuchi K., Kuroda S., Ui M., Iba H., Konishi H., Kikkawa U., Saitoh I., and Fukui Y. (1997). Expression of a constitutively active phosphatidylinositol 3-kinase induces process formation in rat PC12 cells. Use of Cre/loxP recombination system. *J. Biol. Chem.* 272:16089–16092.

Kuroiwa N., Nakamura M., Tagaya M., and Takatsuki A. (2001). Arachidonyltrifluoromethyl ketone, a phospholipase A$_2$ antagonist, induces dispersal of both Golgi stack- and trans Golgi network-resident proteins throughout the cytoplasm. *Biochem. Biophys. Res. Commun.* 281:582–588.

Latorre E., Collado M. P., Fernández I., Aragonés M. D., and Catalán R. E. (2003). Signaling events mediating activation of brain ethanolamine plasmalogen hydrolysis by ceramide. *Eur. J. Biochem.* 270:36–46.

Lauber K., Bohn E., Krober S. M., Xiao Y. J., Blumenthal S. G., Lindemann R. K., Marini P., Wiedig C., Zobywalski A., Baksh S., Xu Y., Autenrieth I. B., Schulze-Osthoff K., Belka C., Stuhler G., and Wesselborg S. (2003). Apoptotic cells induce migration of phagocytes via caspase-3-mediated release of a lipid attraction signal. *Cell* 113:717–730.

Lazarewicz J. W., Wroblewski J. T., and Costa E. (1990). N-methyl-D-aspartate-sensitive glutamate receptors induce calcium-mediated arachidonic acid release in primary cultures of cerebellar granule cells. *J. Neurochem.* 55:1875–1881.

Ledeen R. W. and Wu G. S. (2004). Nuclear lipids: key signaling effectors in the nervous system and other tissues. *J. Lipid Res.* 45:1–8.

Leist M. and Nicotera P. (1998). Apoptosis, excitotoxicity, and neuropathology. *Exp. Cell Res.* 239:183–201.

Lengqvist J., Mata de Urquiza A., Bergman A. C., Willson T. M., Sjövall J., Perlmann T., and Griffiths W. J. (2004). Polyunsaturated fatty acids including docosahexaenoic and arachidonic acid bind to the retinoid X receptor α ligand-binding domain. *Mol. Cell. Proteomics* 3:692–703.

Li L. and Chin L. S. (2003). The molecular machinery of synaptic vesicle exocytosis. *Cell Mol. Life Sci.* 60:942–960.

Linden D. J. and Routtenberg A. (1989). The role of protein kinase C in long-term potentiation: a testable model. *Brain Res. Rev.* 14:279–296.

MacEwan D. J. (1996). Elevated cPLA$_2$ levels as a mechanism by which the p70 TNF and p75 NGF receptors enhance apoptosis. *FEBS Lett.* 379:77–81.

Majno G. and Joris I. (1995). Apoptosis, oncosis, and necrosis: an overview of cell death. *Am. J. Pathol.* 146:3–15.

Manguikian A. D. and Barbour S. E. (2004). Cell cycle dependence of group VIA calcium-independent phospholipase A$_2$ activity. *J. Biol. Chem.* 279:52881–52892.

Marcheselli V. L., Hong S., Lukiw W. J., Tian X. H., Gronert K., Musto A., Hardy M., Gimenez J. M., Chiang N., Serhan C. N., and Bazan N. G. (2003). Novel docosanoids inhibit brain ischemia-reperfusion-mediated leukocyte infiltration and pro-inflammatory gene expression. *J. Biol. Chem.* 278:43807–43817.

Mark R. J., Lovell M. A., Markesbery W. R., Uchida K., and Mattson M. P. (1997). A role for 4-hydroxynonenal, an aldehydic product of lipid peroxidation, in disruption of ion homeostasis and neuronal death induced by amyloid β-peptide. *J. Neurochem.* 68:255–264.

Massicotte G. (2000). Modification of glutamate receptors by phospholipase A2: its role in adaptive neural plasticity. *Cell Mol. Life Sci.* 57:1542–1550.

Masuda S., Murakami M., Takanezawa Y., Aoki J., Arai H., Ishikawa Y., Ishii T., Arioka M., and Kudo I. (2005). Neuronal expression and neuritogenic action of group X secreted phospholipase A$_2$. *J. Biol. Chem.* 280:23203–23214.

Matsuzawa A., Murakami M., Atsumi G., Imai K., Prados P., Inoue K., and Kudo I. (1996). Release of secretory phospholipase A$_2$ from rat neuronal cells and its possible function in the regulation of catecholamine secretion. *Biochem. J.* 318:701–709.

Mayorga L. S., Colombo M. I., Lennartz M., Brown E. J., Rahman K. H., Weiss R., Lennon P. J., and Stahl P. D. (1993). Inhibition of endosome fusion by phospholipase A$_2$ (PLA$_2$) inhibitors points to a role for PLA$_2$ in endocytosis. *Proc. Natl Acad. Sci. USA* 90:10255–10259.

McLean L. R., Hagaman K. A., and Davidson W. S. (1993). Role of lipid structure in the activation of phospholipase A$_2$ by peroxidized phospholipids. *Lipids* 28:505–509.

Ménard C., Patenaude C., and Massicotte G. (2005a). Phosphorylation of AMPA receptor subunits is differentially regulated by phospholipase A$_2$ inhibitors. *Neurosci. Lett.* 389:51–56.

Ménard C., Valastro B., Martel M. A., Chartier T., Marineau A., Baudry M., and Massicotte G. (2005b). AMPA receptor phosphorylation is selectively regulated by constitutive phospholipase A$_2$ and 5-lipoxygenase activities. *Hippocampus* 15:370–380.

Moskowitz N., Schook W., and Puszkin S. (1982). Interaction of brain synaptic vesicles induced by endogenous Ca^{2+}-dependent phospholipase A$_2$. *Science* 216:305–307.

Mukherjee P. K., Marcheselli V. L., Serhan C. N., and Bazan N. G. (2004). Neuroprotectin D1: a docosahexaenoic acid-derived docosatriene protects human retinal pigment epithelial cells from oxidative stress. *Proc. Natl Acad. Sci. USA* 101:8491–8496.

Murakami K. and Routtenberg A. (2003). The role of fatty acids in synaptic growth and plasticity. In: Peet M., Glen L., and Horrobin D. F. (eds.), *Phospholipid Spectrum Disorders in Psychiatry and Neurology*. Marius Press, Carnforth, Lancashire, pp. 77–92.

Ng M. N. P., Kitos T. E., and Cornell R. B. (2004). Contribution of lipid second messengers to the regulation of phosphatidylcholine synthesis during cell cycle re-entry. *Biochim. Biophys. Acta Mol. Cell Biol. Lipids* 1686:85–99.

Nishio H., Takeuchi T., Hata F., and Yagasaki O. (1996). Ca^{2+}-independent fusion of synaptic vesicles with phospholipase A_2-treated presynaptic membranes in vitro. *Biochem. J.* 318:981–987.

Nomura T., Nishizaki T., Enomoto T., and Itoh H. (2001). A long-lasting facilitation of hippocampal neurotransmission via a phospholipase A_2 signaling pathway. *Life Sci.* 68:2885–2891.

Obermeier H., Hrboticky N., and Sellmayer A. (1995). Differential effects of polyunsaturated fatty acids on cell growth and differentiation of premonocytic U937 cells. *Biochim. Biophys. Acta* 1266:179–185.

Oka S. and Arita H. (1991). Inflammatory factors stimulate expression of group II phospholipase A2 in rat cultured astrocytes. Two distinct pathways of the gene expression. *J. Biol. Chem.* 266:9956–9960.

Okada D., Yamagishi S., and Sugiyama H. (1989). Differential effects of phospholipase inhibitors in long-term potentiation in the rat hippocampal mossy fiber synapses and Schaffer/commissural synapses. *Neurosci. Lett.* 100:141–146.

O'Regan M. H., Perkins L. M., and Phillis J. W. (1995a). Arachidonic acid and lysophosphatidylcholine modulate excitatory transmitter amino acid release from the rat cerebral cortex. *Neurosci. Lett.* 193:85–88.

O'Regan M. H., Smith-Barbour M., Perkins L. M., and Phillis J. W. (1995b). A possible role for phospholipases in the release of neurotransmitter amino acids from ischemic rat cerebral cortex. *Neurosci. Lett.* 185:191–194.

O'Regan M. H., Alix S., and Woodbury D. J. (1996). Phospholipase A_2-evoked destabilization of planar lipid membranes. *Neurosci. Lett.* 202:201–203.

Pettus B. J., Bielawski J., Porcelli A. M., Reames D. L., Johnson K. R., Morrow J., Chalfant C. E., Obeid L. M., and Hannun Y. A. (2003). The sphingosine kinase 1/sphingosine-1-phosphate pathway mediates COX-2 induction and PGE_2 production in response to TNF-α. *FASEB J.* 17:1411–1421.

Pettus B. J., Bielawska A., Subramanian P., Wijesinghe D. S., Maceyka M., Leslie C. C., Evans J. H., Freiberg J., Roddy P., Hannun Y. A., and Chalfant C. E. (2004). Ceramide 1-phosphate is a direct activator of cytosolic phospholipase A_2. *J. Biol. Chem.* 279:11320–11326.

Pettus B. J., Kitatani K., Chalfant C. E., Taha T. A., Kawamori T., Bielawski J., Obeid L. M., and Hannun Y. A. (2005). The coordination of prostaglandin E_2 production by sphingosine-1-phosphate and ceramide-1-phosphate. *Mol. Pharmacol.* 68:330–335.

Pirianov G., Danielsson C., Carlberg C., James S. Y., and Colston K. W. (1999). Potentiation by vitamin D analogs of TNFα and ceramide-induced apoptosis in MCF-7 cells is associated with activation of cytosolic phospholipase A_2. *Cell Death Differ.* 6:890–901.

Pittman R. N., Messer A., and Mills J. C. (1998). Asynchronous death as a characteristic feature of apoptosis. In: Koliatsos V. E. and Ratan R. (eds.), *Cell Death and Diseases of the Nervous System*. Humana Press, Inc., Totowa, NJ, pp. 29–43.

Polizotto R. S., de Figueiredo P., and Brown W. J. (1999). Stimulation of Golgi membrane tubulation and retrograde trafficking to the ER by phospholipase A_2 activating protein (PLAP) peptide. *J. Cell Biochem.* 74:670–683.

Reynolds L. J., Hughes L. L., Louis A. I., Kramer R. M., and Dennis E. A. (1993). Metal ion and salt effects on the phospholipase A_2, lysophospholipase, and transacylase activities of human cytosolic phospholipase A$_2$. *Biochim. Biophys. Acta* 1167:272–280.

Robinson B. S., Hii C. S. T., Poulos A., and Ferrante A. (1997). Activation of neutral sphingomyelinase in human neutrophils by polyunsaturated fatty acids. *Immunology* 91:274–280.

Rohrbough J. and Broadie K. (2005). Lipid regulation of the synaptic vesicle cycle. *Nature Rev. Neurosci.* 6:139–150.

Roshak A. K., Capper E. A., Stevenson C., Eichman C., and Marshall L. A. (2000). Human calcium-independent phospholipase A$_2$ mediates lymphocyte proliferation. *J. Biol. Chem.* 275:35692–35698.

Sapirstein A., Saito H., Texel S. J., Samad T. A., O'Leary E., and Bonventre J. V. (2005). Cytosolic phospholipase A$_2$α regulates induction of brain cyclooxygenase-2 in a mouse model of inflammation. *Am. J. Physiol. Regul. Integr. Comp. Physiol.* 288:R1774–R1782.

Sastry P. S. and Rao K. S. (2000). Apoptosis and the nervous system. *J. Neurochem.* 74:1–20.

Sato T., Kageura T., Hashizume T., Hayama M., Kitatani K., and Akiba S. (1999). Stimulation by ceramide of phospholipase A$_2$ activation through a mechanism related to the phospholipase C-initiated signaling pathway in rabbit platelets. *J. Biochem.* (Tokyo) 125:96–102.

Schaeffer E. L. and Gattaz W. F. (2005). Inhibition of calcium-independent phospholipase A$_2$ activity in rat hippocampus impairs acquisition of short- and long-term memory. *Psychopharmacology* (Berl.) 381:392–400.

Schaeffer E. L., Bassi F. J., and Gattaz W. F. (2005). Inhibition of phospholipase A$_2$ activity reduces membrane fluidity in rat hippocampus. *J. Neural Transm.* 112:641–647.

Schmidt A., Wolde M., Thiele C., Fest W., Kratzin H., Podtelejnikov A. V., Witke W., Huttner W. B., and Söling H. D. (1999). Endophilin I mediates synaptic vesicle formation by transfer of arachidonate to lysophosphatidic acid. *Nature* 401:133–141.

Seidenman K. J., Steinberg J. P., Huganir R., and Malinow R. (2003). Glutamate receptor subunit 2 Serine 880 phosphorylation modulates synaptic transmission and mediates plasticity in CA1 pyramidal cells. *J. Neurosci.* 23:9220–9228.

Serhan C. N. (2002). Endogenous chemical mediators in anti-inflammation and pro-resolution. *Curr. Med. Chem. — Anti-Inflammatory Anti-Allergy Agents* 1:177–192.

Serhan C. N. (2005a). Novel eicosanoid and docosanoid mediators: resolvins, docosatrienes, and neuroprotectins. *Curr. Opin. Clin. Nutr. Metab. Care* 8:115–121.

Serhan C. N. (2005b). Novel ω-3-derived local mediators in anti-inflammation and resolution. *Pharmacol. Ther.* 105:7–21.

Serhan C. N., Arita M., Hong S., and Gotlinger K. (2004a). Resolvins, docosatrienes, and neuroprotectins, novel omega-3-derived mediators, and their endogenous aspirin-triggered epimers. *Lipids* 39:1125–1132.

Serhan C. N., Gotlinger K., Hong S., and Arita M. (2004b). Resolvins, docosatrienes, and neuroprotectins, novel omega-3-derived mediators, and their aspirin-triggered endogenous epimers: an overview of their protective roles in catabasis. *Prostaglandins Other Lipid Mediat.* 73:155–172.

Shirai Y., Balsinde J., and Dennis E. A. (2005). Localization and functional interrelationships among cytosolic Group IV, secreted Group V, and Ca^{2+}-independent group VI phospholipase A$_2$s in P388D$_1$ macrophages using GFP/RFP constructs. *Biochim. Biophys. Acta Mol. Cell Biol. Lipids* 1735:119–129.

Slomiany A., Grzelinska E., Kasinathan C., Yamaki K., Palecz D., and Slomiany B. L. (1992). Function of intracellular phospholipase A_2 in vectorial transport of apoproteins from ER to Golgi. *Int. J. Biochem.* 24:1397–1406.

Slomiany A., Nowak P., Piotrowski E., and Slomiany B. L. (1998). Effect of ethanol on intracellular vesicular transport from Golgi to the apical cell membrane: role of phosphatidylinositol 3-kinase and phospholipase A_2 in Golgi transport vesicles association and fusion with the apical membrane. *Alcohol Clin. Exp. Res.* 22:167–175.

Smalheiser N. R., Dissanayake S., and Kapil A. (1996). Rapid regulation of neurite outgrowth and retraction by phospholipase A_2-derived arachidonic acid and its metabolites. *Brain Res.* 721:39–48.

Song I. and Huganir R. L. (2002). Regulation of AMPA receptors during synaptic plasticity. *Trends Neurosci.* 25:578–588.

St-Gelais F., Ménard C., Congar P., Trudeau L. E., and Massicotte G. (2004). Postsynaptic injection of calcium-independent phospholipase A2 inhibitors selectively increases AMPA receptor-mediated synaptic transmission. *Hippocampus* 14:319–325.

Strokin M., Sergeeva M., and Reiser G. (2003). Docosahexaenoic acid and arachidonic acid release in rat brain astrocytes is mediated by two separate isoforms of phospholipase A_2 and is differently regulated by cyclic AMP and Ca^{2+}. *Br. J. Pharmacol.* 139:1014–1022.

Subramanian P., Stahelin R. V., Szulc Z., Bielawska A., Cho W., and Chalfant C. E. (2005). Ceramide 1-phosphate acts as a positive allosteric activator of group IVA cytosolic phospholipase $A_{2\alpha}$ and enhances the interaction of the enzyme with phosphatidylcholine. *J. Biol. Chem.* 280:17601–17607.

Suburo A. and Cei de Job C. (1986). The biphasic effect of phospholipase A_2 inhibitors on axon elongation. *Int. J. Dev. Neurosci.* 4:363–367.

Sun G. Y. and MacQuarrie R. A. (1989). Deacylation-reacylation of arachidonoyl groups in cerebral phospholipids. *Ann. NY Acad. Sci.* 559:37–55.

Tagaya M., Henomatsu N., Yoshimori T., Yamamoto A., Tashiro Y., and Fukui T. (1993). Correlation between phospholipase A_2 activity and intra-Golgi protein transport reconstituted in a cell-free system. *FEBS Lett.* 324:201–204.

Tamagno E., Robino G., Obbili A., Bardini P., Aragno M., Parola M., and Danni O. (2003). H_2O_2 and 4-hydroxynonenal mediate amyloid beta-induced neuronal apoptosis by activating JNKs and p38[MAPK]. *Exp. Neurol.* 180:144–155.

Ueda H. and Fujita R. (2004). Cell death mode switch from necrosis to apoptosis in brain. *Biol. Pharm. Bull.* 27:950–955.

Vanags D. M., Larsson P., Feltenmark S., Jakobsson P. J., Orrenius S., Claesson H. E., and Aguilar-Santelises M. (1997). Inhibitors of arachidonic acid metabolism reduce DNA and nuclear fragmentation induced by TNF plus cycloheximide in U937 cells. *Cell Death Diff.* 4:479–486.

van Rossum G. S. A. T., Bijvelt J. J. M., van den Bosch H., Verkleij A. J., and Boonstra J. (2002). Cytosolic phospholipase A_2 and lipoxygenase are involved in cell cycle progression in neuroblastoma cells. *Cell. Mol. Life Sci.* 59:181–188.

Webb N. R. (2005). Secretory phospholipase A_2 enzymes in atherogenesis. *Curr. Opin. Lipidol.* 16:341–344.

Weber G. F. (1999). Final common pathways in neurodegenerative diseases: regulatory role of the glutathione cycle. *Neurosci. Biobehav. Rev.* 23:1079–1086.

Wei S., Ong W. Y., Thwin M. M., Fong C. W., Farooqui A. A., Gopalakrishnakone P., and Hong W. J. (2003). Differential activities of secretory phospholipase A_2 ($sPLA_2$) in rat brain and effects of $sPLA_2$ on neurotransmitter release. *Neuroscience* 121:891–898.

Williams J. H., Errington M. L., Lynch M. A., and Bliss T. V. P. (1989). Arachidonic acid induces a long-term activity dependent enhancement of synaptic transmission in the hippocampus. *Nature* 341:739–742.

Wissing D., Mouritzen H., Egeblad M., Poirier G. G., and Jäättelä M. (1997). Involvement of caspase-dependent activation of cytosolic phospholipase A_2 in tumor necrosis factor-induced apoptosis. *Proc. Natl Acad. Sci. USA* 94:5073–5077.

Wolf M. J., Izumi Y., Zorumski C. F., and Gross R. W. (1995). Long-term potentiation requires activation of calcium-independent phospholipase A_2. *FEBS Lett.* 377:358–362.

Wullner U., Seyfried J., Groscurth P., Beinroth S., Winter S., Gleichmann M., Heneka M., Loschmann P., Schulz J. B., Weller M., and Klockgether T. (1999). Glutathione depletion and neuronal cell death: the role of reactive oxygen intermediates and mitochondrial function. *Brain Res.* 826:53–62.

Yagami T., Ueda K., Asakura K., Hata S., Kuroda T., Sakaeda T., Takasu N., Tanaka K., Gemba T., and Hori Y. (2002a). Human group IIA secretory phospholipase A_2 induces neuronal cell death via apoptosis. *Mol. Pharmacol.* 61:114–126.

Yagami T., Ueda K., Asakura K., Hayasaki-Kajiwara Y., Nakazato H., Sakaeda T., Hata S., Kuroda T., Takasu N., and Hori Y. (2002b). Group IB secretory phospholipase A_2 induces neuronal cell death via apoptosis. *J. Neurochem.* 81:449–461.

Yagami T., Ueda K., Asakura K., Sakaeda T., Hata S., Kuroda T., Sakaguchi G., Itoh N., Hashimoto Y., and Hori Y. (2003). Porcine pancreatic group IB secretory phospholipase A_2 potentiates Ca^{2+} influx through L-type voltage-sensitive Ca^{2+} channels. *Brain Res.* 960:71–80.

Yagami T., Ueda K., Hata S., Kuroda T., Itoh N., Sakaguchi G., Okamura N., Sakaeda T., and Fujimoto M. (2005). S-2474, a novel nonsteroidal anti-inflammatory drug, rescues cortical neurons from human group IIA secretory phospholipase A_2-induced apoptosis. *Neuropharmacology* 49:174–184.

Yeo J. F., Ong W. Y., Ling S. F., and Farooqui A. A. (2004). Intracerebroventricular injection of phospholipases A_2 inhibitors modulates allodynia after facial carrageenan injection in mice. *Pain* 112:148–155.

Zaleska M. M. and Wilson D. F. (1989). Lipid hydroperoxides inhibit reacylation of phospholipids in neuronal membranes. *J. Neurochem.* 52:255–260.

Zhang J., Hannun Y. A., and Obeid L. M. (1999). A novel assay for apoptotic body formation and membrane release during apoptosis. *Cell Death Differ.* 6:596–598.

Zhao S., Du X. Y., Chai M. Q., Chen J. S., Zhou Y. C., and Song J. G. (2002). Secretory phospholipase A_2 induces apoptosis via a mechanism involving ceramide generation. *Biochim. Biophys. Acta Mol. Cell Biol. Lipids* 1581:75–88.

5
Arachidonic Acid and its Metabolites in Brain

5.1 Introduction

The content, percent distribution, and fatty acid composition of neural membrane phospholipids markedly affect the organization and functional behavior of neurons (Porcellati, 1983; Farooqui and Horrocks, 1985; Farooqui et al., 2000b). Compared to other organs, brain tissue has a considerably higher content of glycerophospholipids. They not only act as precursors for second messengers but also modulate neural membrane fluidity and permeability (Farooqui et al., 2000b). The CNS cannot make most of the polyunsaturated fatty acids used by the brain for neural membrane glycerophospholipid synthesis, so they are transported from the gastrointestinal tract (Horrocks and Yeo, 1999). The liver produces them by synthesis from linoleic and α-linolenic acids, or the diet provides them.

In neural membranes, the saturated fatty acids, palmitic acid or stearic acid, are usually esterified at the sn-1 position of the glycerol backbone and appear to have a role in neuroplasticity (Tone et al., 1987; Wakabayashi et al., 1994), whereas the polyunsaturated fatty acids, arachidonic, adrenic, or docosahexaenoic acids, are esterified at the sn-2 position. These fatty acids not only maintain the orientation of internal membrane domains for interactions among intracellular organelles, but also provide an appropriate environment for the optimal functioning of receptors, membrane-bound enzymes, transporters, and ion channels (Farooqui et al., 2000b). In neural membranes, PtdCho, PtdEtn, PlsEtn, and PtdSer contain high levels of docosahexaenoyl groups at the sn-2 position, whereas PtdIns and PtdH contain high levels of arachidonoyl groups. All subclasses of glycerophospholipids have a high degree of compositional heterogeneity, generally associated with a more diverse acyl group composition at the sn-2 position (Farooqui et al., 2002a). Each subclass of glycerophospholipids exists as a heterogeneous mixture of molecular species. The synthesis of different pools within a glycerophospholipid class appears to be compartmentalized according to the fatty acid composition and the source of the head group (synthesis de novo versus modification and interconversion reactions) (Farooqui et al., 2000b). Neural membrane glycerophospholipids undergo a rapid deacylation–reacylation process involving phospholipases A_2 (PLA_2) and acyltransferases (Sun and MacQuarrie,

1989; Farooqui et al., 2000a), resulting in continuous shuttling of fatty acids between different phospholipid subclasses. The deacylation–reacylation cycle is responsible for the introduction of polyunsaturated fatty acids into glycerophospholipids.

5.2 Incorporation of Arachidonic Acid and Docosahexaenoic Acid into Neural Membranes

The proportions of arachidonic acid (AA) and docosahexaenoic acid (DHA) in neural membrane glycerophospholipids vary considerably in various subclasses. AA is distributed rather evenly in the gray and white matter and among the different cell types in the brain. In contrast, DHA is highly enriched not only in neuronal membranes but also in synaptic membranes. Rat brain synaptosomal membranes contain 31.2% arachidonic acid in PtdIns, 16.5% in PlsEtn, 14.2% in PtdEtn, 6.0% in PtdCho, and 2.3% in PtdSer (Corbin and Sun, 1978). In human brain gray matter, DHA accounts for more than 36% and 24% of the total fatty acids in PtdSer and PtdEtn, respectively (Salem, Jr. et al., 1986). However, the alkenyl groups from the PlsEtn were not included in these percentages. Because 40% of the ethanolamine glycerophospholipids in human gray matter are plasmalogens (Horrocks, 1972), AA and DHA account for only 35 to 40% of the hydrocarbon chains in the gray matter ethanolamine glycerophospholipids (Farooqui and Horrocks, 2001). The photoreceptor cells of the retina are particularly enriched in DHA (Anderson et al., 1976). The myelin sheath contains lower proportions of AA and DHA compared to synaptic plasma membranes. The fatty acid composition of human brains changes rapidly during development (Söderberg et al., 1991; Martínez and Mougan, 1998). The levels of DHA increase with age in PtdEtn and PtdCho, whereas AA levels remain constant. DHA accumulates in glycerophospholipids mainly during the perinatal period. During postnatal development, the levels of DHA increase less markedly than AA, adrenic, and oleic acids in PlsEtn. In PtdSer, oleic acid levels increase dramatically throughout development, but levels of AA and DHA increase only until 6 months of age. After 6 months, DHA remains constant in PtdSer through life, but its percentage decreases due to the accretion of other polyunsaturated fatty acids (Martínez and Mougan, 1998; Akbar and Kim, 2002). Conservation of AA and DHA is important for the brain because these fatty acids are not only constituents of neural membranes, but also precursors for eicosanoids and docosanoids, respectively. Both AA and DHA play critical roles in cell signaling (Farooqui and Horrocks, 2006).

Incubation of [³H]AA with neural membranes in vitro indicates that the bulk of radioactivity is incorporated in PtdCho and PtdIns. After 10-min incubation, the incorporation in PtdIns was 8- to 10-fold higher than in PtdCho. After 35 min, there was no further increase of PtdIns labeling, but that of PtdCho increased significantly by 2-fold. The esterification of AA into PtdIns quickly reaches a steady state, whereas that into PtdCho is not attained so rapidly (Fonlupt et al., 1994).

The incorporation of DHA into PtdIns and PtdCho was similar, but the total incorporation was 5-fold lower than AA. These results are in agreement with earlier results for incorporation in vivo of [^{14}C]AA, which reached maximal at 5 min postinjection in PtdIns both in mass and as a percentage of total phospholipids' radioactivity in awake unanesthetized rats (DeGeorge et al., 1989).

The turnover of AA in brain glycerophospholipids is not uniform. It differs more than 10-fold among PtdIns, PtdCho, PtdSer, and ethanolamine glycerophospholipids (Sun and Su, 1979; Washizaki et al., 1994; Rapoport, 1999), suggesting a separate role for each subclass of glycerophospholipids in the brain tissue. For example, the arachidonic acid half-life in rat and mouse brain PtdIns is one hour and is consistent with the role of polyphosphoinositides in the generation of receptor-mediated second messengers (Washizaki et al., 1994; Rapoport, 1999). In contrast, the arachidonic acid half-life in these brains in PtdEtn is considerably longer, 24 hours, suggesting a structural role in neural membranes (Sun and Su, 1979; Washizaki et al., 1994).

Acyl-CoA synthetase converts free fatty acids into fatty acyl-CoA esters (Cao et al., 2000). Rat tissue has at least five isoforms of acyl-CoA synthetase (Lewin et al., 2001). They are encoded by separate genes and differ from each other in fatty acid preference, subcellular localization, and regulation (Cao et al., 2000; Lewin et al., 2001; Coleman et al., 2000). The incubation of [1-^{14}C]arachidonic acid with brain microsomes in the presence of ATP, CoA, and MgCl$_2$ results in the formation of [1-^{14}C]arachidonyl-CoA. The omission of ATP or CoA results in a 98% decrease in enzymic activity, indicating the absolute requirement of ATP and CoA for the acyl-CoA synthetase reaction (Reddy et al., 1984; Reddy and Bazan, 1984). The addition of unlabeled arachidonic acid and docosahexaenoic acid results in the apparent inhibition of enzymic activity with Ki values of 31 μM for both fatty acids. Based on various kinetic data, a single acyl-CoA synthetase may be involved in fatty acyl-CoA formation. In contrast, other investigators have distinguished acyl-CoA synthetase activities of rat brain microsomes into three forms: very long chain acyl-CoA, long-chain acyl-CoA, and medium-chain acyl-CoA synthetases. These synthetases differ from each other in their physicochemical and kinetic properties. Thus, palmitoyl-CoA synthetase is different from lignoceroyl-CoA and arachidonyl-CoA synthetases (Singh et al., 1988). Some acyl-CoA synthetases have been cloned and characterized from neural and non-neural tissues (Fujino and Yamamoto, 1992; Fujino et al., 1996; Yamashita et al., 1997; Kee et al., 2003; Van Horn et al., 2005).

In addition to being intermediates in fatty acid metabolism in the brain, acyl-CoAs also modulate several cellular mechanisms, including ion fluxes, vesicle trafficking, protein phosphorylation, and gene expression (Faergeman and Knudsen, 1997). Long-chain acyl-CoAs are also involved in long-term potentiation in the hippocampus (Zhang et al., 2000) and in the formation of synaptic vesicle (Schmidt et al., 1999). Different long-chain acyl-CoAs, existing in different cellular compartments, perform these functions. In these compartments, the intracellular concentrations of acyl-CoAs are strictly controlled by the balance among acyl-CoA synthesizing enzymes, acyl-CoA utilizing enzymes (acyl-CoA:

lysophospholipid acyltransferase, and acyl-CoA hydrolases), and fatty acid metabolizing enzymes (Farooqui et al., 2000a).

An acyl-CoA:lysophospholipid acyltransferase was purified 3000-fold from bovine brain microsomes using multiple-column chromatographic procedures. The purified enzyme is highly specific for lyso-PtdCho as the acyl group acceptor (Sun and MacQuarrie, 1989). It uses a variety of unsaturated long-chain acyl-CoAs as substrates. Arachidonoyl-CoA has the highest activity, whereas more saturated and short-chain acyl-CoAs have lower activities (Sun and MacQuarrie, 1989).

Ross and Kish (1994) reported differences in the rate of acylation of different lysophospholipid subclasses by human brain acyl-CoA:lysophospholipid acyltransferase (Ross and Kish, 1994). The rate with lysophosphatidylinositol (lyso-PtdIns) is the highest, followed by lyso-PtdCho, and then by lyso-PtdSer. In contrast, acylation of lyso-PtdEtn is barely detectable. Based on various kinetic and metabolic studies, lyso-PtdCho acyltransferase may compete with acyl-CoA hydrolase and lysophospholipase for acyl-CoA and lyso-PtdCho, respectively.

The brain tissue also contains the CoA-independent transacylation system in microsomes (Ojima et al., 1987; MacDonald and Sprecher, 1991; Yamashita et al., 1997). This system transfers fatty acids from diacyl glycerophospholipids to various phospholipids in the absence of any cofactor. The acyl substrate is a fatty acid esterified at the sn-2 position of a diacyl glycerophospholipid. The only fatty acids transferred by this system are C_{20} and C_{22} polyunsaturated fatty acids. Diacyl glycerophosphocholine is the most preferred substrate. Human brain homogenates possess the ability to transfer fatty acids from lyso-PtdCho to lyso-PtdEtn, but not to lyso-PtdSer or lyso-PtdIns (Ross and Kish, 1994). Furthermore, the incubation of sn-2-labeled PtdEtn with lyso-PtdCho results in the formation of labeled PtdCho. In neuronal membranes, the CoA-independent transacylation system is also involved in the prompt removal of ether-containing lysophospholipids (lysoplasmalogens). This rapid removal of lysoplasmalogens is necessary because ether-containing lysophospholipids are more resistant to lysophospholipase than are their diacyl counterparts. CoA-independent transacylation may modulate the movement of arachidonic acid between glycerophospholipid molecular species in neural membranes (Farooqui et al., 2000a).

5.3 Receptor-Mediated Release of Arachidonic Acid

In primary cell cultures of neuronal and glial origin, several neurotransmitters, including glutamate and its analogs, dopamine, serotonin, endothelin, and ATP, stimulate the release of arachidonic acid by stimulating the multiple forms of $cPLA_2$ (Sanfeliu et al., 1990; Kim et al., 1995; Bruner and Murphy, 1993; Stella et al., 1997; Dumuis et al., 1990; Lazarewicz et al., 1988). This normal and controlled process occurs during receptor stimulation. In neural membranes, $cPLA_2$ is coupled to dopamine, serotonin, P_2-purinergic, endothelin, and glutamate receptors through different coupling mechanisms (Table 5.1). Some receptors

TABLE 5.1. Coupling of PLA_2 isoforms responsible for arachidonic acid release with various receptors in brain tissue.

Receptor type	PLA_2 isoform	Reference
Glutamate receptor	$cPLA_2$, PlsEtn-PLA_2, $iPLA_2$, $sPLA_2$	Lazarewicz et al., 1990; Kolko et al., 1996; Farooqui et al., 2003a
Dopamine receptor	$cPLA_2$	Ross, 2003
Serotonin receptor	$cPLA_2$	Qu et al., 2003a,b, 2005; Kurrasch-Orbaugh et al., 2003
P_2-purinergic receptor	$cPLA_2$	Xing et al., 1994
TNF-α receptor	$cPLA_2$, $sPLA_2$	Atsumi et al., 1998; Jupp et al., 2003
IL-receptor	$cPLA_2$, $sPLA_2$	Xu et al., 2003
Interferon receptor	$cPLA_2$, $sPLA_2$	Xu et al., 2003
Growth factor receptor	$cPLA_2$,	Jupp et al., 2003; Akiyama et al., 2004
Endothelin receptor	$cPLA_2$, $sPLA_2$	Trevisi et al., 2002; Yagami et al., 2005
Muscarinic receptor	$cPLA_2$	Bayón et al., 1997

involve G-proteins (Felder et al., 1991; Audubert et al., 1999; Qu et al., 2003a; Bordayo et al., 2005) and others do not (Lazarewicz et al., 1990).

Glutamate, the major excitatory amino acid neurotransmitter in the mammalian brain, mediates synaptic transmission by interacting with both ionotropic and metabotropic types of glutamate receptors (Farooqui and Horrocks, 1994, 1997). The brain tissue contains huge amounts of glutamate, about 10 mmol/kg, wet weight. Under normal conditions, powerful uptake systems in both glial cells and neurons maintain the concentration of glutamate at a low level, that is, 1 μM, in the extracellular compartment (Danbolt, 1994). Following an ischemic episode or mechanical neural trauma (head injury and spinal cord injury), the extracellular concentration of glutamate increases rapidly (Farooqui and Horrocks, 1991, 1994). However, the sources (neurons vs glia) and molecular mechanisms involved in glutamate release into the extracellular compartment remain controversial. Some studies indicate that a depolarization-induced calcium-dependent exocytic process is responsible for the release and initial accumulation of glutamate in the extracellular compartment (Sánchez-Prieto et al., 1987). However, this type of calcium entry is not sufficient to produce glutamate accumulation responsible for the overstimulation of glutamate receptors (Sánchez-Prieto et al., 1987). Other studies indicate that depolarization-induced reversal of the sodium-dependent, high-affinity, acidic amino acid, plasma membrane transporter causes the release of glutamate (Adam-Vizi, 1992; Szatkowski and Attwell, 1994). The reuptake of glutamate into neurons and glia by this transporter depends on the maintenance of an ATP-driven Na^+ gradient. Decreased ATP during ischemia or mechanical trauma causes the glutamate transporter to malfunction, resulting in the accumulation of glutamate in the extracellular compartment. Phospholipase A_2-mediated plasma membrane disruption for the release of glutamate in the extracellular compartment may be involved (O'Regan et al., 1995; Phillis et al., 1996). Whatever be the mechanism of glutamate release and accumulation in extracellular compartment, it is well established now that abnormally low levels of glutamate can compromise normal levels of excitation, whereas excessive levels can produce toxic effects through the overstimulation of NMDA and non-NMDA types of glutamate receptors (Rothman and Olney, 1986; Lipton and Rosenberg, 1994; Farooqui and Horrocks, 1994).

Two enzymic mechanisms are mainly responsible for AA release from neural membrane glycerophospholipids in the brain tissue. A direct mechanism for AA release involves PLA_2 and an indirect mechanism utilizes the phospholipase C (PLC)/diacylglycerol lipase pathway to release AA (Farooqui et al., 1989). The release of AA within the brain tissue is of considerable physiological importance because this fatty acid is a potent modulator of glutamatergic neurotransmission and a potential mediator of both long-term potentiation and long-term depression. The treatment of cortical, striatal, hippocampal, and hypothalamic neurons and cerebellar granule cells with glutamate, N-methyl-D-aspartate (NMDA), and kainate (KA) results in a dose-dependent increase in PLA_2 activity and arachidonic acid release (Dumuis et al., 1988; Lazarewicz et al., 1990; Farooqui et al., 2003b) (Fig. 5.1). An NMDA antagonist, 2-amino-5-phosphonovalerate (APV); an AMPA receptor antagonist, 6-cyano-7-nitroquinoxaline (CNQX); quinacrine (a nonspecific $cPLA_2$ inhibitor) (Fig. 5.2) (Sanfeliu et al., 1990; Kim et al., 1995; Farooqui et al., 2003b); and also arachidonoyl trifluoromethylketone, a potent inhibitor of $cPLA_2$ (Fig. 5.3); block this release in a dose-dependent manner. These studies strongly suggest that the stimulation of $cPLA_2$ is a glutamate receptor-mediated process in neuronal cultures.

Treatment of astroglial cultures with ATP also evokes AA release in a dose- and time-dependent manner. Thus, PLA_2 activity may be linked to purinergic receptors in astrocytes. This suggestion is supported by studies on the occurrence of various isoforms of PLA_2 in immortalized astrocytes and the astrocytoma cell line 1321N1 and on AA release by various agonists (Sun et al., 2005; Hernández

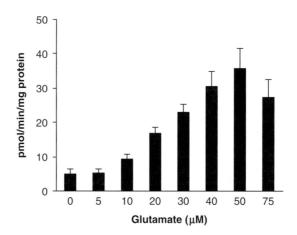

FIG. 5.1. Effects of glutamate on $cPLA_2$ activity in neuron-enriched cultures from rat cerebral cortex. Results are the means ± SEM from three different cultures.

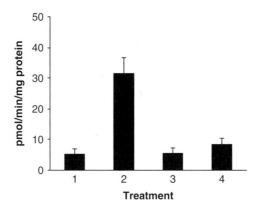

FIG. 5.2. Effects of CNQX on cPLA$_2$ activity in neuron-enriched cultures from rat cerebral cortex. Results are the mean ± SEM from three different cultures. 1. Control, 2. KA, 50 μM, 3. KA + CNQX, 50 μM + 10 μM, 4. CNQX, 10 μM.

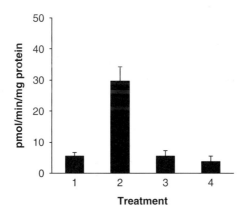

FIG. 5.3. Effects of AACOCF$_3$ on cPLA$_2$ activity in neuron-enriched cultures from rat cerebral cortex. Results are the mean ± SEM from three different cultures. 1. Control, 2. KA, 50 μM, 3. KA + AACOCF$_3$, 50 μM + 1 μM, 4. AACOCF$_3$, 1 μM.

et al., 2000). Astrocytes may be particularly sensitive to the ATP to UTP ratio. These nucleotides act on the P2Y$_2$ receptor and stimulate signaling pathways leading to AA release (Sun et al., 2005). PLA$_2$ inhibitors can prevent this AA release (Sun et al., 2005).

In Chinese hamster ovary (CHO) cells transfected with D$_2$ receptor cDNA, the stimulation of D$_2$ receptors generates AA. The treatment of cultures with antisense oligodeoxynucleotides of cPLA$_2$ blocks the D$_2$-receptor-dependent release of AA, but has no effect on D$_2$-receptor binding or D$_2$-receptor-dependent inhibition of cyclic AMP accumulation (Vial and Piomelli, 1995). These results strongly suggest that cPLA$_2$ activity is coupled to dopamine receptors. In PC12 cells, sPLA$_2$ is coupled to catecholamine secretion. This catecholamine release is inhibited by nonspecific PLA$_2$ inhibitors (Matsuzawa et al., 1996), suggesting a link between biogenic amine receptor and PLA$_2$ activity.

Similarly, stimulation of G-protein-coupled α_2 adrenergic receptors and purinergic receptors also increases AA release (Felder et al., 1991). cPLA$_2$ inhibitors can prevent this release (Audubert et al., 1999). cPLA$_2$ inhibitors and ketanserin, a 5-HT$_{2A}$ receptor antagonist, also block serotonin receptor-mediated release of arachidonic acid in astrocytes and C6 glioma cells (Felder et al., 1990; Garcia and Kim, 1997; Qu et al., 2003a; Kurrasch-Orbaugh et al., 2003), suggesting that cPLA$_2$ is coupled to serotonergic receptors in these cells. In astrocytes and glioma cell cultures, endothelin evokes the release of arachidonic acid through the activation of cPLA$_2$. Mepacrine, a nonspecific PLA$_2$ inhibitor, can prevent this release (Tencé et al., 1992; Dunican et al., 1996). In contrast, endothelin stimulates Ca^{2+}-independent PLA$_2$ in Schwann cell cultures. Bromoenol lactone, a potent and specific inhibitor of iPLA$_2$ activity, blocks this stimulation. In response to cytokines, growth factors, and endotoxin, PLA$_2$ releases AA from neural membranes and immune cell phospholipids (Xu et al., 2003; Tong et al., 1999; Pirianov et al., 1999; Wang et al., 2004; Jupp et al., 2003; Akiyama et al., 2004; Han et al., 2004). Cytokine and growth factor antagonists can prevent the release of AA.

The indirect mechanism of AA release was reported in primary neuronal cell cultures of fetal spinal cord (Farooqui et al., 1993, 2003b). The treatment of neuron-enriched cultures with glutamate or NMDA results in a dose- and time-dependent stimulation of diacylglycerol and monoacylglycerol lipase activities (Figs. 5.4 and 5.5). The NMDA antagonist, dextrorphan, and the diacylglycerol lipase inhibitor, RHC80267, block this increase (Farooqui et al., 1993;, 2003b) (Table 5.2). Unlike glutamate and NMDA, the treatment of neuron-enriched cultures with KA (100 µM) has no effect on diacylglycerol and monoacylglycerol

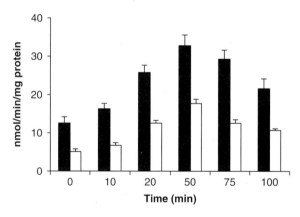

FIG. 5.4. Effects of glutamate on diacylglycerol lipase and monoacylglycerol lipase activities in neuron-enriched cultures from rat cerebral cortex. Results are means ± SEM from three different cultures. Filled bars, monoacylglycerol lipase; open bars, diacylglycerol lipase.

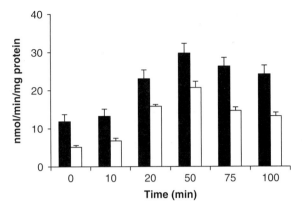

FIG. 5.5. Effects of NMDA on diacylglycerol lipase and monoacylglycerol lipase activities in neuron-enriched cultures from rat cerebral cortex. Results are means ± SEM for three different cultures. Filled bars, monoacylglycerol lipase; open bars, diacylglycerol lipase. The NMDA was 50 μM.

TABLE 5.2. Effects of dextrorphan and RHC 80267 on diacylglycerol lipase and monoacylglycerol lipase activities of neuron-enriched cultures from rat cerebral cortex.

Treatment	Diacylglycerol lipase	Monoacylglycerol lipase
Control	5.27 ± 0.6	12.1 ± 1.9
Glutamate (50 μM)	18.93 ± 1.3	28.7 ± 2.8
Dextrorphan (50 μM)	5.00 ± 0.5	10.6 ± 1.3
Glutamate (50 μM)+Dextrorphan (50 μM)	6.27 ± 0.8	13.7 ± 1.5
Control	5.32 ± 0.6	12.5 ± 1.8
Glutamate (50 μM)	16.73 ± 1.5	27.8 ± 2.3
RHC 80267 (25 μM)	5.53 ± 0.5	12.7 ± 1,5
RHC 80267 (25 μM)+Glutamate (50 μM)	5.39 ± 0.8	12.7 ± 1.9

Diacylglycerol lipase and monoacylglycerol lipase activities are expressed as nmol/min/mg protein. Results are the mean ± SEM for three different cultures.

lipase activities (Farooqui et al., 1993; Farooqui and Horrocks, 1994). The lack of KA effect on diacylglycerol and monoacylglycerol lipases suggests that either KA receptors are not linked to diacylglycerol and monoacylglycerol lipases or that these cultures do not have fully developed KA receptors. Thus, both the $cPLA_2$ pathway and the PLC/diacylglycerol lipase pathway participate in the release of AA in neural cells. However, the relative contributions of these pathways toward AA release are still obscure.

5.4 Neurotrophic Effects of Arachidonic Acid

Under normal conditions, the levels of free AA in the brain tissue are very low (<0.01 mmol/kg). At this concentration, it acts as a second messenger molecule in the nervous system and performs a variety of functions. It regulates the activity of many enzyme proteins, including protein kinase A, protein kinase C, NADPH oxidase, choline acetyltransferase, and caspase-3 (Table 5.3). In addition, AA modulates ion channels, neurotransmitter release, induction of long-term potentiation, and neural cell differentiation (Farooqui et al., 2002b). AA may act as a facilitatory retrograde neuromodulator in glutamatergic synapses (Katsuki and Okuda, 1995), since activation of glutamate receptors releases it. AA modulates acetylcholine release in rat hippocampus (Almeida et al., 1999), and thus modulates LTP and synaptic plasticity (Das, 2003). It also stimulates glucose uptake in cerebral cortical astrocytes. Thus, AA plays a critical role in the regulation of energy metabolism in the cerebral cortex.

In the nucleus, AA also may interact with elements of gene structure (such as promoters, enhancers, suppressors, etc.) in a specific manner that is not shared by eicosanoids or other fatty acids resulting in the modulation of gene expression (Farooqui et al., 1997a). AA has trophic effects in vitro on PC12 cells, hippocampal, and cerebellar neurons. At 1 μM, this fatty acid significantly potentiates the elongation of neurites in hippocampal cultures (Katsuki and Okuda, 1995). The mechanism by which AA affects neurite outgrowth remains unknown. However, this fatty acid is known to activate PKC, an enzyme involved in neuronal plasticity, and differentiation and elongation of neurites (Murakami and Routtenberg, 2003).

The addition of AA to rat dentate gyrus produces a slow onset and persistent increase in synaptic activity accompanied by a marked elevation in the release of glutamate (Lynch and Voss, 1990). AA generated by NMDA receptor stimulation at the postsynaptic level may cross the synaptic cleft to act at the presynaptic level and thus may act as a retrograde messenger for long-term potentiation. Age-dependent suppression of LTP may be a consequence of the decline in AA in the hippocampal dentate gyrus due to long-term exposure of neurons to oxidative stress (McGahon et al., 1997), or to suppression by oxygen free radicals. Supplementation of AA in neural membranes influences both the pre- and postsynaptic membranes through phospholipid metabolic pathways to facilitate the mobility of functional proteins in the plasma membrane due to increased fluidity (McGahon et al., 1997). Collectively these results suggest that low levels of AA are involved in maintaining the structural integrity of neural membranes, determining the fluidity of neural membranes, and thereby regulating neuronal transmission and long-term potentiation.

TABLE 5.3. Effect of arachidonic acid on enzymic activities in neural and non-neural tissues.

Enzyme	Effect	Reference
Protein kinase C	Stimulation	Farooqui et al., 1997a
Diacylglycerol kinase	Stimulation	Rao et al., 1994
Choline acetyltransferase	Stimulation	Chalimoniuk et al., 2004
Protein kinase A	Stimulation	Doolan and Keenan, 1994
NADPH oxidase	Stimulation	Sakata et al., 1987
Nitric oxide synthase	Stimulation	Toborek et al., 2000
Caspase-3	Stimulation	Garrido et al., 2001; Liu et al., 2001

5.5 Neurotoxic Effects of Arachidonic Acid

Under pathological conditions such as ischemia, AA accumulates (0.5 mmol/kg) after its release from membrane phospholipids. At high concentrations, AA produces a variety of detrimental effects on neural cell structure and function. AA causes intracellular acidosis and uncouples oxidative phosphorylation, which results in mitochondrial dysfunction (Schapira, 1996). AA produces mitochondrial swelling in neurons and induces changes in membrane permeability by modulating ion channels (Farooqui et al., 1997a,b). AA has a profound adverse effect on the ATP-producing capacity of mitochondria. It also affects the activity of membrane-bound enzymes, and neurotransmitter release and uptake in neuronal preparations (Schapira, 1996). AA also contributes to the accumulation of glutamate in the synaptic cleft by downregulating glutamate transporters in the brain tissue. AA activates nuclear factor-κB (NF-κB) and decreases neuronal viability (Toborek et al., 1999).

High concentrations of AA and other fatty acids also may act directly on plasma membrane through their detergent-like action (Gamberucci et al., 1997). This involves the formation of micelles, which are aggregates of fatty acid molecules formed because of their poor solubility in aqueous solutions. These micelles disrupt cell membranes and create pores permeable to Na^+ and Ca^{2+} ions (Sawyer and Andersen, 1989). The presence of cations, especially Ca^{2+}, and higher ionic strength enhance the formation of micelles (Tanford, 1980).

The accumulation of AA can also trigger an uncontrolled "arachidonic acid cascade." This sets the stage for increased production of reactive oxygen species (ROS). ROS include oxygen free radicals (superoxide radicals, hydroxyls, and alkoxylradicals, lipid peroxy radicals) and peroxides (hydrogen peroxide and lipid hydroperoxide). At low levels, ROS can function as signaling intermediates in the regulation of fundamental cell activities such as growth and adaptation responses. At higher concentrations, ROS contribute to neural membrane damage when the balance between reducing and oxidizing (redox) forces shifts toward oxidative stress. Free radical scavengers, including superoxide dismutase, catalase, and glutathione, in part control the elimination of ROS.

Other biological targets of ROS may be membrane proteins and DNA (Farooqui et al., 2002b). The reaction between ROS and proteins or unsaturated lipids in the plasma membrane leads to a chemical cross-linking of membrane proteins and lipids, and a reduction in membrane unsaturation. This depletion of unsaturation in membrane lipids is associated with decreased membrane fluidity and decreases in the activity of membrane-bound enzymes, ion channels, and receptors (Ray et al., 1994). ROS may also modulate the expression of cytokines in the nucleus. These cytokines may further stimulate isoforms of PLA_2 in the brain tissue (Farooqui et al., 2002b). Thus, an uncontrolled sustained increase in calcium influx through increased phospholipid degradation can lead to increased membrane permeability and stimulation of many enzymes associated with lipolysis, proteolysis, and disaggregation of microtubules with a disruption of cytoskeleton and membrane structure (Farooqui and Horrocks, 1994).

Free radicals and lipid hydroperoxides generated during the "arachidonic acid cascade" also inhibit reacylation of phospholipids in neuronal membranes (Zaleska and Wilson, 1989). This inhibition may be another mechanism whereby peroxidative processes contribute to irreversible neuronal injury and death.

5.6 Metabolism of Arachidonic Acid in Brain

As stated earlier, free arachidonic acid is either reincorporated into neural membrane phospholipids by reacylation reactions or oxidized by several enzymic mechanisms to various oxygenated metabolites with important neurochemical functions (Wolfe and Horrocks, 1994; Phillis et al., 2006). Thus, cyclooxygenases (COX), lipoxygenases (LOX), and epoxygenases (EPOX) metabolize AA to prostaglandins and thromboxanes, leukotrienes, and epoxyeicosatrienoic acid respectively (Fig. 5.6). These metabolites are known collectively as eicosanoids (from the Greek word *eicosa* for twenty, for 20-carbon fatty acid derivatives). They play important roles in regulating signal transduction and gene transcription processes and also in inducing and maintaining acute inflammatory responses (Wolfe and Horrocks, 1994; Phillis et al., 2006).

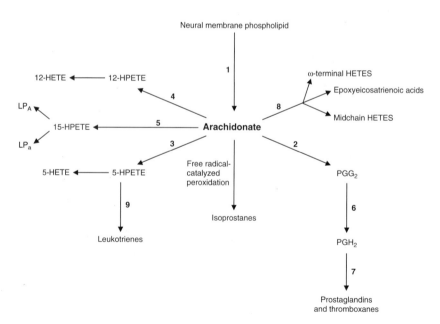

FIG. 5.6. PLA$_2$-mediated release of arachidonic acid and its metabolism by cyclooxygenases, lipoxygenases, and epoxygenases. Phospholipase A$_2$ (1), cyclooxygenase (2), 5-lipoxygenase (3), 12-lipoxygenase (4), 15-lipoxygenase (5), peroxygenase activity of cyclooxygenase (6), prostaglandin and thromboxane synthases (7), cytochrome P450 epoxygenase (8), and leukotriene synthase (9).

Cyclooxygenases are heme-containing bifunctional enzymes with two catalytic centers. One cyclooxygenase center adds 2 oxygen atoms to AA to form the hydroperoxy endoperoxide called PGG_2. The other peroxidase active center reduces PGG_2 to PGH_2. Detailed mechanistic studies reveal a carbon-centered pentadienyl radical at C-11 and a carbon-centered radical at C-8 as the two radical species involved in endoperoxide formation during the cyclooxygenase center-catalyzed reaction. A tyrosyl radical derived from Tyr385 is involved during the peroxidase center-catalyzed reaction. Both activities are functionally coupled: the overall reaction is initiated by the oxidation of the heme group of the peroxidase reaction by low levels of a hydroxyperoxide (PGG_2) to generate a radical intermediate that begins the COX reaction (Patel, 2004). PGH_2 is a precursor to several prostaglandins, thromboxanes (TXA_2), and prostacyclins (PGI_2) (Fig. 5.6). These molecules and their derivatives interact with their specific receptors to modulate cell function (O'Banion, 1999).

Mammalian tissues contain three forms of COX enzymes, designated as COX-1, COX-2, and COX-3. The brain tissue expresses COX-1 constitutively. COX-1 is responsible for the physiological production of prostaglandins (Bazan et al., 1994), is involved in several homeostatic processes, and therefore is called a housekeeping enzyme. COX-2 is normally undetectable in healthy tissues, but inflammatory mediators such as cytokines, growth factors, and bacterial endotoxin induce it rapidly. COX-2 is expressed constitutively in the kidney, stomach, and brain (Hoffmann, 2000). Both isoforms are homodimers with a similar active site and a long substrate channel. However, there are two important structural differences between COX-1 and COX-2. The active site of COX-2 is larger and more accommodating than that of COX-1, and COX-1 displays negative allosterism at low concentrations of arachidonic acid. This property may be responsible for greater eicosanoid production by COX-2 during low arachidonic acid concentrations (Smith et al., 2000). Arachidonic acid is the preferred substrate for both COX-1 and COX-2.

COX-3 is a new member of the COX family. Although different pharmacological properties have been described for COX-3 as compared with COX-1 or COX-2 enzymes, many investigators consider it a splice variant of COX-1 (Chandrasekharan et al., 2002; Davies et al., 2004). In contrast to murine COX-1 and COX-2, analgesic and antipyretic drugs such as acetaminophen, phenacetin, antipyrine, and dipyrone selectively inhibit canine COX-3 activity, and some nonsteroidal anti-inflammatory drugs potently inhibit COX-3 (Kis et al., 2005). Thus, inhibition of COX-3 could represent a primary central mechanism by which these drugs decrease pain and possibly fever (Chandrasekharan et al., 2002).

Lipoxygenases (LOXs) are nonheme, iron-containing dioxygenases that insert molecular oxygen into arachidonic acid. Different LOXs vary in the placement of the hydroxyl group, which determines their name. Thus, 5-LOX catalyzes the synthesis of 5-hydroperoxyeicosatetraenoic acids (5-HPETEs), 12-LOX the formation of 12-HPETEs, 15-LOX generates 15-HPETEs (Watanabe et al., 1993; Phillis et al., 2006), and so on. These HPETEs are unstable intermediates. They are converted to more stable autocrine and paracrine molecules called hydroxyeicosatetraenoic acids (HETEs), either nonenzymically or by peroxidases (Li et al., 1997). These metabolites are then metabolized to leukotrienes (LTs). Unlike prostaglandins that are synthesized in all types of cells, LTs are mainly synthesized in inflammatory cells such as polymorphonuclear leukocytes, macrophages, and mast cells. The brain contains several LOX enzymes (5-LOX, 12-LOX, and 15-LOX). 12-LOX is the predominant LOX isoform in the CNS and its mRNA is present in rat cortical neurons, oligodendrocytes, and astrocytes (Bendani et al., 1995). Rat brain 12-lipoxygenase contains six conserved histidines, characteristic for all cloned lipoxygenases. It has a high degree of identity to porcine leukocyte 12-lipoxygenase (71%) and to human 15-lipoxygenase (75%), but has less resemblance to human platelet 12-lipoxygenase (59%) or rat leukocyte 5-lipoxygenase (41%). The recombinant enzyme is expressed in *Escherichia coli*. A portion of brain 12-lipoxygenase cDNA is used as a probe in Northern blots. Sequencing of parts of the corresponding cDNAs from other rat tissues and their comparison with brain 12-lipoxygenase indicate that mRNAs from different rat tissues are identical (Watanabe et al., 1993).

The action of LOXs on HPETE and HETE also leads to the formation of lipoxins (LXA$_4$ and LXB$_4$), a group of trihydroxytetraene-containing eicosanoids involved in the resolution of acute inflammation by modulating key steps in leukocyte trafficking and preventing neutrophil-mediated acute tissue injury (Serhan, 1994; Serhan and Levy, 2003). Although the occurrence of lipoxins in the brain tissue has been established, detailed investigations on their neurochemical effects and involvement in signal transduction processes are not available (Serhan and Levy, 2003). However, recent work from Serhan's laboratory has indicated that aspirin mediates the generation of lipoxins. These lipoxins are potent anti-inflammatory and proresolving molecules that act through specific G-protein-coupled receptors (ALX receptor) (Norel and Brink, 2004) and regulate cellular activities associated with inflammation and resolution (Serhan, 2005; Chiang et al., 2005). In mouse cornea, LXA$_4$ limits inflammation and promotes wound healing (Gronert, 2005). LXA$_4$ also serves as a "stop signal" that regulates key steps in leukocyte trafficking and prevents neutrophil-mediated tissue injury (Kantarci and Van Dyke, 2003). In periodontal disease, lipoxin generation provides protection against neutrophil-mediated injury (Kantarci and Van Dyke, 2005).

In the presence of NADPH and molecular oxygen, EPOX metabolizes AA to a number of oxygenated metabolites, including (a) four regioisomeric epoxides (5,6; 8,9; 11,12; 14,15 *cis*-epoxyeicosatrienoic acids, EETs), which are subsequently hydrolyzed to the corresponding diol derivatives, (b) six regioisomeric *cis–trans* conjugated mono-hydroxyeicosatetraenoic acid (HETEs), and (c) ω and ω-1 alcohols (Zeldin, 2001). Although the levels of various cytochrome P450 enzymes in brain are low, astrocytes express these enzymes at relatively high levels (Peng et al., 2004). Recent in situ hybridization studies of EPOX mRNA have confirmed its localization in astrocytes, specifically those situated adjacent to blood vessels (Peng et al., 2004). 20-HETE is implicated in the microvascular autoregulatory response. It produces potent constriction of the cerebrovascular bed via inhibition of influx through large conductance K$^+$ channels (Sun et al., 2000) and increased influx through L-type calcium channels (Gebremedhin et al.,

1998). Thus, in cerebral arteries a 6-fold increase in 20-HETE levels occurs under elevated vascular transmural pressure and a 20-HETE inhibitor attenuates pressure-induced arterial autoregulation (Gebremedhin et al., 2000). In addition, the formation of nitric oxide suppresses the synthesis of 20-HETE in isolated cerebral microvessels (Alonso-Galicia et al., 1997, 1999; Sun et al., 2000). Furthermore, astrocyte-generated EETs induce cerebral capillary endothelial cell mitogenesis and tube formation (Munzenmaier and Harder, 2000). Collectively, these studies relate the formation of 20-HETE with the response to nitric oxide generation and autoregulation of microvascular tone.

Studies on astroglial cytochrome P450 expression suggest a putative capacity of these enzymes to metabolize psychoactive or lipophilic xenobiotics that are associated with pharmacological and/or toxicological consequences. Astrocytes appear to be the most active steroidogenic cells in the brain, expressing steroidogenic cytochrome P450 and producing various steroids. EET may contribute to the regulation of the cerebral blood flow and therefore be crucial to cardiovascular homeostasis. These EET-producing enzymes have not been purified and characterized from the brain tissue, so no information is available on the physicochemical properties of these enzymes in brain (Harder et al., 1998).

COX, LOX, and EPOX are important enzymes involved in the generation of oxygenated derivatives of arachidonic acid with second messenger properties. COX enzymes catalyze the conversion of AA into prostaglandins and thromboxanes, LOX generates leukotrienes and lipoxins, and EPOX activity produces eicosatrienoic acids. The ability of the brain tissue to release AA and its metabolites by reactions catalyzed by PLA_2, COX, LOX, and EPOX depends not only on the neural cell type, but also on the region and age of the brain tissue. These enzymes are involved in initiation, maintenance, and modulation of inflammatory processes and also in aging, apoptosis, and synaptic activity (Li et al., 1997; Uz et al., 1998; Chabot et al., 1998; Manev et al., 2000; Maccarrone et al., 2001; Gilroy et al., 2004; Phillis et al., 2006).

5.7 Importance of Eicosanoids in Brain

Eicosanoids differ from other intracellular messengers in one important way. They are not stored in neural cells, but are synthesized rapidly, in response to receptor-mediated stimulation, as modulators of neural cell response. Because of their amphiphilic nature, eicosanoids cross neural cell membranes and leave the cell in which they are generated to act on neighboring cells. This process is observed in all mammalian tissues, including brain, and may be involved in crosstalk and interplay among various neural cells. In the brain tissue, both neurons and glial cells produce prostaglandins, whereas cerebral microvessels and the choroid plexus mainly synthesize thromboxanes. Eicosanoids act through specific superficial or intracellular receptors, modulating signal transduction pathways and gene transcription. Thus, PGD_2 activates the DP receptors, PGE_2 activates the EP receptors, and $PGF_{2\alpha}$, PGI_2, and TXA_2 stimulate the FP, IP, and

TP receptors, respectively (Coleman et al., 1994). Eicosanoid receptors are typically G-protein-coupled receptors with seven transmembrane segments that have an extracellular amino terminus and an intracellular carboxyl terminus. These receptors are involved in the generation of cyclic AMP, diacylglycerol, and phosphatidyl 1,4,5-trisphosphate and the modulation of calcium ion influx. By interacting with eicosanoid receptors on astrocytes, prostaglandins regulate glutamate release into the synaptic cleft (Bazan, 2003). The release of glutamate modulates neuronal excitability and synaptic transmission at the presynaptic level. In contrast, the uptake of glutamate by astrocytes prevents its neurotoxic accumulation in the synaptic cleft.

Some prostaglandins play an important role in neural activity by modulating the release of hormones and neurotransmitters, whereas others are involved in regulating circulatory function (Wolfe and Horrocks, 1994) (Table 5.4). Thromboxane A_2 is a potent vasoconstrictor and produces vasospasm, whereas PGI_2 has opposing effects. At low concentrations, eicosanoids stimulate PKC and other enzymes and have protective effects on cortical neurons against glutamate toxicity (Cazevieille et al., 1994), with the order of protection potency $PGF_{2\alpha} = PGE_2 >$ carba-$TXA_2 >$ $PGE_1 > PGD_2 > PGI_2 +$ carba-$PGI_2 >$ 6-keto-$PGF_{1\alpha}$. The mechanism by which eicosanoids counteract the cytotoxic effect of glutamate remains unknown. However, prostaglandins may interact with EP_2 receptors (a PGE_2 receptor subtype) and suppress the generation of nitric oxide triggered by Ca^{2+} influx through NMDA receptors (Martínez-Cayuela, 1995). Eicosanoids may also be involved in synaptic plasticity related to long-term potentiation and long-term depression. Collective evidence from neural and non-neural cells indicates that low concentrations of eicosanoids induce trophic effects related to normal brain function (Wolfe and Horrocks, 1994).

TABLE 5.4. Roles of cyclooxygenase-, lipoxygenase-, and epoxygenase-generated metabolites of arachidonic acid in brain tissue.

Metabolite	Enzyme	Role	Reference
PGE_2, $PGF_{2\alpha}$, PGI_2, TxA_2	Cyclooxygenase-1	Homeostasis, vasodilation, vasoconstriction, neurotransmitter release, and synaptic plasticity	Vane et al., 1998; Minghetti and Levi, 1998; Smith et al., 2000; Minghetti, 2004
PGE_2, PGI_2	Cyclooxygenase-2	Vasodilation, vasoconstriction, inflammation, and apoptosis	Minghetti, 2004; Simmons et al., 2004
PGA_2, PGJ_2	Cyclooxygenase-2	Cell proliferation	Minghetti and Levi, 1998; Smith et al., 2000
PGD_2	Cyclooxygenase-3	Fever and pain	Chandrasekharan et al., 2002
LTC_4, LTD_4, LTE_4	5-Lipoxygenase	Vasoconstriction, inflammation, monocyte and T-cell trafficking, and apoptosis	Powell and Rokach, 2005; Funk, 1996; Maccarrone et al., 2001
LXA_4, LXB_4	5-Lipoxygenase	Anti-inflammation	Serhan, 1994; Serhan and Levy, 2003
EETs	CytP450 epoxygenase	Gene expression, angiogenesis, and cerebral blood flow	Spector et al., 2004; Wang et al., 2005

The generation and accumulation of eicosanoids under pathological conditions is associated with the modulation of cerebrovascular blood flow. Their active production by circulating cells such as platelets and leukocytes may contribute to the onset of alterations in the microcirculation and ultimately to CNS dysfunction (Wolfe and Horrocks, 1994). High levels of prostaglandins have degenerative effects on differentiated murine neuroblastoma cells in culture (Prasad et al., 1998). In vivo, prostaglandins are involved in the regulation of cytokines and maintenance of the inflammatory cascade. For example, when released from activated microglial cells, PGE_1 and PGE_2 stimulate the expression of interleukin-6 in astrocytes (Fiebich et al., 1997). This process, in turn, initiates the synthesis of additional prostaglandins. Not only activated neutrophils and macrophages, but also astrocytes and oligodendrocytes produce leukotriene B_4. It induces its neurochemical effects by interacting with specific G-protein-coupled receptors. High levels of eicosanoids contribute to the development of cytotoxicity, vasogenic brain edema, as well as neuronal damage (Wolfe and Horrocks, 1994; Phillis et al., 2006).

References

Adam-Vizi V. (1992). External Ca^{2+}-independent release of neurotransmitters. *J. Neurochem.* 58:395–405.

Akbar M. and Kim H. Y. (2002). Protective effects of docosahexaenoic acid in staurosporine-induced apoptosis: involvement of phosphatidylinositol-3 kinase pathway. *J. Neurochem.* 82:655–665.

Akiyama N., Hatori Y., Takashiro Y., Hirabayashi T., Saito T., and Murayama T. (2004). Nerve growth factor-induced up-regulation of cytosolic phospholipase $A_2\alpha$ level in rat PC12 cells. *Neurosci. Lett.* 365:218–222.

Almeida T., Cunha R. A., and Ribeiro J. A. (1999). Facilitation by arachidonic acid of acetylcholine release from the rat hippocampus. *Brain Res.* 826:104–111.

Alonso-Galicia M., Drummond H. A., Reddy K. K., Falck J. R., and Roman R. J. (1997). Inhibition of 20-HETE production contributes to the vascular responses to nitric oxide. *Hypertension* 29:320–325.

Alonso-Galicia M., Hudetz A. G., Shen H., Harder D. R., and Roman R. J. (1999). Contribution of 20-HETE to vasodilator actions of nitric oxide in the cerebral microcirculation. *Stroke* 30:2727–2734.

Anderson R. E., Landis D. J., and Dudley P. A. (1976). Essential fatty acid deficiency and renewal of rod outer segments in the albino rat. *Invest Ophthalmol.* 15:232–236.

Atsumi G., Tajima M., Hadano A., Nakatani Y., Murakami M., and Kudo I. (1998). Fas-induced arachidonic acid release is mediated by Ca^{2+}-independent phospholipase A_2 but not cytosolic phospholipase A_2 which undergoes proteolytic inactivation. *J. Biol. Chem.* 273:13870–13877.

Audubert F., Klapisz E., Berguerand M., Gouache P., Jouniaux A. M., Béréziat G., and Masliah J. (1999). Differential potentiation of arachidonic acid release by rat $\alpha2$ adrenergic receptor subtypes. *Biochim. Biophys. Acta Mol. Cell Biol. Lipids* 1437:265–276.

Bayón Y., Hernández M., Alonso A., Nunez L., Garcia-Sancho J., Leslie C., Crespo M. S., and Nieto M. L. (1997). Cytosolic phospholipase A2 is coupled to muscarinic receptors in the human astrocytoma cell line 1321N1: characterization of the transducing mechanism. *Biochem. J.* 323:281–287.

Bazan N. G. (2003). Synaptic lipid signaling: significance of polyunsaturated fatty acids and platelet-activating factor. *J. Lipid Res.* 44:2221–2233.

Bazan N. G., Fletcher B. S., Herschman H. R., and Mukherjee P. K. (1994). Platelet-activating factor and retinoic acid synergistically activate the inducible prostaglandin synthase gene. *Proc. Natl Acad. Sci. USA* 91:5252–5256.

Bendani M. K., Palluy O., Cook-Moreau J., Beneytout J. L., Rigaud M., and Vallat J. M. (1995). Localization of 12-lipoxygenase mRNA in cultured oligodendrocytes and astrocytes by in situ reverse transcriptase and polymerase chain reaction. *Neurosci. Lett.* 189:159–162.

Bordayo E. Z., Fawcett J. R., Lagalwar S., Svitak A. L., and Frey W. H. I. (2005). Inhibition of ligand binding to G protein-coupled receptors by arachidonic acid. *J. Mol. Neurosci.* 27:185–194.

Bruner G. and Murphy S. (1993). Purinergic P2Y receptors on astrocytes are directly coupled to phospholipase A_2. *Glia* 7:219–224.

Cao Y., Murphy K. J., McIntyre T. M., Zimmerman G. A., and Prescott S. M. (2000). Expression of fatty acid-CoA ligase 4 during development and in brain. *FEBS Lett.* 467:263–267.

Cazevieille C., Muller A., Meynier F., Dutrait N., and Bonne C. (1994). Protection by prostaglandins from glutamate toxicity in cortical neurons. *Neurochem. Int.* 24:395–398.

Chabot C., Gagné J., Giguère C., Bernard J., Baudry M., and Massicotte G. (1998). Bidirectional modulation of AMPA receptor properties by exogenous phospholipase A_2 in the hippocampus. *Hippocampus* 8:299–309.

Chalimoniuk M., King-Pospisil K., Pedersen W. A., Malecki A., Wylegala E., Mattson M. P., Hennig B., and Toborek M. (2004). Arachidonic acid increases choline acetyltransferase activity in spinal cord neurons through a protein kinase C-mediated mechanism. *J. Neurochem.* 90:629–636.

Chandrasekharan N. V., Dai H., Roos K. L., Evanson N. K., Tomsik J., Elton T. S., and Simmons D. L. (2002). COX-3, a cyclooxygenase-1 variant inhibited by acetaminophen and other analgesic/antipyretic drugs: cloning, structure, and expression. *Proc. Natl Acad. Sci. USA* 99:13926–13931.

Chiang N., Arita M., and Serhan C. N. (2005). Anti-inflammatory circuitry: Lipoxin, aspirin-triggered lipoxins and their receptor ALX. *Prostaglandins Leukot. Essent. Fatty Acids* 73:163–177.

Coleman R. A., Smith W. L., and Narumiya S. (1994). International Union of Pharmacology classification of prostanoid receptors: properties, distribution, and structure of the receptors and their subtypes. *Pharmacol. Rev.* 46:205–229.

Coleman R. A., Lewin T. M., and Muoio D. M. (2000). Physiological and nutritional regulation of enzymes of triacylglycerol synthesis. *Annu. Rev. Nutr.* 20:77–103.

Corbin D. R. and Sun G. Y. (1978). Characterization of the enzymic transfer of arachidonoyl groups to 1-acyl-phosphoglycerides in mouse synaptosome fraction. *J. Neurochem.* 30:77–82.

Danbolt N. C. (1994). The high affinity uptake system for excitatory amino acid in brain. *Prog. Neurobiol.* 44:377–396.

Das U. N. (2003). Long-chain polyunsaturated fatty acids in memory formation and consolidation: Further evidence and discussion. *Nutrition* 19:988–993.

Davies N. M., Good R. L., Roupe K. A., and Yanez J. A. (2004). Cyclooxygenase-3: axiom, dogma, anomaly, enigma or splice error?—Not as easy as 1, 2, 3. *J. Pharm. Pharm. Sci.* 7:217–226.

DeGeorge J. J., Noronha J. G., Bell J., Robinson P., and Rapoport S. I. (1989). Intravenous injection of [1-14C]arachidonate to examine regional brain lipid metabolism in unanesthetized rats. *J. Neurosci. Res.* 24:413–423.

Doolan C. M. and Keenan A. K. (1994). Inhibition by fatty acids of cyclic AMP-dependent protein kinase activity in brush border membranes isolated from human placental vesicles. *Br. J. Pharmacol.* 111:509–514.

Dumuis A., Sebben M., Haynes L., Pin J.-P., and Bockaert J. (1988). NMDA receptors activate the arachidonic acid cascade system in striatal neurons. *Nature* 336:68–70.

Dumuis A., Pin P., Oomagari K., Sebben M., and Bockaert J. (1990). Arachidonic acid release from striatal neurons by joint stimulation of ionotropic and metabotropic quisqualate receptors. *Nature* 347:182–184.

Dunican D. J., Griffiths R., Williams D. C., and O'Neill L. A. (1996). Endothelin-1 increases arachidonic acid release in C6 glioma cells through a potassium-modulated influx of calcium. *J. Neurochem.* 67:830–837.

Faergeman N. J. and Knudsen J. (1997). Role of long-chain fatty acyl-CoA esters in the regulation of metabolism and in cell signalling. *Biochem. J.* 323 (Pt 1):1–12.

Farooqui A. A. and Horrocks L. A. (1985). Metabolic and functional aspects of neural membrane phospholipids. In: Horrocks L. A., Kanfer J. N., and Porcellati G. (eds.), *Phospholipids in the Nervous System, Vol. II: Physiological Role.* Raven Press, New York, pp. 341–348.

Farooqui A. A. and Horrocks L. A. (1991). Excitatory amino acid receptors, neural membrane phospholipid metabolism and neurological disorders. *Brain Res. Rev.* 16:171–191.

Farooqui A. A. and Horrocks L. A. (1994). Excitotoxicity and neurological disorders: involvement of membrane phospholipids. *Int. Rev. Neurobiol.* 36:267–323.

Farooqui A. A. and Horrocks L. A. (1997). Excitatory neurotransmitters and their involvement in neurodegeneration. *Encycl. Hum. Biol.* 3:845–851.

Farooqui A. A. and Horrocks L. A. (2001). Plasmalogens, phospholipase A_2, and docosahexaenoic acid turnover in brain tissue. *J. Mol. Neurosci.* 16:263–272.

Farooqui A. A. and Horrocks L. A. (2006). Phospholipase A_2-generated lipid mediators in brain: the good, the bad, and the ugly. *Neuroscientist* 12:245.

Farooqui A. A., Rammohan K. W., and Horrocks L. A. (1989). Isolation, characterization and regulation of diacylglycerol lipases from bovine brain. *Ann. NY Acad. Sci.* 559:25–36.

Farooqui A. A., Anderson D. K., and Horrocks L. A. (1993). Effect of glutamate and its analogs on diacylglycerol and monoacylglycerol lipase activities of neuron-enriched cultures. *Brain Res.* 604:180–184.

Farooqui A. A., Rosenberger T. A., and Horrocks L. A. (1997a). Arachidonic acid, neurotrauma, and neurodegenerative diseases. In: Yehuda S. and Mostofsky D. I. (eds.), *Handbook of Essential Fatty Acid Biology.* Humana Press, Totowa, NJ, pp. 277–295.

Farooqui A. A., Yang H. C., Rosenberger T. A., and Horrocks L. A. (1997b). Phospholipase A_2 and its role in brain tissue. *J. Neurochem.* 69:889–901.

Farooqui A. A., Horrocks L. A., and Farooqui T. (2000a). Deacylation and reacylation of neural membrane glycerophospholipids. *J. Mol. Neurosci.* 14:123–135.

Farooqui A. A., Horrocks L. A., and Farooqui T. (2000b). Glycerophospholipids in brain: their metabolism, incorporation into membranes, functions, and involvement in neurological disorders. *Chem. Phys. Lipids* 106:1–29.

Farooqui A. A., Farooqui T., and Horrocks L. A. (2002a). Molecular species of phospholipids during brain development. Their occurrence, separation and roles. In:

Skinner E. R. (ed.), *Brain Lipids and Disorders in Biological Psychiatry*. Elsevier Science B.V., Amsterdam, pp. 147–158.

Farooqui A. A., Ong W. Y., Lu X. R., and Horrocks L. A. (2002b). Cytosolic phospholipase A$_2$ inhibitors as therapeutic agents for neural cell injury. *Curr. Med. Chem. — Anti-Inflammatory Anti-Allergy Agents* 1:193–204.

Farooqui A. A., Ong W. Y., and Horrocks L. A. (2003a). Plasmalogens, docosahexaenoic acid, and neurological disorders. In: Roels F., Baes M., and de Bies S. (eds.), *Peroxisomal Disorders and Regulation of Genes*. Kluwer Academic/Plenum Publishers, London, pp. 335–354.

Farooqui A. A., Ong W. Y., and Horrocks L. A. (2003b). Stimulation of lipases and phospholipases in Alzheimer disease. In: Szuhaj B. and van Nieuwenhuyzen W. (eds.), *Nutrition and Biochemistry of Phospholipids*. AOCS Press, Champaign, pp. 14–29.

Felder C. C., Kanterman R. Y., Ma A. L., and Axelrod J. (1990). Serotonin stimulates phospholipase a2 and the release of arachidonic acid in hippocampal neurons by a type 2 serotonin receptor that is independent of inositolphospholipid hydrolysis. *Proc. Natl Acad. Sci. USA* 87:2187–2191.

Felder C. C., Williams H. L., and Axelrod J. (1991). A transduction pathway associated with receptors coupled to the inhibitory guanine nucleotide binding protein gi that amplifies atp-mediated arachidonic acid release. *Proc. Natl Acad. Sci. USA* 88:6477–6480.

Fiebich B. L., Hüll M., Lieb K., Gyufko K., Berger M., and Bauer J. (1997). Prostaglandin E$_2$ induces interleukin-6 synthesis in human astrocytoma cells. *J. Neurochem.* 68:704–709.

Fonlupt P., Croset M., and Lagarde M. (1994). Incorporation of arachidonic and docosahexaenoic acids into phospholipids of rat brain membranes. *Neurosci. Lett.* 171:137–141.

Fujino T. and Yamamoto T. (1992). Cloning and functional expression of a novel long-chain acyl-CoA synthetase expressed in brain. *J. Biochem.* (Tokyo) 111:197–203.

Fujino T., Kang M. J., Suzuki H., Iijima H., and Yamamoto T. (1996). Molecular characterization and expression of rat acyl-CoA synthetase 3. *J. Biol. Chem.* 271:16748–16752.

Funk C. D. (1996). The molecular biology of mammalian lipoxygenases and the quest for eicosanoid functions using lipoxygenase-deficient mice. *Biochim. Biophys. Acta Lipids Lipid Metab.* 1304:65–84.

Gamberucci A., Fulceri R., Bygrave F. L., and Benedetti A. (1997). Unsaturated fatty acids mobilize intracellular calcium independent of IP3 generation and VIA insertion at the plasma membrane. *Biochem. Biophys. Res. Commun.* 241:312–316.

Garcia M. C. and Kim H. Y. (1997). Mobilization of arachidonate and docosahexaenoate by stimulation of the 5-HT$_{2A}$ receptor in rat C6 glioma cells. *Brain Res.* 768:43–48.

Garrido R., Mattson M. P., Hennig B., and Toborek M. (2001). Nicotine protects against arachidonic-acid-induced caspase activation, cytochrome c release and apoptosis of cultured spinal cord neurons. *J. Neurochem.* 76:1395–1403.

Gebremedhin D., Lange A. R., Narayanan J., Aebly M. R., Jacobs E. R., and Harder D. R. (1998). Cat cerebral arterial smooth muscle cells express cytochrome P450 4A2 enzyme and produce the vasoconstrictor 20-HETE which enhances L-type Ca^{2+} current. *J. Physiol.* 507(Pt 3):771–781.

Gebremedhin D., Lange A. R., Lowry T. F., Taheri M. R., Birks E. K., Hudetz A. G., Narayanan J., Falck J. R., Okamoto H., Roman R. J., Nithipatikom K., Campbell W. B., and Harder D. R. (2000). Production of 20-HETE and its role in autoregulation of cerebral blood flow. *Circ. Res.* 87:60–65.

Gilroy D. W., Newson J., Sawmynaden P. A., Willoughby D. A., and Croxtall J. D. (2004). A novel role for phospholipase A$_2$ isoforms in the checkpoint control of acute inflammation. *FASEB J.* 18:489–498.

Gronert K. (2005). Lipoxins in the eye and their role in wound healing. Prostaglandins Leukot. Essent. *Fatty Acids* 73:221–229.

Han C., Demetris A. J., Liu Y. H., Shelhamer J. H., and Wu T. (2004). Transforming growth factor-beta (TGF-β) activates cytosolic phospholipase $A_2\alpha$ (cPLA$_2\alpha$)-mediated prostaglandin E_2 (PGE$_2$)/EP$_1$ and peroxisome proliferator-activated receptor-γ (PPAR-γ)/Smad signaling pathways in human liver cancer cells – a novel mechanism for subversion of TGF-β-induced mitoinhibition. *J. Biol. Chem.* 279:44344–44354.

Harder D. R., Roman R. J., Gebremedhin D., Birks E. K., and Lange A. R. (1998). A common pathway for regulation of nutritive blood flow to the brain: arterial muscle membrane potential and cytochrome P450 metabolites. *Acta Physiol. Scand.* 164:527–532.

Hernández M., Nieto M. L., and Sánchez Crespo M. (2000). Cytosolic phospholipase A$_2$ and the distinct transcriptional programs of astrocytoma cells. *Trends Neurosci.* 23:259–264.

Hoffmann C. (2000). COX-2 in brain and spinal cord implications for therapeutic use. *Curr. Med. Chem.* 7:1113–1120.

Horrocks L. A. (1972). Content, composition, and metabolism of mammalian and avian lipids that contain ether groups. In: Snyder F. (ed.), *Ether Lipids: Chemistry and Biology*. Academic Press, New York, pp. 177–272.

Horrocks L. A. and Yeo Y. K. (1999). Health benefits of docosahexaenoic acid (DHA). *Pharmacol. Res.* 40:211–225.

Jupp O. J., Vandenabeele P., and MacEwan D. J. (2003). Distinct regulation of cytosolic phospholipase A$_2$ phosphorylation, translocation, proteolysis and activation by tumour necrosis factor-receptor subtypes. *Biochem. J.* 374:453–461.

Kantarci A. and Van Dyke T. E. (2003). Lipoxins in chronic inflammation. *Crit. Rev. Oral Biol. Med.* 14:4–12.

Kantarci A. and Van Dyke T. E. (2005). Lipoxin signaling in neutrophils and their role in periodontal disease. *Prostaglandins Leukot. Essent. Fatty Acids* 73:289–299.

Katsuki H. and Okuda S. (1995). Arachidonic acid as a neurotoxic and neurotrophic substance. *Prog. Neurobiol.* 46:607–636.

Kee H. J., Koh J. T., Yang S. Y., Lee Z. H., Baik Y. H., and Kim K. K. (2003). A novel murine long-chain acyl-CoA synthetase expressed in brain participates in neuronal cell proliferation. *Biochem. Biophys. Res. Commun.* 305:925–933.

Kim D. K., Rordorf G., Nemenoff R. A., Koroshetz W. J., and Bonventre J. V. (1995). Glutamate stably enhances the activity of two cytosolic forms of phospholipase A$_2$ in brain cortical cultures. *Biochem. J.* 310:83–90.

Kis B., Snipes J. A., and Busija D. W. (2005). Acetaminophen and the cyclooxygenase-3 puzzle: sorting out facts, fictions, and uncertainties. *J. Pharmacol. Exp. Ther.* 315:1–7.

Kolko M., DeCoster M. A., Rodriguez de Turco E. B., and Bazan N. G. (1996). Synergy by secretory phospholipase A$_2$ and glutamate on inducing cell death and sustained arachidonic acid metabolic changes in primary cortical neuronal cultures. *J. Biol. Chem.* 271:32722–32728.

Kurrasch-Orbaugh D. M., Parrish J. C., Watts V. J., and Nichols D. E. (2003). A complex signaling cascade links the serotonin$_{2A}$ receptor to phospholipase A$_2$ activation: the involvement of MAP kinases. *J. Neurochem.* 86:980–991.

Lazarewicz J. W., Wroblewski J. T., Palmer M. E., and Costa E. (1988). Activation of N-methyl-D-aspartate-sensitive glutamate receptors stimulates arachidonic acid release in primary cultures of cerebellar granule cells. *Neuropharmacology* 27:765–769.

Lazarewicz J. W., Wroblewski J. T., and Costa E. (1990). N-methyl-D-aspartate-sensitive glutamate receptors induce calcium-mediated arachidonic acid release in primary cultures of cerebellar granule cells. *J. Neurochem.* 55:1875–1881.

Lewin T. M., Kim J. H., Granger D. A., Vance J. E., and Coleman R. A. (2001). Acyl-CoA synthetase isoforms 1, 4, and 5 are present in different subcellular membranes in rat liver and can be inhibited independently. *J. Biol. Chem.* 276:24674–24679.

Li Y., Maher P., and Schubert D. (1997). A role for 12-lipoxygenase in nerve cell death caused by glutathione depletion. *Neuron* 19:453–463.

Lipton S. A. and Rosenberg P. A. (1994). Excitatory amino acids as a final common pathway for neurologic disorders. *N. Engl. J. Med.* 330:613–622.

Liu D. X., Li L. P., and Augustus L. (2001). Prostaglandin release by spinal cord injury mediates production of hydroxyl radical, malondialdehyde and cell death: a site of the neuroprotective action of methylprednisolone. *J. Neurochem.* 77:1036–1047.

Lynch M. A. and Voss K. L. (1990). Arachidonic acid increases inositol phospholipid metabolism and glutamate release in synaptosomes prepared from hippocampal tissue. *J. Neurochem.* 55:215–221.

Maccarrone M., Melino G., and Finazzi-Agro A. (2001). Lipoxygenases and their involvement in programmed cell death. *Cell Death Diff.* 8:776–784.

MacDonald J. I. S. and Sprecher H. (1991). Phospholipid fatty acid remodeling in mammalian cells. *Biochim. Biophys. Acta* 1084:105–121.

Manev H., Uz T., Sugaya K., and Qu T. Y. (2000). Putative role of neuronal 5-lipoxygenase in an aging brain. *FASEB J.* 14:1464–1469.

Martínez M. and Mougan I. (1998). Fatty acid composition of human brain phospholipids during normal development. *J. Neurochem.* 71:2528–2533.

Martínez-Cayuela M. (1995). Oxygen free radicals and human disease. *Biochimie* 77:147–161.

Matsuzawa A., Murakami M., Atsumi G., Imai K., Prados P., Inoue K., and Kudo I. (1996). Release of secretory phospholipase A_2 from rat neuronal cells and its possible function in the regulation of catecholamine secretion. *Biochem. J.* 318:701–709.

McGahon B., Clements M. P., and Lynch M. A. (1997). The ability of aged rats to sustain long-term potentiation is restored when the age-related decrease in membrane arachidonic acid concentration is reversed. *Neuroscience* 81:9–16.

Minghetti L. (2004). Cyclooxygenase-2 (COX-2) in inflammatory and degenerative brain diseases. *J. Neuropathol. Exp. Neurol.* 63:901–910.

Minghetti L. and Levi G. (1998). Microglia as effector cells in brain damage and repair: focus on prostanoids and nitric oxide. *Prog. Neurobiol.* 54:99–125.

Munzenmaier D. H. and Harder D. R. (2000). Cerebral microvascular endothelial cell tube formation: role of astrocytic epoxyeicosatrienoic acid release. *Am. J. Physiol Heart Circ. Physiol.* 278:H1163–H1167.

Murakami K. and Routtenberg A. (2003). The role of fatty acids in synaptic growth and plasticity. In: Peet M., Glen L., and Horrobin D. F. (eds.), *Phospholipid Spectrum Disorders in Psychiatry and Neurology.* Marius Press, Carnforth, Lancashire, pp. 77–92.

Norel X. and Brink C. (2004). The quest for new cysteinyl-leukotriene and lipoxin receptors: recent clues. *Pharmacol. Ther.* 103:81–94.

O'Banion M. K. (1999). Cyclooxygenase-2: molecular biology, pharmacology, and neurobiology. *Crit Rev. Neurobiol.* 13:45–82.

O'Regan M. H., Perkins L. M., and Phillis J. W. (1995). Arachidonic acid and lysophosphatidylcholine modulate excitatory transmitter amino acid release from the rat cerebral cortex. *Neurosci. Lett.* 193:85–88.

Ojima A., Nakagawa Y., Sugiura T., Masuzawa Y., and Waku K. (1987). Selective transacylation of 1-0-alkylglycerophosphoethanolamine by docosahexaenoate and arachidonate in rat brain microsomes. *J. Neurochem.* 48:1403–1410.

Patel T. B. (2004). Single transmembrane spanning heterotrimeric G protein-coupled receptors and their signaling cascades. *Pharmacol. Rev.* 56:371–385.

Peng X., Zhang C., Alkayed N. J., Harder D. R., and Koehler R. C. (2004). Dependency of cortical functional hyperemia to forepaw stimulation on epoxygenase and nitric oxide synthase activities in rats. *J. Cereb. Blood Flow Metab.* 24:509–517.

Phillis J. W., Smith-Barbour M., and O'Regan M. H. (1996). Changes in extracellular amino acid neurotransmitters and purines during and following ischemias of different durations in the rat cerebral cortex. *Neurochem. Int.* 29:115–120.

Phillis J. W., Horrocks L. A., and Farooqui A. A. (2006). Cyclooxygenases, lipoxygenases, and epoxygenases in CNS: their role and involvement in neurological disorders. *Brain Res. Rev.* (in press).

Pirianov G., Danielsson C., Carlberg C., James S. Y., and Colston K. W. (1999). Potentiation by vitamin D analogs of TNFα and ceramide-induced apoptosis in MCF-7 cells is associated with activation of cytosolic phospholipase A$_2$. *Cell Death Diff.* 6:890–901.

Porcellati G. (1983). Phospholipid metabolism in neural membranes. In: Sun G. Y., Bazan N., Wu J. Y., Porcellati G., and Sun A. Y. (eds.), *Neural Membranes.* Humana Press, New York, pp. 3–35.

Powell W. S. and Rokach J. (2005). Biochemistry, biology and chemistry of the 5-lipoxygenase product 5-oxo-ETE. *Prog. Lipid Res.* 44:154–183.

Prasad K. N., La Rosa F. G., and Prasad J. E. (1998). Prostaglandins act as neurotoxin for differentiated neuroblastoma cells in culture and increase levels of ubiquitin and beta-amyloid. *In Vitro Cell Dev. Biol. Anim.* 34:265–274.

Qu Y., Chang L., Klaff J., Seeman R., Balbo A., and Rapoport S. I. (2003a). Imaging of brain serotonergic neurotransmission involving phospholipase A$_2$ activation and arachidonic acid release in unanesthetized rats. *Brain Res. Protocols* 12:16–25.

Qu Y., Chang L., Klaff J., Seemann R., and Rapoport S. I. (2003b). Imaging brain phospholipase A$_2$-mediated signal transduction in response to acute fluoxetine administration in unanesthetized rats. *Neuropsychopharmacology* 28:1219–1226.

Qu Y., Villacreses N., Murphy D. L., and Rapoport S. I. (2005). 5-HT2A/2C receptor signaling via phospholipase A$_2$ and arachidonic acid is attenuated in mice lacking the serotonin reuptake transporter. *Psychopharmacology* 180:12–20.

Rao K. V., Vaidyanathan V. V., and Sastry P. S. (1994). Diacylglycerol kinase is stimulated by arachidonic acid in neural membranes. *J. Neurochem.* 63:1454–1459.

Rapoport S. I. (1999). In vivo fatty acid incorporation into brain phospholipids in relation to signal transduction and membrane remodeling. *Neurochem. Res.* 24:1403–1415.

Ray P., Ray R., Broomfield C. A., and Berman J. D. (1994). Inhibition of bioenergetics alters intracellular calcium, membrane composition, and fluidity in a neuronal cell line. *Neurochem. Res.* 19:57–63.

Reddy T. S. and Bazan N. G. (1984). Long-chain acyl coenzyme A synthetase activity during the postnatal development of the mouse brain. *Int. J. Dev. Neurosci.* 2:447–450.

Reddy T. S., Sprecher H., and Bazan N. G. (1984). Long-chain acyl-coenzyme A synthetase from rat brain microsomes. Kinetic studies using [1-^{14}C]docosahexaenoic acid substrate. *Eur. J. Biochem.* 145:21–29.

Ross B. M. (2003). Phospholipase A2-associated processes in the human brain and their role in neuropathology and psychopathology. In: Peet M., Glen L., and Horrobin D. F. (eds.), *Phospholipid Spectrum Disorders in Psychiatry and Neurology.* Marius Press, Carnforth, Lancashire, pp. 163–182.

Ross B. M. and Kish S. J. (1994). Characterization of lysophospholipid metabolizing enzymes in human brain. *J. Neurochem.* 63:1839–1848.

Rothman S. M. and Olney J. W. (1986). Glutamate and the pathophysiology of hypoxic-ischemic brain damage. *Ann. Neurol.* 19:105–111.

Sakata A., Ida E., Tominaga M., and Onoue K. (1987). Arachidonic acid acts as an intracellular activator of NADPH-oxidase in Fc gamma receptor-mediated superoxide generation in macrophages. *J. Immunol.* 138:4353–4359.

Salem N., Jr., Kim H. Y., and Yergey J. A. (1986). Docosahexaenoic acid: membrane function and metabolism. In: Simopoulos A. P., Kifer R. R., and Martin R. E. (eds.), *Health Effects of Polyunsaturated Fatty Acids in Seafoods.* Academic Press, Orlando, pp. 263–318.

Sánchez-Prieto J., Sihra T. S., and Nicholls D. G. (1987). Characterization of the exocytotic release of glutamate from guinea-pig cerebral cortical synaptosomes. *J. Neurochem.* 49:58–64.

Sanfeliu C., Hunt A., and Patel A. J. (1990). Exposure to N-methyl-D-aspartate increases release of arachidonic acid in primary cultures of rat hippocampal neurons and not in astrocytes. *Brain Res.* 526:241–248.

Sawyer D. B. and Andersen O. S. (1989). Platelet-activating factor is a general membrane perturbant. *Biochim. Biophys. Acta* 987:129–132.

Schapira A. H. (1996). Oxidative stress and mitochondrial dysfunction in neurodegeneration. *Curr. Opin. Neurol.* 9:260–264.

Schmidt A., Wolde M., Thiele C., Fest W., Kratzin H., Podtelejnikov A. V., Witke W., Huttner W. B., and Söling H. D. (1999). Endophilin I mediates synaptic vesicle formation by transfer of arachidonate to lysophosphatidic acid. *Nature* 401:133–141.

Serhan C. N. (1994). Lipoxin biosynthesis and its impact in inflammatory and vascular events. *Biochim. Biophys. Acta* 1212:1–25.

Serhan C. N. (2005). Lipoxins and aspirin-triggered 15-epi-lipoxins are the first lipid mediators of endogenous anti-inflammation and resolution. *Prostaglandins Leukot. Essent. Fatty Acids* 73:141–162.

Serhan C. N. and Levy B. (2003). Novel pathways and endogenous mediators in anti-inflammation and resolution. *Chem. Immunol. Allergy* 83:115–145.

Simmons D. L., Botting R. M., and Hla T. (2004). Cyclooxygenase isozymes: The biology of prostaglandin synthesis and inhibition. *Pharmacol. Rev.* 56:387–437.

Singh I., Bhuskan A. S., Relan N. K., and Hashimoto T. (1988). Acyl-CoA ligase from rat brain microsome: an immunochemical study. *Biochim. Biophys. Acta* 963:509–514.

Smith W. L., DeWitt D. L., and Garavito R. M. (2000). Cyclooxygenases: structural, cellular, and molecular biology. *Annu. Rev. Biochem.* 69:145–182.

Söderberg M., Edlund C., Kristensson K., and Dallner G. (1991). Fatty acid composition of brain phospholipids in aging and in Alzheimer's disease. *Lipids* 26:421–425.

Spector A. A., Fang X., Snyder G. D., and Weintraub N. L. (2004). Epoxyeicosatrienoic acids (EETs): metabolism and biochemical function. *Prog. Lipid Res.* 43:55–90.

Stella N., Estelles A., Siciliano J., Tencé M., Desagher S., Piomelli D., Glowinski J., and Prémont J. (1997). Interleukin-1 enhances the ATP-evoked release of arachidonic acid from mouse astrocytes. *J. Neurosci.* 17:2939–2946.

Sun G. Y. and MacQuarrie R. A. (1989). Deacylation-reacylation of arachidonoyl groups in cerebral phospholipids. *Ann. NY Acad. Sci.* 559:37–55.

Sun G. Y. and Su K. L. (1979). Metabolism of arachidonoyl phosphoglycerides in mouse brain subcellular fractions. *J. Neurochem.* 32:1053–1059.

Sun C. W., Falck J. R., Okamoto H., Harder D. R., and Roman R. J. (2000). Role of cGMP versus 20-HETE in the vasodilator response to nitric oxide in rat cerebral arteries. *Am. J. Physiol. Heart Circ. Physiol.* 279:H339–H350.

Sun G. Y., Xu J. F., Jensen M. D., Yu S., Wood W. G., Gonzalez F. A., Simonyi A., Sun A. Y., and Weisman G. A. (2005). Phospholipase A$_2$ in astrocytes — responses to oxidative stress, inflammation, and G protein-coupled receptor agonists. *Mol. Neurobiol.* 31:27–41.

Szatkowski M. and Attwell D. (1994). Triggering and execution of neuronal death in brain ischaemia: two phases of glutamate release by different mechanisms. *Trends Neurosci.* 17:359–365.

Tanford C. (1980). The hydrophobic effects: formation of micelles and biological membranes. John Wiley and Sons, New York.

Tencé M., Cordier J., Glowinski J., and Prémont J. (1992). Endothelin-evoked release of arachidonic acid from mouse astrocytes in primary culture. *Eur. J. Neurosci.* 4:993–999.

Toborek M., Malecki A., Garrido R., Mattson M. P., Hennig B., and Young B. (1999). Arachidonic acid-induced oxidative injury to cultured spinal cord neurons. *J. Neurochem.* 73:684–692.

Toborek M., Garrido R., Malecki A., Kaiser S., Mattson M. P., Hennig B., and Young B. (2000). Nicotine attenuates arachidonic acid-induced overexpression of nitric oxide synthase in cultured spinal cord neurons. *Exp. Neurol.* 161:609–620.

Tone O., Miller J. C., Bell J. M., and Rapoport S. I. (1987). Regional cerebral palmitate incorporation following transient bilateral carotid occlusion in awake gerbils. *Stroke* 18:1120–1127.

Tong W., Shah D., Xu J. F., Diehl J. A., Hans A., Hannink M., and Sun G. Y. (1999). Involvement of lipid mediators on cytokine signaling and induction of secretory phospholipase A$_2$ in immortalized astrocytes (DITNC). *J. Mol. Neurosci.* 12:89–99.

Trevisi L., Bova S., Cargnelli G., Ceolotto G., and Luciani S. (2002). Endothelin-1-induced arachidonic acid release by cytosolic phospholipase A$_2$ activation in rat vascular smooth muscle via extracellular signal-regulated kinases pathway. *Biochem. Pharmacol.* 64:425–431.

Uz T., Pesold C., Longone P., and Manev H. (1998). Aging-associated up-regulation of neuronal 5-lipoxygenase expression: putative role in neuronal vulnerability. *FASEB J.* 12:439–449.

Vane J. R., Bakhle Y. S., and Botting R. M. (1998). Cyclooxygenases 1 and 2. *Annu. Rev. Pharmacol. Toxicol.* 38:97–120.

Van Horn C. G., Caviglia J. M., Li L. O., Wang S., Granger D. A., and Coleman R. A. (2005). Characterization of recombinant long-chain rat acyl-CoA synthetase isoforms 3 and 6: identification of a novel variant of isoform 6. *Biochemistry* 44:1635–1642.

Vial D. and Piomelli D. (1995). Dopamine D$_2$ receptors potentiate arachidonate release via activation of cytosolic, arachidonate-specific phospholipase A$_2$. *J. Neurochem.* 64:2765–2772.

Wakabayashi S., Freed L. M., Bell J. M., and Rapoport S. I. (1994). In vivo cerebral incorporation of radiolabeled fatty acids after acute unilateral orbital enucleation in adult hooded Long-Evans rats. *J. Cereb. Blood Flow Metab.* 14:312–323.

Wang X. H., Yan G. T., Wang L. H., Hao X. H., Zhang K., and Xue H. (2004). The mediating role of cPLA$_2$ in IL-1 beta and IL-6 release in LPS-induced HeLa cells. *Cell Biochem. Funct.* 22:41–44.

Wang Y., Wei X., Xiao X., Hui R., Card J. W., Carey M. A., Wang D. W., and Zeldin D. C. (2005). Arachidonic acid epoxygenase metabolites stimulate endothelial cell growth and angiogenesis via mitogen-activated protein kinase and phosphatidylinositol 3-kinase/Akt signaling pathways. *J. Pharmacol. Exp. Ther.* 314:522–532.

Washizaki K., Smith Q. R., Rapoport S. I., and Purdon A. D. (1994). Brain arachidonic acid incorporation and precursor pool specific activity during intravenous infusion of unesterified [^{3}H]arachidonate in the anesthetized rat. *J. Neurochem.* 63:727–736.

Watanabe T., Medina J. F., Haeggstrom J. Z., Radmark O., and Samuelsson B. (1993). Molecular cloning of a 12-lipoxygenase cDNA from rat brain. *Eur. J. Biochem.* 212:605–612.

Wolfe L. S. and Horrocks L. A. (1994). Eicosanoids. In: Siegel G. J., Agranoff B. W., Albers R. W., and Molinoff P. B. (eds.), *Basic Neurochemistry*. Raven Press, New York, pp. 475–490.

Xing M., Wilkins P. L., McConnell B. K., and Mattera R. (1994). Regulation of phospholipase A_2 activity in undifferentiated and neutrophil-like HL60 cells. Linkage between impaired responses to agonists and absence of protein kinase C-dependent phosphorylation of cytosolic phospholipase A_2. *J. Biol. Chem.* 269:3117–3124.

Xu J. F., Yu S., Sun A. Y., and Sun G. Y. (2003). Oxidant-mediated AA release from astrocytes involves cPLA$_2$ and iPLA$_2$. *Free Radic. Biol. Med.* 34:1531–1543.

Yagami T., Ueda K., Sakaeda T., Okamura N., Nakazato H., Kuroda T., Hata S., Sakaguchi G., Itoh N., Hashimoto Y., and Fujimoto M. (2005). Effects of an endothelin B receptor agonist on secretory phospholipase A_2-IIA-induced apoptosis in cortical neurons. *Neuropharmacology* 48:291–300.

Yamashita A., Sugiura T., and Waku K. (1997). Acyltransferases and transacylases involved in fatty acid remodeling of phospholipids and metabolism of bioactive lipids in mammalian cells. *J. Biochem.* (Tokyo) 122:1–16.

Zaleska M. M. and Wilson D. F. (1989). Lipid hydroperoxides inhibit reacylation of phospholipids in neuronal membranes. *J. Neurochem.* 52:255–260.

Zeldin D. C. (2001). Epoxygenase pathways of arachidonic acid metabolism. *J. Biol. Chem.* 276:36059–36062.

Zhang Q., Yoshida S., Sakai K., Liu J., and Fukunaga K. (2000). Changes of free fatty acids and acyl-CoAs in rat brain hippocampal slice with tetraethylammonium-induced long-term potentiation. *Biochem. Biophys. Res. Commun.* 267:208–212.

6
Docosahexaenoic Acid and its Metabolites in Brain

6.1 Location and Turnover of Docosahexaenoic Acid

Docosahexaenoic acid (22:6 n-3, DHA) is an important essential polyunsaturated fatty acid (PUFA). This 22-carbon PUFA contains 6 *cis* double bonds located at positions 4, 7, 10, 13, 16, and 19 (Fig. 6.1). It is highly enriched in excitable neural membranes, constituting approximately 30–40% of the acyl groups in the phospholipids of the cerebral cortex and retina (Lauritzen et al., 2001). The concentration of DHA is particularly high in gray matter of cerebral cortex and in photoreceptor cell. Thus, DHA constitutes >17% of weight of the total fatty acids in the brain of adult rats and >33% of the total fatty acids in the retina (Hamano et al., 1996). This fatty acid is mainly found on the *sn*-2 position of the amino glycerophospholipids, phosphatidylethanolamine (PtdEtn), plasmenylethanolamine (PlsEtn), and phosphatidylserine (PtdSer).

In human brain gray matter, DHA accounts for approximately 24% of total acyl groups in PtdEtn and 37% of total acyl groups in PtdSer. In neural membranes and retina, DHA primarily accumulates during fetal and early postnatal life. Thus, the amount of DHA in the brain increases dramatically during the brain growth spurt, not only because of the growth in brain size, but also because there is an increase in the relative DHA content (Lauritzen et al., 2001). PtdCho contains little DHA at the *sn*-2 position of glycerol moiety, except in the retina.

The turnover of DHA involves a deacylation/reacylation cycle (Farooqui et al., 2000a). This cycle utilizes DHA-selective phospholipase A_2 (plasmalogen-selective phospholipase A_2) and acyltransferase reactions for maintaining the glycerophospholipid composition necessary for the normal function of neural membranes (Farooqui and Horrocks, 2001b; Strokin et al., 2003). DHA can also probably be moved from a diacyl glycerophospholipid to a lysoglycerophospholipid in brain endoplasmic reticulum and plasma membranes by a CoA-independent transacylase. Collective evidence suggests that DHA is used continuously for the biogenesis and maintenance of neuronal and retinal membranes throughout mammalian life. DHA affects many physical properties of membranes, such as bilayer thickness, acyl chain packing, free volume, and phase transition temperature (Mitchell et al., 1998; Wassall et al., 2004). DHA is specifically involved in inducing lateral phase

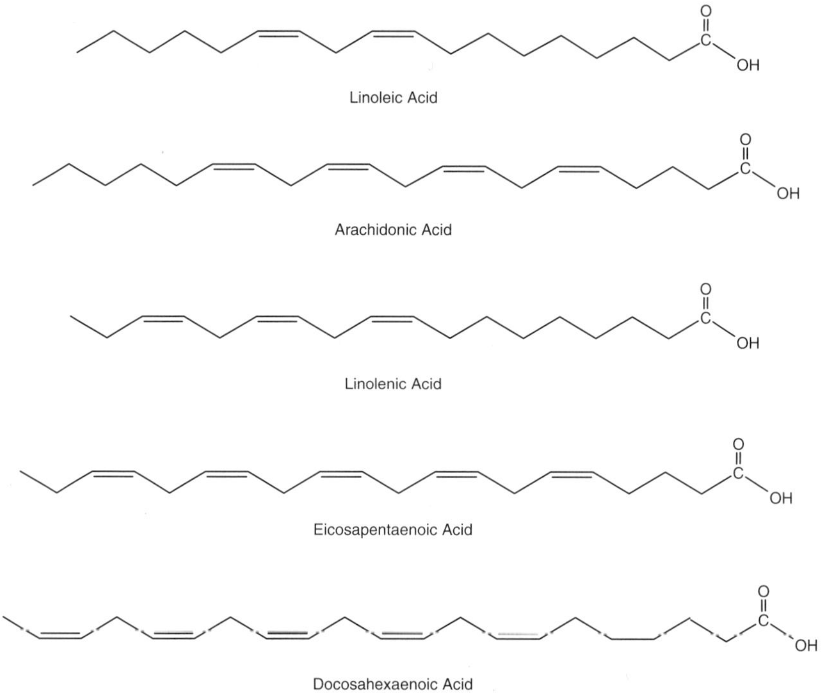

FIG. 6.1. Structures of polyunsaturated fatty acids found in brain. Linoleic acid (18:2n-6), arachidonic acid (20:4n-6), α-linolenic acid (18:3n-3), eicosapentaenoic acid (20:5n-3), and docosahexaenoic acid (22:6n-3).

separations into DHA-rich/cholesterol-poor and DHA-poor/cholesterol-rich lipid microdomains. The relatively low affinity between the DHA acyl chain and cholesterol may promote phase separations (Shaikh et al., 2003, 2004; Wassall et al., 2004). This process may be involved in microdomain (raft) formation in neural membranes. These lipid microdomains play an important role in the compartmentalization and modulation of cell signaling.

DHA-containing bilayers differentiate themselves from AA-containing bilayers by having extremely high water permeability, minimal interaction with cholesterol, and loose acyl chain packing (Mitchell et al., 1998; Stillwell et al., 2005). Collectively, these studies suggest that DHA acyl groups provide neural membranes with lipid microdomains that serve as platforms for compartmentalization, modulation, and integration of signaling (Ma et al., 2004). DHA acyl groups also interact with proteins crucial for the assembly of membrane protein networks (Huster et al., 1998).

For example, rhodopsin, a photoreceptor protein, is loosely bound to glycerophospholipids containing DHA. This DHA-enriched environment may be involved in conformational changes in G protein–coupled photoreceptors inducing modifications in activities of retinal enzymes (Mitchell et al., 1998; Rotstein et al., 2003). Thus, DHA affects retinal cell signaling mechanisms involved in phototransduction (SanGiovanni and Chew, 2005). Studies on G protein–coupled receptor signaling in retinal rod outer segment membranes in DHA-deficient and DHA-adequate rats indicate that second generation DHA-deficient rats have 80% less DHA than DHA-adequate rats. In these rats DHA is replaced by docosapentaenoic acid (22:5n-6). This replacement correlates with desensitization of visual signaling in DHA-deficient retinal rod segments and is related to reduced rhodopsin activation and cGMP phosphodiesterase activity. DHA is associated with signaling cascades that not only modulate rhodopsin regeneration but also activate other membrane-bound retinal proteins (Niu et al., 2004). Thus, DHA insufficiency is involved in alterations of retinal function associated with visual defects.

In brain, DHA-enriched glycerophospholipids containing ethanolamine and serine are associated with specific proteins in phospholipid bilayers. DHA-enriched ethanolamine glycerophospholipids are preferentially located in the intracellular leaflet in acetylcholine receptor-rich membranes. Similarly DHA-enriched PtdSer is also located in the inner lipid bilayer and is an essential cofactor for the activation of protein kinase C and Raf-1 kinase. PtdSer also modulates activities of diacylglycerol kinase, Na^+, K^+-ATPase, and nitric oxide synthase (Ikemoto et al., 2000). Thus, the presence of DHA in neural membranes provides them with an appropriate physical environment for the activity of integral membrane proteins. DHA also modulates ion channels and neurotransmitter receptors (Ferrier et al., 2002; Yehuda et al., 2002). DHA stabilizes neuronal membranes by suppressing voltage-gated Ca^{2+} currents and Na^+ channels (Young et al., 2000). It modulates T-cell activation via protein kinase C-α and -ε and the NF-κB signaling pathway (Denys et al., 2005). DHA also alters the lipid composition of membrane microdomains and suppresses IL-2 receptor signaling that is involved in immunosuppressive effect of DHA (Li et al., 2005).

Neurons lack the enzymes necessary for de novo DHA synthesis. DHA is obtained either directly from the diet or synthesized from its main dietary n-3 precursor, α-linolenic acid (18:3n-3, ALA), primarily in the liver (Scott and Bazan, 1989). Cerebral endothelium synthesizes DHA from dietary precursors via Δ^6-desaturation and retroconversion steps, whereas astrocytes are able to synthesize DHA either from 18-, 20-, and 22-carbon n-3 precursors (via elongation and desaturation steps) or from 24-carbon precursors (Innis and Dyer, 2002). However, the synthesis of DHA in astrocytes is a minor process in quantitative terms as compared with DHA supplied to brain tissue from plasma. It is estimated that between 2% and 8% of DHA in rat brain glycerophospholipids is replaced daily with DHA from the unesterified fatty acid pool in the plasma (Rapoport et al., 2001).

6.2 Incorporation of Docosahexaenoic Acid

DHA incorporation into glycerophospholipids was studied in retina (Stinson et al., 1991) and brain (DeMar et al., 2004) of DHA-deprived and DHA-adequate rats. Injected DHA binds to plasma albumin in the blood. Two factors determine the extent of DHA incorporation in brain and retina: first, the rate of its dissociation from plasma albumin, and second, the esterification of DHA with coenzyme A by long-chain acyl-CoA synthetase (Rapoport, 1999, 2003). In the rat retina, the half-life for loss of DHA from glycerophospholipids has been evaluated by injecting labeled [4,5-^{3}H]DHA into the vitreous humor. The observed half-life of DHA in retinal glycerophospholipids is 19 days (Stinson et al., 1991) because DHA is added at one end of the stack of retinal rods and metabolized at the other end. Apparent half-lives of DHA in individual glycerophospholipids of DHA-adequate rat brain range from 23 to 56 days. These results do not account for the recycling of DHA. About 5% of the brain DHA is lost daily with replacement from the diet (Rapoport, 2003). When recycling is accounted for, half-lives in some regions of the brain are measured in minutes (Rapoport, 2003). Some mechanism must exist in the adult rat brain to minimize a metabolic loss of DHA from neural membrane glycerophospholipids (DeMar et al., 2004). Mice deficient in n-3 fatty acids in their diet are quite slow to recover a more normal fatty acid composition in different areas of their brains (Carrie et al., 2000). Rats deprived of n-3 fatty acids for 15 weeks have 37% less DHA in their brains compared with 89% less DHA in their plasma and have apparent half-lives for DHA at least two-fold greater than in controls (DeMar et al., 2004).

In rat brain after intravenous infusion, 60% and 30% of the [^{3}H]DHA incorporates into synaptosomal and microsomal membrane fractions, respectively. The administration of arecoline, a cholinergic agonist, results in a marked increase in the incorporation of [^{3}H]DHA in the synaptosomal and microsomal fractions. In contrast, arecoline treatment does not affect the incorporation of [^{3}H]palmitic acid. DHA mainly incorporates at the *sn*-2 position of ethanolamine glycerophospholipids, whereas [^{3}H]palmitic acid is mainly esterified at the *sn*-1 position of phosphatidylcholine (Jones et al., 1997; Rapoport, 1999). The differential incorporation of DHA and palmitic acid into various glycerophospholipids may be responsible for better penetration, binding, and packing of neural membrane proteins into lipid bilayers. The location of the acyl groups in glycerophospholipid molecules is important for modulating the water permeability and lateral lipid movement in neural membranes (Mitchell et al., 1998).

Cell bodies and nerve growth cones in PC12 cells preferentially incorporate [^{3}H]DHA (Martin, 1998). In PC12 cells DHA metabolism may compartmentalize (Martin et al., 2000). Furthermore, in PC12 cells [^{3}H]DHA primarily incorporates into the ethanolamine glycerophospholipid fraction, which is enriched in PlsEtn. Collectively, these studies suggest that [^{3}H]DHA-labeled lipids are exclusively synthesized in the cell body and then trafficked to nerve growth cones (Martin, 1998; Martin et al., 2000). This trafficking of DHA from cell bodies to growth cones may be involved in synaptogenesis.

The reincorporation of DHA into membrane glycerophospholipids is catalyzed by acyl-CoA synthetases and acyl-CoA: lysoglycerophospholipid acyltransferases. These enzymes are localized in microsomes (Farooqui et al., 2000a). Acyl-CoA synthetase converts docosahexaenoic acid to docosahexaenoyl-CoA. As with the arachidonyl-CoA synthetase reaction, the omission of ATP and CoA from the reaction mixture results in a 98% decrease in enzymic activity, indicating the absolute requirement for ATP and CoA. Collectively, these studies suggest that the same acyl-CoA synthetase and lysoglycerophospholipid acyl-CoA transferase utilize AA and DHA (Reddy et al., 1984; Reddy and Bazan, 1984), but different PLA$_2$ isoforms (cPLA$_2$ versus PlsEtn-PLA$_2$) may be responsible for the release of AA and DHA in the deacylation/reacylation cycle (Farooqui et al., 2000a).

6.3 Receptor-Mediated Release of Docosahexaenoic Acid from Glycerophospholipids

As stated earlier, DHA and AA are mainly located at the *sn*-2 position of PtdEtn, PlsEtn, and PtdSer. They are released by the action of PLA$_2$ isoforms (Farooqui and Horrocks, 2001b; Strokin et al., 2003; Sergeeva et al., 2005), but the specificity of each isoform of PLA$_2$ is not established. The activity of PLA$_2$ isoforms depends highly upon the structure of its membrane substrate. Subtle variations in the acyl group composition may substantially affect not only the physical state of neural membranes but also activities of membrane-bound enzymes (Martin, 1998), receptors, and ion channels (Poling et al., 1995). The release of AA from the neural membrane glycerophospholipids, PlsEtn, PtdCho, and PtdEtn, is described in Chapters 2 and 5.

The release of DHA from PlsEtn is a receptor-mediated process (Farooqui and Horrocks, 2001a; Farooqui et al., 2003). Thus, the treatment of neuron-enriched cultures with kainate and other glutamate analogs results in a dose- and time-dependent stimulation of PlsEtn-selective PLA$_2$ (Fig. 6.2). A kainate/AMPA antagonist, 6-cyano-7-nitroquinoxaline-2, 3-dione (CNQX), inhibits enzymic activity (Fig. 6.3) and also prevents KA-mediated cell death in neural cell cultures.

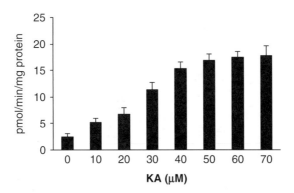

Fig. 6.2. Effect of kainic acid on PlsEtn-selective PLA$_2$ activity of neuron-enriched culture from rat cerebral cortex (Farooqui et al., 2003). Specific activity is expressed as pmol/min/mg protein.

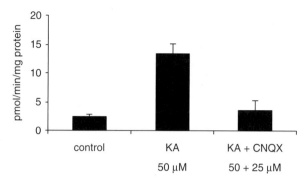

Fɪɢ. 6.3. Effect of CNQX on kainic acid-induced stimulation of PlsEtn-PLA₂ activity of neuron-enriched culture from rat cerebral cortex (Farooqui et al., 2003). Specific activity is expressed as pmol/min/mg protein.

This suggests that the stimulation of PlsEtn-PLA₂ activity is a KA receptor-mediated process. Bromoenol lactone (BEL), a potent inhibitor of iPLA₂ (Farooqui et al., 2003), also prevents both the stimulation of PlsEtn-PLA₂ and neural cell death in neuron-enriched cultures (Lu et al., 2001) (Fig. 6.4). Collectively, these studies suggest that the release of DHA from PlsEtn is a receptor-mediated process catalyzed by PlsEtn-PLA₂.

PtdSer is metabolized to PtdEtn or PtdCho by base-exchange reactions, or to PtdEtn by PtdSer decarboxylation (Porcellati, 1983; Farooqui and Horrocks, 1985; Farooqui et al., 2000b; Mozzi et al., 2003). At present, very little is known about the release of DHA from PtdSer. One study suggests that DHA can be released from PtdSer (Garcia and Kim, 1997). PtdSer in C6 glioma cells contains about 40% of the remaining labeled DHA after 24 h of incubation. Treatment with ROI, a 5-HT₂ₐ receptor agonist, causes the release of [³H]DHA, suggesting the presence of a PLA₂ activity hydrolyzing PtdSer in these C6 glioma cells. *Naja naja* PLA₂ also releases DHA from synaptosomal preparations in a dose- and time-dependent

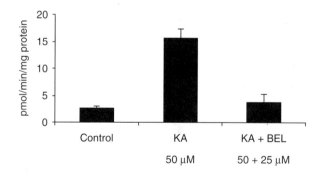

Fɪɢ. 6.4. Effect of bromoenol lactone on kainic acid-induced stimulation of PlsEtn-PLA₂ activity of neuron-enriched culture from rat cerebral cortex (Farooqui et al., 2003). Specific activity is expressed as pmol/min/mg protein.

manner (Kim et al., 1996). The released fatty acids also include AA and oleic acid. However, the rate of DHA release was faster than that of AA or oleic acid.

Low levels of eicosapentaenoic acid (EPA) also occur in neural membranes and play an important role in brain metabolism (Das, 2003; Lonergan et al., 2004), but no information on the release of EPA from neural membrane glycerophospholipids is available at present. EPA and DHA belong to the same family of fatty acids (n-3). They are not only interconverted into each other, but also resemble each other in many biochemical effects, including decreases in production of the key immunoregulatory cytokines (IL-10, TNF-α, and INF-γ) and in prevention of lipopolysaccharide (LPS) toxicity (Zhao et al., 2004; Lonergan et al., 2004; Verlengia et al., 2004b). They differ in effects on the expression of specific genes, and also in many other biochemical and physicochemical effects (Verlengia et al., 2004b). For example, EPA is a substrate for both cyclooxygenase and 5-lipoxygenase giving rise to 3-series prostaglandins, thromboxanes, and 5-series leukotrienes. EPA-derived eicosanoids are less active than AA-derived eicosanoids. In contrast, DHA is not a substrate for cyclooxygenase. EPA is hypotriglyceridemic and hypocholesterolemic, whilst DHA has no effect on plasma triglyceride levels (Hashimoto et al., 1999). DHA is less effective than EPA in inhibiting vascular smooth muscle proliferation. DHA is a more potent inhibitor than EPA of lymphocyte adhesion to endothelial cells (Hashimoto et al., 1999). Furthermore, EPA and DHA differ from each other in their effect on neural membrane capacitance. EPA increases the membrane capacitance of PC12 cells, whereas DHA has no effect (Ong et al., 2006). The reason for the stimulatory effect of EPA on membrane capacitance is not understood. However, it is likely that EPA interacts with the external ion channel domain of PC12 membranes differently than DHA. DHA blocks voltage-activated Na^+ channels, whilst EPA has no effect on membrane excitability and Na^+ channels in hippocampal neurons (Xiao and Li, 1999). Similarly, DHA modulates certain voltage-gated K^+ channels in Chinese hamster ovary cells, whereas EPA has no effect on K^+ channels. EPA modulates DHA synthesis in SH-SY5Y neuroblastoma cell cultures. EPA has antidepressant and antipsychotic activity, but DHA does not. Quantitation of the mRNA levels of genes encoding for several key enzymes of both the endoplasmic reticulum and peroxisomal steps of fatty acid metabolism indicates that EPA downregulates the enzymes involved in DHA synthesis and decreases DHA synthesis from its precursor, α-linolenic acid (Poumès-Ballihaut et al., 2001; Langelier et al., 2005). Collectively, these studies suggest that EPA and DHA differ in their effects on plasma lipid profiles, gene expression, and neural membrane structure.

6.4 Effects of DHA and its Metabolites on Brain Tissue

DHA exerts a direct influence on neuronal activity through several mechanisms. In neural membranes this fatty acid not only alters physicochemical properties, such as fluidity, permeability, fusion behavior, and elastic compressibility (Stillwell and Wassall, 2003), but also modulates the gene expression of many proteins involved in signal transduction and anti-inflammatory processes (Farkas et al., 2000; Kitajka et al., 2002; Puskás et al., 2003; Barceló-Coblijn et al., 2003; Sampath and Ntambi, 2005). To understand how DHA-mediated changes in neural membranes alter neural cell function, it is necessary to understand how DHA-containing glycerophospholipids interact with proteins in neural membranes and how they modulate signal transduction processes associated with various neuronal and glial cell functions.

6.4.1 DHA in Gene Expression, Neurotransmitter Release, and Enzyme Regulation

Feeding DHA to animals results in the overexpression of numerous genes in the brain that control signal transduction, synaptic plasticity, energy metabolism, and membrane trafficking (Kitajka et al., 2002; Puskás et al., 2003). DHA directly binds to and activates transcription factors that upregulate expression of β-oxidation enzymes, while decreasing expression of the desaturases used for the synthesis of DHA from α-linolenic acid (Price et al., 2000; Nakamura and Nara, 2003). Dietary consumption of DHA has numerous beneficial effects on the health of human brain (Horrocks and Yeo, 1999; Horrocks and Farooqui, 2004).

Several unsaturated fatty acids, including DHA, are ligands for the retinoid X receptor (RXR) in brain (de Urquiza et al., 2000; Farooqui et al., 2004; Lengqvist et al., 2004). RXR activation is an obligatory step in signaling to the nucleus and in the regulation of gene expression. RXR may serve as a fatty acid sensor in vivo. A deficiency of DHA reduces the expression of both isoforms of the brain glucose transporter, suggesting that glucose utilization in the cerebral cortex of DHA-deficient rats may be reduced due to post-transcriptional regulation of glucose transporter (Pifferi et al., 2005).

DHA differentially modulates glutamate transporters (GLT1, GLAST, and EAAC1) through different mechanisms (Berry et al., 2005). In the case of GLT1 and EAAC1, DHA stimulates D-[^{3}H]aspartate uptake via a mechanism requiring extracellular Ca^{2+}, CaM kinase II, and protein kinase C, but not protein kinase A. In contrast, the inhibitory effect of DHA on GLAST does not require extracellular Ca^{2+} and does not involve CaM kinase II (Berry et al., 2005). DHA modulates the expression of several gene clusters, including genes for cytokines and related receptors, signal transduction pathways, transcription factors, cell cycle, defense and repair, apoptosis, DNA synthesis, cell adhesion, cytoskeleton, and hormone receptors (Fernstrom, 1999; Farkas et al., 2000; Kim et al., 2000; Akbar and Kim, 2002; Kitajka et al., 2002; Barceló-Coblijn et al., 2003; Nakamura et al., 2004).

Dietary DHA also modulates dopaminergic, noradrenergic, glutamatergic, and serotonergic neurotransmission (Table 6.1) (Chalon et al., 1998; Zimmer et al., 2000; Hogyes et al., 2003), activities of membrane-bound enzymes (Table 6.2), ion channels (Nishikawa et al., 1994; Salem et al., 1988; Xiao and Li, 1999; Yehuda et al., 2002), learning and memory processes (Fujimoto et al., 1989; Fujita et al., 2001), and inflammation and immune function (James et al., 2000; Calder and Grimble, 2002) (Table 6.3). Gene expression and immunity changes are critical for

TABLE 6.1. Effect of DHA on neural and non-neural membrane receptors and signaling.

Receptor	Effect	Reference
Rhodopsin	Stimulated	Litman and Mitchell, 1996; Feller and Gawrisch, 2005
Ca^{2+} channel, Ca^{2+} release, and Ca^{2+} transport proteins	Inhibited	Hirafuji et al., 2003
NMDA receptor	Inhibited	Nishikawa et al., 1994; Young et al., 2000
γ-Aminobutyric type A receptor	Inhibited	Hamano et al., 1996; Nabekura et al., 1998
5-HT$_2$ receptor	Inhibited	Hirafuji et al., 2003
TGF-β receptor	Inhibited	Hirafuji et al., 2003
Retinoid X receptor (RXR)	Stimulated	Farooqui et al., 2004; Lengqvist et al., 2004
TP receptors	Inhibited	Hirafuji et al., 2003

TABLE 6.2. Effect of DHA on enzymic activities associated with signal transduction.

Enzymic activity	Effect	Reference
Phospholipase A$_2$	Inhibited	Farooqui et al., 2006
Protein kinase C	Inhibited	Hirafuji et al., 2003
Cyclooxygenase	Inhibited	Calder, 2003a, 2004
Glutathione peroxidase	Stimulated	Delton-Vandenbroucke et al., 2001; Songur et al., 2004
Tyrosine kinase	Inhibited	Sanderson and Calder, 1998
MAP kinase	Inhibited	Hirafuji et al., 2003
Cyclin-dependent kinase	Inhibited	Hirafuji et al., 2003
Caspase-3	Inhibited	Akbar et al., 2005
Neutral sphingomyelinase	Inhibited	Wu et al., 2005
HMG-CoA reductase	Inhibited	Duncan et al., 2005

TABLE 6.3. Roles of DHA in brain tissue.

Role of DHA	Reference
Modulation of neurotransmitter release	Chalon et al., 1998; Itokazu et al., 2000
Modulation of gene expression	Farkas et al., 2000; Kitajka et al., 2002; Barceló-Coblijn et al., 2003
Modulation of membrane enzymes, ion channels, and receptors	Gerbi et al., 1994; Fernstrom, 1999
Modulation of learning and memory processes	Fujimoto et al., 1989; Fujita et al., 2001; Hashimoto et al., 2002
Modulation of immunity and inflammation	Wu and Meydani, 1998; Calder and Grimble, 2002
Modulation of blood brain barrier	Yehuda et al., 2002
Modulation of apoptosis	Kim et al., 2000

adaptive responses for neural cell survival. Key transcription factors that regulate these adaptive responses include peroxisome proliferator–activated receptors (PPAR), sterol regulatory element binding protein (SREBP), and carbohydrate response element binding protein (ChREBP) (Clarke, 2000; Jump, 2002b; Nakamura et al., 2004). The effect of DHA is sustained as long as the DHA remains in the diet. Thus, DHA acts like a hormone to control the activity of key transcription factors and modulate many signal transduction processes associated with a variety of neural cell functions (Jump, 2002a; Valentine and Valentine, 2004).

6.4.2 DHA and Neurite Outgrowth

Hippocampus and cerebral cortex mediate complex integrative functions, such as abstract reasoning, planning, language, and sensory perception and participate in storage of long-term memory. A deficiency of DHA in the hippocampus decreases neuronal soma size in hippocampus (Ahmad et al., 2002), decreases PtdSer and PlsEtn levels (Hamilton et al., 2000; Farooqui and Horrocks, 2001b), and interferes with learning and memory tasks (Moriguchi et al., 2000). Restoration of memory formation in DHA-deficient animals occurs when these animals were fed a DHA-adequate diet. These observations suggest that DHA plays an important role in development of the hippocampus and cerebral cortex. Formation of neurites and their stabilization is a characteristic feature of developing an adult brain and is critical for synaptic remodeling during memory formation (Cline, 2001). In general, the density and morphology of neuronal dendrites modulates brain responses that are ultimately controlled by certain sets of neurons. In brain tissue, longer neurites and a higher number of dendritic branches bear more synaptic connections (Jan and Jan, 2001, 2003). Supplementation of DHA in cell culture media not only induces neurite outgrowth in PC12 cells (Ikemoto et al., 1997), hippocampal cells (Calderon and Kim, 2004) and rat cortical primary neuronal cultures (Cao et al., 2005), but also promotes branching. Thus, DHA has a role promoting neuronal differentiation (Calderon and Kim, 2004; Cao et al., 2005).

The molecular events associated with DHA-mediated differentiation are not fully understood. However, the overexpression of long-chain acyl-CoA synthetase 6 specifically promotes DHA internalization, activation to DHA-CoA, and accumulation in differentiating PC12 cells (Marszalek et al., 2005). In contrast, oleic acid (OA) and AA internalization and activation to OA-CoA and AA-CoA are only marginally increased by the overexpression of long-chain acyl-CoA synthetase 6. Additionally, the overexpression of long-chain acyl-CoA synthetase 6 increases the level of total cellular glycerophospholipids with the addition of AA and DHA, but not with OA, supporting the view that increased glycerophospholipids may be utilized by neural cells for neurite formation. Furthermore, cultured hippocampal neurons obtained from DHA-deficient rats have decreased neurite outgrowth in comparison to hippocampal neurons from DHA-adequate rats. DHA inclusion in the culture medium increases the neurite length of DHA-deficient neurons to the level of DHA adequate neurons (Calderon and Kim, 2004). Neurite outgrowth requires the synthesis of membrane components, such as phospholipids and proteins (Ikemoto et al., 1999).

Growth-associated protein-43 (GAP-43) or neuromodulin is a neuron-specific protein associated with axon growth and growth cone formation that also modulates neurite outgrowth (Ramakers et al., 1991; Takahata, 1995). It is a substrate for protein kinase C. Cultured neurons with DHA have greater growth-associated protein-43 (GAP-43) immunoreactivity and higher PtdSer and EtnGpl contents but a lower PtdCho content than control neurons (Cao et al., 2005). Fatty acid analyses of DHA-supplemented neurons show significantly increased DHA contents in PtdSer and EtnGpl suggesting that these lipids may be the direct precursors of lipid mediators associated with signal transduction processes involved in the induction of neurite outgrowth in DHA-supplemented cell cultures. Supplementation of serum-free medium with hormones and DHA permits the full development of synapses of cultured mouse fetal hypothalamic cells as attested to by the increase in number and the regular shape and diameter of synaptic vesicles. DHA supplementation also affects the morphology of astrocytes from primary culture.

6.4.3 DHA and Modulation of Learning and Memory

Long-term potentiation (LTP) and long-term depression (LTD) of hippocampal synaptic transmission are two forms of activity-dependent synaptic plasticity that underlie learning and memory. LTP and LTD are modulated by NMDA receptors, glutamate receptors responsible for Ca^{2+} influx into neurons. This increase in the intracellular Ca^{2+} activates ras and extracellular signal related kinase (ERK), via nitric oxide generation by Ca^{2+}-dependent neuronal nitric oxide synthase. Generation of nitric oxide is an important step in the induction of synaptic plasticity, which is essential for memory formation and consolidation (Das, 2003). Intracerebroventricular injections of DHA decrease the excitatory postsynaptic potential (fEPSP) slope in the Schaffer collateral-CA1 neurotransmission, but increase the fEPSP slopes in the perforant path-DG synaptic transmission (Young et al., 2000; Itokazu et al., 2000), suggesting that DHA blocks the induction of CA1 LTP but has no effect on the DG (dentate gyrus) LTP. Thus DHA exerts regionally different effects on hippocampal neurotransmission. Furthermore, in rat brain slices, endogenously released DHA during tetanic stimulation is sufficient to trigger the expression of LTP (Fujita et al., 2001). Addition of glycerophospholipids containing DHA enhances LTP in the rat hippocampal CA1 region (Izaki et al., 1999). Collective evidence suggests that DHA is crucial for the induction of long-term potentiation (LTP).

DHA also blocks the induction of long-term depression (LTD), which requires the activation of NMDA receptors in hippocampal CA1 neurons (Young et al., 1998). The molecular mechanism of this process remains unknown. Based on paired-pulse facilitation profiles, DHA is likely to act on postsynaptic sites (Zucker, 1989). Addition of an NMDA receptor antagonist has no effect on DHA-mediated alterations in LTD; therefore NMDA receptors are not involved in this process (Itokazu et al., 2000). Furthermore, DHA inhibits function of the K^+ channels (Honore et al., 1994; Poling et al., 1995). Since the K^+ channel blocker, tetraethylammonium ion, induces NMDA-independent long-lasting modulation in the Schaffer collateral-CA1 synapses of hippocampal slices (Aniksztejn and Ben Ari, 1991), it is likely that DHA acts through modulation of the K^+ channel. Another possibility is that DHA blocks GABA-induced chloride channel activity and potentiates NMDA responses of dissociated rat substantia nigra neurons (Nabekura et al., 1998). Based on this observation, DHA may improve memory formation by blocking the inhibitory actions of GABA on LTP (Das, 2003). Collectively, these studies suggest that the complete blockade of NMDA receptors prevents both LTP and LTD induction, whereas a moderate concentration of the NMDA antagonist, D-APV, shifts the direction of synaptic plasticity to the induction of LTD (Young et al., 1998).

In transgenic mice overexpressing the Tg2576 gene, a DHA deficiency induced by safflower oil caused decreased NMDA receptor subunits, NR2A and NR2B, in the cortex and hippocampus with no loss of the presynaptic markers, synaptophysin and synaptosomal-associated protein 25. Dietary supplementation with DHA partly protects the mice from NMDA receptor subunit loss. Thus, DHA stabilizes the structure of NMDA receptors (Calon et al., 2005). Collectively, these studies suggest that DHA not only improves cognitive development but also increases neuroplasticity of neural membranes. These processes contribute to synaptogenesis and may be involved in synaptic transmission.

6.4.4 DHA and Apoptotic Cell Death

DHA has antiapoptotic effects in rat retinal photoreceptor cells, HL-60 cells subjected to sphingosine-mediated apoptosis, and Neuro 2A cells subjected to serum starvation-mediated cell death (Rotstein et al., 1997; Kishida et al., 1998; Rotstein et al., 1998; Kim et al., 2000). The molecular mechanism underlying the antiapoptotic effects of DHA remains unknown. However, the translocation of Raf-1 kinase, reduction in caspase-3 activity, and inhibition of the phosphatidylinositol 3-kinase pathway by DHA may be involved in the prevention of apoptotic cell death induced by staurosporine in Neuro 2A cells (Kim et al., 2000; Akbar and Kim, 2002; Akbar et al., 2005). DHA promotes neuronal survival by facilitating membrane translocation/activation of Akt (a serine/threonine kinase involved in cell survival) through its capacity to increase PtdSer. Docosapentaenoic acid (22:5 n-6), which replaces DHA during n-3 deficiency, was less effective in accumulating PtdSer and translocating Akt and thus less effective in preventing apoptotic cell death (Akbar et al., 2005). The extent of the antiapoptotic effect of DHA correlates with a time-dependent increase in the PtdSer content. Treatment of Neuro 2A cells with DHA in serine-free culture medium has no effect on caspase-3 and phosphatidylinositol 3-kinase activities. Thus, an increase in PtdSer content is necessary for staurosporine-induced apoptosis.

In contrast, in non-neural tumor cells and HL-60 cells, DHA increases apoptotic cell death (Siddiqui et al., 2001; Miura et al., 2004). In Jurkat leukemic cells the increase in apoptotic cell death can be blocked by phosphatidic acid (PtdH). PtdH may exert its antiapoptotic effects by inhibiting a protein phosphatase activity. Thus, the activation of protein phosphatase activity is one of the regulatory steps in DHA-mediated apoptosis in Jurkat leukemic cells, and inhibition of this enzyme by PtdH causes increased cell survival by inhibiting the apoptotic process. DHA not only increases ceramide levels, but also reduces the amount of phosphorylated retinoblastoma protein (pRb), a protein involved in the cell cycle and growth. The levels of cyclin A are reduced, while the levels of p21 WAF1 (a cellular inhibitor of cyclin A/cyclin-dependent kinase 2, cdk2) activity are markedly increased in Jurkat leukemic cells (Siddiqui et al., 2003). The net effect of cdk2 inhibition and protein phosphatase activation is apparently an inhibition of pRb phosphorylation and arrest of Jurkat leukemic cell growth (Siddiqui et al., 2001, 2003). Thus, DHA induces cell cycle arrest and apoptosis by activating protein phosphatases. Besides dephosphorylation of retinoblastoma protein, protein phosphatases also interact with bcl2, an apoptotic protein that regulates the release of cytochrome c from mitochondria, and eventually, activation of caspase-3 (Bougnoux, 1999; Siddiqui et al., 2004).

6.4.5 DHA and Generation of Docosanoids

DHA is not a substrate for cyclooxygenase. The action of an enzyme resembling 15-lipoxygenase on DHA produces docosatrienes, resolvins, and protectins (Fig. 6.5) (Hong et al., 2003; Marcheselli et al., 2003; Serhan et al., 2004; Serhan, 2005a). These lipid mediators are collectively called docosanoids. They antagonize the effects of eicosanoids, modulate leukocyte trafficking, and downregulate

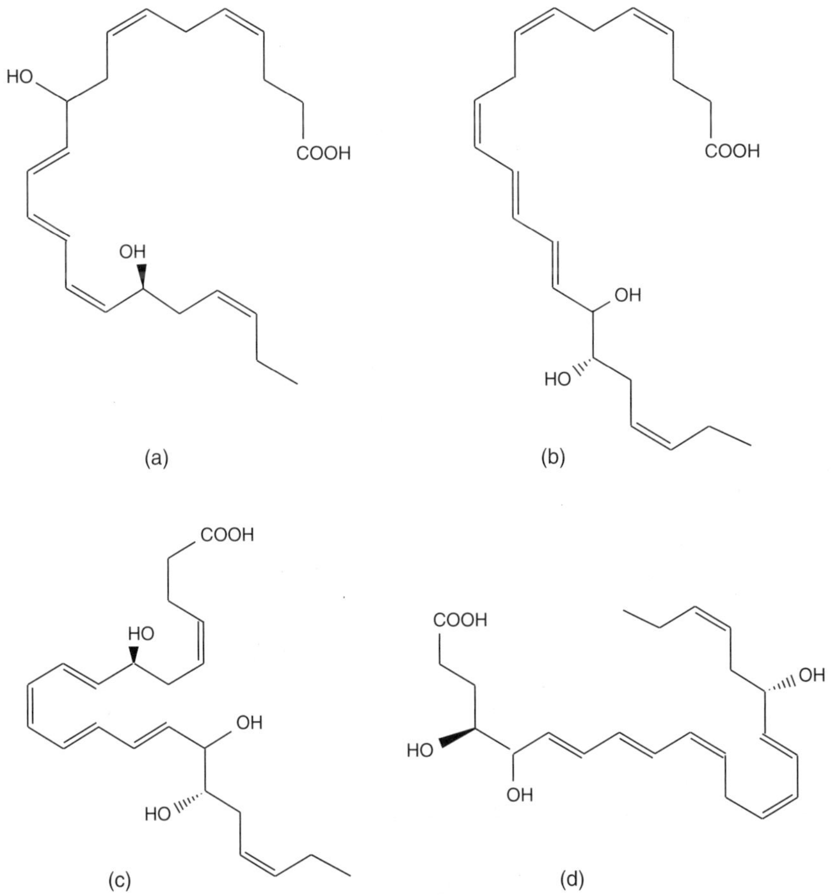

FIG. 6.5. Structures of resolvins and docosatrienes. 10,17 S-Docosatriene (a); 16,17 S-docosatrienes (b); 7S,16,17 S-resolvin (c); and 4S,5,17 S-resolvin (d). These metabolites retard the generation of eicosanoids from arachidonic acid.

the expression of cytokines in glial cells (Hong et al., 2003; Marcheselli et al., 2003; Serhan et al., 2004). Thus docosanoids slow down the inflammatory cycle induced and maintained by the action of cytokines on astrocytes. The neuroprotectins comprise docosatrienes and resolvins of the D series (Serhan, 2005a). The infusion of neuroprotectin D1 (NPD1), following ischemic reperfusion injury or during oxidative stress in cell culture, downregulates oxidative stress and apoptotic DNA damage. NPD1 also upregulates the antiapoptotic Bcl-2 proteins, Bcl-2 and bclxL, and decreases the expression of the proapoptotic proteins, Bax and Bad (Bazan, 2005). Furthermore, this metabolite inhibits caspase-3 activity and blocks IL-1-mediated expression of cyclooxygenase-2. Similarly, in injured mouse corneas, treatment with NPD1 increases the rate of re-epithelialization and attenuates the sequence and effect of thermal injury (Gronert et al., 2005). The cellular mechanism by which NPD1 exerts its effect on wound healing remains unknown. However, NPD1 may have a receptor-mediated effect on epithelial cell proliferation (Gronert et al., 2005). In contrast, the proinflammatory eicosanoids have no impact on corneal re-epithelialization.

Resolvins (RvD1 to RvD6) are generated from DHA, whereas eicosapentaenoic acid is the precursor for resolvin RvE1 (Fig. 6.6). Specific receptors for docosatrienes and resolvins occur in neural and non-neural tissues. These receptors include resolvin D receptors (resoDR1), resolvin E receptors (resoER1), and neuroprotectin D receptors (NPDR). Orphan receptor ChemR23 is a specific G protein–coupled receptor for RvE1 (Flower and Perretti, 2005; Arita et al., 2005). RvE1 dramatically reduces dermal inflammation, peritonitis, dendritic cell migration, and interleukin 12 production (Arita et al., 2005). Characterization of these receptors in brain tissue is in progress (Hong et al., 2003; Marcheselli et al., 2003; Mukherjee et al., 2004; Serhan et al., 2004). The D class resolvins block tumor necrosis factor α-induced interleukin (IL)-1β release from microglial cells and are potent regulators of PMN infiltration in brain (Serhan et al., 2004). Thus, both docosatrienes and resolvins suppress inflammatory reactions by blocking the expression of proinflammatory cytokines and modulating adhesion molecule expression following ischemia and oxidative stress-mediated neural cell injury. In brain tissue, docosanoids not only promote resolution, but also protect neural cells from oxidative stress (Bannenberg et al., 2005; Ariel et al., 2005; Chen and Bazan, 2005; Lukiw et al., 2005). Collectively these studies suggest that the generation of docosanoids may be an internal neuroprotective mechanism for preventing brain damage (Hong et al., 2003; Marcheselli et al., 2003; Mukherjee et al., 2004; Bazan, 2005; Lukiw et al., 2005; Serhan, 2005b).

6.4.6 DHA and the Immune Response

Immune response is a complex host defense mechanism directed against the invading antigens. It involves components of the complement system, synthesis of immunoglobulins, and generation of proinflammatory cytokines by mononuclear phagocytes, astrocytes, and microglial cells. These cells are involved in the clearance of antigens. Low intakes of DHA enhance certain immune functions, whereas high intakes are inhibitory on a wide range of immune functions, such

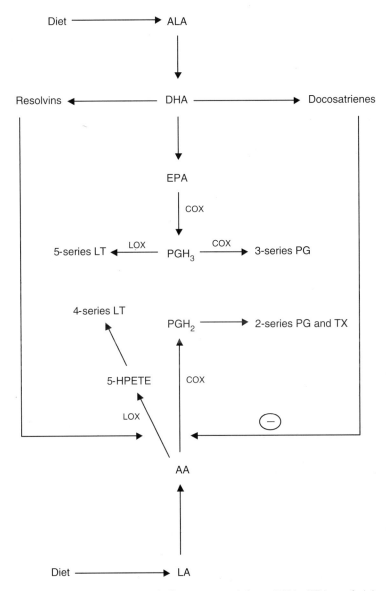

FIG. 6.6. Interactions among metabolites generated from DHA, EPA, and AA. ALA (α–linolenic acid), LA (linoleic acid), DHA (docosahexaenoic acid), EPA (eicosapentaenoic acid), AA (arachidonic acid), COX (cyclooxygenase), LOX (lipoxygenase), PG (prostaglandins), LT (leukotrienes), and 5-HPETE (5-hydroperoxyeicosatetraenoic acid). Resolvins and docosatrienes inhibit the generation of metabolites generated from AA.

as antigen presentation and adhesion molecule expression (Harbige, 2003). DHA also suppresses the production of eicosanoids and cytokines and modulates adhesion molecule expression. These effects occur at the level of altered gene expression (Calder, 1998, 2003b, 2004; Calder and Grimble, 2002).

Intake or administration of DHA decreases AA levels and competitively inhibits the oxygenation of arachidonic acid by cyclooxygenases and suppresses the production of PGE_2 and LTB_4 (Calder, 2003a, 2004) (Fig. 6.6), and proinflammatory cytokines, such as interleukin-1, interleukin-6, and tumor necrosis factor-α (Caughey et al., 1996; Wu and Meydani, 1998). DHA inhibits concanavalin A-induced proliferation and decreases IL-2 and interferon-γ production in Jurkat cells (Verlengia et al., 2004a). DHA alters lipid components of microdomains, which modifies the IL-2-mediated Janus kinase-signal transducer and activator of transcription (STAT) signaling pathway by partially displacing IL-2 receptors from microdomains. It also decreases lymphocyte proliferation and natural killer cell activity, but increases macrophages. DHA regulates lipid homeostasis and shifts the metabolic pathways toward energy supply. This optimizes the function of immune cells. Due to the regulatory impact on different processes of inflammatory and immune cell activation, DHA induces positive effects on various states of immune deficiencies and diseases with hyperinflammatory character (Grimm et al., 2002). Collectively, these studies provide evidence for a functional modification in lipid domains by DHA treatment and explain PUFA-mediated immunosuppressive and autoimmune effects in humans and animals (Horrocks and Farooqui, 2004; Li et al., 2005).

6.4.7 DHA Intake, Oxidative Stress, and Other Side Effects

DHA has 6 *cis* double bonds, which are susceptible to free radical attack and generation of lipid peroxides and aldehyde breakdown products, particularly when the intake of antioxidants such as vitamin E is low. A high intake of encapsulated DHA without concomitant supplementation with vitamin E may exceed the protective capacity of the antioxidant defense systems and can increase plasma indices of oxidative stress (Brown and Wahle, 1990; Nair et al., 1993; Grundt et al., 2003). This can cause myopathies and neuropathies in animals (Combs, Jr. et al., 1975). This is evidenced by an increase in thiobarbituric acid-reactive substances or conjugated diene formation. Contrary to the above view, lipid peroxidation in fetal brain decreases following intra-amniotic administration of ethyl docosahexaenoate in pregnant rats. This finding has been explained by a shift in oxygen utilization via cyclooxygenase and nitric oxide synthase (Green et al., 2001a,b; Mori, 2004). An additional support to the above view comes from studies on aged rats treated with DHA. DHA intake or administration reduces lipid peroxidation and reactive oxygen species in the cerebral cortex and hippocampus of Aβ-infused and aged rats (Hossain et al., 1998, 1999). The preferential incorporation of DHA into PlsEtn, PtdSer, and PtdEtn, which are located in the inner lipid bilayer, may be another plausible antioxidant mechanism to protect DHA in neural membranes from lipid peroxidation. Thus the presence of DHA in neural membranes serves as an antioxidant mechanism in certain regions of rat brain (Hashimoto et al., 2005).

The best sources of DHA are fish and fish oil. High doses of fish oil increase bleeding time, but there is no clinical evidence for increased risk of bleeding in subjects consuming fish oil. The most common adverse effects of fish oil include fishy taste in the mouth, nausea, and gastrointestinal discomfort with belching and bloating (Carroll and Roth, 2002). Although immune responses may be weakened by DHA intake, there is no evidence that intake of DHA is associated with an increased risk of cancer or serious infection (Horrocks and Farooqui, 2004; Li et al., 2005).

In conclusion, DHA modulates membrane fluidity and participates in signal transduction and synaptic plasticity by regulating neurotransmitter release and uptake. DHA also decreases the generation of inflammatory mediators and the expression of adhesion molecules following neural cell injury. In brain, DHA acts through direct as well as indirect mechanisms. The direct mechanism includes the replacement of AA by DHA in neural membranes, thereby limiting the production of AA-generated metabolites. DHA is a substrate for generation of lipid mediators, the docosanoids. These mediators inhibit the activities of cyclooxygenases and lipoxygenases (Corey et al., 1983; Phillis et al., 2006). Indirect mechanisms involve alterations in the expression of inflammatory cytokines and transcription factors. Through these mechanisms, DHA modulates the expression of genes controlling synaptic plasticity, dendrite formation, signal transduction, energy metabolism, and cellular growth.

References

Ahmad A., Moriguchi T., and Salem N. J. (2002). Decrease in neuron size in docosahexaenoic acid-deficient brain. *Pediatr. Neurol.* 26:210–218.

Akbar M., Calderon F., Wen Z. M., and Kim H. Y. (2005). Docosahexaenoic acid: a positive modulator of Akt signaling in neuronal survival. *Proc. Natl Acad. Sci. USA* 102:10858–10863.

Akbar M. and Kim H. Y. (2002). Protective effects of docosahexaenoic acid in staurosporine-induced apoptosis: involvement of phosphatidylinositol-3 kinase pathway. *J. Neurochem.* 82:655–665.

Aniksztejn L. and Ben Ari Y. (1991). Novel form of long-term potentiation produced by a K+ channel blocker in the hippocampus. *Nature* 349:67–69.

Ariel A., Li P. L., Wang W., Tang W. X., Hong S., Gotlinger K. H., and Serhan C. N. (2005). The novel docosatriene, Protectin D1, produced by TH2-polarization promotes human T cell apoptosis via lipid-raft clustering. *Clin. Immunol.* 115:S263.

Arita M., Bianchini F., Aliberti J., Sher A., Chiang N., Hong S., Yang R., Petasis N. A., and Serhan C. N. (2005). Stereochemical assignment, antiinflammatory properties, and receptor for the omega-3 lipid mediator resolvin E1. *J. Exp. Med.* 201:713–722.

Bannenberg G. L., Chiang N., Ariel A., Arita M., Tjonahen E., Gotlinger K. H., Hong S., and Serhan C. N. (2005). Molecular circuits of resolution: formation and actions of resolvins and protectins. *J. Immunol.* 174:4345–4355.

Barceló-Coblijn G., Kitajka K., Puskás L. G., Hõgyes E., Zvara A., Hackler L., Jr., and Farkas T. (2003). Gene expression and molecular composition of phospholipids in rat brain in relation to dietary *n*-6 to *n*-3 fatty acid ratio. *Biochim. Biophys. Acta* 1632:72–79.

Bazan N. G. (2005). Neuroprotectin D1 (NPD1): a DHA-derived mediator that protects brain and retina against cell injury-induced oxidative stress. *Brain Pathol.* 15:159–166.

Berry C. B., Hayes D., Murphy A., Wiessner M., Rauen T., and McBean G. J. (2005). Differential modulation of the glutamate transporters GLT1, GLAST and EAAC1 by docosahexaenoic acid. *Brain Res.* 1037:123–133.

Bougnoux P. (1999). n-3 Polyunsaturated fatty acids and cancer. *Curr. Opin. Clin. Nutr. Metab. Care* 2:121–126.

Brown J. E. and Wahle K. W. J. (1990). Effect of fish-oil and vitamin E supplementation on lipid peroxidation and whole-blood aggregation in man. *Clin. Chim. Acta* 193:147–156.

Calder P. C. (1998). Dietary fatty acids and the immune system. *Nutr. Rev.* 56:S70–S83.

Calder P. C. (2003a). Long-chain n-3 fatty acids and inflammation: potential application in surgical and trauma patients. *Braz. J. Med. Biol. Res.* 36:433–446.

Calder P. C. (2003b). n-3 polyunsaturated fatty acids and inflammation: from molecular biology to the clinic. *Lipids* 38:343–352.

Calder P. C. (2004). n-3 fatty acids, inflammation, and immunity – relevance to postsurgical and critically ill patients. *Lipids* 39:1147–1161.

Calder P. C. and Grimble R. F. (2002). Polyunsaturated fatty acids, inflammation and immunity. *Eur. J. Clin. Nutr.* 56:S14–S19.

Calderon F. and Kim H. Y. (2004). Docosahexaenoic acid promotes neurite growth in hippocampal neurons. *J. Neurochem.* 90:979–988.

Calon F., Lim G. P., Morihara T., Yang F. S., Ubeda O., Salem N. J., Frautschy S. A., and Cole G. M. (2005). Dietary n-3 polyunsaturated fatty acid depletion activates caspases and decreases NMDA receptors in the brain of a transgenic mouse model of Alzheimer's disease. *Eur. J. Neurosci.* 22:617–626.

Cao D. H., Xue R. H., Xu J., and Liu Z. L. (2005). Effects of docosahexaenoic acid on the survival and neurite outgrowth of rat cortical neurons in primary cultures. *J. Nutr. Biochem.* 16:538–546.

Carrie I., Clement M., De Javel D., Frances H., and Bourre J. M. (2000). Specific phospholipid fatty acid composition of brain regions in mice. Effects of n-3 polyunsaturated fatty acid deficiency and phospholipid supplementation. *J. Lipid Res.* 41:465–472.

Carroll D. N. and Roth M. T. (2002). Evidence for the cardioprotective effects of omega-3 fatty acids. *Ann. Pharmacother.* 36:1950–1956.

Caughey G. E., Mantzioris E., Gibson R. A., Cleland L. G., and James M. J. (1996). The effect on human tumor necrosis factor alpha and interleukin 1 beta production of diets enriched in n-3 fatty acids from vegetable oil or fish oil. *Am. J. Clin. Nutr.* 63:116–122.

Chalon S., Delion-Vancassel S., Belzung C., Guilloteau D., Leguisquet A. M., Besnard J. C., and Durand G. (1998). Dietary fish oil affects monoaminergic neurotransmission and behavior in rats. *J. Nutr.* 128:2512–2519.

Chen C. and Bazan N. G. (2005). Lipid signaling: sleep, synaptic plasticity, and neuroprotection. *Prostaglandins Other Lipid Mediat.* 77:65–76.

Clarke S. D. (2000). Polyunsaturated fatty acid regulation of gene transcription: a mechanism to improve energy balance and insulin resistance. *Br. J. Nutr.* 83(Suppl. 1):S59–S66.

Cline H. T. (2001). Dendritic arbor development and synaptogenesis. *Curr. Opin. Neurobiol.* 11:118–126.

Combs G. F., Jr., Noguchi T., and Scott M. L. (1975). Mechanisms of action of selenium and vitamin E in protection of biological membranes. *Fed. Proc.* 34:2090–2095.

Corey E. J., Shih C., and Cashman J. R. (1983). Docosahexaenoic acid is a strong inhibitor of prostaglandin but not leukotriene biosynthesis. *Proc. Natl Acad. Sci. USA* 80:3581–3584.

Das U. N. (2003). Long-chain polyunsaturated fatty acids in memory formation and consolidation: further evidence and discussion. *Nutrition* 19:988–993.

de Urquiza A. M., Liu S., Sjöberg M., Zetterström R. H., Griffiths W., Sjövall J., and Perlmann T. (2000). Docosahexaenoic acid, a ligand for the retinoid X receptor in mouse brain. *Science* 290:2140–2144.

Delton-Vandenbroucke I., Vericel E., Janueli C., Carreras M., Lecomte M., and Lagarde M. (2001). Dual regulation of glutathione peroxidase by docosahexaenoic acid in endothelial cells depending on concentration and vascular bed origin. *Free Radic. Biol. Med.* 30:895–904.

DeMar J. C. J., Ma K. Z., Bell J. M., and Rapoport S. I. (2004). Half-lives of docosahexaenoic acid in rat brain phospholipids are prolonged by 15 weeks of nutritional deprivation of n-3 polyunsaturated fatty acids. *J. Neurochem.* 91:1125–1137.

Denys A., Hichami A., and Khan N. A. (2005). n-3PUFAs modulate T-cell activation via protein kinase C-α and -ε and the NF-κ B signaling pathway. *J. Lipid Res.* 46:752–758.

Duncan R. E., El Sohemy A., and Archer M. C. (2005). Regulation of HMG-CoA reductase in MCF-7 cells by genistein, EPA, and DHA, alone and in combination with mevastatin. *Cancer Lett.* 224:221–228.

Farkas T., Kitajka K., Fodor E., Csengeri I., Lahdes E., Yeo Y. K., Krasznai Z., and Halver J. E. (2000). Docosahexaenoic acid-containing phospholipid molecular species in brains of vertebrates. *Proc. Natl Acad. Sci. USA* 97:6362–6366.

Farooqui A. A., Antony P., Ong W. Y., Horrocks L. A., and Freysz L. (2004). Retinoic acid-mediated phospholipase A$_2$ signaling in the nucleus. *Brain Res. Rev.* 45:179–195.

Farooqui A. A. and Horrocks L. A. (1985). Metabolic and functional aspects of neural membrane phospholipids. In: Horrocks L. A., Kanfer J. N., and Porcellati G. (eds.), *Phospholipids in the Nervous System, Vol. II: Physiological Role*. Raven Press, New York, pp. 341–348.

Farooqui A. A. and Horrocks L. A. (2001a). Plasmalogens, phospholipase A$_2$, and docosahexaenoic acid turnover in brain tissue. *J. Mol. Neurosci.* 16:263–272.

Farooqui A. A. and Horrocks L. A. (2001b). Plasmalogens: workhorse lipids of membranes in normal and injured neurons and glia. *Neuroscientist* 7:232–245.

Farooqui A. A., Horrocks L. A., and Farooqui T. (2000a). Deacylation and reacylation of neural membrane glycerophospholipids. *J. Mol. Neurosci.* 14:123–135.

Farooqui A. A., Horrocks L. A., and Farooqui T. (2000b). Glycerophospholipids in brain: their metabolism, incorporation into membranes, functions, and involvement in neurological disorders. *Chem. Phys. Lipids* 106:1–29.

Farooqui A. A., Ong W. Y., and Horrocks L. A. (2003). Plasmalogens, docosahexaenoic acid, and neurological disorders. In: Roels F., Baes M., and de Bies S. (eds.), *Peroxisomal Disorders and Regulation of Genes*. Kluwer Academic/Plenum Publishers, London, pp. 335–354.

Farooqui A. A., Ong W. Y., and Horrocks L. A. (2006). Inhibitors of brain phospholipase A$_2$ activity: their neuropharmacologic effects and therapeutic importance for the treatment of neurologic disorders. *Pharm. Rev.* (in press).

Feller S. E. and Gawrisch K. (2005). Properties of docosahexaenoic-acid-containing lipids and their influence on the function of rhodopsin. *Curr. Opin. Struct. Biol.* 15:416–422.

Fernstrom J. D. (1999). Effects of dietary polyunsaturated fatty acids on neuronal function. *Lipids* 34:161–169.

Ferrier G. R., Redondo I., Zhu J. Q., and Murphy M. G. (2002). Differential effects of docosahexaenoic acid on contractions and L-type Ca^{2+} current in adult cardiac myocytes. *Cardiovasc. Res.* 54:601–610.

Flower R. J. and Perretti M. (2005). Controlling inflammation: a fat chance? *J. Exp. Med.* 201:671–674.

Fujimoto K., Yao K., Miyazaki T., Hirano H., Nishikawa M., Kimura S., Murayama K., and Nonaka M. (1989). The effect of dietary docosahexaenoate on the learning ability of rats. In: Chandra R. K. (ed.), *Health Effects of Fish and Fish Oils*. ARTS Biomedical, The Netherlands, pp. 275–284.

Fujita S., Ikegaya Y., Nishikawa M., Nishiyama N., and Matsuki N. (2001). Docosahexaenoic acid improves long-term potentiation attenuated by phospholipase A_2 inhibitor in rat hippocampal slices. *Br. J. Pharmacol.* 132:1417–1422.

Garcia M. C. and Kim H. Y. (1997). Mobilization of arachidonate and docosahexaenoate by stimulation of the 5-HT$_{2A}$ receptor in rat C6 glioma cells. *Brain Res.* 768:43–48.

Gerbi A., Zérouga M., Debray M., Durand G., Chanez C., and Bourre J. M. (1994). Effect of fish oil diet on fatty acid composition of phospholipids of brain membranes and on kinetic properties of Na^+, K^+-ATPase isoenzymes of weaned and adult rats. *J. Neurochem.* 62:1560–1569.

Green P., Glozman S., Weiner L., and Yavin E. (2001a). Enhanced free radical scavenging and decreased lipid peroxidation in the rat fetal brain after treatment with ethyl docosahexaenoate. *Biochim. Biophys. Acta Mol. Cell Biol. Lipids* 1532:203–212.

Green P., Glozman S., and Yavin E. (2001b). Ethyl docosahexaenoate-associated decrease in fetal brain lipid peroxide production is mediated by activation of prostanoid and nitric oxide pathways. *Biochim. Biophys. Acta Mol. Cell Biol. Lipids* 1531:156–164.

Grimm H., Mayer K., Mayser P., and Eigenbrodt E. (2002). Regulatory potential of n-3 fatty acids in immunological and inflammatory processes. *Br. J. Nutr.* 87:S59–S67.

Gronert K., Maheshwari N., Khan N., Hassan I. R., Dunn M., and Schwartzman M. L. (2005). A role for the mouse 12/15-lipoxygenase pathway in promoting epithelial wound healing and host defense. *J. Biol. Chem.* 280:15267–15278.

Grundt H., Nilsen D. W., Mansoor M. A., and Nordøy A. (2003). Increased lipid peroxidation during long-term intervention with high doses of n-3 fatty acids (PUFAs) following an acute myocardial infarction. *Eur. J. Clin. Nutr.* 57:793–800.

Hamano H., Nabekura J., Nishikawa M., and Ogawa T. (1996). Docosahexaenoic acid reduces GABA response in substantia nigra neuron of rat. *J. Neurophysiol.* 75:1264–1270.

Hamilton J., Greiner R., Salem N., Jr., and Kim H. Y. (2000). n-3 fatty acid deficiency decreases phosphatidylserine accumulation selectively in neuronal tissues. *Lipids* 35:863–869.

Harbige L. S. (2003). Fatty acids, the immune response, and autoimmunity: a question of n-6 essentiality and the balance between n-6 and n-3. *Lipids* 38:323–341.

Hashimoto M., Hossain M. S., Yamasaki H., Yazawa K., and Masumura S. (1999). Effects of eicosapentaenoic acid and docosahexaenoic acid on plasma membrane fluidity of aortic endothelial cells. *Lipids* 34:1297–1304.

Hashimoto M., Hossain S., Shimada T., Sugioka K., Yamasaki H., Fujii Y., Ishibashi Y., Oka J. I., and Shido O. (2002). Docosahexaenoic acid provides protection from impairment of learning ability in Alzheimer's disease model rats. *J. Neurochem.* 81:1084–1091.

Hashimoto M., Tanabe Y., Fujii Y., Kikuta T., Shibata H., and Shido O. (2005). Chronic administration of docosahexaenoic acid ameliorates the impairment of spatial cognition learning ability in amyloid β-infused rats. *J. Nutr.* 135:549–555.

Hirafuji M., Machida T., Hamaue N., and Minami M. (2003). Cardiovascular protective effects of n-3 polyunsaturated fatty acids with special emphasis on docosahexaenoic acid. *J. Pharmacol. Sci.* 92:308–316.

Hogyes E., Nyakas C., Kiliaan A., Farkas T., Penke B., and Luiten P. G. (2003). Neuroprotective effect of developmental docosahexaenoic acid supplement against excitotoxic brain damage in infant rats. *Neuroscience* 119:999–1012.

Hong S., Gronert K., Devchand P. R., Moussignac R. L., and Serhan C. N. (2003). Novel docosatrienes and 17S-resolvins generated from docosahexaenoic acid in murine brain, human blood, and glial cells – autacoids in anti-inflammation. *J. Biol. Chem.* 278:14677–14687.

Honore E., Barhanin J., Attali B., Lesage F., and Lazdunski M. (1994). External blockade of the major cardiac delayed-rectifier K+ channel (Kv1.5) by polyunsaturated fatty acids. *Proc. Natl Acad. Sci. USA* 91:1937–1941.

Horrocks L. A. and Farooqui A. A. (2004). Docosahexaenoic acid in the diet: its importance in maintenance and restoration of neural membrane function. *Prostaglandins Leukot. Essent. Fatty Acids* 70:361–372.

Horrocks L. A. and Yeo Y. K. (1999). Health benefits of docosahexaenoic acid (DHA). *Pharmacol. Res.* 40:211–225.

Hossain M. S., Hashimoto M., Gamoh S., and Masumura S. (1999). Antioxidative effects of docosahexaenoic acid in the cerebrum versus cerebellum and brainstem of aged hypercholesterolemic rats. *J. Neurochem.* 72:1133–1138.

Hossain M. S., Hashimoto M., and Masumura S. (1998). Influence of docosahexaenoic acid on cerebral lipid peroxide level in aged rats with and without hypercholesterolemia. *Neurosci. Lett.* 244:157–160.

Huster D., Arnold K., and Gawrisch K. (1998). Influence of docosahexaenoic acid and cholesterol on lateral lipid organization in phospholipid mixtures. *Biochemistry* 37:17299–17308.

Ikemoto A., Kobayashi T., Emoto K., Umeda M., Watanabe S., and Okuyama H. (1999). Effects of docosahexaenoic and arachidonic acids on the synthesis and distribution of aminophospholipids during neuronal differentiation of PC12 cells. *Arch. Biochem. Biophys.* 364:67–74.

Ikemoto A., Kobayashi T., Watanabe S., and Okuyama H. (1997). Membrane fatty acid modifications of PC12 cells by arachidonate or docosahexaenoate affect neurite outgrowth but not norepinephrine release. *Neurochem. Res.* 22:671–678.

Ikemoto A., Ohishi M., Hata N., Misawa Y., Fujii Y., and Okuyama H. (2000). Effect of n-3 fatty acid deficiency on fatty acid composition and metabolism of aminophospholipids in rat brain synaptosomes. *Lipids* 35:1107–1115.

Innis S. M. and Dyer R. A. (2002). Brain astrocyte synthesis of docosahexaenoic acid from n-3 fatty acids is limited at the elongation of docosapentaenoic acid. *J. Lipid Res.* 43:1529–1536.

Itokazu N., Ikegaya Y., Nishikawa M., and Matsuki N. (2000). Bidirectional actions of docosahexaenoic acid on hippocampal neurotransmissions in vivo. *Brain Res.* 862:211–216.

Izaki Y., Hashimoto M., and Arita J. (1999). Enhancement by 1-oleoyl-2-docosahexaenoyl phosphatidylcholine of long-term potentiation in the rat hippocampal CA1 region. *Neurosci. Lett.* 260:146–148.

James M. J., Gibson R. A., and Cleland L. G. (2000). Dietary polyunsaturated fatty acids and inflammatory mediator production. *Am. J. Clin. Nutr.* 71:343S–348S.

Jan Y. N. and Jan L. Y. (2001). Dendrites. *Genes Dev.* 15:2627–2641.

Jan Y. N. and Jan L. Y. (2003). The control of dendrite development. *Neuron* 40:229–242.

Jones C. R., Arai T., and Rapoport S. I. (1997). Evidence for the involvement of docosahexaenoic acid in cholinergic stimulated signal transduction at the synapse. *Neurochem. Res.* 22:663–670.

Jump D. B. (2002a). Dietary polyunsaturated fatty acids and regulation of gene transcription. *Curr. Opin. Lipidol.* 13:155–164.

Jump D. B. (2002b). The biochemistry of *n*-3 polyunsaturated fatty acids. *J. Biol. Chem.* 277:8755–8758.

Kim H. Y., Akbar M., Lau A., and Edsall L. (2000). Inhibition of neuronal apoptosis by docosahexaenoic acid (22:6n-3). Role of phosphatidylserine in antiapoptotic effect. *J. Biol. Chem.* 275:35215–35223.

Kim H. Y., Edsall L., and Ma Y. C. (1996). Specificity of polyunsaturated fatty acid release from rat brain synaptosomes. *Lipids* 31(Suppl.):S229–S233.

Kishida E., Yano M., Kasahara M., and Masuzawa Y. (1998). Distinctive inhibitory activity of docosahexaenoic acid against sphingosine-induced apoptosis. *Biochim. Biophys. Acta Lipids Lipid Metab.* 1391:401–408.

Kitajka K., Puskás L. G., Zvara A., Hackler L. J., Barceló-Coblijn G., Yeo Y. K., and Farkas T. (2002). The role of n-3 polyunsaturated fatty acids in brain: modulation of rat brain gene expression by dietary n-3 fatty acids. *Proc. Natl Acad. Sci. USA* 99:2619–2624.

Langelier B., Alessandri J. M., Perruchot M. H., Guesnet P., and Lavialle M. (2005). Changes of the transcriptional and fatty acid profiles in response to n-3 fatty acids in SH-SY5Y neuroblastoma cells. *Lipids* 40:719–728.

Lauritzen L., Hansen H. S., Jorgensen M. H., and Michaelsen K. F. (2001). The essentiality of long chain n-3 fatty acids in relation to development and function of the brain and retina. *Prog. Lipid Res.* 40:1–94.

Lengqvist J., Mata de Urquiza A., Bergman A. C., Willson T. M., Sjövall J., Perlmann T., and Griffiths W. J. (2004). Polyunsaturated fatty acids including docosahexaenoic and arachidonic acid bind to the retinoid X receptor α ligand-binding domain. *Mol. Cell. Proteomics* 3:692–703.

Li Q. R., Wang M., Tan L., Wang C., Ma J., Li N., Li Y. S., Xu G. W., and Li J. S. (2005). Docosahexaenoic acid changes lipid composition and interleukin-2 receptor signaling in membrane rafts. *J. Lipid Res.* 46:1904–1913.

Litman B. J. and Mitchell D. C. (1996). A role for phospholipid polyunsaturation in modulating membrane protein function. *Lipids* 31(Suppl.):S193–S197.

Lonergan P. E., Martin D. S. D., Horrobin D. F., and Lynch M. A. (2004). Neuroprotective actions of eicosapentaenoic acid on lipopolysaccharide-induced dysfunction in rat hippocampus. *J. Neurochem.* 91:20–29.

Lu X. R., Ong W. Y., Halliwell B., Horrocks L. A., and Farooqui A. A. (2001). Differential effects of calcium-dependent and calcium-independent phospholipase A_2 inhibitors on kainate-induced neuronal injury in rat hippocampal slices. *Free Radic. Biol. Med.* 30:1263–1273.

Lukiw W. J., Cui J. G., Marcheselli V. L., Bodker M., Botkjaer A., Gotlinger K., Serhan C. N., and Bazan N. G. (2005). A role for docosahexaenoic acid-derived neuroprotectin D1 in neural cell survival and Alzheimer disease. *J. Clin. Invest.* 115:2774–2783.

Ma D. W. L., Seo J., Switzer K. C., Fan Y. Y., McMurray D. N., Lupton J. R., and Chapkin R. S. (2004). n-3 PUFA and membrane microdomains: a new frontier in bioactive lipid research. *J. Nutr. Biochem.* 15:700–706.

Marcheselli V. L., Hong S., Lukiw W. J., Tian X. H., Gronert K., Musto A., Hardy M., Gimenez J. M., Chiang N., Serhan C. N., and Bazan N. G. (2003). Novel docosanoids inhibit brain ischemia-reperfusion-mediated leukocyte infiltration and pro-inflammatory gene expression. *J. Biol. Chem.* 278:43807–43817.

Marszalek J. R., Kitidis C., DiRusso C. C., and Lodish H. F. (2005). Long-chain acyl-CoA synthetase 6 preferentially promotes DHA metabolism. *J. Biol. Chem.* 280:10817–10826.

Martin R. E. (1998). Docosahexaenoic acid decreases phospholipase A_2 activity in the neurites/nerve growth cones of PC12 cells. *J. Neurosci. Res.* 54:805–813.

Martin R. E., Wickham J. Q., Om A. S., Sanders J., and Ceballos N. (2000). Uptake and incorporation of docosahexaenoic acid (DHA) into neuronal cell body and neurite/nerve growth cone lipids: evidence of compartmental DHA metabolism in nerve growth factor-differentiated PC12 cells. *Neurochem. Res.* 25:715–723.

Mitchell D. C., Gawrisch K., Litman B. J., and Salem N., Jr. (1998). Why is docosahexaenoic acid essential for nervous system function? *Biochem. Soc. Trans.* 26:365–370.

Miura Y., Takahara K., Murata Y., Utsumi K., Tada M., and Takahata K. (2004). Docosahexaenoic acid induces apoptosis via the bax-independent pathway in HL-60 cells. *Biosci. Biotechnol. Biochem.* 68:2415–2417.

Mori T. A. (2004). Effect of fish and fish oil-derived omega-3 fatty acids on lipid oxidation. *Redox Rep.* 9:193–197.

Moriguchi T., Greiner R. S., and Salem N., Jr. (2000). Behavioral deficits associated with dietary induction of decreased brain docosahexaenoic acid concentration. *J. Neurochem.* 75:2563–2573.

Mozzi R., Buratta S., and Goracci G. (2003). Metabolism and functions of phosphatidylserine in mammalian brain. *Neurochem. Res.* 28:195–214.

Mukherjee P. K., Marcheselli V. L., Serhan C. N., and Bazan N. G. (2004). Neuroprotectin D1: a docosahexaenoic acid-derived docosatriene protects human retinal pigment epithelial cells from oxidative stress. *Proc. Natl Acad. Sci. USA* 101:8491–8496.

Nabekura J., Noguchi K., Witt M. R., Nielsen M., and Akaike N. (1998). Functional modulation of human recombinant γ-aminobutyric acid type A receptor by docosahexaenoic acid. *J. Biol. Chem.* 273:11056–11061.

Nair P. P., Judd J. T., Berlin E., Taylor P. R., Shami S., Sainz E., and Bhagavan H. N. (1993). Dietary fish oil-induced changes in the distribution of α-tocopherol, retinol, and β-carotene in plasma, red blood cells, and platelets: modulation by vitamin E. *Am. J. Clin. Nutr.* 58:98–102.

Nakamura M. T., Cheon Y., Li Y., and Nara T. Y. (2004). Mechanisms of regulation of gene expression by fatty acids. *Lipids* 39:1077–1083.

Nakamura M. T. and Nara T. Y. (2003). Essential fatty acid synthesis and its regulation in mammals. *Prostaglandins Leukot. Essent. Fatty Acids* 68:145–150.

Nishikawa M., Kimura S., and Akaike N. (1994). Facilitatory effect of docosahexaenoic acid on N-methyl-D-aspartate response in pyramidal neurones of rat cerebral cortex. *J. Physiol.* (London) 475:83–93.

Niu S. L., Mitchell D. C., Lim S. Y., Wen Z. M., Kim H. Y., Salem N., Jr., and Litman B. J. (2004). Reduced G protein-coupled signaling efficiency in retinal rod outer segments in response to n-3 fatty acid deficiency. *J. Biol. Chem.* 279:31098–31104.

Ong L. W., Jiang B., Tang N., Yeo J. F., Wei S., Farooqui A. A., and Ong W. Y. (2006). Differential effects of polyunsaturated fatty acids on exocytosis in rat pheochromocytoma-12 cells. *Neurochem. Res.* 31:41–48.

Phillis J. W., Horrocks L. A., and Farooqui A. A. (2006). Cyclooxygenases, lipoxygenases, and epoxygenases in CNS: their role and involvement in neurological disorders. *Brain Res. Rev.* (in press).

Pifferi F., Roux F., Langelier B., Alessandri J. M., Vancassel S., Jouin M., Lavialle M., and Guesnet P. (2005). (n-3) polyunsaturated fatty acid deficiency reduces the expression of both isoforms of the brain glucose transporter GLUT1 in rats. *J. Nutr.* 135:2241–2246.

Poling J. S., Karanian J. W., Salem N., Jr., and Vicini S. (1995). Time- and voltage-dependent block of delayed rectifier potassium channels by docosahexaenoic acid. *Mol. Pharmacol.* 47:381–390.

Porcellati G. (1983). Phospholipid metabolism in neural membranes. In: Sun G. Y., Bazan N., Wu J. Y., Porcellati G., and Sun A. Y. (eds.), *Neural Membranes*. Humana Press, New York, pp. 3–35.

Poumès-Ballihaut C., Langelier B., Houlier F., Alessandri J. M., Durand G., Latge C., and Guesnet P. (2001). Comparative bioavailability of dietary alpha-linolenic and docosahexaenoic acids in the growing rat. *Lipids* 36:793–800.

Price P. T., Nelson C. M., and Clarke S. D. (2000). Omega-3 polyunsaturated fatty acid regulation of gene expression. *Curr. Opin. Lipidol.* 11:3–7.

Puskás L. G., Kitajka K., Nyakas C., Barcelo-Coblijn G., and Farkas T. (2003). Short-term administration of omega 3 fatty acids from fish oil results in increased transthyretin transcription in old rat hippocampus. Proc. *Natl Acad. Sci. USA* 100:1580–1585.

Ramakers G. J., Oestreicher A. B., Wolters P. S., Van Leeuwen F. W., De Graan P. N., and Gispen W. H. (1991). Developmental changes in B-50 (GAP-43) in primary cultures of cerebral cortex: B-50 immunolocalization, axonal elongation rate and growth cone morphology. *Int. J. Dev. Neurosci.* 9:215–230.

Rapoport S. I. (1999). In vivo fatty acid incorporation into brain phospholipids in relation to signal transduction and membrane remodeling. *Neurochem. Res.* 24:1403–1415.

Rapoport S. I. (2003). In vivo approaches to quantifying and imaging brain arachidonic and docosahexaenoic acid metabolism. *J. Pediatr.* 143:S26–S34.

Rapoport S. I., Chang M. C. J., and Spector A. A. (2001). Delivery and turnover of plasma-derived essential PUFAs in mammalian brain. *J. Lipid Res.* 42:678–685.

Reddy T. S. and Bazan N. G. (1984). Long-chain acyl coenzyme A synthetase activity during the postnatal development of the mouse brain. Int. J. Dev. Neurosci. 2:447–450.

Reddy T. S., Sprecher H., and Bazan N. G. (1984). Long-chain acyl-coenzyme A synthetase from rat brain microsomes. Kinetic studies using [1-^{14}C]docosahexaenoic acid substrate. *Eur. J. Biochem.* 145:21–29.

Rotstein N. P., Aveldaño M. I., Barrantes F. J., Roccamo A. M., and Politi L. E. (1997). Apoptosis of retinal photoreceptors during development in vitro: protective effect of docosahexaenoic acid. *J. Neurochem.* 69:504–513.

Rotstein N. P., Politi L. E., and Aveldaño M. I. (1998). Docosahexaenoic acid promotes differentiation of developing photoreceptors in culture. *Invest. Ophthalmol. Vis. Sci.* 39:2750–2758.

Rotstein N. P., Politi L. E., German O. L., and Girotti R. (2003). Protective effect of docosahexaenoic acid on oxidative stress-induced apoptosis of retina photoreceptors. *Invest. Ophthalmol. Vis. Sci.* 44:2252–2259.

Salem N., Shingu T., Kim H.-Y., Hullin F., Bougnoux P., and Karanian J. W. (1988). Aberrations in membrane structures and function. In: Karnovsky M. L., Bolis L., and Leaf A. (eds.), *Biological Membranes*. Alan R. Liss, New York, pp. 319–333.

Sampath H. and Ntambi J. M. (2005). Polyunsaturated fatty acid regulation of genes of lipid metabolism. *Annu. Rev. Nutr.* 25:317–340.

Sanderson P. and Calder P. C. (1998). Dietary fish oil appears to prevent the activation of phospholipase C-gamma in lymphocytes. *Biochim. Biophys. Acta* 1392:300–308.

SanGiovanni J. P. and Chew E. Y. (2005). The role of omega-3 long-chain polyunsaturated fatty acids in health and disease of the retina. *Prog. Retinal Eye Res.* 24:87–138.

Scott B. L. and Bazan N. G. (1989). Membrane docosahexaenoate is supplied to the developing brain and retina by the liver. *Proc. Natl Acad. Sci. USA* 86:2903–2907.

Sergeeva M., Strokin M., and Reiser G. (2005). Regulation of intracellular calcium levels by polyunsaturated fatty acids, arachidonic acid and docosahexaenoic acid, in astrocytes: possible involvement of phospholipase A$_2$. *Reprod. Nutr. Dev.* 45:633–646.

Serhan C. N. (2005a). Novel eicosanoid and docosanoid mediators: resolvins, docosatrienes, and neuroprotectins. *Curr. Opin. Clin. Nutr. Metab. Care* 8:115–121.

Serhan C. N. (2005b). Novel ω-3-derived local mediators in anti-inflammation and resolution. *Pharmacol. Ther.* 105:7–21.

Serhan C. N., Arita M., Hong S., and Gotlinger K. (2004). Resolvins, docosatrienes, and neuroprotectins, novel omega-3-derived mediators, and their endogenous aspirin-triggered epimers. *Lipids* 39:1125–1132.

Shaikh S. R., Dumaual A. C., Castillo A., LoCascio D., Siddiqui R. A., Stillwell W., and Wassall S. R. (2004). Oleic and docosahexaenoic acid differentially phase separate from lipid raft molecules: a comparative NMR, DSC, AFM, and detergent extraction study. *Biophys. J.* 87:1752–1766.

Shaikh S. R., Dumaual A. C., LoCassio D., Siddiqui R. A., and Stillwell W. (2003). Acyl chain unsaturation in PEs modulates phase separation from lipid raft molecules. *Biochem. Biophys. Res. Commun.* 311:793–796.

Siddiqui R. A., Jenski L. J., Harvey K. A., Wiesehan J. D., Stillwell W., and Zaloga G. P. (2003). Cell-cycle arrest in Jurkat leukaemic cells: a possible role for docosahexaenoic acid. *Biochem. J.* 371:621–629.

Siddiqui R. A., Shaikh S. R., Sech L. A., Yount H. R., Stillwell W., and Zaloga G. P. (2004). Omega 3-fatty acids: health benefits and cellular mechanisms of action. *Mini-Rev. Medicin. Chem.* 4:859–871.

Siddiqui R. A., Wiesehan J., Stillwel W., Jenski L., and Kovacs R. (2001). Prevention of cytotoxic effects of docosahexaenoic acid in Jurkat leukemic cells by phosphatidic acid. *FASEB J.* 15:A282.

Songur A., Sarsilmaz M., Sogut S., Ozyurt B., Ozyurt H., Zararsiz I., and Turkoglu A. O. (2004). Hypothalamic superoxide dismutase, xanthine oxidase, nitric oxide, and malondialdehyde in rats fed with fish ω-3 fatty acids. *Prog. Neuro-Psychopharmacol. Biol. Psychiat.* 28:693–698.

Stillwell W., Shaikh S. R., Zerouga M., Siddiqui R., and Wassall S. R. (2005). Docosahexaenoic acid affects cell signaling by altering lipid rafts. *Reprod. Nutr. Develop.* 45:559–579.

Stillwell W. and Wassall S. R. (2003). Docosahexaenoic acid: membrane properties of a unique fatty acid. *Chem. Phys. Lipids* 126:1–27.

Stinson A. M., Wiegand R. D., and Anderson R. E. (1991). Fatty acid and molecular species compositions of phospholipids and diacylglycerols from rat retinal membranes. *Exp. Eye Res.* 52:213–218.

Strokin M., Sergeeva M., and Reiser G. (2003). Docosahexaenoic acid and arachidonic acid release in rat brain astrocytes is mediated by two separate isoforms of phospholipase A_2 and is differently regulated by cyclic AMP and Ca^{2+}. *Br. J. Pharmacol.* 139:1014–1022.

Takahata, K. (1995). Effect of DHA on cultured neuronal cells: studies in PC12 cells. *Jpn. J. Pharmacol.* 67:13S.

Valentine R. C. and Valentine D. L. (2004). *Omega*-3 fatty acids in cellular membranes: a unified concept. *Prog. Lipid Res.* 43:383–402.

Verlengia R., Gorjao R., Kanunfre C. C., Bordin S., de Lima T. M., Martins E. F., and Curi R. (2004a). Comparative effects of eicosapentaenoic acid and docosahexaenoic acid on proliferation, cytokine production, and pleiotropic gene expression in Jurkat cells. *J. Nutr. Biochem.* 15:657–665.

Verlengia R., Gorjão R., Kanunfre C. C., Bordin S., Martins de Lima T., Fernandes Martins E., Newsholme P., and Curi R. (2004b). Effects of EPA and DHA on proliferation, cytokine production, and gene expression in Raji cells. *Lipids* 39:857–864.

Wassall S. R., Brzustowicz M. R., Shaikh S. R., Cherezov V., Caffrey M., and Stillwell W. (2004). Order from disorder, corralling cholesterol with chaotic lipids – the role of polyunsaturated lipids in membrane raft formation. *Chem. Phys. Lipids* 132:79–88.

Wu D. and Meydani S. N. (1998). n-3 polyunsaturated fatty acids and immune function. *Proc. Nutr. Soc.* 57:503–509.

Wu M., Harvey K. A., Ruzmetov N., Welch Z. R., Sech L., Jackson K., Stillwell W., Zaloga G. P., and Siddiqui R. A. (2005). Omega-3 polyunsaturated fatty acids attenuate breast cancer growth through activation of a neutral sphingomyelinase-mediated pathway. *Int. J. Cancer* 117:340–348.

Xiao Y. F. and Li X. Y. (1999). Polyunsaturated fatty acids modify mouse hippocampal neuronal excitability during excitotoxic or convulsant stimulation. *Brain Res.* 846:112–121.

Yehuda S., Rabinovitz S., Carasso R. L., and Mostofsky D. I. (2002). The role of polyunsaturated fatty acids in restoring the aging neuronal membrane. *Neurobiol. Aging* 23:843–853.

Young C., Gean P. W., Chiou L. C., and Shen Y. Z. (2000). Docosahexaenoic acid inhibits synaptic transmission and epileptiform activity in the rat hippocampus. *Synapse* 37:90–94.

Young C., Gean P. W., Wu S. P., Lin C. H., and Shen Y. Z. (1998). Cancellation of low-frequency stimulation-induced long-term depression by docosahexaenoic acid in the rat hippocampus. *Neurosci. Lett.* 247:198–200.

Zhao Y., Joshi-Barve S., Barve S., and Chen L. H. (2004). Eicosapentaenoic acid prevents LPS-induced TNF-α expression by preventing NF-κB activation. *J. Am. Coll. Nutr.* 23:71–78.

Zimmer L., Delion-Vancassel S., Durand G., Guilloteau D., Bodard S., Besnard J. C., and Chalon S. (2000). Modification of dopamine neurotransmission in the nucleus accumbens of rats deficient in n-3 polyunsaturated fatty acids. *J. Lipid Res.* 41:32–40.

Zucker R. S. (1989). Short-term synaptic plasticity. *Annu. Rev. Neurosci.* 12:13–31.

7
Nonenzymic Metabolites of Arachidonate and Docosahexaenoate in Brain

7.1 Introduction

Brain tissue is vulnerable to oxidative damage. Brain tissue not only has a large oxidative capacity to use circulating oxygen, but also has low levels of antioxidant enzymic activities. Phospholipids containing polyunsaturated fatty acids, which are especially sensitive to free radical attack because of the presence of active bis-allylic methylene groups, are enriched in brain. The carbon–hydrogen bonds on these activated methylene units have lower bond dissociation energies, making these hydrogen atoms more easily removed in radical reactions (Leonard et al., 2004). Lipid peroxidation begins with oxidative modification of polyunsaturated fatty acid double bonds. Peroxyl radicals abstract a hydrogen atom from the bis-allylic methylene group located between two adjacent double bonds of the hydrocarbon chain. This results in the formation of conjugated double bonds.

Reaction of the fatty acid radical with oxygen yields fatty acid peroxyl radicals that abstract a hydrogen atom from the methylene group of another polyunsaturated fatty acid. The fatty acid is then transformed into a hydroperoxide. These hydroperoxides, in turn, may further breakdown into toxic aldehydes, such as 4-hydroxynonenal, 4-hydroxyhexenal, acrolein, and malondialdehyde. The susceptibility of polyunsaturated fatty acid toward peroxidation increases with an increase in the number of unsaturated sites in the acyl chain. Lipid peroxidation in neural membranes has two broad outcomes. First is the structural damage to neural membranes and second is the generation of oxidized glycerophospholipids and their products. Some of these products are chemically reactive and are capable of covalently modifying neural membrane proteins. Oxidized glycerophospholipids and their breakdown products are major effectors of tissue damage following lipid peroxidation.

7.2 Reactive Oxygen Species

As stated in Chapters 5 and 6, besides COX, LOX, and EPOX-generated lipid mediators (prostaglandins, leukotrienes, and thromboxanes) (Fig. 7.1), the oxidation of AA also generates reactive oxygen species (ROS). ROS include oxygen

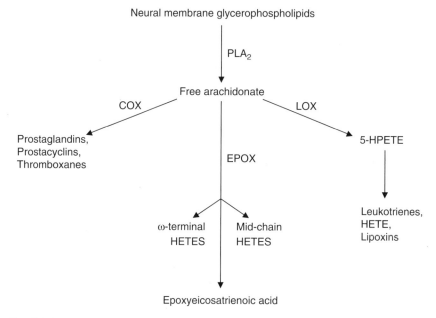

FIG. 7.1. Generation of eicosanoids from free AA in brain tissue. The action of PLA$_2$ on neural membrane glycerophospholipids generates AA. The metabolism of AA via cyclooxygenase (COX) generates prostaglandins, prostacyclins, thromboxanes. Lipoxygenase (LOX) acts on AA to form leukotrienes, HETE (hydroxyeicosatetraenoic acid), and lipoxins. The EPOX pathway produces ω-terminal HETES, mid-chain HETES, and epoxyeicosatrienoic acid.

free radicals (superoxide, hydroxyl, and alkoxyl radicals), and peroxides (hydrogen peroxide and lipid hydroperoxides). ROS are very reactive and have a very short half-life. Mitochondria are the most important cellular sources of ROS production. Among the neural cells, astrocytes are most resistant to ROS attack. Astrocytes protect neurons from oxidative stress because they have higher glutathione content than other neural cells. During scavenging of ROS, the reduced form of glutathione is oxidized.

At low levels, ROS function as signaling intermediates in the regulation of fundamental cell activities, such as growth and adaptation responses. At this concentration, ROS are required not only for receptor kinase activation, but they also modulate phosphorylation of transcription factors, such as AP-1 and NFκB (Leonard et al., 2004). At higher concentrations, ROS contribute to neural membrane damage when the balance between reducing and oxidizing (redox) forces shifts toward oxidative stress. The biological targets of ROS include membrane proteins, unsaturated lipids, and DNA (Berlett and Stadtman, 1997; Dean et al., 1997; Valko et al., 2005). Oxidative modifications of amino acid side chains and ROS-mediated peptide cleavage are indicators of protein oxidation. The increase in carbonyl groups in proteins is another index of protein oxidation and

ROS-mediated damage (Fiez, 1996). The reaction between ROS and proteins or unsaturated lipids in the plasma membrane leads to chemical cross-linking of membrane proteins and lipids and a reduction in membrane unsaturation. The depletion of unsaturation in membrane lipids is associated with decreased membrane fluidity and decreased activity of membrane-bound enzymes, ion channels, and receptors (Ray et al., 1994; Choe et al., 1995; Fernstrom, 1999).

ROS also attack DNA bases causing damage through hydroxylation, ring opening, and fragmentation (Buisson et al., 1993). This attack generates 8-hydroxy-2′-deoxyguanosine (8-OHdGua), and 2, 6-diamino-4-hydroxy-5-formamidopyrimidine (FapyGua) (Jenkinson et al., 1999) (Fig. 7.2). ROS may also attack the sugar

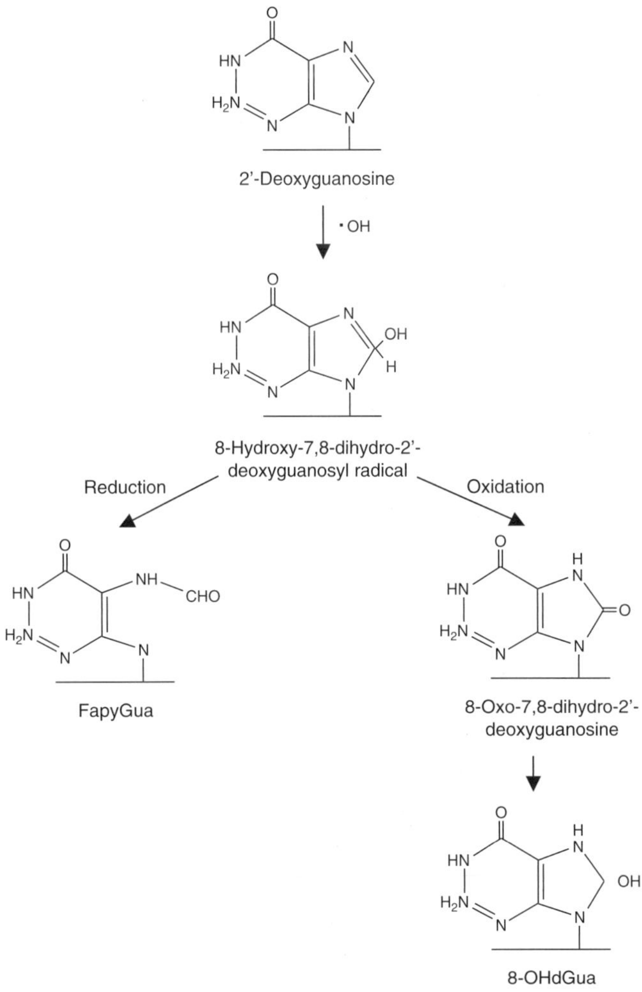

FIG. 7.2. Generation of 8-hydroxy-2′-deoxyguanosine (8-OHdGua) and 2,6-diamino-4-hydroxy-5-formamidopyrimidine (fapyGua) via the action of ROS on DNA.

phosphate backbone of DNA, producing apurinic sites in which the base has been removed by an oxidant-mediated reaction (Halliwell, 1994). An indication of this DNA damage comes from the presence of free bases in urine. Abstraction of hydrogen by ROS at the C-4 position of the sugar moiety also produces single-strand breaks in DNA. This couples with a second sugar oxidation on the complementary strand, causing a double strand break in DNA. These reactions may be responsible for the mutagenic effects of ROS in brain tissue (Buisson et al., 1993).

Brain tissue contains specific enzymes to deal with the ROS. Superoxide dismutase converts the superoxide anion radical into hydrogen peroxide, which can readily diffuse through neural membranes. Hydrogen peroxide itself is not a free radical, but is a major source for generation of the hydroxyl radicals formed in the Fenton reaction catalyzed by iron and copper. Glutathione peroxidase and catalase remove the hydrogen peroxide. The glutathione-dependent system not only works as a ROS scavenger, but also regulates the redox state of brain tissue. Activities of these enzymes are quite low in brain tissue compared with liver and other tissues. Collectively, these studies suggest that the oxidation of glycerophospholipids, chemical cross-linking of neural membrane proteins, and oxidation of neural cell DNA are significant chemical events associated with oxidative stress and disruption of ion homeostasis during lipid peroxidation. All these processes are related to oxidative stress-mediated neurodegeneration (Fig. 7.3) in acute neural trauma and neurodegenerative diseases (Farooqui et al., 2000b).

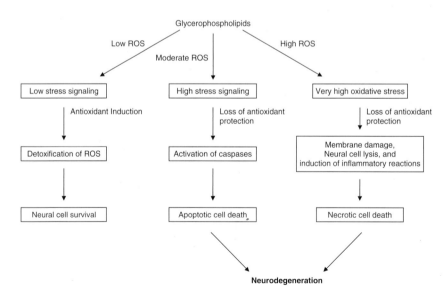

FIG. 7.3. Effect of low, moderate, and high oxidative stress on neural cell survival and neurodegeneration through apoptotic and necrotic cell death.

7.3 Lipid Hydroperoxides

Lipid hydroperoxides are oxidants that can amplify the initial oxidative insult. Unlike ROS, lipid hydroperoxides have a longer half-life. They can migrate from their points of origin to other brain regions that are rich in iron (Cleland and James, 1997). This movement of lipid hydroperoxides can be spontaneous or facilitated by lipid transfer proteins. These lipid hydroperoxides have major effects on membrane structure and function. In the presence of iron and other transition metal ions, lipid hydroperoxides are converted into lipid alkoxyl and peroxyl radicals. These radicals can initiate further lipid peroxidation chain reactions. The termination of lipid peroxidation occurs via the coupling of any two radicals to form nonradical products, which are stable and unable to propagate lipid peroxidation chains (Heinle et al., 2000).

Lipid hydroperoxides are also formed enzymically during oxidative stress from reactions catalyzed by 5-LOX, 15-LOX, COX-1, and COX-2. Both 15-LOX and COX-2 convert linoleic acid into 13(S)-hydroperoxyoctadecadienoic acid (13-HPODE), the prototypic n-6 PUFA hydroperoxide. The homolytic decomposition of 13-HPODE produces a bifunctional electrophilic aldehyde (Schneider et al., 2004). Two quite distinct pathways are involved in the generation of these aldehydes. One pathway, which involves the intermediate formation of hydroperoxide-derived alkoxy radicals, results in the formation of 4,5-epoxy-2(E)-decenal through an α-cleavage reaction. The other pathway involves the intermediate formation of the potential genotoxin, 4-hydroperoxy-2-nonenal (4-HPNE), which then decomposes to 4-oxo-2-nonenal (ONE) and 4-hydroxy-2-nonenal (4-HNE) (West et al., 2004) (also see below).

The detoxification of glycerophospholipid hydroperoxides can be accomplished through the combination enzymic activity of PLA_2 and reduction of the resultant fatty acid hydroperoxides with glutathione peroxidase (van Kuijk et al., 1987). The latter enzyme acts on membranes and reduces glycerophospholipid hydroperoxides to the nontoxic hydroxyl derivatives (Fisher et al., 1999). The restoration of membrane integrity is achieved by the reinsertion of the nonoxidized fatty acyl group by the deacylation/reacylation cycle (Farooqui et al., 2000a). The presence of DHA at the sn-1 position of PtdEtn or PtdCho protects against formation of hydroperoxides (Lyberg et al., 2005).

The oxidized glycerophospholipids generated by ROS attacks on membranes are better substrates for PLA_2 than are the native glycerophospholipids (McLean et al., 1993; Murakami et al., 1997). Very little is known about oxidized glycerophospholipids in brain, but much information is available about them in nonneural tissues (Leitinger, 2003; Furnkranz and Leitinger, 2004). These lipids include oxidized 1-palmitoyl-2-arachidonoyl-sn-glycero-3-phosphocholine, 1-palmitoyl-2-(5) oxovaleroyl-sn-glycero-3-phosphocholine, 1-palmitoyl-2-glutaroyl-sn-glycero-3-phosphocholine, and 1-palmitoyl-2-epoxyisoprostane-sn-glycero-3-phosphocholine. Oxidized glycerophospholipids are proinflammatory agonists. They promote chronic inflammation and their effects are mediated by inflammatory cytokines, such as monocyte chemotactic protein-1 (MCP-1) and interleukin-8 (IL-8) (Yeh et al., 2001). The transcription factor PPARα plays an important role in the induction of MCP-1 and IL-8 mediated by oxidized glycerophospholipids (Lee et al., 2000a).

The cellular response to oxidized glycerophospholipids depends on not only their concentration, but also on the extent of their oxidation. Lower concentrations of moderately oxidized glycerophospholipids do not induce cell death, but instead induce an adaptive response to the stress of a subsequent exposure to ROS. These oxidized glycerophospholipids act through G protein–coupled receptors and upregulate cAMP/protein kinase-mediated pathways (Leitinger, 2003). The oxidized glycerophospholipids also induce monocyte-endothelial cell interactions that are independent of platelet-activating factor receptors (Leitinger et al., 1997; Leitinger, 2003). These glycerophospholipids may also be involved in the induction of vascular endothelial growth factor expression (McIntyre et al., 1999; Leitinger, 2005). In non-neural cells, high concentrations of fully oxidized glycerophospholipids and their metabolites produce neural degeneration (Farooqui et al., 1997).

At low levels, ROS not only act as second messengers, but are also associated with gene regulation (Allen and Tresini, 2000). Under these conditions, induction of antioxidant enzymes and other antioxidants, such as glutathione, vitamin E, and ascorbic acid, prevent peroxidative damage by detoxifying ROS resulting in neural cell survival (Fig. 7.3). Moderate ROS levels may cause sublethal oxidative stress. This results in the loss of antioxidant protection, decreased ATP levels, and activation of specific proteolytic enzymes, such as caspases. This process produces neurodegeneration through apoptotic cell death (Farooqui et al., 2004). Under these circumstances, even though neural cell damage exceeds the repair capacity, the damage can be repaired through endogenous defenses (Duffy et al., 1998). High levels of ROS not only produce rapid loss of antioxidant protection and decreased ATP levels, but also cause membrane damage, loss of ion homeostasis, alterations in cellular redox, neural cell lysis, and initiation of inflammatory reactions, resulting in the necrotic type of cell death (Farooqui et al., 2004).

7.4 Isoprostanes, Isofurans, Isothromboxanes, Isoleukotrienes, and Neuroprostanes

7.4.1 Isoprostanes

Isoprostanes are prostaglandin-like mediators formed nonenzymically by free radical-catalyzed peroxidation of esterified AA in vivo (Figs. 7.4 and 7.5). The minimum requirement for the generation of an isoprostane is a polyunsaturated fatty acid with three contiguous, methylene-interrupted double bonds (Basu, 2004). The mechanism by which isoprostanes are formed is analogous to the formation of prostaglandins by COX enzymes (Morrow et al., 1999). Unlike prostaglandins, the formation of isoprostanes in situ initially takes place at the esterified AA on the glycerophospholipid molecule (Fam and Morrow, 2003).

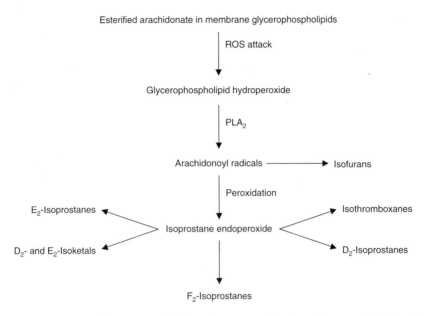

FIG. 7.4. Synthesis of isoprostanes, isothromboxanes, and isofurans from arachidonic acid.

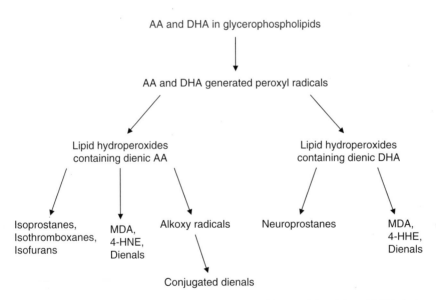

FIG. 7.5. Nonenzymic degradation of glycerophospholipids containing AA and DHA during oxidative stress. Phospholipids containing AA produce isoprostanes, isothromboxanes, isofurans, and 4-HNE (4-hydroxynonenal), whereas glycerophospholipids containing DHA generate neuroprostanes and 4-HHE (4-hydroxyhexenal). MDA (malonaldehyde) and conjugated dienes are common products of the non-enzymic oxidation of AA and DHA.

Nonenzymic synthesis of the family of F_2-isoprostanes (Fig. 7.6) involves the formation of positional peroxyl radical isomers of arachidonic acid, which undergo endocyclization to form PGG_2-like compounds. These compounds are reduced to PGF_2-like compounds. F_2-Isoprostane (F_2-IsoP) is subsequently released in free form by the action of PLA_2 (Morrow et al., 1992; Fam and Morrow, 2003). The structural difference between isoprostanes and prostaglandins is that in isoprostanes the side chains are *cis* to the cyclopentane ring, whereas in prostaglandins they have the *trans* orientation. The administration of carbon tetrachloride to a rat in vivo can induce the formation of F_2-IsoP in liver within 15 min. Isoprostanes are increased about 200-fold after the oxidant injury inflicted by carbon tetrachloride. F_2-IsoP appears first in the circulation and after several hours is excreted in rat urine. Isoprostanes are attractive indices of lipid peroxidation because of the specificity of their formation, their chemical stability, and the development of sensitive and specific methods for their measurement using mass spectrometry and radioimmunoassay (Fam and Morrow, 2003).

Because isoprostane endoperoxides rearrange to form D- and E-rings, the formation of D_2/E_2 and 8-epi-$PGF_{2\alpha}$ isoprostanes also takes place in vivo (Fig. 7.6). Like F_2-IsoP, they are esterified to glycerophospholipids and are released in tissues in free form through the action of PLA_2. It is not known how long the esterified F_2-IsoP may persist in the membrane and which isoform of PLA_2 releases F_2-IsoP from neural membranes. In rat tissues the levels of D_2/E_2-IsoP are one-third to one-fourth of the levels of F_2-IsoP (Fam and Morrow, 2003).

Normal human urine contains 400–500 pg isoprostane/mg creatinine. Isoprostanes are also formed in human placenta during storage at −20°C. Their concentrations are higher than those of prostaglandins produced by isoforms of COX (Morrow et al., 1990). The concentration of isoprostanes is also increased

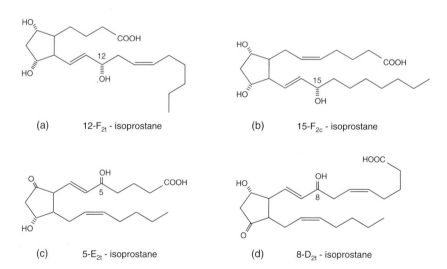

(a)   12-F_{2t} - isoprostane

(b)   15-F_{2c} - isoprostane

(c)   5-E_{2t} - isoprostane

(d)   8-D_{2t} - isoprostane

Fig. 7.6. Structures of isoprostanes with F, E, and D rings.

in rat exposed to oxidative stress-associated neurological disorders (Morrow et al., 1991). Injections of LPS into the mouse brain also increase levels of iso-prostanes that can be abrogated by genetic deletion of the NFκB p50 subunit or the NFκB-responsive gene-inducible nitric oxide synthase (Montine et al., 2002; Milatovic et al., 2003), suggesting a link between NFκB activation and iso-prostane formation.

Isoprostanes act through prostaglandin and thromboxane-like receptors and their effects can be blocked by thromboxane receptor antagonists (Takahashi et al., 1992; Morrow et al., 1996; Opere et al., 2005). Thromboxane receptors, like prostaglandin receptors, are linked to different sets of G proteins resulting in distinct biological effects on brain and other body tissues (Lahaie et al., 1998). The occurrence of IsoP receptors in smooth muscle cells has also been proposed (Fig. 7.7), but no information is available on their structure and characterization (Habib and Badr, 2004). Molecular cloning strategies are required to provide unequivocal proof of the existence of a unique isoprostane receptor. Isoprostanes induce contraction in vascular smooth muscle. They trigger activation of phospholipase C (Fukunaga et al., 1993), protein kinase C, and calcium channels. The elevation of cytosolic calcium has also been demonstrated in endothelial cells in response to isoprostanes (Lahaie et al., 1998). Isoprostanes also modulate the cellular growth and DNA synthesis in both vascular smooth muscle cells and endothelial cells (Yura et al., 1999). SQ29548, a TXA_2 receptor antagonist, partially blocks the effects.

Isoprostanes are very potent vasoconstrictors in brain microvasculature. F_2-IsoP exerts its action in vascular beds by facilitating binding between endothelial cells and monocytes (Lahaie et al., 1998; Fam and Morrow, 2003). Binding

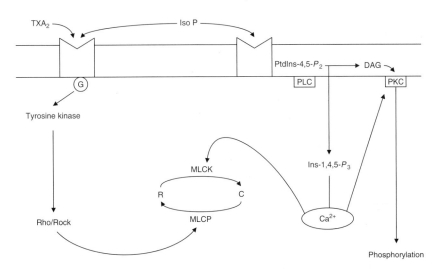

Fig. 7.7. A hypothetical diagram showing the interaction between isoprostane and thromboxane receptors involved in muscle contraction.

between endothelial cells and monocytes is the key initial event in atherogenesis. Isoprostane-mediated monocyte adhesion is VCAM-1 independent but involves protein kinase A and mitogen-activated protein kinase kinase 1. F_2-IsoP also modulates the p38 MAPK pathway during monocyte adhesion (Cracowski, 2004). Thus F_2-IsoP also not only affects vascular and bronchial smooth muscles function, but also modulates cellular proliferation (Fam and Morrow, 2003). These processes may relate to inflammation and atherosclerosis. Collectively, these studies suggest that IsoP are not only negative feedback regulators of associated inflammation, but also induce vasoconstriction, mitogenesis, and monocyte adhesion (Cracowski, 2004).

7.4.2 Isothromboxanes

Isoprostanes are prostaglandin-like compounds. Studies in vivo and in vitro indicate that isoprostane endoperoxide rearranges to thromboxane-like compounds, isothromboxanes (IsoTXB$_2$), in rat liver (Morrow et al., 1996). The levels of IsoTXB$_2$ in liver are similar to the levels of D$_2$/E$_2$-isoprostanes.

The formation of isoketals also occurs through the rearrangement of H$_2$-IsoP endoperoxides (Fig. 7.8). Unlike the F$_2$-IsoP, the isoketals result in modification of biologically important proteins rather than activation of specific receptors (Davies et al., 2004). Isoketals are highly reactive γ-ketoaldehydes that form pyrrole adducts with the ε-amino group of lysine residues on protein (Davies et al.,

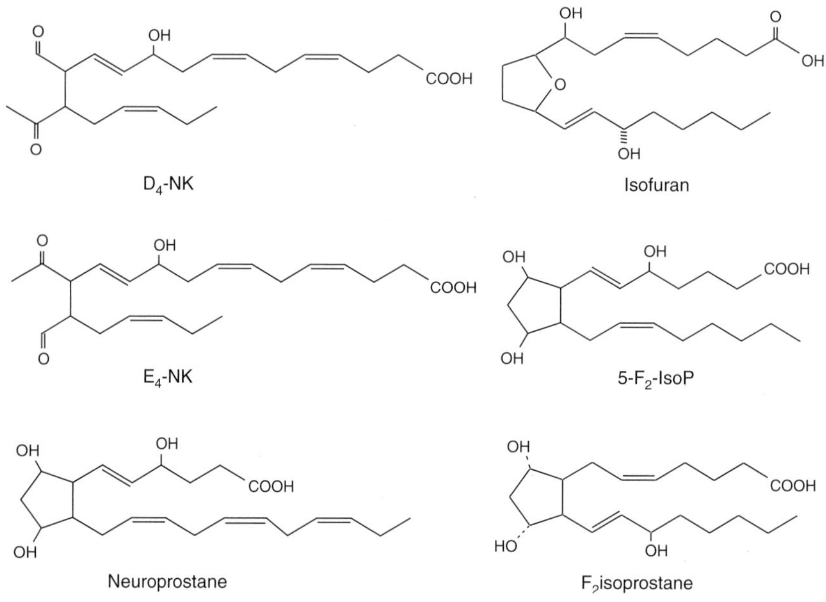

FIG. 7.8. Structures of isoketals, neuroketals, and other toxic aldehydes.

2004). Isoketals inhibit the activity of proteasomes in glial cells with an IC_{50} of 330 nM and induce cell death with an IC_{50} of 670 nM. Intrahemispheric injections of 15-E_2-IsoK disrupt the blood-brain barrier. Isoketals have been detected in tissues as well as biological fluids.

7.4.3 Isofurans

During lipid peroxidation studies under high oxygen tension, substituted tetrahydrofuran derivatives were found (Fessel et al., 2002). These compounds are isofurans (IsoF) (Fig. 7.9). Based on labeling studies, two mechanisms are proposed for the formation of IsoF: a cyclic peroxide cleavage pathway and an epoxide hydrolysis pathway. Oxygen concentration affects the formation of isofurans. As oxygen concentrations increase, the formation of isofurans is favored, whereas the formation of isoprostanes becomes disfavored. The oxygen concentration differentially modulates the formation of isoprostanes and isofurans. Isoprostanes may thus not provide an accurate measure of free radical reactions that occur in the presence of high oxygen concentrations. The isofuran/isoprostane ratio is a useful index and an important measure of steady state tissue oxygenation. The generation of isofurans is not only a useful index for assessing the role of ROS at high oxygen concentration, but also an important parameter for evaluating the effectiveness of antioxidant therapies (Roberts, II et al., 2005). Levels of IsoF increase significantly in the substantia nigra of Parkinson disease patients when compared with age-matched controls. The formation of IsoF may be due to

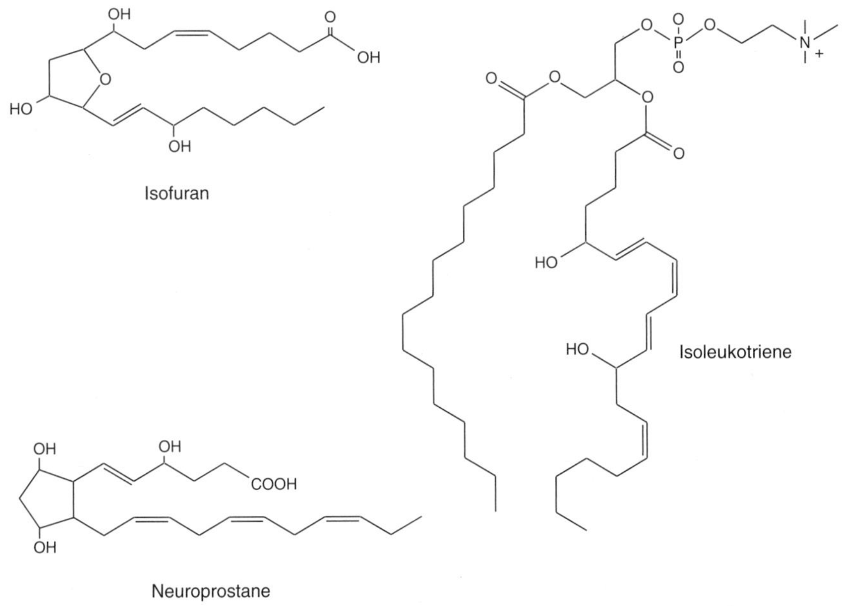

FIG. 7.9. Structures of isofurans, isoleukotrienes, and neuroprostanes.

altered oxygen tension and mitochondrial dysfunction in Parkinson disease (Pratico et al., 2004). Elevated levels of F_2-IsoP have been reported to occur in cerebrospinal fluid from Huntington disease, Creutzfeldt-Jakob disease, traumatic brain injury, and multiple sclerosis (Musiek et al., 2005).

7.4.4 Isoleukotrienes

Free radical attack on 1-hexadecanoyl-2-arachidonyl-*sn*-glycero-3-phosphocholine also results in formation of B_4-isoleukotrienes (Harrison and Murphy, 1995). B_4-Isoleukotrienes (Fig. 7.9) induce their effect by binding to the high-affinity LTB_4 receptors that express on inflammatory cells, such as neutrophils, eosinophils, and macrophages. B_4-isoleukotriene elevates intracellular calcium ions in Indo-1-loaded human polymorphonuclear leukocytes and this increase in calcium ions can be blocked LY223982, a leukotriene B_4 receptor antagonist, suggesting that isoleukotrienes act through leukotrienes B_4 receptors.

7.4.5 Neuroprostanes

DHA undergoes nonenzymic oxidation. Compounds generated by this process are called neuroprostanes (NP) (Roberts, II et al., 1998; Nourooz-Zadeh et al., 1999; Roberts, II and Fessel, 2004; Yin et al., 2005). Similarly, nonenzymic oxidation of eicosapentaenoic acid (EPA) results in formation of F_3 isoprostane (Nourooz-Zadeh et al., 1997). As stated in Chapter 6, levels of this fatty acid are very low in humans, unless they consume a large amount of fish. AA is evenly distributed in all neural cell types in brain. DHA is highly enriched in neurons, so the formation of NP can be used as an important index of neuronal damage. NP have 22 carbons and 4 double bonds and are analogous to isoprostanes (Fig. 7.9). During the formation of NP, oxygen-mediated DHA radicalization results in the generation of peroxyl radicals. These radicals undergo endocyclization followed by the addition of molecular oxygen and reduction to form the F ring of NP. It is likely that glycerophospholipids containing esterified NP alter the fluidity and permeability of neuronal membranes causing impairment in normal neuronal function (Fam and Morrow, 2003; Yin et al., 2005).

Nothing is known about the PLA_2 activity involved in the release of NP from glycerophospholipids esterified with NP. F_4-NP is the first characterized neuroprostane. The occurrence of F_4-NP can be detected in cerebrospinal fluid (CSF) from normal individuals. The levels of F_4-NP are significantly increased in CSF from patients with Alzheimer disease (Reich et al., 2001). The occurrence of E_4-NP and D_4-NP has also been reported in normal rat and human brain (Reich et al., 2000). Levels of E_4/D_4-NP in normal brain were one-third compared with the levels of F_4-NP (Roberts, II and Fessel, 2004).

7.4.5 Neuroketals

Nonenzymic oxidation of DHA also produces neuroketals (NK) (Bernoud-Hubac et al., 2001). Like IsoK, NK are very reactive. They form not only lactam and

Schiff base adducts, but also generate lysine adducts suggesting that these metabolites may be involved in protein–protein cross-linking in brain tissue under oxidative stress. The collective evidence suggests that AA and DHA undergo nonenzymic oxidation with the generation of isoprostanes, isofurans, and neuroprostanes. These compounds could have neurochemical effects intensifying oxidative stress, and may be involved in acute neural trauma and neurodegenerative diseases (Roberts, II and Fessel, 2004; Roberts, II et al., 2005; Farooqui and Horrocks, 2006). High levels of isoprostanes and neuroprostanes are reliable indices of oxidative stress in vivo (Roberts, II et al., 1998, 2005; Fam and Morrow, 2003).

7.5 Generation of 4-HNE and its Effect on Brain Metabolism

7.5.1 4-HNE is a Signaling Molecule

Nonenzymic peroxidation of linoleic acid (LA), AA, and DHA generates 4-oxo-2-nonenal (4-ONE), 4-hydroxynonenal (4-HNE), and 4-hydroxyhexenal (4-HHE), respectively (Fig. 7.10). These reactive aldehydes are important mediators of neural cell damage because of their ability to covalently modify biomolecules with disruption of important cellular function (Esterbauer et al., 1991; Lin et al., 2005; Farooqui and Horrocks, 2006). 4-HNE, a nine-carbon α, β-unsaturated aldehyde, at low concentration (0.8–2.8 μM), modulates cellular signaling in brain tissue (Keller and Mattson, 1998). After treatment of cell samples with 4-HNE, results of microarray analysis show alteration of intracellular redox status, cytotoxicity through 4-HNE's ability to damage proteins, and activation of numerous cellular stress signaling responses that ultimately alter gene expression and cell viability

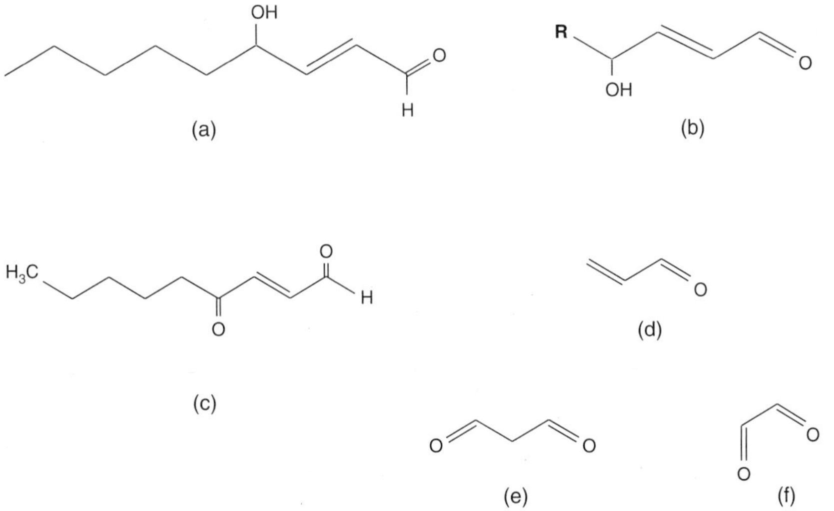

FIG. 7.10. Structures of 4-hydroxy-2-nonenal (4-HNE) (a), 4-hydroxy-2-alkenal (4-HAE) (b), 4-oxo-2-nonenal (4-ONE) (c), acrolein (d), malondialdehyde (MDA) (e), and glyoxal (f).

(West and Marnett, 2005). 4-HNE affects signaling pathways through increased basal and GTP-stimulated phospholipase C and adenylate cyclase activities and decreased ornithine decarboxylase activities (Rossi et al., 1993) (Table 7.1). In addition, 4-HNE has been reported to activate signaling via c-jun N-terminal kinase and to inhibit other regulatory mechanisms, such as NF-κB and the proteasomal degradation pathway (Page et al., 1999).

In dentate granule cells, 4-HNE modulates L-type Ca^{2+} channels and plays an important role in physiological processes associated with neuroplasticity (Akaishi et al., 2004). In non-neural cells at low levels (i.e., < 1.00 μM), 4-HNE can differentially modulate cell cycle signaling (Barrera et al., 2004). It not only orchestrates the expression of the c-myc gene involved in cell proliferation, but also decreases cyclins D_1, D_2, and A in the G_0/G_1 phase of the cell cycle. 4-HNE at and below 1.00 μM reduces E_2F transcription activity by modifying a number of genes involved in regulation of the pRb/E_2F pathway (Barrera et al., 2004). It also activates the antioxidant response triggered by nuclear translocation of transcription factor Nrf2 (Numazawa et al., 2003). This transcription factor regulates a battery of genes that protect against oxidative injury. The collective evidence suggests that 4-HNE may be an important signaling molecule for the regulation of cell proliferation and differentiation. Factors that contribute to 4-HNE neurotoxicity include its relative stability and ability to easily pass among subcellular compartments and to interact with a multitude of different enzymes associated with signal transduction processes.

7.5.2 Neurotoxic Effects

4-HNE not only reacts with lysine, cysteine, and histidine residues in proteins, but also with free amino acids, deoxyguanosine, and aminoglycerophospholipids (Esterbauer et al., 1991; Guichardant et al., 2002). The C3 position of 4-HNE is a highly reactive site that undergoes a Michael addition reaction with cellular thiols and hence readily forms adducts with glutathione or protein-containing

TABLE 7.1. Effect of 4-HNE on enzymic activities of neural and non-neural tissues.

Enzyme	Effect	Reference
Na^+,K^+-ATPase	Inhibited	Kadoya et al., 2003
Ca^{2+}-ATPase	Inhibited	Mark et al., 1997
Protein kinase C	Stimulated	Chiarpotto et al., 1999
Phospholipase C	Stimulated	Rossi et al., 1993
Phospholipase D	Stimulated	Natarajan et al., 1993
Adenylate cyclase	Stimulated	Paradisi et al., 1985
c-jun-N-terminal kinase	Stimulated	Tamagno et al., 2003
Aldolase reductase	Inhibited	Del Corso et al., 1998
Glucose 6-phosphate dehydrogenase	Inhibited	Friguet et al., 1994
Cysteine ligase	Stimulated	Dickinson et al., 2002
Caspase-3	Stimulated	Ji et al., 2001
iNOS	Stimulated	Lee et al., 2004a
Flippase	Inhibited	Castegna et al., 2004

thiol groups. 4-HNE may cause a number of deleterious effects in cells, including inhibition of DNA and RNA synthesis, disturbance in calcium homeostasis, and inhibition of mitochondrial respiration.

The modification of the adenine nucleotide translocator by 4-HNE leads not only to the inhibition of enzymic activities, but also to suppression of ADP and ATP transport through the inner mitochondrial membrane (Picklo et al., 1999). These events play a substantial role in the disruption of the energy-producing capacity of mitochondria. It is estimated that the localized concentration of 4-HNE can increase to as high as 4.5 mM within a peroxidizing membrane bilayer (Esterbauer et al., 1991). Also, suppression of the adenine nucleotide translocator by 4-HNE suppresses ADP and ATP transport through the inner mitochondrial membrane. These processes additionally disrupt the energy-producing functions of mitochondria (Chen et al., 1995).

4-HNE participates in protein cross-linking chemistry via pyrrole formation and Michael adduct-imine formation. 4-HNE exerts its neurotoxicity through several different pathways, but all share protein modification and subsequent dysfunction as the fundamental mechanism. In brain tissue, 4-HNE alters the function of key membrane proteins, including glucose transporter, glutamate transporter, and sodium, potassium ATPases (Mark et al., 1997; Lauderback et al., 2001). Inhibition of sodium, potassium ATPase by 4-HNE can result in the depolarization of neuronal membranes leading to the opening of NMDA receptor channels and the influx of additional calcium ions into the cell (Kadoya et al., 2003). This calcium entry can be very harmful for neurons.

4-HNE also exerts a biphasic effect on NMDA current. In hippocampal neurons after 4-HNE exposure, an early enhancement of NMDA current within the first 30 to 120 min is followed at 6 h by a delayed decrease in current that is significantly less than the basal current (Lu et al., 2001). The molecular mechanism of this biphasic action of 4-HNE on NMDA current is unknown. However, the early enhancement of NMDA current may involve increased phosphorylation of the NR1, an NMDA receptor subunit, and the delayed suppression of NMDA current by 4-HNE may be due to the depletion of ATP resulting in impairment of NMDA receptor channel function (Lu et al., 2001). In cortical neurons, 4-HNE disrupts G-protein-linked muscarinic cholinergic receptors (mAChR) and metabotropic glutamate receptors (mGluR). The disruption of these receptors by 4-HNE may result in alterations in the activity of phospholipase C indicating that 4-HNE modulates signal transduction processes in brain tissue.

4-HNE binds covalently to phosphatidylethanolamine (PtdEtn) and plasmenylethanolamine (PlsEtn). It does not bind to phosphatidylserine. The Michael adduct, 4-HNE-PtdEtn, is a poor substrate for $sPLA_2$ and is not cleaved by PLD (Guichardant et al., 2002; Bacot et al., 2003). PlsEtn also forms a complex with 4-HNE, but is further degraded only at its sn-1 position, the alkenyl chain, which might affect the antioxidant potential of PlsEtn molecules (Farooqui and Horrocks, 2001). The targeting of various classes of ethanolamine glycerophospholipids by 4-HNE produces different degrees of toxicity in neural cells (Guichardant et al., 2002; Bacot et al., 2003).

4-HNE also increases the permeability of the blood-brain barrier (Mertsch et al., 2001). During excitotoxicity, increases in $cPLA_2$ activity and immunoreactivity (Farooqui et al., 2000c) are accompanied by a decrease in the level of the antioxidant glutathione (Ong et al., 2000) in rat hippocampus indicating alterations in cellular redox status. The decrease in glutathione levels may be due to either the formation of 4-HNE-glutathione adducts or the decrease in cysteine uptake due to kainate-mediated neurotoxicity (Farooqui et al., 2001). Both processes increase the vulnerability of neurons to oxidative stress. 4-HNE inhibits rat brain mitochondrial respiration, blocks neurite outgrowth, disrupts neuronal microtubules, and modifies cellular tubulin, which may contribute to the cytoskeletal changes in neurons undergoing a neurodegenerative process (Neely et al., 1999; Farooqui et al., 2004). Also, 4-HNE decreases cellular ATP levels by impairing glucose transport and by depressing mitochondrial function (Keller et al., 1997).

4-HNE induces apoptotic cell death in PC12 cells and rat hippocampal neurons in primary cultures (Kruman et al., 1997). The mechanism of 4-HNE-mediated apoptosis remains unknown. However, 4-HNE may induce apoptosis by altering mitochondrial function, releasing cytochrome c, and subsequently activating the caspase cascade (West et al., 2004). These processes ultimately lead to the activation of caspases and to fragmentation of nucleosomal DNA, resulting in apoptotic cell death. In SH-SY5Y neuroblastoma cells, 4-HNE produces apoptosis by activating the Fas/FasL signaling pathway mediated by p53 (Uchida, 2003). Apoptotic cell death is known to occur in neurodegenerative diseases and neurotraumatic situations, such as ischemia, spinal cord trauma, and head injury (Subramaniam et al., 1997; Selley et al., 2002; Farooqui et al., 2004) in which high levels of 4-HNE are present. Apparently, 4-HNE triggers an oxidative stress response, disrupts mitochondrial function, and blocks numerous cellular "housekeeping" and signal transduction-mediating enzymes (Table 7.1). These processes may lead to oxidative stress and apoptosis.

The balance between neurotrophic and neurotoxic concentrations of 4-HNE is governed not only by its rate of production, but also by its metabolic detoxification. The major route of 4-HNE metabolism in non-neural tissue is the conjugation of 4-HNE with glutathione. Glutathione transferase catalyzes this reaction. The activity of this enzyme in brain tissue is very low compared with liver and kidney (Uchida, 2003). In addition, brain aldehyde dehydrogenase oxidizes 4-HNE to 4-hydroxynonenoic acid (Picklo et al., 2001). This metabolite is an endogenous ligand for the γ-hydroxybutyrate receptor in rat and human cerebral cortices. It may be involved in cross-talk between γ-hydroxybutyrate receptors and receptors that modulate PLA_2 activity and generate 4-HNE in brain tissue. Not only 4-HNE, but also its metabolites, may act as signaling molecules in brain tissue.

7.6 Effects of Acrolein in Brain

Besides 4-HNE, nonenzymic peroxidation of AA also generates acrolein (2-propenal) (Fig. 7.10), another α, β unsaturated aldehyde (Esterbauer et al., 1991). The pronounced toxicity of acrolein reflects its ability to alkylate nucleophilic centers in macromolecules. In contrast to 4-HNE, acrolein has a half-life of 7 to 10 days and is 100 times more reactive than 4-HNE. Like 4-HNE, acrolein binds to proteins, DNA, and glycerophospholipids, and disrupts the functions of these molecules. Acrolein reacts with cysteine, histidine, and lysine residues of proteins. Its incorporation into proteins generates carbonyl derivatives (Uchida, 2003). It also reacts with nucleophilic sites in DNA. This reaction results in modification of DNA bases through the formation of exocyclic adducts. Acrolein produces toxic effects in brain tissue by binding to proteins and inducing mitochondrial oxidative stress (Luo and Shi, 2004). Thus, acrolein inhibits state 3 respiration with an IC_{50} of approx. 0.4 µmol/mg protein. However, there is no reduction in the activity of complexes I–V. Glutathione and N-acetylcysteine can prevent this inhibition.

Acrolein binds to synaptosomal membrane proteins in a dose-dependent manner and increases the levels of protein carbonyl groups. However, pretreatment of synaptosomes with glutathione ethyl ester (GEE) significantly ameliorated both the conformational alterations and protein carbonyls induced by acrolein (Pocernich et al., 2001). Similarly, an in vivo increase in glutathione levels by intraperitoneal injections of N-acetylcysteine decreases carbonyl levels in synaptosomes isolated from acrolein-injected animals compared with synaptosomes from control animals (Pocernich et al., 2001). Acrolein does not alter mitochondrial calcium transporter activity or induce cytochrome c release. Acrolein is a potent inhibitor of brain mitochondrial respiration (Picklo and Montine, 2001). Acrolein-mediated toxicity is accompanied by significant impairment of adenine nucleotide translocase activity (Luo and Shi, 2004) and of glucose and glutamate uptake in primary neuronal cultures (Lovell et al., 2000). It remains to be seen whether acrolein and 4-HNE bind to the same protein or different proteins following peroxidation of AA. However, it is known that acrolein is 100-fold more reactive than 4-HNE toward nucleophiles (Kehrer and Biswal, 2000).

7.7 Generation of DHA Metabolites and Their Effect on Brain Metabolism

7.7.1 Neurotrophic Effects of DHA

DHA affects the physicochemical properties (fluidity, permeability, fusion behavior, and elastic compressibility) of neural membranes (Stillwell and Wassall, 2003), and modulates gene expression of many enzymes involved in signal transduction processes (Horrocks and Farooqui, 2004). Thus, DHA increases dopaminergic, noradrenergic, glutamatergic, and serotonergic neurotransmission, activities of membrane-bound enzymes, ion channels, and receptors, learning and memory processes, inflammation and immunity, apoptosis, and gene expression (Horrocks and Farooqui, 2004). The effect of DHA continues as long as the DHA remains in the diet. DHA acts like a hormone to control the activity of key transcription factors. As stated in Chapter 6, the action of 15-LOX on DHA produces 10, 17S-docosatrienes and 17S-resolvins (Marcheselli et al., 2003). Docosanoids is the collective name for these second messengers. These metabolites not only antagonize the effects of eicosanoids, but also modulate leukocyte trafficking as well as downregulating the expression of cytokines (Marcheselli et al., 2003).

7.7.2 Neurotoxic Effects of DHA

At high levels without sufficient antioxidants, DHA may induce lipid peroxidation because this fatty acid possesses a high degree of unsaturation. This may result in generation of lipid peroxides and aldehyde breakdown products with pro-oxidant properties. Like AA and 4-HNE, DHA is oxidized to 4-hydroxyhexenal (4-HHE) (Fig. 7.10). 4-HHE has a conjugated double bond between the α and β carbon, the γ carbon of 4-HHE is electron deficient and reacts readily with nucleophiles, such as thiols and amines, whilst the carbonyl group forms Schiff bases with amino groups, such as the N-termini of proteins and the ϵ-amino group of lysine.

In spite of the structural similarity between 4-HNE and 4-HHE, the biological actions and efficacies of these aldehydes vary greatly. For example, 4-HHE acts more effectively on mitochondrial permeability transition than 4-HNE (Kristal et al., 1996). 4-HHE more effectively inhibits the mitochondrial ATP translocator than does 4-HNE (Picklo et al., 1999). Recent studies indicate that 4-HHE modulates endothelial nitric oxide synthase (iNOS) through NF-κB activation (Lee et al., 2004a). In contrast, 4-HNE inhibits NF-κB activation. These studies suggest that peroxidation of AA and DHA generates end products that have different effects on transcription factor activities of neural and non-neural tissues (Camandola et al., 2000; Lee et al., 2004a).

Like 4-HNE, 4-HHE induces apoptotic cell death in endothelial cells. The molecular mechanism associated with 4-HHE-mediated cell death remains unknown. However, 4-HHE does trigger apoptotic cell death by inducing apoptotic Bax coupled with a decrease in antiapoptotic Bcl-2 (Lee et al., 2004b). Cell death mediated by 4-HHE involves ROS, nitric oxide, and ONOO⁻ generation, leading to redox imbalance leading to vascular dysfunction. Furthermore, 4-HHE-mediated apoptosis can be blocked by the antioxidant *N*-acetylcysteine, a ROS scavenger, and penicillamine, a ONOO⁻ scavenger. This suggests that 4-HHE-mediated apoptotic cell death involves alterations in redox status and oxidative stress.

7.8 Effects of Nonenzymic Degradation of LA on Brain Metabolism

Similar to the nonenzymic lipid peroxidation of AA and DHA, the nonenzymic lipid peroxidation of LA results in formation of linoleic acid hydroperoxide. This hydroperoxide decomposes to form alkoxy and peroxy free radicals as well as an α,β-unsaturated aldehyde, 4-oxo-2-nonenal (4-ONE) (West et al., 2004). Peroxidized glycerophospholipids perturb the structure of neural membranes and increase intracellular calcium ion concentrations. The binding of calcium to peroxidized glycerophospholipids facilitates the action of PLA_2 on neural membranes (Farooqui et al., 2004). 4-ONE reacts with the 2'-deoxyguanosine, 2'-deoxyadenosine, and 2'-deoxycytidine bases of DNA and His, Cys, and Lys residues of proteins more rapidly than do 4-HNE and 4-HHE (Lee et al., 2000b; Lin et al., 2005). Thus, compared with 4-HNE, 4-ONE efficiently induces apoptotic cell death through the activation of the cascade of caspases and fragmentation of nucleosomal DNA (West et al., 2004; Schneider et al., 2004).

Collectively, these studies suggest that the neurotoxicity of 4-ONE, 4-HNE, and 4-HHE is caused by a combination of noncovalent and covalent chemical reactions with macromolecules. Although their neurotoxic end point is rapidly achieved through irreversible covalent modification of proteins associated with signal transduction, the reversible effects of 4-ONE, 4-HNE, and 4-HHE may also play a substantial role in altering signaling processes associated with neurotoxicity. Their reactivity toward proteins associated with signal transduction modulates the toxicity of these electrophilic aldehydes. For example, 4-oxo-2-nonenal (ONE), an aldehyde derived from the peroxidation of linoleoyl chains of fatty acids, is more reactive than 4-HNE, not only in Michael addition chemistry toward cysteine and histidine, but also in Schiff base formation with lysine. Differences in chemical reactivity of these aldehydes also translate into their biological activity. The exposure of two different neuronal cell lines to 4-ONE and 4-HNE indicates that 4-ONE is more neurotoxic than 4-HNE (Lin et al., 2005). This suggests that among 4-ONE, 4-HNE, and 4-HHE, 4-ONE is the most toxic product of lipid peroxidation.

References

Akaishi T., Nakazawa K., Sato K., Ohno Y., and Ito Y. (2004). 4-Hydroxynonenal modulates the long-term potentiation induced by L-type Ca^{2+} channel activation in the rat dentate gyrus in vitro. *Neurosci. Lett.* 370:155–159.

Allen R. G. and Tresini M. (2000). Oxidative stress and gene regulation. *Free Radic. Biol. Med.* 28:463–499.

Bacot S., Bernoud-Hubac N., Baddas N., Chantegrel B., Deshayes C., Doutheau A., Lagarde M., and Guichardant M. (2003). Covalent binding of hydroxy-alkenals 4-HDDE, 4-HHE, and 4-HNE to ethanolamine phospholipid subclasses. *J. Lipid Res.* 44:917–926.

Barrera G., Pizzimenti S., and Dianzani M. U. (2004). 4-Hydroxynonenal and regulation of cell cycle: effects on the pRb/E2F pathway. *Free Radic. Biol. Med.* 37:597–606.

Basu S. (2004). Isoprostanes: novel bioactive products of lipid peroxidation. *Free Radic. Res.* 38:105–122.

Berlett B. S. and Stadtman E. R. (1997). Protein oxidation in aging, disease, and oxidative stress. *J. Biol. Chem.* 272:20313–20316.

Bernoud-Hubac N., Davies S. S., Boutaud O., Montine T. J., and Roberts L. J., II (2001). Formation of highly reactive gamma-ketoaldehydes (Neuroketals) as products of the neuroprostane pathway. *J. Biol. Chem.* 276:30964–30970.

Buisson A., Lakhmeche N., Verrecchia C., Plotkine M., and Boulu R. G. (1993). Nitric oxide: an endogenous anticonvulsant substance. *NeuroReport* 4:444–446.

Camandola S., Poli G., and Mattson M. P. (2000). The lipid peroxidation product 4-hydroxy-2,3-nonenal increases AP-1-binding activity through caspase activation in neurons. *J. Neurochem.* 74:159–168.

Castegna A., Lauderback C. M., Mohmmad-Abdul H., and Butterfield D. A. (2004). Modulation of phospholipid asymmetry in synaptosomal membranes by the lipid peroxidation products, 4-hydroxynonenal and acrolein: implications for Alzheimer's disease. *Brain Res.* 1004:193–197.

Chen J. J., Bertrand H., and Yu B. P. (1995). Inhibition of adenine nucleotide translocator by lipid peroxidation products. *Free Radic. Biol. Med.* 19:583–590.

Chiarpotto E., Domenicotti C., Paola D., Vitali A., Nitti M., Pronzato M. A., Biasi F., Cottalasso D., Marinari U. M., Dragonetti A., Cesaro P., Isidoro C., and Poli G. (1999). Regulation of rat hepatocyte protein kinase C beta isoenzymes by the lipid peroxidation product 4-hydroxy-2,3-nonenal: a signaling pathway to modulate vesicular transport of glycoproteins. *Hepatology* 29:1565–1572.

Choe M., Jackson C., and Yu B. P. (1995). Lipid peroxidation contributes to age-related membrane rigidity. *Free Radic. Biol. Med.* 18:977–984.

Cleland L. G. and James M. J. (1997). Rheumatoid arthritis and the balance of dietary n-6 and n-3 essential fatty acids. *Br. J Rheumatol.* 36:513–514.

Cracowski J. L. (2004). Isoprostanes: an emerging role in vascular physiology and disease? *Chem. Phys. Lipids* 128:75–83.

Davies S. S., Amarnath V., and Roberts L. J., II (2004). Isoketals: highly reactive gamma-ketoaldehydes formed from the H-2-isoprostane pathway. *Chem. Phys. Lipids* 128:85–99.

Dean R. T., Fu S., Stocker R., and Davies M. J. (1997). Biochemistry and pathology of radical-mediated protein oxidation. *Biochem. J.* 324:1–18.

Del Corso A., Dal Monte M., Vilardo P. G., Cecconi I., Moschini R., Banditelli S., Cappiello M., Tsai L., and Mura U. (1998). Site-specific inactivation of aldose reductase by 4-hydroxynonenal. *Arch. Biochem. Biophys.* 350:245–248.

Dickinson D. A., Iles K. E., Watanabe N., Iwamoto T., Zhang H., Krzywanski D. M., and Forman H. J. (2002). 4-Hydroxynonenal induces glutamate cysteine ligase through JNK in HBE1 cells. *Free Radic. Biol. Med.* 33:974–987.

Duffy S., So A., and Murphy T. H. (1998). Activation of endogenous antioxidant defenses in neuronal cells prevents free radical-mediated damage. *J. Neurochem.* 71:69–77.

Esterbauer H., Schaur R. J., and Zollner H. (1991). Chemistry and biochemistry of 4-hydroxynonenal, malonaldehyde and related aldehydes. *Free Radic. Biol. Med.* 11:81–128.

Fam S. S. and Morrow J. D. (2003). The isoprostanes: unique products of arachidonic acid oxidation – a review. *Curr. Med. Chem.* 10:1723–1740.

Farooqui A. A. and Horrocks L. A. (2001). Plasmalogens: workhorse lipids of membranes in normal and injured neurons and glia. *Neuroscientist* 7:232–245.

Farooqui A. A. and Horrocks L. A. (2006). Phospholipase A_2-generated lipid mediators in brain: the good, the bad, and the ugly. *Neuroscientist* 12:245.

Farooqui A. A., Yang H.-C., and Horrocks L. A. (1997). Involvement of phospholipase A_2 in neurodegeneration. *Neurochem. Int.* 30:517–522.

Farooqui A. A., Horrocks L. A., and Farooqui T. (2000a). Deacylation and reacylation of neural membrane glycerophospholipids. *J. Mol. Neurosci.* 14:123–135.

Farooqui A. A., Horrocks L. A., and Farooqui T. (2000b). Glycerophospholipids in brain: their metabolism, incorporation into membranes, functions, and involvement in neurological disorders. *Chem. Phys. Lipids* 106:1–29.

Farooqui A. A., Ong W. Y., Horrocks L. A., and Farooqui T. (2000c). Brain cytosolic phospholipase A_2: localization, role, and involvement in neurological diseases. *Neuroscientist* 6:169–180.

Farooqui A. A., Ong W. Y., Lu X. R., Halliwell B., and Horrocks L. A. (2001). Neurochemical consequences of kainate-induced toxicity in brain: involvement of arachidonic acid release and prevention of toxicity by phospholipase A_2 inhibitors. *Brain Res. Rev.* 38:61–78.

Farooqui A. A., Ong W. Y., and Horrocks L. A. (2004). Biochemical aspects of neurodegeneration in human brain: involvement of neural membrane phospholipids and phospholipases A_2. *Neurochem. Res.* 29:1961–1977.

Fernstrom J. D. (1999). Effects of dietary polyunsaturated fatty acids on neuronal function. *Lipids* 34:161–169.

Fessel J. P., Porter N. A., Moore K. P., Sheller J. R., and Roberts L. J., II (2002). Discovery of lipid peroxidation products formed in vivo with a substituted tetrahydrofuran ring (isofurans) that are favored by increased oxygen tension. *Proc. Natl Acad. Sci. USA* 99:16713–16718.

Fiez J. A. (1996). Cerebellar contributions to cognition. *Neuron* 16:13–15.

Fisher A. B., Dodia C., Manevich Y., Chen J. W., and Feinstein S. I. (1999). Phospholipid hydroperoxides are substrates for non-selenium glutathione peroxidase. *J. Biol. Chem.* 274:21326–21334.

Friguet B., Stadtman E. R., and Szweda L. I. (1994). Modification of glucose-6-phosphate dehydrogenase by 4-hydroxy-2-nonenal. *J. Biol. Chem.* 269:21639–21643.

Fukunaga M., Makita N., Roberts L. J., Morrow J. D., Takahashi K., and Badr K. F. (1993). Evidence for the existence of F2-isoprostane receptors on rat vascular smooth muscle cells. *Am. J. Physiol.* 264:C1619–C1624.

Furnkranz A. and Leitinger N. (2004). Regulation of inflammatory responses by oxidized phospholipids structure–function relationships. *Curr. Pharm. Des.* 10:915–921.

Guichardant M., Bernoud-Hubac N., Chantegrel B., Deshayes C., and Lagarde M. (2002). Aldehydes from n-6 fatty acid peroxidation. Effects on aminophospholipids. *Prostaglandins Leukot. Essent. Fatty Acids* 67:147–149.

Habib A. and Badr K. F. (2004). Molecular pharmacology of isoprostanes in vascular smooth muscle. *Chem. Phys. Lipids* 128:69–73.

Halliwell B. (1994). Free radicals and antioxidants: a personal view. *Nutr. Rev.* 52:253–265.

Harrison K. A. and Murphy R. C. (1995). Isoleukotrienes are biologically active free radical products of lipid peroxidation. *J. Biol. Chem.* 270:17273–17278.

Heinle H., Gugeler N., Felde R., Okech D., and Spiteller G. (2000). Oxidation of plasmalogens produces highly effective modulators of macrophage function. *Z. Naturforsch.* [C] 55:115–120.

Horrocks L. A. and Farooqui A. A. (2004). Docosahexaenoic acid in the diet: its importance in maintenance and restoration of neural membrane function. *Prostaglandins Leukot. Essent. Fatty Acids* 70:361–372.

Jenkinson A. M., Collins A. R., Duthie S. J., Wahle K. W. J., and Duthie G. G. (1999). The effect of increased intakes of polyunsaturated fatty acids and vitamin E on DNA damage in human lymphocytes. *FASEB J.* 13:2138–2142.

Ji C., Amarnath V., Pietenpol J. A., and Marnett L. J. (2001). 4-Hydroxynonenal induces apoptosis via caspase-3 activation and cytochrome c release. *Chem. Res. Toxicol.* 14:1090–1096.

Kadoya A., Miyake H., and Ohyashiki T. (2003). Contribution of lipid dynamics on the inhibition of bovine brain synaptosomal Na^+–K^+-ATPase activity induced by 4-hydroxy-2-nonenal. *Biol. Pharm. Bull.* 26:787–793.

Kehrer J. P. and Biswal S. S. (2000). The molecular effects of acrolein. *Toxicol. Sci.* 57:6–15.

Keller J. N. and Mattson M. P. (1998). Roles of lipid peroxidation in modulation of cellular signaling pathways, cell dysfunction, and death in the nervous system. *Rev. Neurosci.* 9:105–116.

Keller J. N., Mark R. J., Bruce A. J., Blanc E., Rothstein J. D., Uchida K., Wäg G., and Mattson M. P. (1997). 4-Hydroxynonenal, an aldehydic product of membrane lipid peroxidation, impairs glutamate transport and mitochondrial function in synaptosomes. *Neuroscience* 80:685–696.

Kristal B. S., Park B. K., and Yu B. P. (1996). 4-Hydroxyhexenal is a potent inducer of the mitochondrial permeability transition. *J. Biol. Chem.* 271:6033–6038.

Kruman I., Bruce-Keller A. J., Bredesen D., Wäg G., and Mattson M. P. (1997). Evidence that 4-hydroxynonenal mediates oxidative stress-induced neuronal apoptosis. *J. Neurosci.* 17:5089–5100.

Lahaie I., Hardy P., Hou X., Hassessian H., Asselin P., Lachapelle P., Almazan G., Varma D. R., Morrow J. D., Roberts L. J., II, and Chemtob S. (1998). A novel mechanism for vasoconstrictor action of 8-isoprostaglandin $F_{2\alpha}$ on retinal vessels. *Am. J. Physiol.* 274:R1406–R1416.

Lauderback C. M., Hackett J. M., Huang F. F., Keller J. N., Szweda L. I., Markesbery W. R., and Butterfield D. A. (2001). The glial glutamate transporter, GLT-1, is oxidatively modified by 4-hydroxy-2-nonenal in the Alzheimer's disease brain: the role of $A\beta1–42$. *J. Neurochem.* 78:413–416.

Lee H., Shi W., Tontonoz P., Wang S., Subbanagounder G., Hedrick C. C., Hama S., Borromeo C., Evans R. M., Berliner J. A., and Nagy L. (2000a). Role for peroxisome proliferator-activated receptor α in oxidized phospholipid-induced synthesis of monocyte chemotactic protein-1 and interleukin-8 by endothelial cells. *Circ. Res.* 87:516–521.

Lee S. H., Rindgen D., Bible R. H., Jr., Hajdu E., and Blair I. A. (2000b). Characterization of 2′-deoxyadenosine adducts derived from 4-oxo-2-nonenal, a novel product of lipid peroxidation. *Chem. Res. Toxicol.* 13:565–574.

Lee J. Y., Je J. H., Jung K. J., Yu B. P., and Chung H. Y. (2004a). Induction of endothelial iNOS by 4-hydroxyhexenal through NF-κB activation. *Free Radic. Biol. Med.* 37:539–548.

Lee J. Y., Je J. H., Kim D. H., Chung S. W., Zou Y., Kim N. D., Yoo M. A., Baik H. S., Yu B. P., and Chung H. Y. (2004b). Induction of endothelial apoptosis by 4-hydroxyhexenal. *Eur. J. Biochem.* 271:1339–1347.

Leitinger N. (2003). Oxidized phospholipids as modulators of inflammation in atherosclerosis. *Curr. Opin. Lipidol.* 14:421–430.

Leitinger N. (2005). Oxidized phospholipids as triggers of inflammation in atherosclerosis. *Mol. Nutr. Food Res.* 49:1063–1071.

Leitinger N., Watson A. D., Faull K. F., Fogelman A. M., and Berliner J. A. (1997). Monocyte binding to endothelial cells induced by oxidized phospholipids present in minimally oxidized low density lipoprotein is inhibited by a platelet activating factor receptor antagonist. *Adv. Exp. Med. Biol.* 433:379–382.

Leonard S. S., Harris G. K., and Shi X. (2004). Metal-induced oxidative stress and signal transduction. *Free Radic. Biol. Med.* 37:1921–1942.

Lin D., Lee H. G., Liu Q., Perry G., Smith M. A., and Sayre L. M. (2005). 4-Oxo-2-nonenal is both more neurotoxic and more protein reactive than 4-hydroxy-2-nonenal. *Chem. Res. Toxicol.* 18:1219–1231.

Lovell M. A., Xie C., and Markesbery W. R. (2000). Acrolein, a product of lipid peroxidation, inhibits glucose and glutamate uptake in primary neuronal cultures. *Free Radic. Biol. Med.* 29:714–720.

Lu C., Chan S. L., Haughey N., Lee W. T., and Mattson M. P. (2001). Selective and biphasic effect of the membrane lipid peroxidation product 4-hydroxy-2,3-nonenal on *N*-methyl-D-aspartate channels. *J. Neurochem.* 78:577–589.

Luo H. and Shi R. Y. (2004). Acrolein induces axolemmal disruption, oxidative stress, and mitochondrial impairment in spinal cord tissue. *Neurochem. Int.* 44:475–486.

Lyberg A. M., Fasoli E., and Adlercreutz P. (2005). Monitoring the oxidation of docosahexaenoic acid in lipids. *Lipids* 40:969–979.

Marcheselli V. L., Hong S., Lukiw W. J., Tian X. H., Gronert K., Musto A., Hardy M., Gimenez J. M., Chiang N., Serhan C. N., and Bazan N. G. (2003). Novel docosanoids inhibit brain ischemia-reperfusion-mediated leukocyte infiltration and pro-inflammatory gene expression. *J. Biol. Chem.* 278:43807–43817.

Mark R. J., Lovell M. A., Markesbery W. R., Uchida K., and Mattson M. P. (1997). A role for 4-hydroxynonenal, an aldehydic product of lipid peroxidation, in disruption of ion homeostasis and neuronal death induced by amyloid β-peptide. *J. Neurochem.* 68:255–264.

McIntyre T. M., Zimmerman G. A., and Prescott S. M. (1999). Biologically active oxidized phospholipids. *J. Biol. Chem.* 274:25189–25192.

McLean L. R., Hagaman K. A., and Davidson W. S. (1993). Role of lipid structure in the activation of phospholipase A_2 by peroxidized phospholipids. *Lipids* 28:505–509.

Mertsch K., Blasig I., and Grune T. (2001). 4-Hydroxynonenal impairs the permeability of an in vitro rat blood–brain barrier. *Neurosci. Lett.* 314:135–138.

Milatovic D., Zaja-Milatovic S., Montine K. S., Horner P. J., and Montine T. J. (2003). Pharmacologic suppression of neuronal oxidative damage and dendritic degeneration following direct activation of glial innate immunity in mouse cerebrum. *J. Neurochem.* 87:1518–1526.

Montine T. J., Milatovic D., Gupta R. C., Valyi-Nagy T., Morrow J. D., and Breyer R. M. (2002). Neuronal oxidative damage from activated innate immunity is EP2 receptor-dependent. *J. Neurochem.* 83:463–470.

Morrow J. D., Harris T. M., and Roberts L. J., II (1990). Noncyclooxygenase oxidative formation of a series of novel prostaglandins: analytical ramifications for measurement of eicosanoids. *Anal. Biochem.* 184:1–10.

Morrow J. D., Hill K. E., Burk R. F., Nammour T. M., Badr K. F., and Roberts L. J. (1991). Formation of unique biologically active prostaglandins in vivo by a non-cyclooxygenase free radical catalyzed mechanism. *Adv. Prostaglandin Thromboxane Leukot. Res.* 21A:125–128.

Morrow J. D., Awad J. A., Boss H. J., Blair I. A., and Roberts L. J., II (1992). Non-cyclooxygenase-derived prostanoids (F2-isoprostanes) are formed *in situ* on phospholipids. *Proc. Natl Acad. Sci. USA* 89:10721–10725.

Morrow J. D., Awad J. A., Wu A., Zackert W. E., Daniel V. C., and Roberts L. J., II (1996). Nonenzymatic free radical-catalyzed generation of thromboxane-like compounds (isothromboxanes) in vivo. *J. Biol. Chem.* 271:23185–23190.

Morrow J. D., Tapper A. R., Zackert W. E., Yang J., Sanchez S. C., Montine T. J., and Roberts L. J., II (1999). Formation of novel isoprostane-like compounds from docosahexaenoic acid. *Adv. Exp. Med. Biol.* 469:343–347.

Murakami M., Nakatani Y., Atsumi G., Inoue K., and Kudo I. (1997). Regulatory functions of phospholipase A_2. *Crit. Rev. Immunol.* 17:225–283.

Musiek E. S., Milne G. L., McLaughlin B., and Morrow J. D. (2005). Cyclopentenone eicosanoids as mediators of neurodegeneration: a pathogenic mechanism of oxidative stress-mediated and cyclooxygenase-mediated neurotoxicity. *Brain Pathol.* 15:149–158.

Natarajan V., Scribner W. M., and Taher M. M. (1993). 4-Hydroxynonenal, a metabolite of lipid peroxidation, activates phospholipase D in vascular endothelial cells. *Free Radic. Biol. Med.* 15:365–375.

Neely M. D., Sidell K. R., Graham D. G., and Montine T. J. (1999). The lipid peroxidation product 4-hydroxynonenal inhibits neurite outgrowth, disrupts neuronal microtubules, and modifies cellular tubulin. *J. Neurochem.* 72:2323–2333.

Nourooz-Zadeh J., Halliwell B., and Änggård E. E. (1997). Evidence for the formation of F3-isoprostanes during peroxidation of eicosapentaenoic acid. Biochem. *Biophys. Res. Commun.* 236:467–472.

Nourooz-Zadeh J., Liu E. H. C., Yhlen B., Änggård E. E., and Halliwell B. (1999). F_4-isoprostanes as specific marker of docosahexaenoic acid peroxidation in Alzheimer's disease. *J. Neurochem.* 72:734–740.

Numazawa S., Ishikawa M., Yoshida A., Tanaka S., and Yoshida T. (2003). Atypical protein kinase C mediates activation of NF-E2-related factor 2 in response to oxidative stress. *Am. J. Physiol. Cell Physiol.* 285:C334–C342.

Ong W. Y., Hu C. Y., Hjelle O. P., Ottersen O. P., and Halliwell B. (2000). Changes in glutathione in the hippocampus of rats injected with kainate: depletion in neurons and upregulation in glia. *Exp. Brain Res.* 132:510–516.

Opere C. A., Zheng W. D., Huang J. F., Adewale A., Kruglet M., and Ohia S. E. (2005). Dual effect of isoprostanes on the release of [^{3}H]D-aspartate from isolated bovine retinae: role of arachidonic acid metabolites. *Neurochem. Res.* 30:129–137.

Page S., Fischer C., Baumgartner B., Haas M., Kreusel U., Loidl G., Hayn M., Ziegler-Heitbrock H. W., Neumeier D., and Brand K. (1999). 4-Hydroxynonenal prevents NF-κB activation and tumor necrosis factor expression by inhibiting IκB phosphorylation and subsequent proteolysis. *J. Biol. Chem.* 274:11611–11618.

Paradisi L., Panagini C., Parola M., Barrera G., and Dianzani M. U. (1985). Effects of 4-hydroxynonenal on adenylate cyclase and 5′-nucleotidase activities in rat liver plasma membranes. *Chem. Biol. Interact.* 53:209–217.

Picklo M. J. and Montine T. J. (2001). Acrolein inhibits respiration in isolated brain mitochondria. *Biochim. Biophys. Acta* 1535:145–152.

Picklo M. J., Amarnath V., McIntyre J. O., Graham D. G., and Montine T. J. (1999). 4-Hydroxy-2(*E*)-nonenal inhibits CNS mitochondrial respiration at multiple sites. *J. Neurochem.* 72:1617–1624.

Picklo M. J., Olson S. J., Markesbery W. R., and Montine T. J. (2001). Expression and activities of aldo–keto oxidoreductases in Alzheimer disease. *J. Neuropathol. Exp. Neurol.* 60:686–695.

Pocernich C. B., Cardin A. L., Racine C. L., Lauderback C. M., and Butterfield D. A. (2001). Glutathione elevation and its protective role in acrolein-induced protein damage in synaptosomal membranes: relevance to brain lipid peroxidation in neurodegenerative disease. *Neurochem. Int.* 39:141–149.

Pratico D., Rokach J., Lawson J., and FitzGerald G. A. (2004). F-2-isoprostanes as indices of lipid peroxidation in inflammatory diseases. *Chem. Phys. Lipids* 128:165–171.

Ray P., Ray R., Broomfield C. A., and Berman J. D. (1994). Inhibition of bioenergetics alters intracellular calcium, membrane composition, and fluidity in a neuronal cell line. *Neurochem. Res.* 19:57–63.

Reich E. E., Markesbery W. R., Roberts L. J., II, Swift L. L., Morrow J. D., and Montine T. J. (2001). Brain regional quantification of F-ring and D-/E-ring isoprostanes and neuroprostanes in Alzheimer's disease. *Am. J. Pathol.* 158:293–297.

Roberts L. J., II and Fessel J. P. (2004). The biochemistry of the isoprostane, neuroprostane, and isofuran pathways of lipid peroxidation. *Chem. Phys. Lipids* 128:173–186.

Roberts L. J., II, Montine T. J., Markesbery W. R., Tapper A. R., Hardy P., Chemtob S., Dettbarn W. D., and Morrow J. D. (1998). Formation of isoprostane-like compounds (neuroprostanes) *in vivo* from docosahexaenoic acid. *J. Biol. Chem.* 273:13605–13612.

Roberts L. J., II, Fessel J. P., and Davies S. S. (2005). The biochemistry of the isoprostane, neuroprostane, and isofuran pathways of lipid peroxidation. *Brain Pathol.* 15:143–148.

Rossi M. A., Di Mauro C., and Dianzani M. U. (1993). Action of lipid peroxidation products on phosphoinositide specific phospholipase C. *Mol. Aspects Med.* 14:273–279.

Schneider C., Porter N. A., and Brash A. R. (2004). Autoxidative transformation of chiral ω6 hydroxy linoleic and arachidonic acids to chiral 4-hydroxy-2E-nonenal. *Chem. Res. Toxicol.* 17:937–941.

Selley M. L., Close D. R., and Stern S. E. (2002). The effect of increased concentrations of homocysteine on the concentration of (E)-4-hydroxy-2-nonenal in the plasma and cerebrospinal fluid of patients with Alzheimer's disease. *Neurobiol. Aging* 23:383–388.

Stillwell W. and Wassall S. R. (2003). Docosahexaenoic acid: membrane properties of a unique fatty acid. *Chem. Phys. Lipids* 126:1–27.

Subramaniam R., Roediger F., Jordan B., Mattson M. P., Keller J. N., Wäg G., and Butterfield D. A. (1997). The lipid peroxidation product, 4-hydroxy-2-trans-nonenal, alters the conformation of cortical synaptosomal membrane proteins. *J. Neurochem.* 69:1161–1169.

Takahashi K., Nammour T. M., Fukunaga M., Ebert J., Morrow J. D., Roberts L. J., Hoover R. L., and Badr K. F. (1992). Glomerular actions of a free radical-generated novel prostaglandin, 8-epi-prostaglandin F2α, in the rat. Evidence for interaction with thromboxane A2 receptors. *J. Clin. Invest.* 90:136–141.

Tamagno E., Robino G., Obbili A., Bardini P., Aragno M., Parola M., and Danni O. (2003). H_2O_2 and 4-hydroxynonenal mediate amyloid beta-induced neuronal apoptosis by activating JNKs and p38[MAPK]. *Exp. Neurol.* 180:144–155.

Uchida K. (2003). 4-Hydroxy-2-nonenal: a product and mediator of oxidative stress. *Prog. Lipid Res.* 42:318–343.

Valko M., Morris H., and Cronin M. T. (2005). Metals, toxicity and oxidative stress. *Curr. Med. Chem.* 12:1161–1208.

van Kuijk F. J. G. M., Sevanian A., Handelman G. J., and Dratz E. A. (1987). A new role for phospholipase A_2: protection of membranes from lipid peroxidation damage. *Trends Biochem. Sci.* 12:31–34.

West J. D. and Marnett L. J. (2005). Alterations in gene expression induced by the lipid peroxidation product, 4-hydroxy-2-nonenal. *Chem. Res. Toxicol.* 18:1642–1653.

West J. D., Ji C., Duncan S. T., Amarnath V., Schneider C., Rizzo C. J., Brash A. R., and Marnett L. J. (2004). Induction of apoptosis in colorectal carcinoma cells treated with 4-hydroxy-2-nonenal and structurally related aldehydic products of lipid peroxidation. *Chem. Res. Toxicol.* 17:453–462.

Yeh M., Leitinger N., de Martin R., Onai N., Matsushima K., Vora D. K., Berliner J. A., and Reddy S. T. (2001). Increased transcription of IL-8 in endothelial cells is differentially regulated by TNF-alpha and oxidized phospholipids. *Arterioscler. Thromb. Vasc. Biol.* 21:1585–1591.

Yin H. Y., Musiek E. S., Gao L., Porter N. A., and Morrow J. D. (2005). Regiochemistry of neuroprostanes generated from the peroxidation of docosahexaenoic acid in vitro and in vivo. *J. Biol. Chem.* 280:26600–26611.

Yura T., Fukunaga M., Khan R., Nassar G. N., Badr K. F., and Montero A. (1999). Free-radical-generated F2-isoprostane stimulates cell proliferation and endothelin-1 expression on endothelial cells. *Kidney Int.* 56:471–478.

8
Lyso-Glycerophospholipids

8.1 Introduction

Lyso-glycerophospholipids are metabolic intermediates in glycerophospholipid metabolism. They consist of one long hydrophobic acyl chain and one hydrophilic polar head group attached to a glycerol backbone. In unstimulated neural cells, they occur at low levels (0.5 to 3%). They are transiently produced during the remodeling of glycerophospholipids (Farooqui et al., 2000). Lyso-glycerophospholipids interact with the lipid and protein moieties of neural membranes and modulate the function of neural membrane proteins, such as enzymes and growth factors (Kern et al., 2001). Lyso-glycerophospholipids include lyso-phosphatidylcholines (lyso-PtdCho), lyso-phosphatidylethanolamines (lyso-PtdEtn), lyso-phosphatidylserines (lyso-PtdSer), lyso-phosphatidylinositols (lyso-PtdIns), and lyso-plasmalogens (lyso-PlsEtn and lyso-PlsCho) (Fig. 8.1). In addition, other lyso-glycerophospholipids, such as lyso-phosphatidic acid (lyso-PtdH) and lyso-platelet-activating factor (lyso-PAF), are also generated during glycerophospholipid metabolism.

The metabolism and roles of lyso-PtdH and lyso-PAF (Anliker and Chun, 2004; Farooqui and Horrocks, 2004b) are discussed in Chapters 2 and 9, respectively. Lyso-PtdCho, lyso-PtdEtn, lyso-PtdSer, and the lyso-plasmalogens, lyso-PlsEtn and lyso-PlsCho, are generated along with free fatty acids during glycerophospholipid hydrolysis by phospholipases A_1 (PLA_1), phospholipases A_2 (PLA_2), and plasmalogen-selective phospholipase A_2 ($PlsEtn-PLA_2$) (Farooqui and Horrocks, 2001; Farooqui and Horrocks, 2004a). High-performance liquid chromatography, liquid chromatography–mass spectrometry–mass spectrometry (LC–MS–MS) and electrospray ionization mass spectrometry are used to separate and quantify them (Lesnefsky et al., 2000; Han et al., 2001). Synthesis of these lyso-glycerophospholipids also occurs during the reacylation/deacylation cycle that maintains the acyl group composition of neural membranes (Sun and MacQuarrie, 1989; Farooqui et al., 2000, 2006).

The presence of the hydrophilic head group in relation to the hydrocarbon tail makes lyso-glycerophospholipids pack in the form of highly curved structures that cannot form bilayers. Lyso-glycerophospholipids are nonbilayer-forming lipids (Fuller and Rand, 2001). At low concentrations, lyso-glycerophospholipids

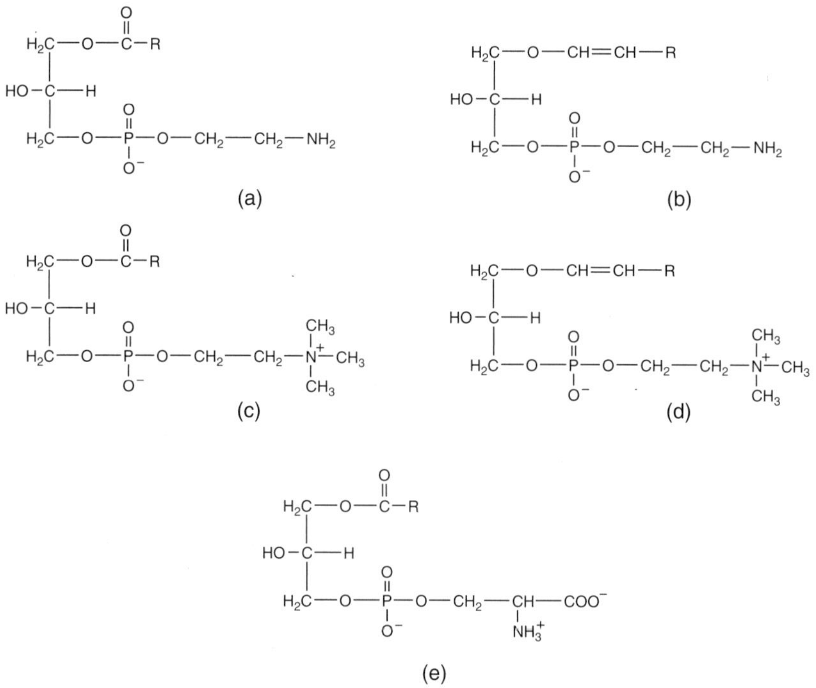

Fig. 8.1. Chemical structures of lyso-glycerophospholipids. Lyso-phosphatidylethanolamine (a); Lyso-plasmenylethanolamine (b); Lyso-phosphatidylcholine (c); Lyso-plasmenylcholine (d); and Lyso-phosphatidylserine (e).

form micelles, but at higher concentrations, they tend to form cylindrical hexagonal phases. At high concentrations, they disorganize structural arrays, alter membrane permeability, and disturb osmotic equilibrium. In lipid bilayers, lyso-glycerophospholipids affect the gating kinetics of several membrane channels, including gramicidin channels (Lundbaek and Andersen, 1994). They stabilize dimer formation between two peptide helices in apposing monolayers, forming an open channel. Because of their detergent-like properties lyso-glycerophospholipids are potentially toxic to cells (Weltzien, 1979; Farooqui et al., 1997). The levels of lyso-glycerophospholipids are strictly controlled. High levels of lyso-glycerophospholipids under pathological situations perturb neural membrane structure, affect many membrane-bound enzymes related to signal transduction, and cause cell lysis (Farooqui and Horrocks, 2006).

1-Acyl-2-lyso-*sn*-Gro*P*Cho is the major lyso-glycerophospholipid of neural membranes, generated by the action of cPLA$_2$ or iPLA$_2$ on PtdCho. 1-Acyl-2-lyso-*sn*-Gro*P*Cho is either hydrolyzed to fatty acid and glycerophosphocholine by lyso-phospholipases (Farooqui et al., 1985) or reacylated to the native glycerophospholipid by CoA-dependent or CoA-independent acyltransferase reactions (Fig. 8.2) (Farooqui et al., 2000; Balsinde, 2002). Thus, 1-acyl-2-lyso-*sn*-Gro*P*Cho accepts an acyl group in the deacylation/reacylation cycle. Lyso-

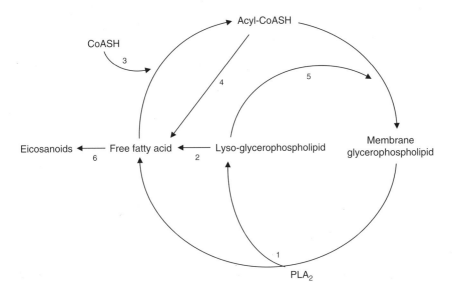

FIG. 8.2. The deacylation–reacylation cycle in brain. Phospholipase A$_2$ (1); lysophospholipase (2); acyl-CoA synthase (3); acyl-CoA hydrolase (4); acyl-CoA:lysophospholipid acyltransferase (5); cyclooxygenase and lipoxygenase (6).

glycerophospholipid: lyso-glycerophospholipid transferase also regulates lysophospholipid levels in neural membranes. Acetylation of 1-alkyl-2-lyso-*sn*-GroPCho produces platelet-activating factor (PAF), a potent proinflammatory lipid mediator, involved in many pathological processes. 1-Acyl-2-lyso-*sn*-GroPEtn, 1-acyl-2-lyso-*sn*-GroPSer, and 1-acyl-2-lyso-*sn*-GroPIns are minor lyso-glycerophospholipids of neural membranes. Like 1-acyl-2-lyso-*sn*-GroPCho, they are formed through the action of isoforms of PLA$_2$ on PtdEtn, PtdSer, and PtdIns. The occurrence of PLA$_2$ isoforms hydrolyzing PtdEtn, PtdSer, and PtdIns has been reported in mammalian tissues, but detailed investigations on isolation and characterization of these isoforms have not been performed (Farooqui and Horrocks, 2004a). Similarly, the hydrolysis of ethanolamine or choline plasmalogens by PlsEtn-selective or PlsCho-selective PLA$_2$ generates lyso-PlsEtn or lyso-PlsCho in brain tissue. These lyso-glycerophospholipids may be involved in modulating signal transduction processes.

8.2 Effects of Lyso-Glycerophospholipids on Neural Membrane Metabolism

8.2.1 1-Acyl-2-lyso-sn-GroPCho (Lyso-PtdCho)

Lyso-PtdCho is an amphiphilic phospholipid present in a variety of mammalian tissues. It acts on neural membranes in several ways. Its incorporation into neural membranes causes significant perturbation of the orderly packed glycerophospholipid molecules in the lipid bilayer. Lyso-PtdCho can interact directly with ion channels (Corr et al., 1995) and alter their activity. Finally, it may participate in signal transduction processes and modulate cellular function (Farooqui and Horrocks, 2006). Thus in model and biological membrane systems, the incorporation of lyso-PtdCho not only changes physicochemical properties of membranes, but also produces changes in their molecular dynamics. Added lyso-PtdCho lowers the electrical resistance of model membranes and increases the permeability. The addition of lyso-PtdCho to a mixture of other lipids causes significant changes in their assembly and organizes them into a structure with greater curvature (Chernomordik et al., 1995). In vitro studies also indicate that the effect of lyso-PtdCho depends on its location in the bilayer, outer, inner monolayer, or symmetrically. Thus exogenous lyso-PtdCho and arachidonic acid differentially affect the fusion of vesicles to planar bilayers depending on their location (Chernomordik et al., 1995). Lyso-PtdCho in lipid bilayers induces membrane tension or stress that influences the conformation and activities of membrane-bound proteins.

Injections of lyso-PtdCho into brain result in acute inflammatory demyelination at the injection site, breakdown of the blood–brain barrier, and interstitial edema around the injection site (Ousman and David, 2000; Lovas et al., 2000; Degaonkar et al., 2002, 2005). Similarly, lyso-PtdCho injections into adult mouse spinal cord produce an early and transient influx of T cells and neutrophils. This is accompanied by rapid recruitment and activation of monocytes, followed by stimulation of microglial cells. In addition, injections of lyso-PtdCho also produce increased expression of the vascular cell adhesion molecule (VCAM-1) and the intracellular vascular molecule (ICAM-1) in blood vessels (Ousman and David, 2000). Treatment of cerebellar slices with lyso-PtdCho also causes demyelination in vitro (Birgbauer et al., 2004). A single dose of lyso-PtdCho in the striatum results in the accumulation of dopamine and reduction in levels of 3,4-dihydroxyphenylacetic acid (DOPAC) and homovanillic acid (HVA) in this region (Lee et al., 2004, 2005). Lyso-PtdCho interferes with dopaminergic neurotransmission, such as release, binding to postsynaptic receptors, uptake, or metabolism, resulting in retarding dopamine turnover and inducing bradykinesia in animals (Lee et al., 2005). This process may also relate to an impairment of locomotor activities in rats. Lyso-PtdCho may act as a ligand to its own receptors (Zhu et al., 2001). It is likely that modulation of dopamine receptor function by lyso-PtdCho may be due to an interaction between dopaminergic receptor and lyso-PtdCho receptor (Lee et al., 2004).

Intracerebroventricular injections of lyso-PtdCho increase behavioral responses and allodynia in acute and chronic models of inflammatory pain mediated by carrageenan (Vahidi et al., 2006), suggesting that lyso-PtdCho is involved in the modulation of neuronal plasticity in nociceptive neurons (Ji et al., 2003). The administration of PLA_2 inhibitors prevents behavioral responses and allodynia (Yeo et al., 2004). In contrast, lyso-PtdEtn shows no significant increase or decrease in behavioral responses. Lyso-PtdCho also inhibits N-methyl-D-aspartate (NMDA) responses, both in nucleated patches taken from cultured neurons and in cells expressing recombinant NMDA receptors. This inhibition is reversible, voltage independent, and stronger at nonsaturating doses of agonist. It is not linked to the charge on the polar head and is not mimicked by lyso-PtdH or PtdCho (Casado and Ascher, 1998), suggesting that the lyso-PtdCho effect requires insertion into the lipid bilayer. The slow time course of its effect probably reflects the time required for its passage from the extracellular solution into the membrane and back (Casado and Ascher, 1998).

In brain, lyso-PtdCho also reversibly blocks exocytosis (Poole et al., 1970) at a stage between triggering and membrane merger (Vogel et al., 1993). Collectively these studies suggest that in mammalian tissues lyso-PtdCho not only regulates membrane-bound enzymes, receptors, and ion channels, but also modulates signal transduction, and platelet aggregation (Oishi et al., 1988; Sakai et al., 1994; Yuan et al., 1996). Lyso-PtdCho stimulates the transcription of cytokines, chemokines, and adhesion molecules in vitro (Murugesan et al., 2003).

Lyso-PtdCho promotes the activation of microglia and other immune cells and induces the deramification of murine microglia (Schilling et al., 2004). The deramification of microglial cells can be prevented by inhibition of nonselective cation channels and K^+– Cl^- co-transporters. Deramification results in the complete retraction of cell extensions and an increased size of cell bodies with amoeboid morphology. Lyso-PtdCho also stimulates cell motility and releases proinflammatory cytokines. Lyso-PtdCho modulates ion channel permeability in various brain preparations, but the mechanism is not known. At least three different mechanisms are possible. Firstly, by incorporating into neural membranes, it can perturb the orderly packing of glycerophospholipid bilayers inducing alterations of the normal conformation of integral membrane proteins, such as ion channels. Secondly, lyso-PtdCho can directly interact with ion channel proteins, and finally, lyso-PtdCho can modulate ion channels by modulating signal transduction processes. Thus in neurons, lyso-PtdCho produces prolonged membrane hyperpolarization of K^+ channels (Maingret et al., 2000). Under certain conditions, lyso-PtdCho also causes cell fusion indicating that lyso-PtdCho may be involved in cell–cell and membrane–membrane interactions. This suggests that lyso-PtdCho may be involved in neurotransmitter release. Lyso-PtdCho may act as a physiological carrier of DHA to the brain tissue by facilitating DHA transport through the blood–brain barrier (Bernoud et al., 1999). Thus in neural and non-neural tissues, at low concentrations lyso-PtdCho may not only modulate signal transduction processes associated with normal brain metabolism, but also be involved in neurotransmitter release and DHA transport into the brain.

Another important effect of lyso-PtdCho is its ability to activate protein kinases, such as protein kinase C, protein kinase A, c-jun terminal kinase, and tyrosine kinase (Table 8.1). Other enzymes, such as nitric oxide synthase and cyclooxygenase-2, are stimulated by lyso-PtdCho, whereas CTP-phosphocholine cytidylyltransferases are inhibited (Boggs et al., 1995; Gómez-Muñoz et al., 1999). Lyso-PtdCho stimulates phospholipases A_2 and D (Cox and Cohen, 1996; Fang et al., 1997). In contrast, other lyso-glycerophospholipids, such as lyso-PtdEtn and lyso-PtdSer, markedly inhibit phospholipase D activity (Ryu and Palta, 2000).

TABLE 8.1. Effect of lyso-phosphatidylcholine on enzymic activities in neural and non-neural tissues.

Enzyme	Effect	Reference
Protein kinase C	Stimulation	Bassa et al., 1999
Tyrosine kinase	Stimulation	Légrádi et al., 2004
c-jun N-terminal kinase	Stimulation	Fang et al., 1997
Phospholipase D	Stimulation	Cox and Cohen, 1996
Adenylate cyclase	Stimulation	Yuan et al., 1996
Cyclooxygenase	Stimulation	Rikitake et al., 2001
Nitric oxide synthase	Inhibition	Durante et al., 1997
Calpain	Stimulation	Chaudhuri et al., 2003
MAP kinase	Stimulation	Bassa et al., 1999
HMG-CoA reductase	Stimulation	Muir et al., 1996
Na^+, K^+-ATPase	Inhibition	Fink and Gross, 1984
Arginase	Stimulation	Durante et al., 1997

Lyso-PtdCho also regulates guanylate and adenylate cyclase activities (Yuan et al., 1996), inhibits insulin receptor autophosphorylation and signaling, and increases the expression of adhesion molecules on endothelial cells. Low concentrations of lyso-PtdCho inhibit Na^+, K^+-ATPase (Lundbaek and Andersen, 1994), whereas high concentrations lead to enhanced ion permeability via increased membrane fluidity and the formation of actual ion pores (Bao et al., 2004). Many effects induced by lyso-PtdCho are mediated by protein kinase C. In addition, lyso-PtdCho not only modulates ion current activity but also amplifies the oxidative state in non-neural membranes (Leitinger, 2005).

The effect of lyso-PtdCho on the Na^+–H^+ exchanger remains controversial. Earlier studies indicate that this lyso-phospholipid inhibits the Na^+–H^+ exchanger, but recent studies provide evidence that lyso-PtdCho has no effect (Goel et al., 2003). Lyso-PtdCho also enhances cellular responses for proliferation and differentiation when other second messengers like diacylglycerols and calcium ions are present in the medium. Lyso-PtdCho also regulates the expression of nuclear factor kappa B (NFκB), heparin-binding epidermal growth factor-like growth factor, and cellular adhesion molecule-1 (Kume et al., 1992; Nakano et al., 1994; Kume and Gimbrone, Jr., 1994; Zembowicz et al., 1995) (Table 8.2). It also modulates the ICAM promoter (Zhu et al., 1997).

As stated earlier, in non-neural cells lyso-PtdCho acts as an agonist for certain G-protein-coupled receptors. For example, it induces insulin secretion from pancreatic β-cells. The molecular mechanism involved in this secretory process remains elusive. An orphan G-protein-coupled receptor GPR119, predominantly expressed in the pancreas, plays a pivotal role in this event (Soga et al., 2005). Lyso-PtdCho potently enhances insulin secretion in response to high concentrations of glucose in the perfused rat pancreas via stimulation of adenylate cyclase, and dose dependently induces intracellular cAMP accumulation and insulin secretion in a mouse pancreatic beta-cell line, NIT-1. GPR119-specific siRNA significantly blocks lyso-PtdCho-induced insulin secretion from NIT-1 cells. This

interact with high-affinity NGF receptors of the TrkA-type and modulate PtdCho-selective phospholipase (PLD). This enzyme may be involved in exocytotic signaling pathways in rat peritoneal mast cells (Seebeck et al., 2001). The broad-spectrum serine/threonine kinase inhibitor staurosporine potently inhibits exocytosis and PLD activity, whereas the protein kinase C (PKC)-activator PMA, phorbol-12-myristate-13-acetate, activates exocytosis and PLD activity, suggesting a role for PKC as mediator for the activation of PLD induced by NGF/lyso-PtdSer.

Lyso-PtdSer also stimulates an intracellular calcium ion increase in L2071 mouse fibroblast cells. 1-[6-((17β-3-Methoxyestra-1,3,5(10)-trien-17-yl)amino) hexyl]-1H-pyrrole-2,5-dione (U-73122) blocks this increase, but pertussis toxin does not, suggesting that lyso-PtdSer stimulates calcium signaling via G-protein-coupled receptor-mediated phospholipase C activation (Park et al., 2006). Moreover, the lyso-phosphatidic acid receptor antagonist, (S)-phosphoric acid mono-(2-octadec-9-enoylamino-3-[4-(pyridine-2-ylmethoxy)-phenyl]-propyl) ester (VPC 32183), does not block lyso-PtdSer-induced calcium mobilization, indicating that lyso-PtdSer binds to its own receptor. In L2071 cells, lyso-PtdSer stimulates two types of mitogen-activated protein kinase, namely, extracellular signal-regulated protein kinase (ERK) and p38 kinase. Pertussis toxin inhibits the activation of both ERK and p38 kinase, indicating the association of pertussis toxin-sensitive G-proteins in the stimulatory process. In L2071 cells, lyso-PtdSer stimulates chemotactic migration. Pertussis toxin completely inhibits this process, indicating the involvement of pertussis toxin-sensitive Gi protein(s). This chemotaxis of L2071 cells induced by lyso-PtdSer is also dramatically blocked by 2-(4-morpholinyl)-8-phenyl-4H-1-benzopyran-4-one (LY294002) and by 2'-amino-3'-methoxyflavone (PD98059). Collectively, these studies demonstrate that lyso-PtdSer stimulates at least two different signaling cascades, one involving a pertussis toxin-insensitive but phospholipase C-dependent intracellular calcium ion increase, and the other, a pertussis toxin-sensitive chemotactic migration mediated by phosphoinositide 3-kinase and ERK (Park et al., 2006). Lyso-PtdSer also stimulates intracellular release of calcium in human leukemic THP-1 cells but not in normal human peripheral blood mononuclear cells (Park et al., 2005), indicating that the lyso-PtdSer receptor may be associated with leukemia. Lyso-PtdSer also stimulates the intracellular calcium ion, $[Ca^{2+}]_i$, increase in leukemic cells, but not in normal human peripheral blood mononuclear cells. This $[Ca^{2+}]_i$ increase stimulated by lyso-PtdSer can be blocked by U-73122, but not by U-73343. Lyso-PtdSer also stimulated the generation of inositol phosphates in THP-1 cells, indicating that lyso-PtdSer stimulates calcium ion signaling via PLC activation. Moreover, pertussis toxin (PTX) completely prevents the $[Ca^{2+}]_i$ increase by Lyso-PtdSer, indicating the involvement of PTX-sensitive G-proteins. Furthermore, the $[Ca^{2+}]_i$ increase mediated by lyso-PtdSer can be completely prevented by suramin, indicating G-protein-coupled receptor activation. Based on these pharmacological studies, it is proposed that lyso-PtdSer specifically stimulates $[Ca^{2+}]_i$ increase in leukemic cells through a lyso-PtdSer receptor linked to phospholipase C via PTX-sensitive G-proteins (Park et al., 2005, 2006).

8.2.4 Lyso-PtdIns

In neural membranes the deacylation of PtdIns by a PtdIns-specific PLA_1 produces lyso-PtdIns (Ueda et al., 1993; Tsutsumi et al., 1994). Lyso-PtdIns is also generated by the reverse reaction of lyso-PtdIns acyltransferase (Yamashita et al., 2003). In synaptic membranes, lyso-PtdIns is hydrolyzed by a PLC specific for lyso-PtdIns (Kobayashi et al., 1996). In Ras-transformed cells, a PtdIns-specific PLA_2 catalyzes lyso-PtdIns synthesis. Lyso-PtdIns enhances phosphoinositide breakdown, mobilizes cytosolic Ca^{2+}, and stimulates arachidonic acid release, suggesting that it enhances both PLC and PLA_2 activities. Pretreatment of cells with pertussis toxin blocks none of these effects. Instead, tyrphostins AG18 and AG561, tyrosine kinase inhibitors, completely block the mitogenic action of lyso-PtdIns. The effects of lyso-PtdIns are distinguishable from those of the well-known mitogen lyso-PtdH, which affects the signaling pathways differently. These results suggest that the mitogenic activity of lyso-PtdIns is associated with the activation of PLC and PLA_2 and is relatively specific for ras-transformed cells (Falasca et al., 1995). The treatment of H-Ras-transformed fibroblasts with ionophore A23187 causes a 10-fold increase in the levels of this lysolipid in the extracellular medium (Falasca et al., 1998), suggesting the stimulation of PLA_2 activity. In H-Ras-transformed fibroblasts, extracellular lyso-PtdIns can be hydrolyzed rapidly to inositol 1:2-cyclic phosphate. The formation and release of lyso-PtdIns may function as an autocrine mechanism that participates in the Ras-dependent stimulation of cell growth (Falasca et al., 1998). Collectively these studies suggest that in non-neural tissues lyso-PtdIns is not only associated with autocrine mechanisms, but also with an important component of the CoA-dependent transacylation system that modulates polyphosphoinositide homeostasis in rat liver microsomes (Yamashita et al., 2003).

8.2.5 Lyso-PlsEtn and Lyso-PlsCho

Plasmalogen-selective phospholipase A_2 (PlsEtn-PLA_2) generates ethanolamine and choline lyso-plasmalogens (Farooqui and Horrocks, 2001). In brain tissue they are either rapidly reacylated to maintain normal levels of plasmalogens in neural membranes or hydrolyzed by a lyso-plasmalogenase (Jurkowitz-Alexander et al., 1989). Lyso-plasmalogens can also be converted to an acetylated platelet-activating factor analog either by a CoA-independent transacetylase activity or via acetyl transferase activity (Lee, 1998). Like lyso-PtdCho, lyso-PlsEtn and lyso-PlsCho are amphiphilic molecules. They act as detergents and affect the integrity of neural membranes by interacting with individual proteins or by affecting the biophysical properties of neural membranes. Lyso-PlsEtn and lyso-PlsCho increase membrane fluidity (Han and Gross, 1991) and modulate activities of various enzymes. Thus lyso-PlsCho activates cAMP-dependent protein kinase, PKA (Williams and Ford, 1997), suggesting that this lyso-plasmalogen may be involved in a signal transduction process. The activation of PKA mediated by lyso-plasmalogens suggests that these lyso-glycerophospholipids may be crucial in turning off PKA activation, similar to the inactivation of PKC by diacylglyc-erol lipase. Other lyso-glycerophospholipids, such as lyso-PlsEtn and lyso-PtdSer, have no effect on cAMP-dependent protein kinase activity. By altering the action potential and inducing depolarization, high levels of lyso-plasmalogens in heart tissue produce spontaneous contraction, which may cause arrhythmia (Caldwell and Baumgarten, 1998).

8.3 Lyso-Phospholipases in Brain

Lyso-phospholipases are enzymes that catalyze the hydrolysis of the carboxyl ester bonds of lyso-glycerophospholipids and generate fatty acids and water-soluble glycerophosphocholine or glycerophosphoethanolamine. They are widely distributed and exist in a number of isoforms (Wang and Dennis, 1999). Lyso-phospholipases are classified into large molecular weight and low molecular weight isoforms. Large isoform enzymes (mol mass: 60 kDa and above) have not only hydrolase activity, but also transacylase activity, whereas small isoform enzymes (mol mass: 16.5 to 28 kDa) show only hydrolytic activity. We purified a lyso-phospholipase activity from bovine brain acetone powder using a multiple column chromatographic procedure (Farooqui et al., 1985). The purified enzyme migrates as a single band on SDS-polyacryamide gel electrophoresis and has mol mass of 36 kDa. It shows optimal activity at pH 7.0–7.5. The variation of sub-strate concentration at a fixed enzyme concentration resulted in a double recipro-cal plot with an apparent Km value of 18.0 μM and a Vmax value of 0.55 μmol/min/mg (Table 8.3). Nonionic detergents like Triton-X-100 and Tween-20 above 0.2% strongly inhibit the lyso-phospholipase activity. Purified lyso-phospholipase hydrolyzes PtdCho and PtdEtn at similar rates (Farooqui et al., 1985). Another lyso-phospholipase was purified from bovine brain cytosol using a multiple column chromatographic procedure (Pete and Exton, 1996). This enzyme shows selectivity for arachidonoyl-substituted lyso-PtdCho and hydrolyzes this glycerophospholipid at pH 7.4–8.0. MgCl$_2$ stimulates it. The puri-fied enzyme shows a single band on SDS-gel electrophoresis (mol mass: 95 kDa). It contains PLA$_2$ activity and hydrolyzes PtdCho at a 5-fold lower rate than lyso-PtdCho. A variety of lower mol mass lyso-phospholipase activities (mol mass: 20 to 28 kDa) have been purified from non-neural tissues (Garsetti et al., 1992). These have lower activity compared with the 95-kDa bovine lyso-phospholipase.

Purified cPLA$_2$ (mol mass: 85 kDa) also displays lyso-phospholipase and CoA-independent transacylase activities (Wang and Dennis, 1999). Like cPLA$_2$ activity, the lyso-phospholipase activity is stimulated by PIP$_2$ and glycerol. A similarly purified preparation of cPLA$_2$ from the macrophage cell line RAW 264.7 also exhibits lyso-phospholipase activity (Leslie, 1991). This enzyme has a mol mass of 100 kDa and moves as a single band on polyacryamide gels. At pH 6.0 this lyso-phospholipase exhibits apparent Km and Vmax values of 25 μM and 1.5 μmol/min/mg, respectively (Table 8.3). Thus, the hydrolysis of PtdCho by cPLA$_2$ generates the substrate for its lyso-phospholipase activity that hydrolyzes

TABLE 8.3. Kinetic parameters of neural and non-neural lyso-phospholipases and lyso-plasmalogenases.

Source	Substrate	pH optimum	Km value (μM)	Vmax (μmol/min/mg)	Reference
Bovine brain acetone powder	Lyso-phospholipid thioester	7.0–7.5	18.0	0.55	Farooqui et al., 1985
Bovine brain cytosol	1-Arachidonoyl-2-lyso-sn-GroPCho	7.5	–	70.00	Pete and Exton, 1996
Macrophage cell line RAW 264.7	1-Palmitoyl-2-lyso-sn-GroPCho	6.0–8.0	25	1.50	Leslie, 1991
Human brain (cloned)	1-Palmitoyl-2-lyso-sn-GroPCho	8.0	12.7	1.13	Wang et al., 1999
Human brain (membranes)	1-Palmitoyl-2-lyso-sn-GroPCho	8.0	19.3	18.3	Ross and Kish, 1994
Human brain (cytosol)	1-Palmitoyl-2-lyso-sn-GroPCho	8.0	8.1	19.7	Ross and Kish, 1994
Rat liver microsomes	Lyso-PlsCho	6.6	5.5	11.7	Jurkowitz-Alexander et al., 1989
Rat liver microsomes	Lyso-PlsEtn	7.1	42.0	13.6	Jurkowitz-Alexander et al., 1989
Rat intestine	Lyso-PlsEtn	6.8	40.0	70.0	Jurkowitz et al., 1999
Rat intestine	Lyso-PlsCho	7.4	66.0	50	Jurkowitz et al., 1999

fatty acid from the sn-1 position indicating that cPLA$_2$ can hydrolyze lyso-glycerophospholipids as they accumulate in membranes and protect tissue from toxic effects of lyso-glycerophospholipids.

Purified iPLA$_2$ from P388D$_1$ macrophage cells also has a lyso-phospholipase activity, which is inhibited by Triton-X-100 and stimulated by glycerol (Wang and Dennis, 1999). Thus, the broad substrate specificity of PLA$_2$ and lyso-phospholipases and strong immunological identity between the 95-kDa lyso-phospholipase and recombinant cPLA$_2$ suggest that these enzymes are structurally related and may be involved in not only maintaining signal transduction processes and glycerophospholipid homeostasis in neural membranes, but also protecting neural cells from the toxic effects of lyso-glycerophospholipids. Other lyso-phospholipase activities with low mol mass appear to be different proteins as suggested by their structural differences (Wang and Dennis, 1999). Thus, elucidation of the function of various lyso-phospholipases is complicated by the occurrence of multiple forms of these enzymes in brain tissue. Multiple forms of lyso-phospholipases may not function interchangeably but act in parallel on different pools of lyso-glycerophospholipids in various types of neural cells, neurons, astrocytes, oligodendrocytes, and microglial cells, located in different regions of brain tissue. Coordination and integration of various lipid mediators in various subcellular compartments of different neural cells is necessary for optimal functioning of lyso-phospholipase-mediated signal transduction processes. This suggests that a tight and differential regulation of lyso-phospholipases is important for normal brain function specifically during pathological situations (Farooqui et al., 1985).

8.4 Lyso-Plasmalogenase in Brain

Lyso-plasmalogenase cleaves the alkenyl ether bond in lyso-plasmalogens and generates water-soluble glycerophosphoethanolamine (GroPEtn) or glycerophosphocholine (GroPCho) and a fatty aldehyde (Jurkowitz-Alexander et al., 1989) (Fig. 8.3). This enzyme has no activity toward monoacyl- or monoalkyl-lysoglycerophospholipids. It occurs in brain microsomes, but its activity is 700-fold less in brain microsomes than in liver microsomes. It has been partially purified and characterized from rat liver microsomes (Jurkowitz-Alexander et al., 1989).

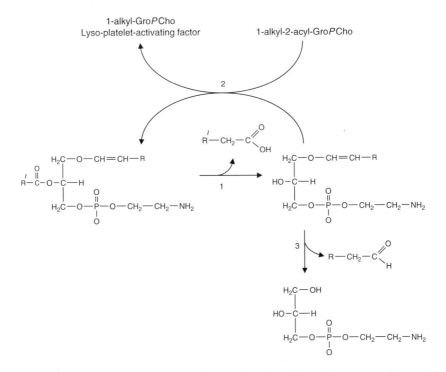

FIG. 8.3. Metabolism of lysoplasmalogens in brain. Phospholipase A_2 (1); acyl-CoA:lysophospholipid acyltransferase (2); and lysoplasmalogenase (3).

This enzyme is inhibited by nonionic (Triton-X-100 and octyl glucoside) and anionic (deoxycholate) detergents. Sulfhydryl-blocking reagents, such as iodoacetate and p-chloromercuribenzoate, also inhibit lyso-plasmalogenase activity in a dose- and time-dependent manner. Divalent metal ions have no effect on lyso-plasmalogenase activity. The role of lyso-plasmalogenase in brain tissue is not fully understood. However, it is proposed that this enzyme, together with PlsEtn-PLA$_2$, may be involved in modulating the levels of lyso-plasmalogen needed for the maintenance of signal transduction process associated with cell differentiation (Jurkowitz et al., 1999).

8.5 Concluding Remarks

Lyso-glycerophospholipids have emerged as important lipid mediators for normal brain function. In brain they are not only involved in the modulation of neurotransmitter release and regulation of activities of membrane-bound enzymes, but also in transport of docosahexaenoic acid through the blood–brain barrier, microglial cell activation, signal transduction processes associated with neuroinflammation, and modulation of many genes, including those involved in neural cell differentiation and oxidative stress. Under pathological conditions, their accumulation produces demyelination and neural cell injury. In neural membranes, their levels are controlled not only by their reacylation, but also through activities of lyso-phospholipases as well as PLA$_2$. In neural and non-neural cells, lyso-glycerophospholipids also induce morphological changes in neural membranes, including membrane fusion and lysis. They also induce secretion of hormones, growth factors, and other lipid mediators that modulate the homeostasis and dynamics of membrane glycerophospholipids.

References

Anliker B. and Chun J. (2004). Cell surface receptors in lysophospholipid signaling. *Semin. Cell Dev. Biol.* 15:457–465.

Aoki J., Nagai Y., Hosono H., Inoue K., and Arai H. (2002). Structure and function of phosphatidylserine-specific phospholipase A$_1$. *Biochim. Biophys. Acta Mol. Cell Biol. Lipids* 1582:26–32.

Balsinde J. (2002). Roles of various phospholipases A$_2$ in providing lysophospholipid acceptors for fatty acid phospholipid incorporation and remodelling. *Biochem. J.* 364:695–702.

Bao S. Z., Miller D. J., Ma Z. M., Wohltmann M., Eng G., Ramanadham S., Moley K., and Turk J. (2004). Male mice that do not express group VIA phospholipase A$_2$ produce spermatozoa with impaired motility and have greatly reduced fertility. *J. Biol. Chem.* 279:38194–38200.

Bassa B. V., Roh D. D., Vaziri N. D., Kirschenbaum M. A., and Kamanna V. S. (1999). Lysophosphatidylcholine activates mesangial cell PKC and MAP kinase by PLCγ-1 and tyrosine kinase-Ras pathways. *Am. J. Physiol.* 277:F328–F337.

Bernoud N., Fenart L., Molière P., Dehouck M. P., Lagarde M., Cecchelli R., and Lecerf J. (1999). Preferential transfer of 2-docosahexaenoyl-1-lysophosphatidylcholine through an in vitro blood–brain barrier over unesterified docosahexaenoic acid. *J. Neurochem.* 72:338–345.

Birgbauer E., Rao T. S., and Webb M. (2004). Lysolecithin induces demyelination in vitro in a cerebellar slice culture system. *J. Neurosci. Res.* 78:157–166.

Boggs K. P., Rock C. O., and Jackowski S. (1995). Lysophosphatidylcholine and 1-*O*-octadecyl-2-*O*-methyl-*rac*-glycero-3-phosphocholine inhibit the CDP-choline pathway of phosphatidylcholine synthesis at the CTP: phosphocholine cytidylyltransferase step. *J. Biol. Chem.* 270:7757–7764.

Bruni A., Bigon E., Boarato E., Mietto L., Leon A., and Toffano G. (1982). Interaction between nerve growth factor and lysophosphatidylserine on rat peritoneal mast cells. *FEBS Lett.* 138:190–192.

Bruni A., Bigon E., Battistella A., Boarato E., Mietto L., and Toffano G. (1984). Lysophosphatidylserine as histamine releaser in mice and rats. *Agents Actions* 14:619–625.

Bruni A., Monastra G., Bellini F., and Toffano G. (1988). Autacoid properties of lyso-phosphatidylserine. *Prog. Clin. Biol. Res.* 282:165–179.

Caldwell R. A. and Baumgarten C. M. (1998). Plasmalogen-derived lysolipid induces a depolarizing cation current in rabbit ventricular myocytes. *Circ. Res.* 83:533–540.

Casado M. and Ascher P. (1998). Opposite modulation of NMDA receptors by lyso-phospholipids and arachidonic acid: common features with mechanosensitivity. *J. Physiol.* 513(Pt 2):317–330.

Chaudhuri P., Colles S. M., Damron D. S., and Graham L. M. (2003). Lysophosphatidylcholine inhibits endothelial cell migration by increasing intracellular calcium and activating calpain. *Arterioscler. Thromb. Vasc. Biol.* 23:218–223.

Chernomordik L., Chanturiya A., Green J., and Zimmerberg J. (1995). The hemifusion intermediate and its conversion to complete fusion: regulation by membrane composition. *Biophys. J.* 69:922–929.

Corr P. B., Yamada K. A., Creer M. H., Wu J., McHowat J., and Yan G. X. (1995). Amphipathic lipid metabolites and arrythmias during ischemia. In: Zipes D. P. and Jalife J. (eds.), *Cardiac Electrophysiology: From Cell to Bedside.* W. B. Saunders, Philadelphia, pp. 182–203.

Cox D. A. and Cohen M. L. (1996). Lysophosphatidylcholine stimulates phospholipase D in human coronary endothelial cells: Role of PKC. *Am. J. Physiol. Heart Circ. Physiol.* 271:H1706–H1710.

Degaonkar M. N., Khubchandhani M., Dhawan J. K., Jayasundar R., and Jagannathan N. R. (2002). Sequential proton MRS study of brain metabolite changes monitored during a complete pathological cycle of demyelination and remyelination in a lysophosphatidyl choline (LPC)-induced experimental demyelinating lesion model. *NMR Biomed.* 15:293–300.

Degaonkar M. N., Raghunathan P., Jayasundar R., and Jagannathan N. R. (2005). Determination of relaxation characteristics during preacute stage of lysophosphatidyl choline-induced demyelinating lesion in rat brain: an animal model of multiple sclerosis. *Magn. Reson. Imaging* 23:69–73.

Durante W., Liao L., Peyton K. J., and Schafer A. I. (1997). Lysophosphatidylcholine regulates cationic amino acid transport and metabolism in vascular smooth muscle cells. Role in polyamine biosynthesis. *J. Biol. Chem.* 272:30154–30159.

Falasca M., Silletta M. G., Carvelli A., Di Francesco A. L., Fusco A., Ramakrishna V., and Corda D. (1995). Signalling pathways involved in the mitogenic action of lyso-phosphatidylinositol. *Oncogene* 10:2113–2124.

Falasca M., Iurisci C., Carvelli A., Sacchetti A., and Corda D. (1998). Release of the mitogen lysophosphatidylinositol from H-Ras-transformed fibroblasts; a possible mechanism of autocrine control of cell proliferation. *Oncogene* 16:2357–2365.

Fang X., Gibson S., Flowers M., Furui T., Bast R. C., Jr., and Mills G. B. (1997). Lysophosphatidylcholine stimulates activator protein 1 and the c-Jun N-terminal kinase activity. *J. Biol. Chem.* 272:13683–13689.

Farooqui A. A. and Horrocks L. A. (2001). Plasmalogens: workhorse lipids of membranes in normal and injured neurons and glia. *Neuroscientist* 7:232–245.

Farooqui A. A. and Horrocks L. A. (2004a). Brain phospholipases A_2: a perspective on the history. *Prostaglandins Leukot. Essent. Fatty Acids* 71:161–169.

Farooqui A. A. and Horrocks L. A. (2004b). Plasmalogens, platelet activating factor, and other ether lipids. In: Nicolaou A. and Kokotos G. (eds.), *Bioactive Lipids*. Oily Press, Bridgwater, England, pp. 107–134.

Farooqui A. A. and Horrocks L. A. (2006). Phospholipase A_2-generated lipid mediators in brain: the good, the bad, and the ugly. *Neuroscientist* 12:245.

Farooqui A. A., Pendley C. E., II, Taylor W. A., and Horrocks L. A. (1985). Studies on diacylglycerol lipases and lysophospholipases of bovine brain. In: Horrocks L. A., Kanfer J. N., and Porcellati G. (eds.), *Phospholipids in the Nervous System, Vol. II: Physiological Role*. Raven Press, New York, pp. 179–192.

Farooqui A. A., Yang H. C., Rosenberger T. A., and Horrocks L. A. (1997). Phospholipase A_2 and its role in brain tissue. *J. Neurochem.* 69:889–901.

Farooqui A. A., Horrocks L. A., and Farooqui T. (2000). Deacylation and reacylation of neural membrane glycerophospholipids. *J. Mol. Neurosci.* 14:123–135.

Farooqui A. A., Horrocks L. A., and Farooqui T. (2006). Choline and ethanolamine glycerophospholipids. In: Tettamanti G. and Goracci G. (eds.), *Handbook of Neurochemistry*. Springer, New York.

Fink K. L. and Gross R. W. (1984). Modulation of canine myocardial sarcolemmal membrane fluidity by amphiphilic compounds. *Circ. Res.* 55:585–594.

Flemming P. K., Dedman A. M., Xu S. Z., Li J., Zeng F., Naylor J., Benham C. D., Bateson A. N., Muraki K., and Beech D. J. (2006). Sensing of lysophospholipids by TRPC5 calcium channel. *J. Biol. Chem.* 281:4977–4982.

Fuller N. and Rand R. P. (2001). The influence of lysolipids on the spontaneous curvature and bending elasticity of phospholipid membranes. *Biophys. J.* 81:243–254.

Garsetti D. E., Ozgur L. E., Steiner M. R., Egan R. W., and Clark M. A. (1992). Isolation and characterization of three lysophospholipases from the murine macrophage cell line WEHI 265.1. *Biochim. Biophys. Acta Lipids Lipid Metab.* 1165:229–238.

Goel D. P., Ford D. A., and Pierce G. N. (2003). Lysophospholipids do not directly modulate Na^+–H^+ exchange. *Mol. Cell. Biochem.* 251:3–7.

Gómez-Muñoz A., O'Brien L., Hundal R., and Steinbrecher U. P. (1999). Lysophosphatidylcholine stimulates phospholipase D activity in mouse peritoneal macrophages. *J. Lipid Res.* 40:988–993.

Han X. and Gross R. W. (1991). Proton nuclear magnetic resonance studies on the molecular dynamics of plasmenylcholine/cholesterol and phosphatidylcholine/cholesterol bilayers. *Biochim. Biophys. Acta Biomembr.* 1063:129–136.

Han X. L., Holtzman D. M., and McKeel D. W., Jr. (2001). Plasmalogen deficiency in early Alzheimer's disease subjects and in animal models: molecular characterization using electrospray ionization mass spectrometry. *J. Neurochem.* 77:1168–1180.

Horigome K., Tamori-Natori Y., Inoue K., and Nojima S. (1986). Effect of serine phospholipid structure on the enhancement of concanavalin A-induced degranulation in rat mast cells. *J. Biochem.* (Tokyo) 100:571–579.

Horigome K., Hayakawa M., Inoue K., and Nojima S. (1987). Purification and character-ization of phospholipase A2 released from rat platelets. *J. Biochem.* (Tokyo) 101:625–631.

Horigome K., Pryor J. C., Bullock E. D., and Johnson E. M., Jr. (1993). Mediator release from mast cells by nerve growth factor. neurotrophin specificity and receptor mediation. *J. Biol. Chem.* 268:14881–14887.

Hosono H., Aoki J., Nagai Y., Bandoh K., Ishida M., Taguchi R., Arai H., and Inoue K. (2001). Phosphatidylserine-specific phospholipase A_1 stimulates histamine release from rat peritoneal mast cells through production of 2-acyl-1-lysophosphatidylserine. *J. Biol. Chem.* 276:29664–29670.

Ikeda Y., Fukuoka S., and Kito M. (1997). Increase in lysophosphatidylethanolamine in the cell membrane upon the regulated exocytosis of pancreatic acinar AR42J cells. *Biosci. Biotechnol. Biochem.* 61:207–209.

Ikeuchi Y., Nishizaki T., and Matsuoka T. (1995). Lysophosphatidylcholine inhibits NMDA-induced currents by a mechanism independent of phospholipase A_2-mediated protein kinase C activation in hippocampal glial cells. *Biochem. Biophys. Res. Commun.* 217:811–816.

Ikeuchi Y., Nishizaki T., Matsuoka T., and Sumikawa K. (1997). Long-lasting enhance-ment of ACh receptor currents by lysophospholipids. *Brain Res. Mol. Brain Res.* 45:317–320.

Inoue K., Kobayashi T., and Kudo I. (1989). Function and metabolism of lysophos-phatidylserine in rat mast cell activation. In: Bazan N. G., Horrocks L. A., and Toffano G. (eds.), *Phospholipids in the Nervous System, Biochemical and Molecular Pathology.* Liviana Press, Padova, pp. 225–231.

Iwata H., Ohta A., and Baba A. (1986). Stimulatory effect of veratridine on lysophos-phatidylethanolamine formation in rat brain synaptosomes. *Jpn J. Pharmacol.* 41:293–297.

Ji R. R., Kohno T., Moore K. A., and Woolf C. J. (2003). Central sensitization and LTP: do pain and memory share similar mechanisms? *Trends Neurosci.* 26:696–705.

Jurkowitz M. S., Horrocks L. A., and Litsky M. L. (1999). Identification and characteri-zation of alkenyl hydrolase (lysoplasmalogenase) in microsomes and identification of a plasmalogen-active phospholipase A_2 in cytosol of small intestinal epithelium. *Biochim. Biophys. Acta Lipids Lipid Metab.* 1437:142–156.

Jurkowitz-Alexander M., Ebata H., Mills J. S., Murphy E. J., and Horrocks L. A. (1989). Solubilization, purification, and characterization of lysoplasmalogen alkenylhydrolase (lysoplasmalogenase) from rat liver microsomes. *Biochim. Biophys. Acta* 1002:203–212.

Kern R., Joseleau-Petit D., Chattopadhyay M. K., and Richarme G. (2001). Chaperone-like properties of lysophospholipids. Biochem. *Biophys. Res. Commun.* 289:1268–1274.

Kobayashi T., Kishimoto M., and Okuyama H. (1996). Phospholipases involved in lysophosphatidylinositol metabolism in rat brain. *J. Lipid Mediat. Cell Signal.* 14:33–37.

Kume N. and Gimbrone M. A., Jr. (1994). Lysophosphatidylcholine transcriptionally induces growth factor gene expression in cultured human endothelial cells. *J. Clin. Invest.* 93:907–911.

Kume N., Cybulsky M. I., and Gimbrone M. A., Jr. (1992). Lysophosphatidylcholine, a com-ponent of atherogenic lipoproteins, induces mononuclear leukocyte adhesion molecules in cultured human and rabbit arterial endothelial cells. *J. Clin. Invest.* 90:1138–1144.

Lambert I. H. and Falktoft B. (2000). Lysophosphatidylcholine induces taurine release from HeLa cells. *J. Membr. Biol.* 176:175–185.

Lee T. C. (1998). Biosynthesis and possible biological functions of plasmalogens. *Biochim. Biophys. Acta Lipids Lipid Metab.* 1394:129–145.

Lee E. S. Y., Chen H. T., Shepherd K. R., Lamango N. S., Soliman K. F. A., and Charlton C. G. (2004). Inhibitory effects of lysophosphatidylcholine on the dopaminergic system. *Neurochem. Res.* 29:1333–1342.

Lee E. S. Y., Soliman K. F. A., and Charlton C. G. (2005). Lysophosphatidylcholine decreases locomotor activities and dopamine turnover rate in rats. *Neurotoxicology* 26:27–38.

Légrádi A., Chitu V., Szukacsov V., Fajka-Boja R., Szücs K. S., and Monostori E. (2004). Lysophosphatidylcholine is a regulator of tyrosine kinase activity and intracellular Ca^{2+} level in Jurkat T cell line. *Immunol. Lett.* 91:17–21.

Leitinger N. (2005). Oxidized phospholipids as triggers of inflammation in atherosclerosis. *Mol. Nutr. Food Res.* 49:1063–1071.

Leslie C. C. (1991). Kinetic properties of a high molecular mass arachidonoyl-hydrolyzing phospholipase A_2 that exhibits lysophospholipase activity. *J. Biol. Chem.* 266:11366–11371.

Lesnefsky E. J., Stoll M. S. K., Minkler P. E., and Hoppel C. L. (2000). Separation and quantitation of phospholipids and lysophospholipids by high-performance liquid chromatography. *Anal. Biochem.* 285:246–254.

Lourenssen S. and Blennerhassett M. G. (1998). Lysophosphatidylserine potentiates nerve growth factor-induced differentiation of PC12 cells. *Neurosci. Lett.* 248:77–80.

Lovas G., Palkovits M., and Komoly S. (2000). Increased c-Jun expression in neurons affected by lysolecithin-induced demyelination in rats. *Neurosci. Lett.* 292:71–74.

Lundbaek J. A. and Andersen O. S. (1994). Lysophospholipids modulate channel function by altering the mechanical properties of lipid bilayers. *J. Gen. Physiol.* 104:645–673.

Maingret F., Patel A. J., Lesage F., Lazdunski M., and Honoré E. (2000). Lysophospholipids open the two-pore domain mechano-gated K^+ channels TREK-1 and TRAAK. *J. Biol. Chem.* 275:10128–10133.

Mazurek N., Weskamp G., Erne P., and Otten U. (1986). Nerve growth factor induces mast cell degranulation without changing intracellular calcium levels. *FEBS Lett.* 198:315–320.

Mietto L., Boarato E., Toffano G., and Bruni A. (1987). Lysophosphatidylserine-dependent interaction between rat leukocytes and mast cells. *Biochim. Biophys. Acta* 930:145–153.

Muir L. V., Born E., Mathur S. N., and Field F. J. (1996). Lysophosphatidylcholine increases 3-Hydroxy-3-methylglutaryl-coenzyme A reductase gene expression in CaCo-2 cells. *Gastroenterology* 110:1068–1076.

Murugesan G., Rani M. R. S., Gerber C. E., Mukhopadhyay C., Ransohoff R. M., Chisolm G. M., and Kottke-Marchant K. (2003). Lysophosphatidylcholine regulates human microvascular endothelial cell expression of chemokines. *J. Mol. Cell Cardiol.* 35:1375–1384.

Nagai Y., Aoki J., Sato T., Amano R., Matsuda Y., Arai H., and Inoue K. (1999). An alternative splicing form of phosphatidylserine-specific phospholipase A_1 that exhibits lysophosphatidylserine-specific lysophospholipase activity in humans. *J. Biol. Chem.* 274:11053–11059.

Nakano T., Raines E. W., Abraham J. A., Klagsbrun M., and Ross R. (1994). Lysophosphatidylcholine upregulates the level of heparin-binding epidermal growth factor-like growth factor mRNA in human monocytes. *Proc. Natl Acad. Sci. USA* 91:1069–1073.

Oishi K., Raynor R. L., Charp P. A., and Kuo J. F. (1988). Regulation of protein kinase C by lysophospholipids. Potential role in signal transduction. *J. Biol. Chem.* 263:6865–6871.

Ousman S. S. and David S. (2000). Lysophosphatidylcholine induces rapid recruitment and activation of macrophages in the adult mouse spinal cord. *Glia* 30:92–104.

Park K. S., Lee H. Y., Kim M. K., Shin E. H., and Bae Y. S. (2005). Lysophosphatidylserine stimulates leukemic cells but not normal leukocytes. *Biochem. Biophys. Res. Commun.* 333:353–358.

Park K. S., Lee H. Y., Kim M. K., Shin E. H., Jo S. H., Kim S. D., Im D. S., and Bae Y. S. (2006). Lysophosphatidylserine stimulates L2071 mouse fibroblast chemotactic migration via a process involving pertussis toxin-sensitive trimeric G-proteins. *Mol. Pharmacol.* 69:1066–1073.

Pete M. J. and Exton J. H. (1996). Purification of a lysophospholipase from bovine brain that selectively deacylates arachidonoyl-substituted lysophosphatidylcholine. *J. Biol. Chem.* 271:18114–18121.

Poole A. R., Howell J. I., and Lucy J. A. (1970). Lysolecithin and cell fusion. *Nature* 227:810–814.

Rikitake Y., Hirata K., Kawashima S., Takeuchi S., Shimokawa Y., Kojima Y., Inoue N., and Yokoyama M. (2001). Signaling mechanism underlying COX-2 induction by lysophosphatidylcholine. *Biochem. Biophys. Res. Commun.* 281:1291–1297.

Ross B. M. and Kish S. J. (1994). Characterization of lysophospholipid metabolizing enzymes in human brain. *J. Neurochem.* 63:1839–1848.

Ryu S. B. and Palta J. P. (2000). Specific inhibition of rat brain phospholipase D by lysophospholipids. *J. Lipid Res.* 41:940–944.

Sakai M., Miyazaki A., Hakamata H., Sasaki T., Yui S., Yamazaki M., Shichiri M., and Horiuchi S. (1994). Lysophosphatidylcholine plays an essential role in the mitogenic effect of oxidized low density lipoprotein on murine macrophages. *J. Biol. Chem.* 269:31430–31435.

Schilling T., Lehmann F., Ruckert B., and Eder C. (2004). Physiological mechanisms of lysophosphatidylcholine-induced de-ramification of murine microglia. *J. Physiol.* (Lond.) 557:105–120.

Seebeck J., Westenberger K., Elgeti T., Ziegler A., and Schutze S. (2001). The exocytotic signaling pathway induced by nerve growth factor in the presence of lyso-phos-phatidylserine in rat peritoneal mast cells involves a type D phospholipase. *Regul. Pept.* 102:93–99.

Soga T., Ohishi T., Matsui T., Saito T., Matsumoto M., Takasaki J., Matsumoto S., Kamohara M., Hiyama H., Yoshida S., Momose K., Ueda Y., Matsushime H., Kobori M., and Furuichi K. (2005). Lysophosphatidylcholine enhances glucose-dependent insulin secretion via an orphan G-protein-coupled receptor. *Biochem. Biophys. Res. Commun.* 326:744–751.

Sun G. Y. and MacQuarrie R. A. (1989). Deacylation–reacylation of arachidonoyl groups in cerebral phospholipids. *Ann. NY Acad. Sci.* 559:37–55.

Tsutsumi T., Kobayashi T., Ueda H., Yamauchi E., Watanabe S., and Okuyama H. (1994). Lysophosphoinositide-specific phospholipase C in rat brain synaptic plasma membranes. *Neurochem. Res.* 19:399–406.

Ueda H., Kobayashi T., Kishimoto M., Tsutsumi T., and Okuyama H. (1993). A possible pathway of phosphoinositide metabolism through EDTA-insensitive phospholipase A_1 followed by lysophosphoinositide-specific phospholipase C in rat brain. *J. Neurochem.* 61:1874–1881.

Vahidi W. H., Ong W. Y., Farooqui A. A., and Yeo J. F. (2006). Pronociceptive effect of central nervous lysophospholipids in a mouse model of orofacial pain. *Exp. Brain Res.* (in press).

Vogel S. S., Leikina E. A., and Chernomordik L. V. (1993). Lysophosphatidylcholine reversibly arrests exocytosis and viral fusion at a stage between triggering and membrane merger. *J. Biol. Chem.* 268:25764–25768.

Wang A. and Dennis E. A. (1999). Mammalian lysophospholipases. *Biochim. Biophys. Acta* 1439:1–16.

Wang A., Yang H. C., Friedman P., Johnson C. A., and Dennis E. A. (1999). A specific human lysophospholipase: cDNA cloning, tissue distribution and kinetic characterization. *Biochim. Biophys. Acta* 1437:157–169.

Weltzien H. U. (1979). Cytolytic and membrane-perturbing properties of lyso-phosphatidylcholine. *Biochim. Biophys. Acta* 559:259–287.

Williams S. D. and Ford D. A. (1997). Activation of myocardial cAMP-dependent protein kinase by lysoplasmenylcholine. *FEBS Lett.* 420:33–38.

Yamashita A., Watanabe M., Sato K., Miyashita T., Nagatsuka T., Kondo H., Kawagishi N., Nakanishi H., Kamata R., Sugiura T., and Waku K. (2003). Reverse reaction of lysophosphatidylinositol acyltransferase — functional reconstitution of coenzyme A-dependent transacylation system. *J. Biol. Chem.* 278:30382–30393.

Yeo J. F., Ong W. Y., Ling S. F., and Farooqui A. A. (2004). Intracerebroventricular injection of phospholipases A_2 inhibitors modulates allodynia after facial carrageenan injection in mice. *Pain* 112:148–155.

Yuan Y., Schoenwaelder S. M., Salem H. H., and Jackson S. P. (1996). The bioactive phospholipid, lysophosphatidylcholine, induces cellular effects via G-protein-dependent activation of adenylyl cyclase. *J. Biol. Chem.* 271:27090–27098.

Zembowicz A., Jones S. L., and Wu K. K. (1995). Induction of cyclooxygenase-2 in human umbilical vein endothelial cells by lysophosphatidylcholine. *J. Clin. Invest.* 96:1688–1692.

Zhu Y., Lin J. H. C., Liao H. L., Verna L., and Stemerman M. B. (1997). Activation of ICAM-1 promoter by lysophosphatidylcholine: possible involvement of protein tyrosine kinases. *Biochim. Biophys. Acta Lipids Lipid Metab.* 1345:93–98.

Zhu K., Baudhuin L. M., Hong G., Williams F. S., Cristina K. L., Kabarowski J. H., Witte O. N., and Xu Y. (2001). Sphingosylphosphorylcholine and lysophosphatidylcholine are ligands for the G protein-coupled receptor GPR4. *J. Biol. Chem.* 276:41325–41335.

9
Lysophosphatidic Acid and its Metabolism in Brain

9.1 Functions of Lysophosphatidic Acid in Brain

Lysophosphatidic acid (lyso-PtdH, 1-O-acyl-2-hydroxy-sn-glycerol-3-phosphate) belongs to the lysophospholipid family and deserves discussion here because it has a glycerol backbone and PLA$_2$ generates it. Another lysophospholipid lipid mediator, sphingosine 1-phosphate, which has a sphingosine backbone, is not discussed here because PLA$_2$ does not generate it. Its mechanism of action and biological function are described elsewhere (Heringdorf et al., 2002). In some molecular species of lyso-PtdH, the long-chain substituent at the sn-1 position can be an alkyl or alkenyl group, generating 1-O-alkyl-sn-glycero-3-phosphate, 1-O-cis-alk-1-enyl-sn-glycero-3-phosphate. Other variants have cyclic phosphate linkages to form 1-acyl-sn-glycerol-2,3-cyclic phosphates. Common molecular species of lyso-PtdH isolated from brain and serum include arachidonoyl (20:4), oleoyl (18:1), palmitoyl (16:0), and stearoyl (18:0) acyl groups. Structural–activity relationship studies have indicated that a phosphate monoester and a long-chain of greater than 12 carbons are required for the biological activity of lyso-PtdH (Lynch and MacDonald, 2001, 2002).

Lyso-PtdH is the simplest phospholipid that is not only an intermediate in intracellular phospholipid metabolism, but also acts as a growth-factor-like extracellular mediator. It has various effects on neural and non-neural cells. Thus it induces proliferation in fibroblasts, differentiation in keratinocytes, platelet aggregation, mitogenesis in clonal cell lines and primary cell cultures, activation of ion currents in *Xenopus oocytes*, muscle contraction in smooth muscles, and remodeling of actin cytoskeleton (Tigyi and Miledi, 1992; Tokumura et al., 1994; Snitko et al., 1997; Nishiuchi et al., 1997; Carroll et al., 1997; Takuwa et al., 2002; Anliker and Chun, 2004). Besides these effects in non-neural cells, lyso-PtdH stimulates mitogenesis, protects from apoptosis, induces actin cytoskeletal reorganization and cell shape changes, chemotaxis, and stimulates tumor cell invasion (Takuwa et al., 2002). In fibroblasts, lyso-PtdH induces the hydrolysis of phosphoinositides by PLC, increases intracellular Ca^{2+}, and activates the Ras/Raf MAP-kinase cascade. LysoPtdH is a normal constituent of serum. Activated platelets release it during blood clotting. It is transported in the blood stream bound to albumin. Its concentration in serum can reach 1 to 5 µM. The lyso-PtdH concentration is low in mammalian cerebrospinal fluid. However, this concentration reaches serum levels following brain injury. A high concentration of lyso-PtdH may disrupt the blood–brain barrier (Tigyi et al., 1995). Lyso-PtdH and its homologues are also present in aqueous humor where it is involved in maintaining the integrity of the normal cornea and in promoting cellular regeneration of the injured cornea (Liliom et al., 1998b).

In neural cells, lyso-PtdH induces several responses including stimulation of the release of noradrenaline from cerebral cortical synaptosomes, inhibition of glutamate uptake by astrocytes, elevation of neuronal intracellular calcium, and stimulation of dopamine release from PC12 cells (Nishikawa et al., 1989; Tigyi and Miledi, 1992; Shiono et al., 1993; Tigyi et al., 1994, 1996a,b; Keller et al., 1996; Holtsberg et al., 1997; Ye et al., 2002; Anliker and Chun, 2004; Moolenaar et al., 2004). Glial tumor-derived cells also respond to lyso-PtdH. Lyso-PtdH blocks β-adrenergic-mediated shape change and stimulates forskolin-induced elevation in cyclic AMP levels in glial cells (Kreps et al., 1993; Koschel and Tas, 1993). Lyso-PtdH is a potent inducer of growth cone collapse and neurite retraction in neuroblastoma and PC12 cells and in primary neurons and cortical neuroblasts. Lyso-PtdH also mediates the reversal of stellation in astrocytes (Ramakers and Moolenaar, 1998). In brain-derived endothelial cells, lyso-PtdH increases tight-junction permeability implicating this lipid mediator in the modulation of blood–brain barrier function (Schulze et al., 1997). Lyso-PtdH enhances the chemokinetic migration of murine microglial cells through the activation of Ca^{2+}-activated K^+ currents (Schilling et al., 2004). Lyso-PtdH also has a neurogenic effect on mouse embryonic cortical hemispheres. It causes them to expand and fold up into a structure that resembles a primate brain (Kingsbury et al., 2003). Collectively, these studies indicate that lyso-PtdH is a lipid mediator with growth factor-like activities. Because of its hydrophilic structure lyso-PtdH acts as an intracellular messenger in a paracrine/autocrine manner (Xie et al., 2002). It modulates neurite retraction, cytoskeleton reorganization, neurogenesis, neural migration, myelination, apoptosis, and neurotransmitter release (Fukushima, 2004) (Fig. 9.1).

9.2 Synthesis and Degradation of lyso-PtdH

Brain contains the highest concentration of lyso-PtdH (Das and Hajra, 1989). The hydrolysis of pre-existing phospholipids and their metabolites through several enzymic reactions generates lyso-PtdH (Fig. 9.2). Lyso-PtdH is synthesized by the acylation of *sn*-glycerol-3-phosphate by acyl CoA in the membranes of endoplasmic reticulum and mitochondria. This reaction is catalyzed by glycerophosphate acyltransferase (Pages et al., 2001). Alternatively, lyso-PtdH can be generated by the phosphorylation of a monoacylglycerol. Lyso-PtdH is also generated by the action of phosphatidic acid specific PLA_2 on phosphatidic acid (PtdH) (Thomson and Clark, 1994, 1995). Lyso-PtdH is also synthesized by PLD-mediated hydrolysis

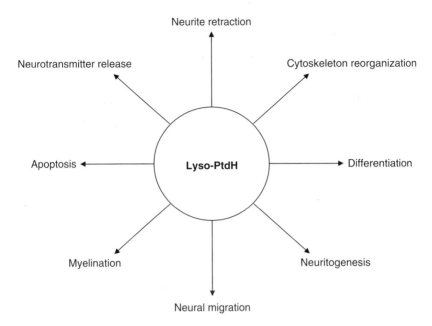

FIG. 9.1. Proposed roles of lysophosphatidic acid in brain.

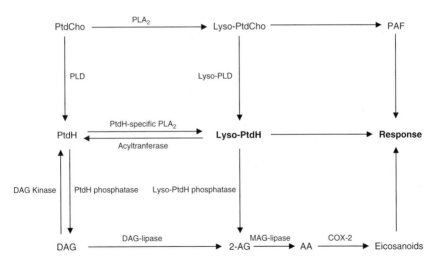

FIG. 9.2. Metabolism of lysophosphatidic acid and phosphatidic acid in brain. Phosphatidylcholine (PtdCho); lysophosphatidylcholine (lyso-PtdCho), lysophosphatidic acid (Lyso-PtdH); phosphatidic acid (PtdH); diacylglycerol (DAG); 2-arachidonoyl-glycerol (2-AG); platelet activating factor (PAF); phospholipase A₂ (PLA₂); phospholipase D (PLD), and cyclooxygenase-2 (COX-2).

of lyso-PtdCho (Pages et al., 2001; Moolenaar et al., 2004). Several enzymes participate in lyso-PtdH catabolism. Thus, lyso-PtdH is converted to PtdH by a lyso-PtdH-acyltransferase (Pages et al., 2001; Aoki, 2004). This enzyme is localized in microsomes and plasma membranes. It is crucial for de novo synthesis of glycerophospholipids. Lyso-PtdH can also be converted into monoacylglycerol by lysophosphatidate phosphohydrolase (lysophosphatidic acid phosphatase) (Brindley et al., 2002). The dephosphorylation of lyso-PtdH is the major pathway that terminates signaling processes mediated by lyso-PtdH. Although brain tissue has multiple pathways of synthesis and degradation of lyso-PtdH, their relative contributions to intracellular and extracellular lyso-PtdH production are not known because specific inhibitors for many of the enzymes involved in its metabolism are not available.

9.3 LPA Receptors and Lyso-PtdH-Mediated Signaling in Brain

Lyso-PtdH elicits its biological functions through three types of G protein-coupled receptors called LPA receptors (Fig. 9.3). These receptors have an apparent mol mass of 38–40 kDa. LPA receptors have been classified into at least three groups, namely LPA_1 (earlier name Edg-2), LPA_2 (Edg-4), and LPA_3 (Edg-7) (Chun, 1999; Fukushima et al., 2001; Ye et al., 2002) (Table 9.1). The LPA_1 receptor has seven putative transmembrane domains, 364 amino acids, and apparent molecular mass of 41 kDa. Most body tissues express it. Mice lacking the LPA_1 receptor show partial lethality due to defective sucking and olfactory dysfunction. The survivors have reduced body mass and head/facial deformities and increased Schwann cell death. These mice have markedly decreased signaling mediated by lyso-PtdH in cerebral cortical neuroprogenitor cells and in embryonic fibroblasts. LPA_2 contains 351 amino acids (human) and 348 amino acids (mouse) with an apparent molecular mass of 39 kDa. Embryonic and neonatal mouse brain express the LPA_2 receptor but adult mouse brain does not. It is barely detectable in adult human brain (Ye et al., 2002; Anliker and Chun, 2004). Mice lacking the LPA_2 receptor look phenotypically normal but show reduced signaling mediated by lyso-PtdH, including decreased PLC activation and Ca^{2+} mobilization, and no inhibition of adenylate cyclase. The LPA_3 receptor has a gene structure containing the conserved intron in transmembrane domain 6. Human LPA_3 receptor has 353 amino acids with an apparent molecular mass of 40 kDa. LPA_3 receptor expression is developmentally regulated in mouse brain (Ye et al., 2002). Unlike LPA_1 and LPA_2 receptors, the LPA_3 receptor is not coupled to the $G_{12/13}$ type of G-proteins and has a more restricted expression.

By RNA analysis, the LPA_1 receptor is restricted to oligodendrocytes and Schwann cells. The mRNA encoding the LPA_2 receptor is absent from adult brain, but can be detected in developing brain. LPA_2 receptor expression is most prominent in leukocytes. The LPA_3 receptor mRNA is found in extracts of kidney, lungs, and heart. A low amount of LPA_3 receptor transcript was reported in

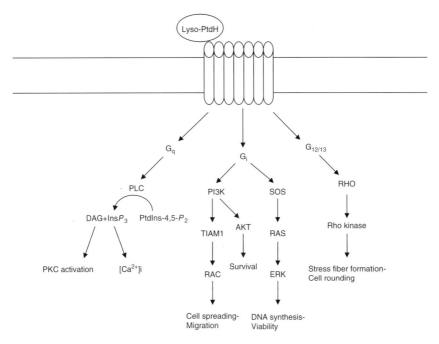

FIG. 9.3. Coupling of lysophosphatidic acid receptor with G-proteins is associated with signal transduction pathways involved in many cellular responses.

TABLE 9.1. Classification and properties of lyso-PtdH receptors.

IUPHAR nomenclature	Edg nomenclature	G-protein coupling	Ligand	Antagonists	Reference
LPA$_1$	Edg-2	Gi, Gq, G$_{12/13}$	Lyso-PtdH	VPC12249 DGPP 8:0 FAP-12	Heise et al., 2001; Anliker and Chun, 2004
LPA$_2$	Edg-4	Gi, Gq, G$_{12/13}$	Lyso-PtdH	–	Heise et al., 2001; Anliker and Chun, 2004
LPA$_3$	Edg-7	Gi, Gq	Lyso-PtdH	VPC12249 DGPP 8:0 FAP-12	Heise et al., 2001; Anliker and Chun, 2004

Edg is an acronym for endothelial differentiation gene.

brain tissue (Contos et al., 2000; Fukushima et al., 2001). The three LPA receptors have about 50% sequence similarity with each other. Recently a new receptor, LPA$_4$ (P2Y9/GPR23) was identified in ovary. This receptor shares only 20% to 24% homology with other LPA receptors. Peroxisome proliferator-activator receptor γ (PPARγ), a nuclear transcription factor, is an intracellular receptor for lyso-PtdH (McIntyre et al., 2003; Tsukahara et al., 2006). Collectively, these studies suggest that all LPA receptors are expressed in brain tissue, but there is a variation of both spatial and temporal expression patterns. For example, LPA$_1$ receptors are expressed in neuroblasts during embryonic development (Hecht et al., 1996), but in oligodendrocytes and Schwann cells at later ages (Weiner et al., 1998). Other developmental and spatial patterns of expression occur for both LPA$_2$ and LPA$_3$. The occurrence of multiple LPA receptors and their different spatial patterns of expression provide brain with signaling processes essential for proper brain development (Fukushima, 2004; Kingsbury et al., 2004).

LPA receptors undergo rapid ligand-induced internalization from the plasma membrane (Van Leeuwen et al., 2003). Phosphorylation of Ser/Thr residues at the C-terminal end accompanies ligand-mediated internalization and desensitization of LPA receptors. The fate of internalized LPA receptors is not yet known, but like other G protein-coupled receptors they probably undergo degradation and recycling processes (Ye et al., 2002; Moolenaar et al., 2004). Lyso-PtdH and its receptors modulate activities of many enzyme systems (Table 9.2). Neurochemical signaling that mediates the cellular effects of lyso-PtdH includes stimulation of phospholipases, mobilization of intracellular Ca^{2+}, inhibition of adenylyl cyclase, activation of phosphatidylinositol 3-kinase, and activation of the Ras-Raf—MAP-kinase and Rho GTPases (Ishii et al., 2000; Moolenaar et al., 2004). All these processes involve the participation of G-proteins. LPA$_1$ is mostly associated with activation of G$_{i\alpha}$ pathways and is expressed in oligodendrocytes and peripheral tissues, whereas LPA$_2$ and LPA$_3$ are coupled mostly with G$_{q/11\alpha}$ pathways (Bandoh et al., 1999). LPA$_2$ is expressed in embryonic brain and LPA$_3$ has a restricted expression in brain tissue.

Lyso-PtdH stimulates the release of arachidonic acid from astrocytes (Pébay et al., 1999; Rao et al., 2003), indicating the involvement of PLA$_2$. The PLA$_2$ inhibitor, quinacrine, partially blocks this response, which is reduced strongly in

TABLE 9.2. Effect of lysophosphatidic acid on various enzymic activities in neural and non-neural tissues.

Enzyme	Effect	Reference
PLD	Stimulation	Tou and Gill, 2005
Lipid phosphate phosphatase	Stimulation	Brindley et al., 2002; Brindley, 2004
PLC	Stimulation	Takuwa et al., 2002
Lysophospholipase	Inhibition	Baker and Chang, 2000
Lipoprotein lipase	Stimulation	Pulinilkunnil et al., 2005
Cyclooxygenase-2	Induction	Symowicz et al., 2005
Lipoxygenase	Stimulation	Willard et al., 2001
MAP-kinase	Stimulation	Cai et al., 2005
Ras-MEK kinase-1	Stimulation	Bian et al., 2004
Extracellular signal regulated kinase (ErK)	Stimulation	Pébay et al., 1999
Transglutaminase	Stimulation	Yoo et al., 2005
Ornithine decarboxylase	Induction	Facchini et al., 2005
Metalloproteinase	Induction	Symowicz et al., 2005
Na$^+$, K$^+$-ATPase	Inhibition	Nishikawa et al., 1988

the absence of calcium ions. Furthermore, RG80267, a PLC inhibitor, does not affect the release of arachidonic acid induced by lyso-PtdH, suggesting the lack of involvement of the PLC/diacylglycerol lipase pathway in this release of arachidonic acid. Quantitative differences exist in arachidonic acid release by lyso-PtdH. Pretreatment with PTX completely blocks arachidonic acid release mediated by lyso-PtdH in cells expressing the LPA_3 receptor, but not in cells expressing LPA_1 and LPA_2. Thus, the LPA_3 receptor preferentially utilizes Gi/o for arachidonic acid release, whereas LPA_1 and LPA_2 receptors use PTX-insensitive G-proteins for their signal transduction (Ishii et al., 2000). Most striking differences in cell morphology are observed during LPA receptor expression. Expression of LPA_1 and LPA_2 produces a rounding effect in B103 cells, whereas the expression of LPA_3 receptor in B103 cells has no such effect (Ishii et al., 2000). Rho-mediated signaling induces the morphological changes in B103 cells. Similar morphological changes occur in cultured astrocytes following lyso-PtdH treatment (Steiner et al., 2002). In these astrocytes, lyso-PtdH stimulates ROS synthesis, activates multiple protein kinases, upregulates c-fos and c-jun expression, inhibits glutamate uptake, and induces cytokine expression (Steiner et al., 2002). Lyso-PtdH also upregulates nerve growth factor expression in astrocytes (Eddleston and Mucke, 1993). The release of nerve growth factor and inhibition of glutamate uptake may have a significant impact on survival of neurons in brain tissue.

9.4 Agonists and Antagonists of LPA Receptors

Although lyso-PtdH and its receptors modulate signaling in brain tissue, very little information is available on the effects of LPA receptor agonists and antagonists on neurons, astrocytes, oligodendrocytes, and microglial cells. Most of the information on their effects was obtained on non-neural cells (Anliker and Chun, 2004). The major limitation on pharmacological studies of LPA receptors has been the lack of receptor subtype-specific agonists and antagonists. Structure–activity relationship studies on lyso-PtdH indicate a strong requirement for the phosphate group. Replacement of the phosphate group with an alcohol causes a decrease in ligand potency (Lynch and MacDonald, 2001). Attempts have been made to synthesize lyso-PtdH analogs with improved potency and receptor selectivity. Several analogs, such as 1-oleoyl-2-O-methyl-rac-glycero-3-phosphothionate (OMPT) and palmitoyl-hydroxydioxazaphosphocanes (DOXP-OH) have been synthesized and tested for lyso-PtdH-like activity (Gueguen et al., 1999; Hasegawa et al., 2003) (Fig. 9.4). OMPT binds to the LPA_3 receptor in mammalian cells and elicits multiple responses, such as activation of G-proteins, Ca^{2+} mobilization, and activation of mitogen-activated protein kinases. Thus, OMPT offers a powerful probe for the dissection of LPA signaling events in mammalian systems. Similarly, fatty alcohol phosphates (FAP) containing saturated hydrocarbon chains from 4 to 22 carbons in length have been synthesized. Decyl and dodecyl FAP (FAP-10 and FAP-12) (Fig 9.5) are specific agonists for the LPA_2 receptor (EC_{50} 3700 and 700 nM, respectively) yet selective antagonists

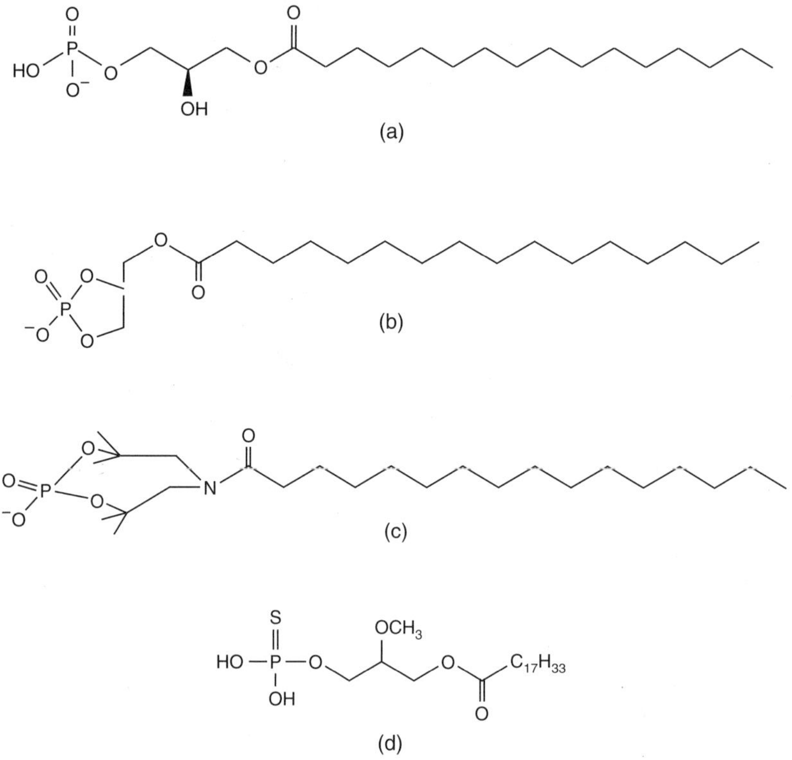

(a)

(b)

(c)

(d)

FIG. 9.4. Chemical structures of LPA receptor agonists. Lysophosphatidic acid (18:0) (a); cyclic phosphatidic acid (b); palmitoyl hydroxydioxazaphosphocanes (DOXP-OH) (c); and 1-oleoyl-2-O-methyl-*rac*-glycero-3-phosphothionate (OMPT) (d).

of the LPA$_3$ receptor (Ki 90 nM) (Table 9.3) and FAP-12 is a weak antagonist of the LPA$_1$ receptor. Neither LPA$_1$ nor LPA$_3$ receptors are activated by FAP, but the LPA$_2$ receptor is activated by FAP with carbon chains between 10 and 14 (Virag et al., 2003). The glycerol backbone is important, but can be substituted with ethanolamine, serine or tyrosine. *N*-Acyl serine phosphoric acid and *N*-acyl tyrosine phosphoric acid (Fig. 9.5) analogs inhibit platelet aggregation mediated by lyso-PtdH, oscillatory Cl⁻ currents, and neutrophil adhesion to endothelial cells (Sugiura et al., 1994; Liliom et al., 1996; Hooks et al., 1998). Thus, these compounds have LPA receptor antagonistic activity. A propanoic acid derivative, 3-(4-[4-([1-(2-chlorophenyl)ethoxy]carbonyl amino)-3-methyl-5-isoxazolyl] benzylsulfanyl) propanoic acid (Ki16425) (Fig. 9.6) is a potent antagonist for LPA$_1$ and LPA$_3$ receptors (Palomaki and Laitinen, 2006). It may be useful in evaluating the role of LPA and its receptor subtypes involved in biological actions. Ki16425 inhibits responses induced by lyso-PtdH in the decreasing order of LPA$_1$ ≥ LPA$_3$ >> LPA$_2$.

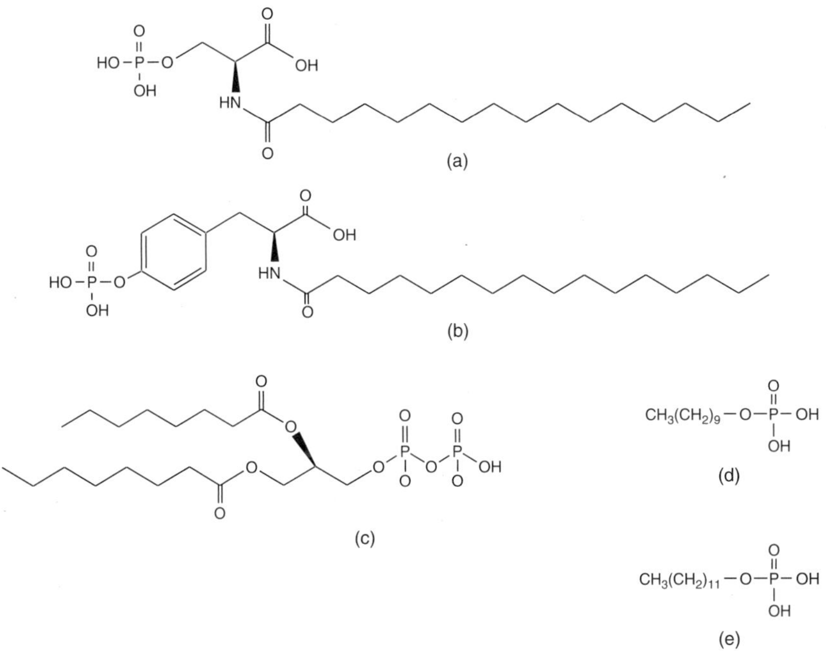

FIG. 9.5. Chemical structures of first-generation LPA receptor antagonists. *N*-Palmitoyl-L-serine-phosphoric acid (NP-Ser-PA) (a); *N*-palmitoyl-L-tyrosine-phosphoric acid (NP-Tyr-PA) (b); diacylglycerol pyrophosphate (DGPP 8:0) (c); FAP-10 (d); and FAP-12 (e).

TABLE 9.3. Antagonists and their Ki values for LPA receptor subtypes.

Antagonist	LPA receptor subtype	Ki (nM)	Reference
NP-Ser-PA	All	805	Liliom et al., 1996
NP-Tyr-PA	All	330	Liliom et al., 1996
NAE-PA	LPA$_1$	137	Sardar et al., 2002
NAE-PA	LPA$_3$	428	Sardar et al., 2002
DGPP 18:0	LPA$_1$	6600	Fischer et al., 2001
DGPP 18:0	LPA$_3$	106	Fischer et al., 2001
VPC 12249	LPA$_1$	137	Heise et al., 2001
VPC 12249	LPA$_3$	428	Heise et al., 2001
1,2-Dioctanoyl-glycerothiophosphate	LPA$_3$	5.00	Durgam et al., 2006
1,2-Dioctyl serine diamide phosphate	LPA$_3$	–	Durgam et al., 2006
Fatty alcohol phosphate-12	LPA$_3$	90	Virag et al., 2003
Tetradecyl phosphonate	LPA$_3$	17	Durgam et al., 2005

Ki values cannot be compared to determine the relative efficacy of the antagonists because these values have been obtained using different assays for LPA receptors in various types of cells.

Attempts have been made to synthesize 2-substituted lyso-PtdH analogs (Heise et al., 2001). Starting with an *N*-acyl ethanolamine phosphate analog of lyso-PtdH, a series of compounds with substitution at the second carbon were synthesized and tested for several biochemical parameters. These compounds are VPC

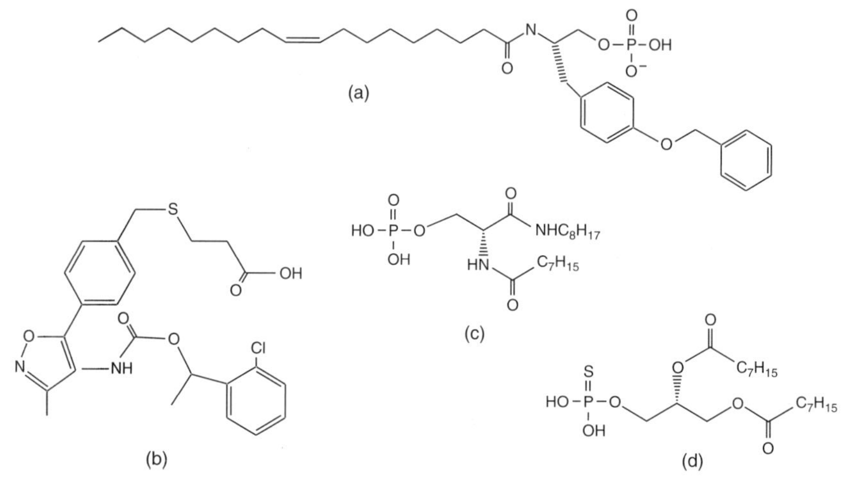

FIG. 9.6. Chemical structures of second-generation LPA receptor antagonists. *N*-oleoylethanolamide phosphate substituted at the second carbon with a benzyl-4-oxybenzyl moiety (VPC12249) (a); Ki16425, (3-(4-[4-([1-(2-chlorophenyl)ethoxy] carbonyl amino)-3-methyl-5-isoxazolyl] benzylsulfanyl) propanoic acid) (b); 1,2-dioctyl serinediamide phosphate (c); and 1,2-dioctanoyl-glycerothiophosphate (d).

compounds (Fig. 9.6) (Heise et al., 2001). Out of 13 VPC compounds, only one compound, VPC12084, has slight efficacy for the LPA$_1$ receptor. VPC 32179 is devoid of agonist activity at the human LPA$_2$ and LPA$_3$ receptors and behaves as a competitive antagonist at the LPA$_3$ receptor. However, VPC 32179 has partial agonist activity in a cell migration assay; most likely due to activity at the LPA$_1$ receptor. VPC 32183 is another competitive antagonist at the LPA$_1$ and LPA$_3$ receptors. Another VPC compound, VPC12249, has a potent competitive antagonistic activity. The Ki value for inhibiting Ca^{2+} mobilization in HEK293T cells is 130 nM. These cells express both LPA$_1$ and LPA$_2$ receptors.

Two short-chain PtdH derivatives, dioctanoyl-glycerol-pyrophosphate (DGPP 8:0) and dioctyl-PtdH 8:0, are selective and potent antagonists (Fischer et al., 2001) (Table 9.3). They can be used to identify LPA$_1$ and LPA$_3$ receptors. Neither molecule affects the LPA$_2$ receptor. The Ki value for DGPP 8:0 for the LPA$_3$ receptor is 106 nM. It is a poor antagonist of the LPA$_1$ receptor with a Ki value of 6.6 μM. The replacement of the phosphate headgroup by thiophosphate in a series of fatty alcohol phosphates improves agonist and antagonist activities at LPA receptors (Fig. 9.6) (Durgam et al., 2005). Short chain PtdH 8:0 analogs also have LPA receptor subtype antagonistic activity. Thus dioctyl PtdH 8:0 shows stereospecific responses towards LPA receptors. (R)-Isomers of dioctyl PtdH 8:0 series have agonistic activity, whereas (S)-isomers have antagonistic activity for LPA receptors (Durgam et al., 2006).

The mechanism of the antagonistic effects of above compounds is not known. However, modeling and docking studies (Sardar et al., 2002) on DGPP indicate that DGPP binds to LPA receptors through interactions with cationic amino acids in transmembrane helices III and VII. However, a very different interaction exists between DGPP and the extracellular loops (Sardar et al., 2002). Docking studies with benzyl-4-oxybenzyl NAEPA indicate that this antagonist interacts with the extracellular loops in a manner similar to DGPP. Thus more studies are required on the mechanism of other antagonists before these compounds can be used as potential therapeutic agents for various diseases involving LPA receptors (see below).

9.5 Lyso-PtdH and its Receptors in Neurological Diseases

Normal brain astrocytes display a stellate process-bearing morphology. Following brain injury, to protect brain tissue, astrocytes proliferate and undergo reactive gliosis resulting in scar formation. Lyso-PtdH may play an important role in this process. Levels of lyso-PtdH are increased after brain injury, such as hemorrhagic injury (Tigyi et al., 1995) and cerebral ischemia (Sun et al., 1992). High levels of lyso-PtdH induce neurite retraction in cultured cells of neuronal and glial origin, a crucial process that occurs during brain development and neurodegeneration. It is proposed that lyso-PtdH acts through Rho-mediated signaling to induce contraction-related cytoskeleton changes to reorganize astrocytic morphology (Tigyi et al., 1996a,b; Ramakers and Moolenaar, 1998). Lyso-PtdH also induces changes in tubulin pools and increases in the phosphorylation levels of microtubule-associated proteins (MAP) (Yoshida and Ueda, 2001). Collective evidence suggests that lyso-PtdH-mediated reorganization of the cytoskeleton is an important event in the process of neurite retraction.

An increase in site-specific tau phosphorylation, resembling Alzheimer disease, during lyso-PtdH-induced neurite retraction was demonstrated in differentiated SY-SH5Y human neuroblastoma cells. Based on the effect of kinase inhibitors, this phosphorylation may be mediated by glycogen synthase kinase-3 (GSK-3). These results support the hypothesis that activation of GSK-3 occurs in the Rho pathway and may represent an important link between microtubule and microfilament dynamics during neuritogenesis and in pathological situations, such as Alzheimer disease (Sayas et al., 1999, 2002).

Neurological and behavioral analysis of mice homozygous for a targeted deletion at the LPA$_1$ receptor locus has indicated a marked deficit in prepulse inhibition, widespread changes in the levels and turnover of the neurotransmitter 5-HT, a brain region-specific alteration in levels of amino acids, and a craniofacial dysmorphism in these mice. The loss of LPA$_1$ receptors generates defects resembling those found in psychiatric diseases (Harrison et al., 2003). Alterations in LPA receptors may occur in psychiatric disorders.

LysoPtdH and its receptors are also involved in the pathophysiology of pain (Renback et al., 1999; Inoue et al., 2004; Vahidi et al., 2006). Intraplantar injections of lyso-PtdH in the hind limb of mice produce dose-dependent nociceptive flexor responses (Renback et al., 1999). Repeated challenges with lyso-PtdH produce constant responses. Pretreatment with pertussis toxin (PTX) markedly reduces these responses mediated by lyso-PtdH. In addition, intraplantar application of CP-99994, a substance P (NK1) receptor antagonist, markedly lowers the lyso-PtdH responses. These observations suggest that lyso-PtdH has a nociceptive effect on sensory neurons through G(i/o) activation and this process is accompanied by substance P released from nociceptor endings (Renback et al., 1999). Similarly, intracerebroventricular injections of lyso-PtdH increase allodynia (Vahidi et al., 2006). These findings are consistent with the report that mice that lack LPA receptors have increased resistance to pain (Inoue et al., 2004). Thus wild-type mice with a nerve injury develop behavioral allodynia and hyperalgesia accompanied with demyelination in the dorsal root and increased expression of both protein kinase Cγ within the spinal cord dorsal horn and the α_2 and δ_1 calcium channel subunit in dorsal root ganglia (Inoue et al., 2004). Intrathecal injections of lyso-PtdH induce behavioral, morphological, and neurochemical changes similar to those observed after nerve ligation. In contrast, mice lacking LPA$_1$ receptors associated with the activation of Rho–Rho kinase pathway do not develop signs of neuropathic pain after peripheral nerve injury. Inhibitors of Rho and Rho kinase also block signs of neuropathic pain (Inoue et al., 2004). Collectively these studies suggest that pathophysiological conditions, such as neuropathic pain following brain injury may involve components of the signaling cascade downstream of LPA receptors, in particular those involving Ras or Rho. In addition, up- or down-regulation of LPA receptor subtypes, alteration of their ratio, and increased availability of the lysophospholipid ligands at sites of injury or inflammation, likely contribute to disease and may be important targets for therapeutic intervention (Renback et al., 1999; Inoue et al., 2004; Vahidi et al., 2006).

Lyso-PtdH and its homologues are physiological constituents of the biologic fluids bathing the cornea. It is generated in increased amounts after eye injury in aqueous humor and lacrimal gland fluid. Lyso-PtdH and its homologues may be involved in maintaining the integrity of the control cornea and in promoting the regeneration of the injured cornea through the Rho/Rho kinase-signaling pathway (Liliom et al., 1998a; Mettu et al., 2004). Furthermore, the bioactivity of lyso-PtdH in modulating the trabecular meshwork function and the potential involvement of lyso-PtdH in the regulation of the conventional outflow pathway (Vasantha Rao et al., 2001) may open new approaches to develop a better understanding, not only of the physiology and pathophysiology of primary open-angle glaucoma, but also of potential novel therapeutic interventions for glaucomatous disease.

9.6 Lyso-PtdH and its Receptors in Non-Neural Diseases

As stated earlier, in non-neural tissues, lyso-PtdH contributes to a number of fundamental cellular functions, which include proliferation, differentiation, survival, migration, adhesion, invasion, and morphogenesis. These functions influence many biological processes that include angiogenesis, wound healing, immunity, and carcinogenesis (Ishii et al., 2004). Abnormalities in these processes are associated with the pathogenesis of cancer, autoimmunity, immunodeficiency, atherosclerosis, and ischemia–reperfusion injury (Chun and Rosen, 2006; Gardell et al., 2006).

Lyso-PtdH levels are elevated in ascitic fluid from ovarian cancer patients. In experimental models of ovarian cancer, lyso-PtdH promotes cancer cell invasion/metastasis by up-regulating protease expression, elevating protease activity, and enhancing angiogenic factor expression. The effect of lyso-PtdH on ovarian cancer migration is an essential component of cancer cell invasion. Lyso-PtdH stimulates both chemotaxis and chemokinesis of ovarian cancer cells (Al-Rasheed et al., 2004). Moreover, constitutively active H-Ras enhances ovarian cancer cell migration, whereas dominant negative H-Ras blocks lyso-PtdH-stimulated cell migration, suggesting that Ras works downstream of Gi to mediate cell migration stimulated by lyso-PtdH. Collective evidence suggests that the Gi-Ras-MEKK1 signaling pathway mediates LPA-stimulated ovarian cancer cell migration by facilitating focal adhesion kinase redistribution to focal contacts (Al-Rasheed et al., 2004). Although controversial, levels of specific lysophospholipids including lyso-PtdH may be altered in the blood of cancer patients, providing a potential mechanism for early diagnosis.

Several of the enzymes involved in the metabolism of lysophospholipids are aberrant in ovarian and other cancers (Umezu-Goto et al., 2004). Although the underlying mechanisms associated with this pathophysiology remain elusive, aberrations in the production and degradation of lyso-PtdH have been identified in cancer cells and in cancer patients. In combination with alterations in LPA receptor expression and function, lyso-PtdH appears to be an important mediator in the pathophysiology of cancer. Therefore, LPA receptors have emerged as drug targets for therapeutic intervention (Brindley, 2004).

LPA receptors are expressed at the apical surface of intestinal epithelial cells, where they form a macromolecular complex with Na^+/H^+ exchanger regulatory factor-2 and cystic fibrosis transmembrane conductance regulator (CFTR) through a PSD95/Dlg/ZO-1-based interaction (Li et al., 2005). Lyso-PtdH prevents CFTR-dependent iodide efflux through the Gi pathway mediated by lyso-PtdH. Furthermore, lyso-PtdH not only blocks CFTR-mediated short-circuit currents in a compartmentalized fashion, but also reduces cholera toxin-induced CFTR-dependent intestinal fluid secretion, suggesting that LPA receptors are associated with intestinal epithelial cell function. Collectively these studies suggest that lyso-PtdH also plays a vital role in a variety of conditions involving gastrointestinal wound repair, apoptosis, inflammatory bowel disease, and diarrhea (Li et al., 2005).

Neointimal lesions are characterized by accumulation of cells within the arterial wall and are a prelude to atherosclerotic disease. A brief exposure of cells to alkyl ether analogs of the growth factor-like phospholipid lyso-PtdH generates oxidative modification of low-density lipoprotein and also induces a progressive formation of neointimal lesions in vivo in a rat carotid artery model (Zhang et al.,

2004). This effect is completely blocked by the PPARγ antagonist GW9662 and mimicked by PPARγ agonists, rosiglitazone and 1-*O*-hexadecyl-2-azeleoyl-Gro*P*Cho (Zhang et al., 2004). It is not known how lyso-PtdH enters the nucleus and acts as a physiological agonist for PPARγ. Collectively these studies indicate that selected lyso-PtdH analogs are important novel endogenous PPARγ ligands capable of mediating vascular remodeling and that activation of the nuclear transcription factor PPARγ is both necessary and sufficient for neointima formation by components of oxidized low-density lipoprotein.

References

Al-Rasheed N. M., Chana R. S., Baines R. J., Willars G. B., and Brunskill N. J. (2004). Ligand-independent activation of peroxisome proliferator-activated receptor-γ by insulin and C-peptide in kidney proximal tubular cells — dependent on phosphatidylinositol 3-kinase activity. *J. Biol. Chem.* 279:49747–49754.

Anliker B. and Chun J. (2004). Cell surface receptors in lysophospholipid signaling. *Semin. Cell Dev. Biol.* 15:457–465.

Aoki J. (2004). Mechanisms of lysophosphatidic acid production. *Semin. Cell Dev. Biol.* 15:477–489.

Baker R. R. and Chang H. Y. (2000). A metabolic path for the degradation of lysophosphatidic acid, an inhibitor of lysophosphatidylcholine lysophospholipase, in neuronal nuclei of cerebral cortex. *Biochim. Biophys. Acta Mol. Cell Biol. Lipids* 1483:58–68.

Bandoh K., Aoki J., Hosono H., Kobayashi S., Kobayashi T., Murakami-Murofushi K., Tsujimoto M., Arai H., and Inoue K. (1999). Molecular cloning and characterization of a novel human G-protein-coupled receptor, EDG7, for lysophosphatidic acid. *J. Biol. Chem.* 274:27776–27785.

Bian D., Su S., Mahanivong C., Cheng R. K., Han Q., Pan Z. K., Sun P., and Huang S. (2004). Lysophosphatidic acid stimulates ovarian cancer cell migration via a Ras-MEK kinase 1 pathway. *Cancer Res.* 64:4209–4217.

Brindley D. N. (2004). Lipid phosphate phosphatases and related proteins: signaling functions in development, cell division, and cancer. *J. Cell. Biochem.* 92:900–912.

Brindley D. N., English D., Pilquil C., Buri K., and Ling Z. C. (2002). Lipid phosphate phosphatases regulate signal transduction through glycerolipids and sphingolipids. *Biochim. Biophys. Acta Mol. Cell Biol. Lipids* 1582:33–44.

Cai W., Xu Y., Chen J. Z., Huang S. R., Lu Z. Y., and Wang Z. K. (2005). Yangxueqingnao particles inhibit rat vascular smooth muscle cell proliferation induced by lysophosphatidic acid. *J. Zejiang Univ. Sci.* B 6:892–896.

Carroll R. C., Wang X. F., Lanza F., Steiner B., and Kouns W. C. (1997). Blocking platelet aggregation inhibits thromboxane A2 formation by low dose agonists but does not inhibit phosphorylation and activation of cytosolic phospholipase A2. *Thromb. Res.* 88:109–125.

Chun J. (1999). Lysophospholipid receptors: implications for neural signaling. *Crit. Rev. Neurobiol.* 13:151–168.

Chun J. and Rosen H. (2006). Lysophospholipid receptors as potential drug targets in tissue transplantation and autoimmune diseases. *Curr. Pharm. Des.* 12:161–171.

Contos J. J. A., Ishii I., and Chun J. (2000). Lysophosphatidic acid receptors. *Mol. Pharmacol.* 58:1188–1196.

Das A. K. and Hajra A. K. (1989). Quantification, characterization and fatty acid composition of lysophosphatidic acid in different rat tissues. *Lipids* 24:329–333.

Durgam G. G., Virag T., Walker M. D., Tsukahara R., Yasuda S., Liliom K., van Meeteren L. A., Moolenaar W. H., Wilke N., Siess W., Tigyi G., and Miller D. D. (2005). Synthesis, structure–activity relationships, and biological evaluation of fatty alcohol phosphates as lysophosphatidic acid receptor ligands, activators of PPARγ, and inhibitors of autotaxin. *J. Med. Chem.* 48:4919–4930.

Durgam G. G., Tsukahara R., Makarova N., Walker M. D., Fujiwara Y., Pigg K. R., Baker D. L., Sardar V. M., Parrill A. L., Tigyi G., and Miller D. D. (2006). Synthesis and pharmacological evaluation of second-generation phosphatidic acid derivatives as lysophosphatidic acid receptor ligands. *Bioorg. Med. Chem. Lett.* 16:633–640.

Eddleston M. and Mucke L. (1993). Molecular profile of reactive astrocytes — implications for their role in neurologic disease. *Neuroscience* 54:15–36.

Facchini A., Borzi R. M., and Flamigni F. (2005). Induction of ornithine decarboxylase in T/C-28a2 chondrocytes by lysophosphatidic acid: signaling pathway and inhibition of cell proliferation. *FEBS Lett.* 579:2919–2925.

Fischer D. J., Nusser N., Virag T., Yokoyama K., Wang D. A., Baker D. L., Bautista D., Parrill A. L., and Tigyi G. (2001). Short-chain phosphatidates are subtype-selective antagonists of lysophosphatidic acid receptors. *Mol. Pharmacol.* 60:776–784.

Fukushima N. (2004). LPA in neural cell development. J. Cell. Biochem. 92:993–1003.

Fukushima N., Ishii I., Contos J. J. A., Weiner J. A., and Chun J. (2001). Lysophospholipid receptors. *Annu. Rev. Pharmacol. Toxicol.* 41:507–534.

Gardell S. E., Dubin A. E., and Chun J. (2006). Emerging medicinal roles for lysophospholipid signaling. *Trends Mol. Med.* 12:65–75.

Gueguen G., Gaige B., Grevy J. M., Rogalle P., Bellan J., Wilson M., Klaebe A., Pont F., Simon M. F., and Chap H. (1999). Structure–activity analysis of the effects of lysophosphatidic acid on platelet aggregation. *Biochemistry* 38:8440–8450.

Harrison S. M., Reavill C., Brown G., Brown J. T., Cluderay J. E., Crook B., Davies C. H., Dawson L. A., Grau E., Heidbreder C., Hemmati P., Hervieu G., Howarth A., Hughes Z. A., Hunter A. J., Latcham J., Pickering S., Pugh P., Rogers D. C., Shilliam C. S., and Maycox P. R. (2003). LPA1 receptor-deficient mice have phenotypic changes observed in psychiatric disease. *Mol. Cell Neurosci.* 24:1170–1179.

Hasegawa Y., Erickson J. R., Goddard G. J., Yu S., Liu S., Cheng K. W., Eder A., Bandoh K., Aoki J., Jarosz R., Schrier A. D., Lynch K. R., Mills G. B., and Fang X. (2003). Identification of a phosphothionate analogue of lysophosphatidic acid (LPA) as a selective agonist of the LPA$_3$ receptor. *J. Biol. Chem.* 278:11962–11969.

Hecht J. H., Weiner J. A., Post S. R., and Chun J. (1996). Ventricular zone gene-1 (vzg-1) encodes a lysophosphatidic acid receptor expressed in neurogenic regions of the developing cerebral cortex. *J. Cell Biol.* 135:1071–1083.

Heise C. E., Santos W. L., Schreihofer A. M., Heasley B. H., Mukhin Y. V., MacDonald T. L., and Lynch K. R. (2001). Activity of 2-substituted lysophosphatidic acid (LPA) analogs at LPA receptors: discovery of a LPA1/LPA3 receptor antagonist. *Mol. Pharmacol.* 60:1173–1180.

Heringdorf D. M. Z., Himmel H. M., and Jakobs K. H. (2002). Sphingosylphosphorylcholine-biological functions and mechanisms of action. *Biochim. Biophys. Acta Mol. Cell Biol. Lipids* 1582:178–189.

Holtsberg F. W., Steiner M. R., Furukawa K., Keller J. N., Mattson M. P., and Steiner S. M. (1997). Lysophosphatidic acid induces a sustained elevation of neuronal intracellular calcium. *J. Neurochem.* 69:68–75.

Hooks S. B., Ragan S. P., Hopper D. W., Honemann C. W., Durieux M. E., MacDonald T. L., and Lynch K. R. (1998). Characterization of a receptor subtype-selective lysophosphatidic acid mimetic. *Mol. Pharmacol.* 53:188–194.

Inoue M., Rashid M. H., Fujita R., Contos J. J. A., Chun J., and Ueda H. (2004). Initiation of neuropathic pain requires lysophosphatidic acid receptor signaling. *Nat. Med.* 10:712–718.

Ishii I., Contos J. J. A., Fukushima N., and Chun J. (2000). Functional comparisons of the lysophosphatidic acid receptors, LP_{A1}/VZG-1/EDG-2, LP_{A2}/EDG-4, and LP_{A3}/EDG-7 in neuronal cell lines using a retrovirus expression system. *Mol. Pharmacol.* 58:895–902.

Ishii I., Fukushima N., Ye X. Q., and Chun J. (2004). Lysophospholipid receptors: signaling and biology. *Annu. Rev. Biochem.* 73:321–354.

Keller J. N., Steiner M. R., Mattson M. P., and Steiner S. M. (1996). Lysophosphatidic acid decreases glutamate and glucose uptake by astrocytes. *J. Neurochem.* 67:2300–2305.

Kingsbury M. A., Rehen S. K., Contos J. J. A., Higgins C. M., and Chun J. (2003). Non-proliferative effects of lysophosphatidic acid enhance cortical growth and folding. *Nat. Neurosci.* 6:1292–1299.

Kingsbury M. A., Rehen S. K., Ye X., and Chun J. (2004). Genetics and cell biology of lysophosphatidic acid receptor-mediated signaling during cortical neurogenesis. *J. Cell. Biochem.* 92:1004–1012.

Koschel K. and Tas P. W. L. (1993). Lysophosphatidic acid reverts the beta-adrenergic agonist-induced morphological response in C6 rat glioma cells. *Exp. Cell Res.* 206:162–166.

Kreps D. M., Whittle S. M., Hoffman J. M., and Toews M. L. (1993). Lysophosphatidic acid mimics serum-induced sensitization of cyclic AMP accumulation. *FASEB J.* 7:1376–1380.

Li C., Dandridge K. S., Di A., Marrs K. L., Harris E. L., Roy K., Jackson J. S., Makarova N. V., Fujiwara Y., Farrar P. L., Nelson D. J., Tigyi G. J., and Naren A. P. (2005). Lysophosphatidic acid inhibits cholera toxin-induced secretory diarrhea through CFTR-dependent protein interactions. *J. Exp. Med.* 202:975–986.

Liliom K., Bittman R., Swords B., and Tigyi G. (1996). N-palmitoyl-serine and N-palmitoyl-tyrosine phosphoric acids are selective competitive antagonists of the lysophosphatidic acid receptors. *Mol. Pharmacol.* 50:616–623.

Liliom K., Fischer D. J., Virág T., Sun G., Miller D. D., Tseng J. L., Desiderio D. M., Seidel M. C., Erickson J. R., and Tigyi G. (1998a). Identification of a novel growth factor-like lipid, 1-*O-cis*-alk-1'-enyl-2-lyso-*sn*-glycero-3-phosphate (alkenyl-GP) that is present in commercial sphingolipid preparations. *J. Biol. Chem.* 273:13461–13468.

Liliom K., Guan Z., Tseng J. L., Desiderio D. M., Tigyi G., and Watsky M. A. (1998b). Growth factor-like phospholipids generated after corneal injury. *Am. J. Physiol.* 274:C1065–C1074.

Lynch K. R. and MacDonald T. L. (2001). Structure—activity relationships of lysophospholipid mediators. *Prostaglandins Other Lipid Mediat.* 64:33–45.

Lynch K. R. and MacDonald T. L. (2002). Structure–activity relationships of lysophosphatidic acid analogs. *Biochim. Biophys. Acta Mol. Cell Biol. Lipids* 1582:289–294.

McIntyre T. M., Pontsler A. V., Silva A. R., St Hilaire A., Xu Y., Hinshaw J. C., Zimmerman G. A., Hama K., Aoki J., Arai H., and Prestwich G. D. (2003). Identification of an intracellular receptor for lysophosphatidic acid (LPA): LPA is a transcellular PPARγ agonist. *Proc. Natl Acad. Sci. USA* 100:131–136.

Mettu P. S., Deng P. F., Misra U. K., Gawdi G., Epstein D. L., and Rao P. V. (2004). Role of lysophospholipid growth factors in the modulation of aqueous humor outflow facility. *Invest. Ophthalmol. Vis. Sci.* 45:2263–2271.

Moolenaar W. H., van Meeteren L. A., and Giepmans B. N. (2004). The ins and outs of lysophosphatidic acid signaling. *BioEssays* 26:870–881.

Nishikawa T., Tomori Y., Yamashita S., and Shimizu S. (1988). Inhibition of synaptosomal $(Na^+ + K^+)$-ATPase activity by lysophosphatidic acid: its possible role in membrane depolarization. *Jpn J. Pharmacol.* 47:143–150.

Nishikawa T., Tomori Y., Yamashita S., and Shimizu S. (1989). Inhibition of Na^+,K^+-ATPase activity by phospholipase A_2 and several lysophospholipids: possible role of phospholipase A_2 in noradrenaline release from cerebral cortical synaptosomes. *J. Pharm. Pharmacol.* 41:450–458.

Nishiuchi T., Hamada T., Kodama H., and Iba K. (1997). Wounding changes the spatial expression pattern of the Arabidopsis plastid omega-3 fatty acid desaturase gene (FAD7) through different signal transduction pathways. *Plant Cell* 9:1701–1712.

Pages C., Simon M. F., Valet P., and Saulnier-Blache J. S. (2001). Lysophosphatidic acid synthesis and release. *Prostaglandins Other Lipid Mediat.* 64:1–10.

Palomaki V. A. and Laitinen J. T. (2006). The basic secretagogue compound 48/80 activates G proteins indirectly via stimulation of phospholipase D-lysophosphatidic acid receptor axis and 5-HT$_{1A}$ receptors in rat brain sections. *Br. J. Pharmacol.* 147:596–606.

Pébay A., Torrens Y., Toutant M., Cordier J., Glowinski J., and Tencé M. (1999). Pleiotropic effects of lysophosphatidic acid on striatal astrocytes. *Glia* 28:25–33.

Pulinilkunnil T., An D., Ghosh S., Qi D., Kewalramani G., Yuen G., Virk N., Abrahani A., and Rodrigues B. (2005). Lysophosphatidic acid-mediated augmentation of cardiomyocyte lipoprotein lipase involves actin cytoskeleton reorganization. *Am. J. Physiol. Heart Circ. Physiol.* 288:H2802–H2810.

Ramakers G. J. and Moolenaar W. H. (1998). Regulation of astrocyte morphology by RhoA and lysophosphatidic acid. *Exp. Cell Res.* 245:252–262.

Rao T. S., Lariosa-Willingham K. D., Lin F. F., Palfreyman E. L., Yu N., Chun J., and Webb M. (2003). Pharmacological characterization of lysophospholipid receptor signal transduction pathways in rat cerebrocortical astrocytes. *Brain Res.* 990:182–194.

Renback K., Inoue M., and Ueda H. (1999). Lysophosphatidic acid-induced, pertussis toxin-sensitive nociception through a substance P release from peripheral nerve endings in mice. *Neurosci. Lett.* 270:59–61.

Sardar V. M., Bautista D. L., Fischer D. J., Yokoyama K., Nusser N., Virag T., Wang D. A., Baker D. L., Tigyi G., and Parrill A. L. (2002). Molecular basis for lysophosphatidic acid receptor antagonist selectivity. *Biochim. Biophys. Acta* 1582:309–317.

Sayas C. L., Moreno-Flores M. T., Avila J., and Wandosell F. (1999). The neurite retraction induced by lysophosphatidic acid increases Alzheimer's disease-like Tau phosphorylation. *J. Biol. Chem.* 274:37046–37052.

Sayas C. L., Avila J., and Wandosell F. (2002). Regulation of neuronal cytoskeleton by lysophosphatidic acid: role of GSK-3. *Biochim. Biophys. Acta* 1582:144–153.

Schilling T., Stock C., Schwab A., and Eder C. (2004). Functional importance of Ca^{2+}-activated K^+ channels for lysophosphatidic acid-induced microglial migration. *Eur. J. Neurosci.* 19:1469–1474.

Schulze C., Smales C., Rubin L. L., and Staddon J. M. (1997). Lysophosphatidic acid increases tight junction permeability in cultured brain endothelial cells. *J. Neurochem.* 68:991–1000.

Shiono S., Kawamoto K., Yoshida N., Kondo T., and Inagami T. (1993). Neurotransmitter release from lysophosphatidic acid stimulated PC12 cells: involvement of lysophosphatidic acid receptors. *Biochem. Biophys. Res. Commun.* 193:667–673.

Snitko Y., Yoon E. T., and Cho W. H. (1997). High specificity of human secretory class II phospholipase A2 for phosphatidic acid. *Biochem. J.* 321:737–741.

Steiner M. R., Urso J. R., Klein J., and Steiner S. M. (2002). Multiple astrocyte responses to lysophosphatidic acids. *Biochim. Biophys. Acta Mol. Cell Biol. Lipids* 1582:154–160.

Sugiura T., Tokumura A., Gregory L., Nouchi T., Weintraub S. T., and Hanahan D. J. (1994). Biochemical characterization of the interaction of lipid phosphoric acids with human platelets: comparison with platelet activating factor. *Arch. Biochem. Biophys.* 311:358–368.

Sun G. Y., Lu F. L., Lin S. E., and Ko M. R. (1992). Decapitation ischemia-induced release of free fatty acids in mouse brain. Relationship with diacylglycerols and lysophospholipids. *Mol. Chem. Neuropathol.* 17:39–50.

Symowicz J., Adley B. P., Woo M. M., Auersperg N., Hudson L. G., and Stack M. S. (2005). Cyclooxygenase-2 functions as a downstream mediator of lysophosphatidic acid to promote aggressive behavior in ovarian carcinoma cells. *Cancer Res.* 65:2234–2242.

Takuwa Y., Takuwa N., and Sugimoto N. (2002). The Edg family G protein-coupled receptors for lysophospholipids: their signaling properties and biological activities. *J. Biochem.* (Tokyo) 131:767–771.

Thomson F. J. and Clark M. A. (1994). Purification of a lysophosphatidic acid-hydrolysing lysophospholipase from rat brain. *Biochem. J.* 300:457–461.

Thomson F. J. and Clark M. A. (1995). Purification of a phosphatidic-acid-hydrolysing phospholipase A_2 from rat brain. *Biochem. J.* 306:305–309.

Tigyi G. and Miledi R. (1992). Lysophosphatidates bound to serum albumin activate membrane currents in Xenopus oocytes and neurite retraction in PC12 pheochromocytoma cells. *J. Biol. Chem.* 267:21360–21367.

Tigyi G., Dyer D. L., and Miledi R. (1994). Lysophosphatidic acid possesses dual action in cell proliferation. *Proc. Natl Acad. Sci. USA* 91:1908–1912.

Tigyi G., Hong L., Yakubu M., Parfenova H., Shibata M., and Leffler C. W. (1995). Lysophosphatidic acid alters cerebrovascular reactivity in piglets. *Am. J. Physiol.* 268:H2048–H2055.

Tigyi G., Fischer D. J., Seboek A., Marshall F., Dyer D. L., and Miledi R. (1996a). Lysophosphatidic acid-induced neurite retraction in PC12 cells: neurite-protective effects of cyclic AMP signaling. *J. Neurochem.* 66:549–558.

Tigyi G., Fischer D. J., Seboek A., Yang C., Dyer D. L., and Miledi R. (1996b). Lysophosphatidic acid-induced neurite retraction in PC12 cells: control by phosphoinositide-Ca2+ signaling and Rho. *J. Neurochem.* 66:537–548.

Tokumura A., Iimori M., Nishioka Y., Kitahara M., Sakashita M., and Tanaka S. (1994). Lysophosphatidic acids induce proliferation of cultured vascular smooth muscle cells from rat aorta. *Am. J. Physiol.* 267:C204–C210.

Tou J. S. and Gill J. S. (2005). Lysophosphatidic acid increases phosphatidic acid formation, phospholipase D activity and degranulation by human neutrophils. *Cell Signal.* 17:77–82.

Tsukahara T., Tsukahara R., Yasuda S., Makarova N., Valentine W. J., Allison P., Yuan H. B., Baker D. L., Li Z. G., Bittman R., Parrill A., and Tigyi G. (2006). Different residues mediate recognition of 1-*O*-oleyl-lysophosphatidic acid and rosiglitazone in the ligand binding domain of peroxisome proliferator-activated receptor γ. *J. Biol. Chem.* 281: 3398–3407.

Umezu-Goto M., Tanyi J., Lahad J., Liu S. Y., Yu S. X., Lapushin R., Hasegawa Y., Lu Y. L., Trost R., Bevers T., Jonasch E., Aldape K., Liu J. S., James R. D., Ferguson C. G., Xu Y., Prestwich G. D., and Mills G. B. (2004). Lysophosphatidic acid production and action: Validated targets in cancer? *J. Cell. Biochem.* 92:1115–1140.

Vahidi W. H., Ong W. Y., Farooqui A. A., and Yeo J. F. (2006). Effect of central nervous system free fatty acids and lysophospholipids on allodynia in a mouse model of orofacial pain. *Exp Brain Res.* (in press).

Van Leeuwen F. N., Olivo C., Grivell S., Giepmans B. N., Collard J. G., and Moolenaar W. H. (2003). Rac activation by lysophosphatidic acid LPA1 receptors through the guanine nucleotide exchange factor Tiam1. *J. Biol. Chem.* 278:400–406.

Vasantha Rao P., Deng P. F., Kumar J., and Epstein D. L. (2001). Modulation of aqueous humor outflow facility by the Rho kinase-specific inhibitor Y-27632. *Invest. Ophthalmol. Vis. Sci.* 42:1029–1037.

Virag T., Elrod D. B., Liliom K., Sardar V. M., Parrill A. L., Yokoyama K., Durgam G., Deng W., Miller D. D., and Tigyi G. (2003). Fatty alcohol phosphates are subtype-selective agonists and antagonists of lysophosphatidic acid receptors. *Mol. Pharmacol.* 63:1032–1042.

Weiner J. A., Hecht J. H., and Chun J. (1998). Lysophosphatidic acid receptor gene vzg-1/lpA1/edg-2 is expressed by mature oligodendrocytes during myelination in the postnatal murine brain. *J. Comp. Neurol.* 398:587–598.

Willard F. S., Berven L. A., and Crouch M. F. (2001). Lysophosphatidic acid activates the 70-kDa S6 kinase via the lipoxygenase pathway. *Biochem. Biophys. Res. Commun.* 287:607–613.

Xie Y. H., Gibbs T. C., and Meier K. E. (2002). Lysophosphatidic acid as an autocrine and paracrine mediator. *Biochim. Biophys. Acta Mol. Cell Biol. Lipids* 1582:270–281.

Ye X. Q., Fukushima N., Kingsbury M. A., and Chun J. (2002). Lysophosphatidic acid in neural signaling. *NeuroReport* 13:2169–2175.

Yoo J. O., Yi S. J., Choi H. J., Kim W. J., Kim Y. M., Han J. A., and Ha K. S. (2005). Regulation of tissue transglutaminase by prolonged increase of intracellular Ca^{2+}, but not by initial peak of transient Ca^{2+} increase. *Biochem. Biophys. Res. Commun.* 337:655–662.

Yoshida A. and Ueda H. (2001). Neurobiology of the Edg2 lysophosphatidic acid receptor. *Jpn. J. Pharmacol.* 87:104–109.

Zhang C. X., Baker D. L., Yasuda S., Makarova N., Balazs L., Johnson L. R., Marathe G. K., McIntyre T. M., Xu Y., Prestwich G. D., Byun H. S., Bittman R., and Tigyi G. (2004). Lysophosphatidic acid induces neointima formation through PPARγ activation. *J. Exp. Med.* 199:763–774.

10
Involvement of Phospholipids and Phospholipases A₂ in Neurological Disorders

10.1 Introduction

Brain has a very high metabolic rate that it must maintain for its normal function. This requires an uninterrupted supply of both glucose and oxygen, which brain tissue uses for producing ATP that maintains the high metabolic rate. Underlying this unusual high-energy demand is the need for not only maintaining the appropriate ionic gradients across the neural membranes, but also creating the proper cellular redox potentials. Full and transient deficits in glucose and oxygen can rapidly compromise ATP generation and threaten cellular integrity by either not maintaining or abnormally modulating ion homeostasis and cellular redox. The initial response to a transient insufficiency of energy is depolarization resulting in Na^+ influx into axons. Prolonged energy insufficiency results in a massive influx of Ca^{2+} that facilitates neural cell death.

Neurological disorders are characterized by neural injury or death caused by many different factors, including, but not limited to, inherited genetic abnormalities, problems in the immune system, and metabolic or mechanical insults to the brain or spinal cord tissues. These disorders include acute neural trauma and neurodegenerative diseases. Under both pathological situations, due to compromised ATP generation, neural cells lose their ability to maintain normal ion homeostasis and cellular redox. This can lead to neural cell injury and death in brain tissue and spinal cord (Siesjö, 1978).

10.2 Similarities and Differences Between Acute Neural Trauma and Neurodegenerative Diseases

Ischemia and traumatic head and spinal cord injuries fall within acute neural injury but they arise from very different kinds of initial insult to brain and spinal cord tissues. Ischemia is a metabolic insult caused by severe reduction or blockade in cerebral blood flow. This blockade not only decreases oxygen and glucose delivery to brain tissue but also results in the build-up of potentially toxic products in brain. Because neurons do not store energy-generating substances, there is a rapid decrease in ATP production causing marked impaired ion homeostasis, glutamate release and excitotoxic cascade, and free radical generation resulting in neuronal injury and cell death (Siesjö, 1988a,b; Farooqui and Horrocks, 1994). Neurons undergoing severe ischemia die rapidly (minutes to hours) by necrotic cell death at the core of ischemic injury, whereas penumbral region neurons display delayed vulnerability and die through apoptotic cell death (Farooqui et al., 2004a).

In contrast, mechanical impact and shear forces cause traumatic head and spinal injuries (McIntosh et al., 1998). The traumatic injury to head and spinal cord consists of two broadly defined components: a primary component, attributable to the mechanical insult itself, and a secondary component, attributable to the series of systemic and local neurochemical and pathophysiological changes that occur in brain and spinal cord after the initial traumatic insult (Klussmann and Martin-Villalba, 2005). The primary injury causes a rapid deformation of brain and spinal cord tissues, leading to rupture of neural cell membranes, release of intracellular contents, and disruption of blood flow and breakdown of the blood–brain barrier. In contrast, many neurochemical alterations characterize secondary injury to brain and spinal cord, including glial cell reactions involving both activated microglia and astroglia and demyelination involving oligodendroglia (Beattie et al., 2000). Neurochemically, secondary injury is characterized by the release of glutamate from intracellular stores (Demediuk et al., 1988; Panter et al., 1990; Sundström and Mo, 2002), excitotoxicity, and over-expression of cytokines (Hayes et al., 2002; Ahn et al., 2004).

Excitotoxicity (a process by which high levels of glutamate excite neurons and bring about their demise), neuroinflammation (a neuroprotective mechanism whose prolonged presence is injurious to neurons), and oxidative stress (cytotoxic consequences produced by oxygen free radicals) are major components and central to the pathogenesis of ischemic, traumatic brain, and spinal cord injuries. Like ischemia in head injury and spinal cord trauma, neurons die rapidly (hours to days) at the injury core by necrotic cell death, whereas in the surrounding area neurons undergo apoptotic cell death (several days to months) (McIntosh et al., 1998; Farooqui et al., 2004a). Furthermore, cerebral ischemia, head trauma, and spinal cord injuries trigger similar auto-protective mechanisms including the induction of heat shock proteins, anti-inflammatory cytokines, and production of endogenous antioxidants (Leker and Shohami, 2002).

Neurodegenerative diseases are a complex group of neurological disorders that involve site-specific premature and slow death of certain neuronal populations in brain tissue (Graeber and Moran, 2002). For example in Alzheimer disease (AD), neuronal degeneration occurs in the nucleus basalis, whereas in Parkinson disease (PD), neurons in the substantia nigra die. The most severely affected neurons in Huntington disease (HD) are striatal medium spiny neurons. The most important risk factors for neurodegenerative diseases are old age and a positive family history. The onset of neurodegenerative diseases is often subtle and usually occurs in mid- to late-life and their progression depends not only on genetic, but also on environmental factors (Graeber and Moran, 2002). These diseases lead to progressive cognitive and motor disabilities with devastating consequences to their patients.

Although each neurodegenerative disease has a separate etiology with distinct morphological and pathophysiological characteristics, they may also share the same terminal neurochemical common processes, such as excitotoxicity, oxidative stress, and inflammation (Farooqui and Horrocks, 1994). It remains controversial whether these processes are the cause or consequence of neurodegeneration (Andersen, 2004; Juranek and Bezek, 2005). Similarly, very little information is available on the rate of neurodegeneration and clinical expression of neurodegenerative diseases with age. Although the molecular mechanism of neurodegeneration in neurodegenerative diseases remains unknown, however, neuronal death takes place via apoptosis as well as necrosis (Farooqui et al., 2004a). Thus discovering the molecular mechanisms in neurodegenerative diseases remains a most challenging area of neuroscience research (Graeber and Moran, 2002).

10.3 Involvement of Excitotoxicity and Glycerophospholipid Degradation Mediated by PLA_2 in Acute Neural Trauma and Neurodegenerative Diseases

Excitotoxicity is defined as a process by which high levels of glutamate and its analogs excite neurons and bring about their demise (Olney et al., 1979; Choi, 1988).

Glutamate and its analogs exert their effect by interacting with glutamate receptors (excitatory receptors). These receptors include N-methyl-D-aspartate (NMDA), α-amino-3-hydroxy-5-methyl-4-isoxazole propionate (AMPA), kainate, L-2-amino-4-phosphonobutanoate (L-AP4), and *trans*-1-amino-cyclopentyl-1, 3-dicarboxylate (*trans*-ACPD) receptors. Excitotoxicity is mediated by calcium influx that initiates a cascade of events involving free radical generation, mito-chondrial dysfunction, and activation of many enzymes including those involved in the generation and metabolism of arachidonic acid (Farooqui and Horrocks, 1991, 1994; Farooqui et al., 2001; Wang et al., 2005). These enzymes include iso-forms of PLA_2, cyclooxygenase-2 (COX-2), lipoxygenases (LOX), and epoxyge-nases (EPOX) (Phillis et al., 2006). Accumulation of oxygenated arachidonic acid metabolites along with abnormal homeostasis, and lack of energy generation is associated with neural cell injury and cell death in acute neural trauma (ischemia, epilepsy, head injury, and spinal cord trauma) and neurodegenerative diseases, such as Alzheimer disease (AD), Parkinson disease (PD), multiple sclerosis (MS), and prion diseases like Creutzfeldt–Jakob disease (CJD).

Glutamate can damage glial cells by mechanisms that do not involve glutamate receptor activation, but rather glutamate uptake (Oka et al., 1993; Matute et al., 2006). Glutamate uptake from the extracellular space by specific glutamate trans-porters is essential for maintaining excitatory postsynaptic currents (Auger and Attwell, 2000) and for blocking excitotoxic death due to overstimulation of glu-tamate receptors (Rothstein et al., 1996). Out of five glutamate transporters cloned from brain tissue, at least two transporters, namely excitatory amino acid transporter E1 (EAAT1) and excitatory amino acid transporter E2 (EAAT2), are expressed in astrocytes, oligodendrocytes, and microglial cells (Matute et al., 2006). Exposure of astroglial, oligodendroglial, and microglial cell cultures to glutamate produces glial cell demise by a transporter-related mechanism involving the inhibition of cystine uptake, which causes a decrease in glutathione and makes glial cells vulnerable to toxic free radicals (Oka et al., 1993; Matute et al., 2006).

Injections of glutamate and its analogs and ischemic injury produce a marked increase in cPLA$_2$ isoform mRNA and protein levels (Kim et al., 1995; Sandhya et al., 1998; Ong et al., 2003). This increase in PLA$_2$ can be prevented not only by glutamate receptor antagonists (Sanfeliu et al., 1990; Kim et al., 1995), but also by PLA$_2$ inhibitors (Ong et al., 2003), indicating that generation of arachidonic acid is a receptor-mediated process.

Prostaglandins and leukotrienes, the oxygenated products of arachidonic acid, modulate glutamate receptors in the hippocampus (Chabot et al., 1998). These studies suggest cross talk among glutamate, prostaglandin, leukotriene, and thromboxane receptors. Under normal conditions, this cross talk refines communication among glutamate, prostaglandin, leukotriene, and thromboxane receptors, but under pathological situations, it promotes neuronal injury that depends on the magnitude of PLA$_2$ expression and generation of arachidonic acid metabolites. It is likely that increased activities of PLA$_2$ isoforms and high levels of their reaction products are involved in extending excitotoxicity and oxidative stress during neurodegeneration (Farooqui and Horrocks, 2006b). The participation of the indirect mechanism of arachidonic acid release involving the PLC/diacylglycerol pathway may also potentiate neurodegeneration (Farooqui et al., 1993).

The neurochemical consequences of increased activities of PLA$_2$ isoforms and high levels of arachidonic acid oxygenated products include not only the generation of highly reactive oxygen free radical species with their potent damaging effects on neural membrane phospholipids, proteins, and DNA (oxidative stress), but also induction of inflammatory reactions (Farooqui and Horrocks, 2006b). Our emphasis on the interplay among glutamate receptors, activities of PLA$_2$, oxidative stress, and neuroinflammation does not rule out the participation of other mechanisms involved in neural cell injury. However, it is timely and appropriate to apply the concept of interplay among glutamate, PLA$_2$-generated products, oxidative stress, and neuroinflammation to neural cell injury in acute neural trauma and neurodegenerative diseases. Lack of coordination among the above parameters may control the time taken by neural cells to die. For example, in ischemic, traumatic brain, and spinal cord injuries, neuronal cell death occurs within hours to days, whereas in neurodegenerative diseases, neuronal damage takes years to develop. For ischemia and traumatic brain and spinal cord injuries, there is a therapeutic window of 4 to 6 h (Leker and Shohami, 2002) for partial restoration of many body functions. In contrast, there is no therapeutic window for neurodegenerative diseases and drug intervention starts as soon as first symptoms of the disease appear.

There are many neurochemical similarities between acute neural trauma and neurodegenerative diseases. For example, in acute neural trauma and neurodegenerative diseases, neuronal and glial cells generate ROS and activities of specific mitochondrial enzymic complexes, such as cytochrome oxidase, are also reduced (Fiskum et al., 1999). Furthermore, activated microglia and astrocytes impose inflammation on neurons by virtue of their production of cytokines, such as tumor necrosis factor-α (TNF-α) that may have paracrine effects on neurons. Elevated cytokine production is a characteristic feature of acute neural trauma and neurodegenerative diseases (McGeer and McGeer, 1998; Bramlett and Dietrich, 2004; Farooqui and Horrocks, 2006a). The consequences of lack of oxygen and mitochondrial dysfunction in acute neural trauma also include failure of ATP production, rapid generation of ROS, exacerbation of excitotoxicity, and induction of apoptosis through the release of cytochrome c (Farooqui et al., 2004a). These processes result in a rapid loss of ion homeostasis and neuronal demise.

In neurodegenerative diseases, on the other hand, glucose metabolism slows down, but mitochondria, in spite of their dysfunction, are still capable of generating some ATP for maintaining ion homeostasis to a limited extent. This process results in a cumulative and slow brain damage that takes a much longer time to develop. Thus, many neurodegenerative diseases occur later in life and their onset is consistent with prolonged exposure to excitotoxicity, oxidative stress, and neuroinflammation. Importantly, neurogenesis, a process associated with birth and maturation of functional new hippocampal neurons, is impaired by interplay among excitotoxicity, oxidative stress, and neuroinflammation accounting for brain atrophy in patients with neurodegenerative diseases.

Furthermore, in neurodegenerative diseases, neurons increase their defenses by developing compensatory responses (oxidative strength) (Numazawa et al., 2003; Moreira et al., 2005a) aimed to avoid or at least reduce cellular damage caused by the interplay among excitotoxicity, oxidative stress, and neuroinflammation. These studies are supported by the view that Aβ deposition may not be the initiator of AD pathogenesis, but rather a downstream protective adaptation mechanism developed by cells in response to coordinated and upregulated interplay among excitotoxicity, oxidative stress, and neuroinflammation (Numazawa et al., 2003; Lee et al., 2004; Moreira et al., 2005a,b). This protective role of Aβ explains why many aged individuals, despite having a high number of senile plaques in their brain, show little or no cognitive loss.

10.3.1 PLA$_2$ Activity in Neurological Disorders

Activities of PLA$_2$ isoforms are upregulated in acute neural trauma, ischemia, spinal cord injury, head injury, and many neurodegenerative diseases (Tables 10.1 and 10.2) with substantial inflammatory and oxidative components, such as AD, PD, and MS (Sun et al., 2004; Phillis and O'Regan, 2004; Kalyvas and David, 2004). Premature neurodegeneration in specific populations of neurons in brain tissue characterizes all these neurological disorders. Levels of glycerophospholipids,

TABLE 10.1. Status of PLA$_2$ reaction products, oxidative stress, and inflammation in acute neural trauma (ischemia, head injury, and spinal cord trauma).

Neurochemical parameter	Ischemia	Head injury	Spinal cord injury	Reference
Glycerophospholipid metabolism	Enhanced	Enhanced	Enhanced	DeMedio et al., 1980; Demediuk et al., 1985c; Bazan et al., 1986; Farooqui et al., 2004a
PLA$_2$ activity	Increased	Increased	Increased	Edgar et al., 1982; Taylor, 1988; Shohami et al., 1989; Schapira, 1996
Free fatty acids	Increased	Increased	Increased	Bazan, 1970; Bazan et al., 1971; Wei et al., 1982; Demediuk et al., 1985b, 1987; Bazan et al., 1986; Shohami et al., 1989
Eicosanoids	Increased	Increased	Increased	Ellis et al., 1981; Griffiths et al., 1983; Saunders and Horrocks, 1987; Shohami et al., 1987; Xu et al., 1990; Liu et al., 2001
Lipid peroxides	Increased	Increased	Increased	Anderson and Means, 1985; Demediuk et al., 1985a; Bazan, 1989
Ca^{2+} influx	Increased	Increased	Increased	Stokes et al., 1983; Dienel, 1984; Stokes and Somerson, 1987; Hayes et al., 1992; Beer et al., 2000
4-Hydroxynonenal	Increased	Increased	Increased	Springer et al., 1997; Zhang et al., 1999; McKracken et al., 2001
Oxidative stress	Increased	Increased	Increased	Hall, 1996; Farooqui et al., 2004a
Neuroinflammation	Increased	Increased	Increased	Graham and Chen, 2001; Farooqui et al., 2004a
Apoptotic cell death	Increased	Increased	Increased	Springer et al., 1999; McIntosh et al., 1998; Beattie et al., 2000; Graham and Chen, 2001; Raghupathi, 2004

such as PtdCho, PlsEtn, and PtdIns are markedly decreased in neural membranes from different regions of human brain of patients with acute neural trauma, ischemia, spinal cord injury, and head injury (Edgar et al., 1982; Taylor, 1988; Shohami et al., 1989; Rordorf et al., 1991; Clemens et al., 1996), and neurodegenerative diseases, such as AD and PD (Stokes and Hawthorne, 1987; Söderberg et al., 1990; Wells et al., 1995; Guan et al., 1999; Han et al., 2001; Pettegrew et al., 2001). An elevation of glycerophospholipid degradation metabolites, such as phosphodiesters, phosphomonoesters, fatty acids, prostaglandins, isoprostanes, 4-hydroxynonenals, and other lipid mediators generated by lipid peroxidation accompanies this decrease in glycerophospholipid levels (Farooqui and Horrocks, 2006b). Physicochemical and pathological consequences of disturbed glycerophospholipid metabolism in neural membranes include alterations in membrane

TABLE 10.2. Status of PLA_2-generated reaction products, oxidative stress, and inflammation in neurodegenerative diseases.

Neurochemical parameter	Alzheimer disease	Parkinson disease	Prion diseases	Multiple sclerosis and EAE	Reference
Glycerophos-pholipid metabolism	Enhanced	Decreased	No change/ enhanced	Increased	Pettegrew et al., 1995; Husted et al., 1994; Guan et al., 1996; Prasad et al., 1998; Ross et al., 1998; Jin et al., 2005
PLA_2 activity	Increased	Decreased	Increased	Increased	Huterer et al., 1995; Stephenson et al., 1999; Yoshinaga et al., 2000; Stewart et al., 2001; Farooqui et al., 2003b; Kalyvas and David, 2004; Bate et al., 2004
Free fatty acid composition	Altered	–	–	Altered	Söderberg et al., 1991; Wilson and Tocher, 1991; Pamplona et al., 2005
Eicosanoids	Increased	Increased	Increased	Increased	Pasinetti and Aisen, 1998; Minghetti et al., 2000; Bazan et al., 2002; Neu et al., 2002; Teismann et al., 2003
Lipid peroxides	Increased	Increased	Increased	Increased	Newcombe et al., 1994; Farooqui and Horrocks, 1998; Arlt et al., 2002
Ca^{2+} influx	Increased	–	Decreased	–	Peterson et al., 1985; Peterson and Goldman, 1986; Kristensson et al., 1993
4-Hydroxy-nonenal	Increased	Increased	Increased	Increased	Newcombe et al., 1994; Selley et al., 2002; Zarkovic, 2003
Oxidative stress	Increased	Increased	Increased	Increased	Gorman et al., 1996; Syburra and Passi, 1999; Brown, 2005; Farooqui and Horrocks, 2006b
Neuroinfla-mmation	Increased	Increased	Increased	Increased	Eikelenboom et al., 2002; Kalyvas and David, 2004; Tsutsui et al., 2004; Nagatsu and Sawada, 2005
Apoptotic cell death	Increased	Increased	Increased	–	Lev et al., 2003; Saresella et al., 2005; LeBlanc, 2005; Kristiansen et al., 2005

fluidity and permeability, alterations in ion homeostasis, and changes in activities of membrane-bound enzymes, receptors, and ion channels, and in oxidative stress. Many of these lipid mediators are pro-inflammatory. Their effects are accompanied by the activation of astrocytes and microglia and the release of inflammatory cytokines. These cytokines in turn propagate and intensify neuroinflammation by a number of mechanisms including further upregulation of PLA$_2$ isoforms, generation of platelet-activating factor, stimulation of nitric oxide synthase, and calpain activation (Farooqui and Horrocks, 1991, 2006b; Farooqui et al., 2000, 2002; Ray et al., 2003). Collectively, these studies suggest that increased glycerophospholipid degradation through the activation of PLA$_2$ isoforms can lead to changes in membrane permeability and stimulation of many enzymes associated with lipolysis, proteolysis, and disaggregation of microtubules with a disruption of cytoskeleton and membrane structure (Farooqui and Horrocks, 1994, 2006b).

The stimulation of PLA$_2$ isoforms and accumulation of free fatty acids under pathological situations also sets the stage for increased production of reactive oxygen species (ROS) through the arachidonic acid cascade (Farooqui et al., 1997b). ROS include oxygen free radicals (superoxide radicals, hydroxyl, and alkoxyl radicals, lipid peroxy radicals) and peroxides (hydrogen peroxide and lipid hydroperoxide). At low levels, ROS can function as signaling intermediates in the regulation of fundamental cell activities, such as growth and adaptation responses. At higher concentrations, ROS contribute to neural membrane damage when the balance between reducing and oxidizing (redox) forces shifts toward oxidative stress. Thus, oxidative stress refers to the cytotoxic consequences caused by oxygen free radicals (such as superoxide anion, hydrogen peroxide, and hydroxyl ion) generated as byproducts of pathologic metabolic processes. The imbalance between free radical production and cellular defense mechanisms causes the destruction of neural cells (Juranek and Bezek, 2005). Free radical scavengers including superoxide dismutase, catalase, and glutathione control, in part, the elimination of ROS. Membrane proteins and DNA may be other biological targets of ROS (Refsgaard et al., 2000; Farooqui et al., 2002). The reaction between ROS and proteins or unsaturated lipids in the plasma membrane leads to a chemical cross-linking of membrane proteins and lipids and a reduction in membrane unsaturation (Fig. 10.1). This depletion of unsaturation in membrane

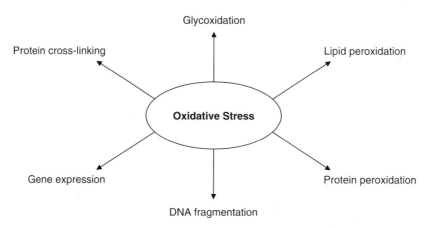

FIG. 10.1. Consequences of oxidative stress in brain tissue.

lipids is associated with decreased membrane fluidity and decreases in the activity of membrane-bound enzymes, ion-channels, and receptors (Ray et al., 1994). ROS also upregulates the gene expression of cytokines through transcription factors in the nucleus (Schneider et al., 1999; Gabriel et al., 1999) (Fig. 10.2). This process leads to the intensification of neural injury.

10.3.2 PLA₂ in Ischemic Injury

Ischemic injury produces the stimulation of cPLA₂, PlsEtn-PLA₂, and PLC in brain tissue (Edgar et al., 1982; Rordorf et al., 1991; Clemens et al., 1996; Phillis and O'Regan, 2004). The stimulation of these enzymes results in a massive release of free fatty acids in brain, the Bazan effect (Bazan, 1970; Farooqui et al., 1994). The Bazan effect also produces the loss of essential glycerophospholipids and the accumulation of lyso-glycerophospholipids (Sun and Foudin, 1984; Hirashima et al., 1984; Abe et al., 1987). During early stages of ischemia (within 1 min), inositol-containing glycerophospholipids are the main source of the increase in free fatty acid and diacylglycerol (Ikeda et al., 1986). At a longer time, ischemic injury

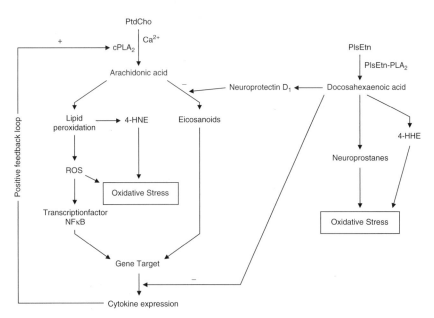

Fig. 10.2. Release of arachidonic acid (AA) and docosahexaenoic acid (DHA) by PLA₂ isoforms and crosstalk between AA and DHA-generated lipid mediators. Phosphatidylcholine (PtdCho); ethanolamine plasmalogen (PlsEtn); cytosolic phospholipase A₂ (cPLA₂); plasmalogen-selective phospholipase A₂ (PlsEtn-PLA₂); 4-hydroxynonenal (4-HNE); 4-hydroxyhexenal (4-HHE); upregulation (+); and down-regulation (−). Notice the modulations of cytokine gene expression by DHA and of cPLA₂ activity by cytokines.

produces changes in the levels of other glycerophospholipids. For example, levels of plasmalogens are markedly decreased in endothelin-1-induced ischemia in synaptosomal membranes from rat striatum (Zhang and Sun, 1995; Viani et al., 1995). This is due to stimulation of PlsEtn-selective PLA$_2$. Collective evidence suggests that the accumulation of free fatty acids, depletion of ATP, alterations in ion homeostasis, and loss of cellular redox induce neural membrane dysfunction. Furthermore, the hydrolysis of cardiolipin by mitochondrial sPLA$_2$ disrupts the mitochondrial electron transport chain and increases ROS production (Adibhatla and Hatcher, 2006). The stimulation of other PLA$_2$ isoforms and reperfusion injury also results in excessive ROS levels producing oxidative stress (Adibhatla and Hatcher, 2006). Mitochondrial inhibitors such as rotenone block ROS production during ischemic reperfusion injury. Marked increases in intracellular [Ca^{2+}] and [Na$^+$] result from energy failure and excitotoxicity. They inhibit complex 1 and generate more superoxide anions. A combination of the above processes can produce neuronal membrane dysfunction and neurodegeneration following ischemic injury (Farooqui and Horrocks, 1991; Adibhatla and Hatcher, 2006).

The stimulation of PlsEtn-PLA$_2$ may occupy a proximal position in the injury pathway, initiating neural cell injury, whereas cPLA$_2$ may participate by hydrolyzing PtdCho and amplifying the injury process (Sapirstein and Bonventre, 2000; Farooqui et al., 2003b, 2004b). The stimulation of PLA$_2$ isoforms in ischemic injury is well known (Edgar et al., 1982; Rordorf et al., 1991; Clemens et al., 1996), but the cell type (neurons, astrocyte, or microglia) in which this stimulation occurs remains controversial. Some studies indicate that upregulation of cPLA$_2$ activity and immunoreactivity occurs in astrocytes of the CA1 hippocampal region at 72 h after ischemic injury (Clemens et al., 1996). Thus, reactive astrocytes are associated with delayed neuronal death. In contrast, studies on unilateral hypoxic–ischemic injury in immature rat brain indicate that the increased cPLA$_2$ immunoreactivity is mainly located in microglia (Walton et al., 1997), although astrocytic induction of cPLA$_2$ was not ruled out. These studies are also in conflict with studies on the expression of cPLA$_2$ mRNA, which does not occur in the CA1 region after ischemia (Owada et al., 1994). According to these studies, dentate granule cells express cPLA$_2$ mRNA.

Studies on transient focal cerebral ischemia induced in rats by occlusion of the middle cerebral artery indicate that sPLA$_2$ group IIA mRNA expression is a biphasic process following 60 min of ischemia-reperfusion. An early phase of sPLA$_2$ group IIA mRNA expression occurs at 30 min after injury and a second increase in that expression takes place at a late phase between 12 h and 14 days (Lin et al., 2004). In situ hybridization studies indicate that the early-phase increase in sPLA$_2$ group IIA mRNA is associated with changes in ischemic cortex, whereas the late-phase increase occurs in the penumbral area. No increase in cPLA$_2$ occurs in the penumbral area at 3 days after ischemia-reperfusion, suggesting that the reactive astrocytic sPLA$_2$ group IIA activity is closely associated with inflammatory processes.

The stimulation of isoforms of PLA$_2$ in ischemic injury may occur through several mechanisms. Thus, one possibility is covalent modification, such as phosphorylation of cPLA$_2$ (Edgar et al., 1982). Another possibility is increased expression of cPLA$_2$ mRNA and sPLA$_2$ mRNA mediated by cytokines (Sun et al., 2004; Lin et al., 2004). Yet another possibility through which cPLA$_2$ stimulation can occur is its cleavage by caspase-3 (Wissing et al., 1997). Caspase-3-mediated stimulation of cPLA$_2$ takes place during apoptotic cell death. This type of cell death occurs in brain tissue after ischemic injury (Sapirstein and Bonventre, 2000; Farooqui et al., 2004a).

The role of cPLA$_2$ in neuronal damage is strongly supported by studies on cPLA$_2$-knockout mice (Bonventre et al., 1997; Sapirstein and Bonventre, 2000; Tabuchi et al., 2003). Following transient middle cerebral artery occlusion, cPLA$_2$-knockout mice develop smaller infarcts, less brain edema, and less neurological deficits than control mice, indicating a reduced susceptibility of cPLA$_2$-knockout mice to ischemic neurodegeneration. Studies on brain lipid metabolism in cPLA$_2$-knockout mice have indicated that there is no net change in unesterified arachidonic acid. However, a 50% reduction in esterified arachidonic acid in phosphatidylcholine supports the involvement of cPLA$_2$ (Rosenberger et al., 2003). cPLA$_2$-knockout mice also show a 62% reduction in the rate of formation of prostaglandin E$_2$, once again suggesting a coupling between cPLA$_2$ and cyclooxygenase activities (Murakami et al., 1997; Bosetti and Weerasinghe, 2003). A patient with a genetic mutation deficiency of cPLA$_2$-α has reduced prostaglandin metabolites in the urine, with serum TxB$_2$ production at 4.6% of normal controls and serum 12-HETE at 1.3% of normal controls (Adler et al., 2006). Primary neural cell cultures prepared from cPLA$_2$-deficient mice also generate significantly smaller amounts of prostaglandins and leukotrienes (Uozumi and Shimizu, 2002). This suggests that the cPLA$_2$ deletion contributes to a decrease in arachidonic acid supply to cyclooxygenase-2 and a resultant decrease in synthesis of prostaglandins.

Significant information is available on the modulation of cPLA$_2$-α activity through post-translational phosphorylation and calcium binding (Hernández et al., 2000), but little is known about the specifics of its transcriptional control. The cPLA$_2$-α promoter consists of a novel AAGGAG motif at −30 to −35 bp, which is bound by a TATA-box binding protein (TBP) and is critical for basal transcriptional activity (Cowan et al., 2004). DNA sequencing analysis of the cPLA$_2$ promoter also suggests a distal cluster of potential hypoxia-inducible factor-1-DNA binding sites homologous to 5′-NCGTG-3′, located between −1087 and −996 bp of the major start of transcription at +1bp (Genbank U08374) (Alexandrov et al., 2006). Detailed investigations using gel shift assay analysis indicate strong hypoxia-inducible factor-1-DNA binding to only one site within this cluster. Promoter deletion analysis indicates the functional importance of this chromatin domain in conveying oxygen sensitivity to cPLA$_2$ gene transcription (Alexandrov et al., 2006). Collectively, these studies suggest that the hypoxia-sensitive domain may promote oxygen sensitivity via transcription factor clustering or Circe effects.

cPLA$_2$-α plays an important role in hypoxic pulmonary vasoconstriction injury in mice. Hypoxic injury induced by occlusion of the left main stem bronchus increases left lung pulmonary vascular resistance in cPLA$_2$-α(+/+) mice but not in cPLA$_2$-α(−/−) mice. cPLA$_2$-α(+/+) mice can maintain better systemic oxygenation during left main stem bronchus occlusion than cPLA$_2$-α(−/−) mice (Ichinose et al., 2002). Administration of AACOCF$_3$ prevents the increase in left lung pulmonary vascular resistance in cPLA$_2$-α(+/+) mice mediated by left main stem bronchus occlusion, whereas exogenous arachidonic acid restores hypoxic pulmonary vasoconstriction in cPLA$_2$-α(−/−) mice. These studies suggest that cPLA$_2$-α activity is associated with the murine pulmonary vasoconstrictor response to hypoxia and augmenting pulmonary vascular tone restores hypoxic pulmonary vasoconstriction in the absence of cPLA$_2$-α activity (Ichinose et al., 2002).

10.3.3 PLA$_2$ in Alzheimer Disease

Activities of cPLA$_2$ (Fig 10.3) and PlsEtn-PLA$_2$ (Fig. 10.4) are markedly increased in the nucleus basalis and hippocampal regions of AD brain when compared with age-matched control brains (Stephenson et al., 1996, 1999; Farooqui et al., 1997a, 2003a,b). COX-2 activity increases similarly in the hippocampal neurons of AD patients when compared with age-matched controls (Sugaya et al., 2000). This elevation produces an increase in levels of prostaglandins in brain

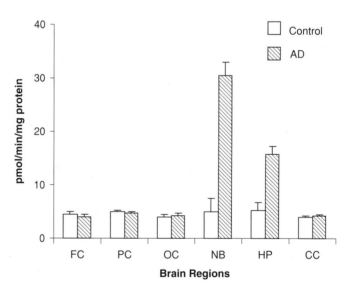

Fig. 10.3. cPLA$_2$ activity in cytosol obtained from different regions of brains from Alzheimer disease patients. Activities of cPLA$_2$ are shown in different regions of brains from normal subjects and AD patients. Open bars and filled bars represent cPLA$_2$ activity in controls and AD patients, respectively. Frontal cortex (FC); parietal cortex (PC); occipital cortex (OC); nucleus basalis (NB); hippocampus (HP); and corpus callosum (CC). Specific activity is expressed as pmol/min/mg protein. Data are modified from (Farooqui et al., 2003a,b).

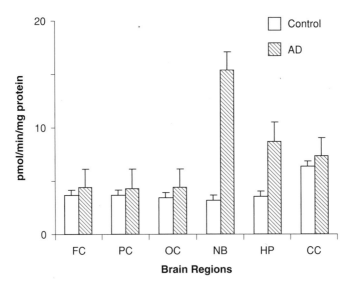

Fig. 10.4. PlsEtn-PLA$_2$ activity in the cytosol obtained from different regions of brains from Alzheimer disease patients. Open bars and filled bars represent PlsEtn-PLA$_2$ activity in controls and AD patients, respectively. Frontal cortex (FC); parietal cortex (PC); occipital cortex (OC); nucleus basalis (NB); hippocampus (HP); and corpus callosum (CC). Specific activity is expressed as pmol/min/mg protein. Data are modified from (Farooqui et al., 2003a,b).

tissues and CSF from AD patients (Montine et al., 1999). Interactions between increased PGE$_2$ synthesis and γ-secretase activity not only modulate more β-amyloid deposition, but also induce neuroinflammation in AD brain (Gasparini et al., 2004; Boutaud et al., 2005). Other investigators reported decreased activities of cPLA$_2$ and iPLA$_2$ in AD (Gattaz et al., 1995, 2004). This discrepancy is not fully understood. However, differences in methodology for PLA$_2$ determination, time between death and autopsy, and handling of human brain samples for enzyme preparation may account for this discrepancy. Human brain samples were used as obtained within 2 to 3 hours after death (Farooqui et al., 2003b), whereas other investigators (Gattaz et al., 1995, 2004) obtained brain samples at a longer time period after death. Thus, more determinations are required on the activities of PLA$_2$ isoforms, not only in membrane and cytosolic fractions from different regions of AD brain, but also at various stages of AD (initial stage, moderately advanced stage, and advanced AD) in human populations. It should be kept in mind that the progress of neurodegeneration varies considerably during the development of AD. This process is influenced not only by diet and genetic factors, but also by environmental factors (Kidd, 2005).

The elevation of glycerophospholipid degradation metabolites, phosphomonoesters and phosphodiesters, in AD brain supports our finding of increased cPLA$_2$ and PlsEtn-PLA$_2$ activities. The increase in phosphomonoesters and phosphodiesters correlates with pathologic markers of AD, such as neurofibrillary tangles and senile plaques (Pettegrew, 1989). Glycerophosphocholine, glycerophosphoethanolamine, and glycero-3-phosphate augment the aggregation of Aβ. This indicates that increased concentrations of glycerophospholipid metabolites may be associated with the deposition of Aβ in normal aging and the even greater deposition of Aβ in AD patients (Klunk et al., 1997). Changes in brain glycerophospholipid and high-energy phosphate metabolism occur before any clinical manifestation of AD (Pettegrew et al., 1995), suggesting abnormal signal transduction due to disturbed glycerophospholipid metabolism may be an important feature of AD. Progressive neurodegeneration in AD may also involve reactive oxygen species (ROS), including superoxide anion, hydrogen peroxide, and hydroxyl radical, inducing cell degeneration (Farooqui and Horrocks, 2006b). Glycerophospholipids in general and plasmalogens in particular are good substrates for lipid peroxidation. This process provides a steady supply of free radicals, such as alkyl and peroxyl radicals that attack cellular components, such as proteins and DNA.

Stimulation of PlsEtn-PLA$_2$ activity in the hippocampal and nucleus basalis regions of AD brain releases DHA from plasmalogens. This fatty acid protects neural cells against Aβ toxicity and accumulation (Corey et al., 1983). An enzyme resembling 15-lipoxygenase acts on DHA. This produces neuroprotectin D1, a 10, 17S-docosatriene (Lukiw et al., 2005). This metabolite of DHA represses Aβ-mediated activation of proinflammatory genes and upregulates anti-apoptotic genes encoding Bcl-2, Bc-xl, and Bfl-1(A1), indicating that neuroprotectin D1 promotes neural cell survival in AD brain (Lukiw et al., 2005; Farooqui and Horrocks, 2006b).

The aldehydic products of arachidonic acid and DHA metabolism, 4-HNE and 4-HHE, which accumulate in AD brain, co-localize with intraneuronal neurofibrillary tangles and may contribute to the cytoskeletal derangement found in AD. Although neurotoxic consequences of the overproduction of 4-HNE and 4-HHE have been highlighted in AD and other neurodegenerative diseases (Farooqui and Horrocks, 2006b), it is noteworthy that these reactive aldehydes are also generated at low levels in neural cells and participate in normal physiological signaling (Barrera et al., 2004; Akaishi et al., 2004). Another class of nonenzymic lipid peroxidation products was also recently identified. It includes F4-isoprostanes and γ-ketoaldehyde isoketals, and neuroketals (Nourooz-Zadeh et al., 1999; Montine and Morrow, 2005). These lipid peroxidation products are more reactive than 4-HNE and 4-HHE. Unlike enzymic products derived from AA and DHA, isoketals and neuroketals remain esterified to glycerophospholipids. They form pyrrole and Schiff base adducts with PtdEtn (Bernoud-Hubac et al., 2004). At present, very little is known about their toxicity in normal and AD brain.

Alterations in glycerophospholipid metabolism may be closely associated with the loss of synapses and neurons and the formation of senile plaques and neurofibrillary tangles in AD (Pettegrew, 1989; Farooqui and Horrocks, 1994). The loss of synapses in AD may be specifically related to the lower levels of plasmalogens in autopsy brain samples (Wells et al., 1995; Ginsberg et al., 1998;

Guan et al., 1999; Han et al., 2001; Pettegrew et al., 2001), indicating that plasmalogen deficiency may be related to the stimulation of PlsEtn-PLA$_2$ activity and loss of DHA from neural membranes (Farooqui et al., 1997a). The plasmalogen deficiency can lead to neuronal membrane destabilization with alterations in membrane fluidity and permeability (Farooqui et al., 1997a), causing Ca^{2+} influx and mitochondrial membrane depolarization that can initiate a cascade of neurochemical reactions resulting in apoptotic and necrotic cell death (Farooqui et al., 2004a). The decrease in plasmalogen levels may produce membrane destabilization by changing the critical temperature necessary for maintaining the stability of the lipid bilayer (Ginsberg et al., 1998). Based on fluorescent probe studies, plasmalogen deficiency increases membrane lipid mobility, resulting in relocation of cholesterol to more hydrophobic areas in the lipid bilayer (Maeba and Ueta, 2003) and exposing many glycerophospholipids containing polyunsaturated fatty acids to peroxidation. These processes may be closely associated with the loss of synapses and impairment of cognitive function in AD patients.

The cause of increased cPLA$_2$ and PlsEtn-PLA$_2$ activities in AD brain is not fully understood. However, there are several possibilities. β-Amyloid peptide (Aβ), which accumulates in AD, may activate cPLA$_2$ activity (Lehtonen et al., 1996; Kanfer et al., 1998). Thus, the treatment of cortical cultures with Aβ stimulates cPLA$_2$ activity in a dose-dependent manner and this stimulation is blocked by cPLA$_2$ antisense oligonucleotides (ODN) (Kriem et al., 2004), strongly suggesting the involvement of cPLA$_2$ in the pathogenesis of AD (Kriem et al., 2004). Aβ deposition may not be the initiator of AD pathogenesis, but a protective adaptation response to coordinated interplay among excitotoxicity, oxidative stress, and neuroinflammation (Numazawa et al., 2003; Lee et al., 2004; Moreira et al., 2005a). The second possibility is that the activation of astrocytes and microglia in AD may result in expression of the cytokines, TNF-α, IL-1β, and IL-6, that are known to stimulate cPLA$_2$ activity (Xu et al., 2003; Rosales-Corral et al., 2004). Another mechanism of cPLA$_2$ activation may involve the proteolytic cleavage of cPLA$_2$ by caspase-3 (Wissing et al., 1997; Beer et al., 2000). A specific tetrapeptide inhibitor of caspase-3 (acetyl-Asp-Glu-Val-Asp-aldehyde) blocks this activation of cPLA$_2$, indicating that caspase-mediated proteolysis of cPLA$_2$ retards cell injury and death. Finally, the Aβ-mediated influx of calcium ions promotes the activation and translocation of cPLA$_2$ from cytosol to neural membranes. This results in breakdown of the membranes and abnormal signal transduction in AD (Farooqui and Horrocks, 1994). Changes in calcium ion signaling mediated by β-amyloid underlie its action on long-term potentiation and also on many calcium-dependent enzymes (Farooqui and Horrocks, 1994), which may render neurons vulnerable to neurodegenerative process. At this stage, we do not know whether elevation of cPLA$_2$ and PlsEtn-PLA$_2$ activities is the cause or the consequence of the neurodegenerative process and whether changes in the activities of PLA$_2$ isoforms are primary or secondary. Thus, more studies are required on the involvement of PLA$_2$ isoforms in the pathogenesis of AD.

Activities of lysophospholipases are also increased in cytosolic fractions from the nucleus basalis and hippocampal regions of AD patients when compared with the same regions of age-matched control brain (Farooqui et al., 1988, 1990) (Fig. 10.5), as well as in cytosolic and membrane preparations of whole brain homogenate (Ross and Kish, 1994). The increased activity of lysophospholipase in AD brain may represent an efficient mechanism for the removal of toxic lysoglycerophospholipids from brain tissue. This supports the view that lysophospholipases may be involved in maintaining low levels of lysoglycerophospholipids within brain tissue. Furthermore, two glycerophospholipid degradation products, glycerophosphocholine and glycerophosphoethanolamine, at a relatively high concentration also inhibit lysophospholipase activity (Fallbrook et al., 1999). Thus, brain tissue has efficient mechanisms to maintain the homeostasis of membrane glycerophospholipids in normal and AD brain tissues.

10.3.4 PLA$_2$ in Parkinson Disease (PD) and its Animal Models

Parkinson disease (PD) is a neurodegenerative disorder characterized by a dramatic loss of dopaminergic neurons in the substantia nigra (SN). Among the many pathogenic mechanisms thought to contribute to the demise of these cells, mitochondrial dysfunction along with ATP depletion and oxidative stress (ROS generation) are pivotal processes that occur relatively earlier during neurodegeneration

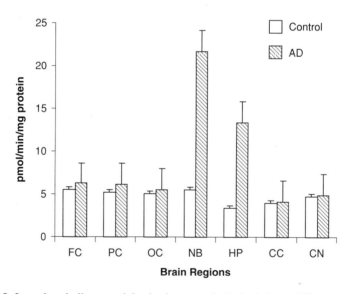

FIG. 10.5. Lysophospholipase activity in the cytosol obtained from different regions of brains from Alzheimer disease patients. Open bars and filled bars represent lysophospholipase activity in controls and AD patients, respectively. Frontal cortex (FC); parietal cortex (PC); occipital cortex (OC); nucleus basalis (NB); hippocampus (HP); and corpus callosum (CC); and caudate nucleus (CN). Specific activity is expressed as nmol/min/mg protein. Data are modified from (Farooqui et al., 1988, 1990).

in PD. Polyunsaturated fatty acids are the major targets for ROS attack on neural membrane glycerophospholipids. In early stages of PD, levels of polyunsaturated fatty acids are reduced in the substantia nigra, whereas levels of malondialdehyde-lysine (MDAL), 4-hydroxynonenal-lysine (HNE), and other lipid peroxides are markedly increased in the substantia nigra, amygdala, and frontal cortex (Farooqui and Horrocks, 1998; Dalfo et al., 2005). ROS also stimulate PLA_2 resulting in neurodegeneration in PD (Han et al., 2003). This stimulation causes the generation of more ROS and accumulation of lipid peroxidation products, resulting in a redox imbalance that overwhelms the protective defense mechanism of neural cells. Factors such as dopamine, and transition metals may, under certain circumstances, also contribute to the formation of ROS. Determination of the activities of calcium-dependent and calcium-independent PLA_2 in different regions of PD brain indicate that the substantia nigra has lower enzymic activity when compared with the temporal cortex and hippocampal regions (Ross et al., 1998). It is proposed that a low PLA_2 activity and a low rate of membrane glycerophospholipid synthesis in the substantia nigra along with slow detoxification of oxidized glycerophospholipids are important for peroxidative injury in the substantia nigra of PD patients (Ross et al., 2001).

Mice deficient in $cPLA_2$ activity are resistant to methyl-4-phenyl-1,2,3, 6-tetrahydropyridine (MPTP) neurotoxicity. This strongly suggests that $cPLA_2$ is closely associated with the pathophysiology of PD (Klivenyi et al., 1998). In brain, MPTP is converted to its toxic metabolite, 1-methyl-4-phenylpyridinium ion (MPP^+) in the presence of monoamine oxidase B. MPP^+ is actively taken up into nigrostriatal neurons where it inhibits mitochondrial oxidative phosphorylation leading to neuronal cell death (Singer et al., 1987). MPP^+-mediated toxicity in GH3 cell cultures supports the involvement of $cPLA_2$ in PD pathogenesis (Yoshinaga et al., 2000). The stimulation of PLA_2 and arachidonic acid release in GH3 cells accompanies neurodegeneration mediated by MPP^+. Arachidonoyl trifluoromethyl ketone ($AACOCF_3$), a specific inhibitor of $cPLA_2$, can block this release of arachidonic acid. Once again, this suggests the involvement of $cPLA_2$ in MPP^+-mediated neurodegeneration.

10.3.5 PLA_2 in Multiple Sclerosis (MS) and Experimental Autoimmune Encephalomyelitis (EAE)

MS and EAE, an animal model for MS, are inflammatory demyelinating diseases of the brain and spinal cord that result in motor and sensory deficits. Myelin and oligodendrocytes are considered the major targets of injury caused by a cell-mediated immune response. Proposed pathophysiological mechanisms include immune-mediated inflammation, oxidative stress, and excitotoxicity (Fig. 10.6). The risk of developing MS may include an increased dietary intake of saturated fatty acids. These fatty acids may not only exert immunosuppressive actions through their incorporation in immune cells, but may also affect cell functions within the brain tissue. PLA_2 activity is markedly higher in brain tissue from MS patients than in controls (Huterer et al., 1995). $cPLA_2$ is highly expressed in EAE

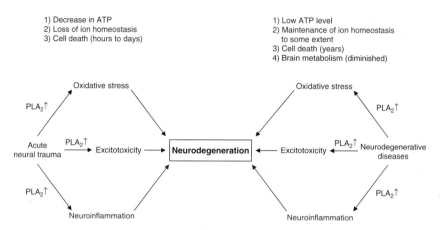

FIG. 10.6. Interplay among excitotoxicity, oxidative stress, and neuroinflammation in acute neural trauma and neurodegenerative diseases. The upward arrow near PLA$_2$ indicates the upregulation of isoforms of PLA$_2$.

lesions (Trigueros et al., 2003; Phillis and O'Regan, 2004; Kalyvas and David, 2004) and inhibition of this enzyme results in a remarkable reduction in the onset and progression of EAE. The reduction in EAE severity correlates with cPLA$_2$ activity and its downstream mediators, such as COX-2, LTB$_4$, and various chemokines and cytokines (Kalyvas and David, 2004). Furthermore, the determination of eicosanoids in the CFS from MS patients indicates that levels of LTB$_4$ are markedly increased indicating the importance of this lipid mediator in MS (Neu et al., 2002). These studies strongly support the view that cPLA$_2$ and its downstream eicosanoids may be involved in the induction and maintenance of neuroinflammation in MS patients.

MS plaques has increased percentages of saturated fatty acids, n–6, n–3, and total polyunsaturated fatty acids, whereas the percentages of monoenes and alk-l-enyl ethers are decreased in comparison to normal brains (Wilson and Tocher, 1991). These results are consistent with increased cellularity and astrogliosis associated with MS plaques. However, analysis of plaque glycerophospholipids shows that the fatty acid changes observed in total lipids are not simply due to the increased proportion of glycerophospholipids and decreased myelin lipids, but that the fatty acid composition of the individual glycerophospholipids was different.

Myelin oligodendrocyte glycoprotein is an agent causing EAE in wild type mice (cPLA$_2$-$\alpha^{+/-}$). cPLA$_2$-$\alpha^{-/-}$ deficient mice are resistant to EAE after injection of this glycoprotein (Marusic et al., 2005). Microscopic examination of the brain and spinal cord indicated remarkable differences between the cPLA$_2$-$\alpha^{+/-}$ and cPLA$_2$-$\alpha^{-/-}$ mice. The cPLA$_2$-$\alpha^{+/-}$ mice show numerous multifocal to coalescing inflammatory cell infiltrations in the brain and spinal cord. These inflammatory cell infiltrates, consisting of mononuclear cells, primarily lymphocytes, macrophages, and glial cells, are present in the leptomeninges, around blood vessels in the leptomeninges and white matter, and in the parenchyma of the white matter. In contrast, brains from cPLA$_2$-$\alpha^{-/-}$ mice show very little or no inflammatory cell infiltration, indicating that the cPLA$_2$-α deficient mice are resistant to EAE development (Marusic et al., 2005). Two explanations are suggested for the resistance of cPLA$_2$-α deficient mice against EAE. First, it is possible that in the cPLA$_2$-α deficient mouse, the number of encephalitogenic cells or their function is not adequate for the full development of EAE. Secondly, it is possible that encephalitogenic T-cells, once in the brain, are not able to mediate full EAE development. In the second case, resistance to EAE induction in the cPLA$_2$-α deficient mouse can be caused by a defective effector phase of EAE (Marusic et al., 2005). Also, lysoglycerophospholipids, generated by cPLA$_2$-α, can be converted to platelet-activating factor. It may play an important role during the effector phase of EAE by acting as a strong chemoattractant and increasing the permeability of the blood–brain barrier, and thereby facilitating the entry of proinflammatory cells into brain tissue (Marusic et al., 2005). This suggestion is supported by studies on mice deficient in PAF-receptors. They have a reduced incidence and severity of EAE (Kihara et al., 2005).

sPLA$_2$ activity is also elevated in EAE and following LPS-mediated neurotoxicity (Pinto et al., 2003). An extracellular sPLA$_2$ inhibitor, N-derivatized phosphatidylethanolamine linked to a polymeric carrier, blocks CNS inflammation under both in vivo and in vitro conditions. These interesting observations suggest that more studies are required on the involvement of PLA$_2$ isoforms in neurodegenerative processes in MS.

10.3.6 PLA$_2$ in Prion Diseases

Prion diseases include scrapie, found in goats and sheep, bovine spongiform encephalopathy (mad cow disease) in cattle, and fetal familial insomnia, Creutzfeldt–Jakob disease (CJD), kuru, and Gerstmann–Sträussler–Scheinker syndrome in humans (Prusiner, 2001; Grossman et al., 2003). Neuronal loss, spongiform degeneration, and glial cell proliferation are the pathological hallmarks of prion diseases. Human prion protein (PrP^c) contains 209 amino acids, a disulfide bridge between residues 179 and 214, a glycosylphosphatidylinositol (GPI) anchor, and two sites of nonobligatory N-linked glycosylation at amino acids 181 and 197 (DeArmond and Prusiner, 2003). In prion diseases soluble PrP^c, which consists of α-helix and random coil structures, is refolded into a β-pleated sheet containing insoluble protease resistant isoform, PrP^{sc} (DeArmond and Prusiner, 2003). The accumulation of PrP^{sc} in the cytoplasm, in secondary lysosomes, and in the neuronal plasmalemma and synaptic regions may be responsible for the loss of cognitive function in prion diseases (Jeffrey et al., 1992).

PrPsc and PrP106-126 (a neurotoxic prion peptide) stimulate NMDA receptor and this stimulation is blocked by MK-801, memantine, and flupirtine (Muller et al., 1993; Perovic et al., 1995; Peyrin et al., 1999). PrP106-126 peptide-mediated stimulation of the NMDA receptor is accompanied with the release of arachidonic acid in cerebellar granule neurons suggesting the association of PLA$_2$ isoforms in the pathogenesis of prion diseases (Stewart et al., 2001). The involvement of PLA$_2$ in the pathogenesis of prion diseases is also supported by recent neuronal cell culture studies (Bate and Williams, 2004). In a tissue culture model of prion disease, neuronal PLA$_2$ is activated by GPI isolated from PrP^c or PrP^{sc}. The ability of GPI to activate PLA$_2$ is lost by either the removal of acyl chains or the cleavage of the phosphatidylinositol-glycan linkage and inhibited by a monoclonal antibody that recognizes phosphatidylinositol (Bate and Williams, 2004). Furthermore, the treatment of neuronal cultures with inositol monophosphate or sialic acid provides resistance to the toxic effects of prion neurotoxic peptides.

These observations strongly implicate PLA$_2$ in the pathogenesis of prion diseases. It is not known whether the involvement of PLA$_2$ in prion-mediated diseases is a primary event or a secondary effect due to an abnormal signal transduction process related to inflammation and oxidative stress in degenerating neurons. However, studies on the use of quinacrine, an acridine-based PLA$_2$ antagonist, indicate that this drug inhibits PrP^{sc} formation, with an IC50 value of 300 nM, and can be used for the treatment of the human prion disease, Creutzfeldt–Jakob disease (CJD) (Doh-ura et al., 2000; Korth et al., 2001; Love, 2001; Follette, 2003; May et al., 2003; Rossi et al., 2003).

10.3.7 PLA$_2$ in Spinal Cord Injury

Traumatic injury to spinal cord consists of two broadly defined components: a primary component, attributable to the mechanical insult itself, and a secondary component, attributable to the series of systemic and local neurochemical and pathophysiological changes that occur in spinal cord after the initial traumatic insult (Klussmann and Martin-Villalba, 2005). The primary injury causes a rapid deformation of brain and spinal cord tissues, leading to rupture of neural cell membranes, release of intracellular contents, disruption of blood flow, and breakdown of the blood–brain barrier.

In contrast, secondary injury to the spinal cord is characterized by many neurochemical alterations, glial cell reactions involving both activated microglia and astroglia, and demyelination involving oligodendroglia (Beattie et al., 2000). Excitotoxicity, inflammatory reactions, and oxidative stress are major components of secondary injury. They play a central role in regulating the pathogenesis of spinal cord trauma. Other neurochemical changes include a rise in glutamate, intracellular calcium, degradation of membrane glycerophospholipids with generation of free fatty acids, diacylglycerols, eicosanoids, and lipid peroxides (Demediuk et al., 1985b), and activation of phospholipases and lipases (Anderson et al., 1985; Taylor, 1988).

During the first minute of compression trauma to spinal cord, 10% of the PlsEtn is lost with an overall loss of 18% found at 30 min after the compression injury (Horrocks et al., 1985). Similar results have been reported in another model of spinal cord injury in rabbits (Lukácová et al., 1996). The loss of PlsEtn after compression and ischemic injuries can be explained by the stimulation of PlsEtn-PLA$_2$ due to shear stress (Taylor, 1988). Stimulation of the PlsEtn-PLA$_2$ may result in changes in membrane fluidity and permeability resulting in increased Ca^{2+} influx, impaired mitochondrial function, and the subsequent generation of ROS. Low levels of ROS act as second messengers and produce neurodegeneration by apoptosis, whereas high levels of ROS produce irreversible damage to cellular components and cause cell death by necrosis (Denecker et al., 2001). Necrosis normally occurs at the core of injury site, whereas neural cells, including oligodendroglia, undergo apoptosis several hours or days after injury in the surrounding area. Secondary injury in spinal cord trauma is modulated by the interplay among excitotoxicity, oxidative stress, and neuroinflammation.

10.3.8 PLA$_2$ in Head Injury

The neurochemical changes in head injury are accompanied by widespread neuronal depolarization, accumulation of glutamate in extracellular space, and increased levels of arachidonic acid, eicosanoids and leukotrienes (McIntosh et al., 1998; Schuhmann et al., 2003). The release of arachidonic acid and its metabolites is due to the activation of cPLA$_2$ (Shohami et al., 1989), as well as the PLC/DAG-lipase pathway (Wei et al., 1982). This also results in generation and accumulation of ROS, which causes oxidative stress. The pathological consequences of alterations in glycerophospholipid metabolism in neural trauma and neurodegenerative diseases may include release of glutamate, stimulation of PLA$_2$ and diacylglycerol lipase activities, generation of eicosanoids, free radical damage, energy failure, and alteration in membrane fluidity and permeability. This may influence the pattern of membrane-bound enzymes, receptors, and ion channels (Farooqui and Horrocks, 1994). Inflammation and edema are also prominent components in the brain's response to traumatic injury. Thus, interplay among excitotoxicity, oxidative stress, and neuroinflammation seems to be involved in head injury.

10.3.9 PLA$_2$ in Epilepsy

Epileptic seizures stimulate cPLA$_2$ activity and expression with the accumulation of arachidonic acid (Visioli et al., 1994; Kajiwara et al., 1996). Levels of free fatty acids (FFA) and diacylglycerols (DAG) in rat brain rise rapidly with the onset of epileptic seizures indicating the activation of PLA$_2$ and PLC (Visioli et al., 1994). However, the ictal/interictal accumulation of FFA attenuates as recurrent seizures continue. FFA and DAG levels were compared in rat cerebral cortex during recurrent ictal periods as a function of associated levels of interictal activity. The rise in rat cortical FFA levels during early seizures for 20:4, 22:6, and 18:0 is 3.6-, 2.5-, and 2.2-fold greater, respectively, than for DAG, when adjacent interictal activity is intense as compared to weak activity. During late seizures, this difference drops to 2.2-fold for 20:4, the only FFA that has a significantly higher value between robust versus weak interictal activity. In contrast, accumulation of DAG during early and late seizures is observed only when adjacent interictal activity is high (Visioli et al., 1994). The cortical accumulation of FFA and DAG during ictal periods of similar intensity and duration depends upon the electrocortical activity during adjacent interictal periods. Studies on the pentylenetetrazol (PTZ)-induced model of epilepsy in rat brain also indicate significant elevations in sPLA$_2$ activity in cortical, hippocampal, and cerebellar regions when compared with the control group. The increase in sPLA$_2$ activity is more pronounced in hippocampal and cortical regions than in the cerebellar region (Yegin et al., 2002). At present, information on activities of PLA$_2$ isoforms is not available in different regions of epileptic human brain. More studies are needed on the involvement of PLA$_2$ isoforms in the pathogenesis of epilepsy.

10.4 Excitotoxicity-Mediated Neurodegeneration Involves PLA$_2$ Activation, Generation of Lipid Mediators, Oxidative Stress, and Neuroinflammation

In brain tissue, excitotoxicity is a major process that produces PLA$_2$-mediated enhancement of glycerophospholipid metabolism, oxidative stress, and inflammation in acute neural trauma, including ischemia, head injury, spinal cord trauma, and epilepsy, as well as in neurodegenerative diseases, AD, PD, MS, and prion diseases (Farooqui and Horrocks, 1994). This enhancement in glycerophospholipid metabolism results in markedly increased levels of lipid mediators, such as free fatty acids, eicosanoids, 4-HNE, isoprostanes, and lipid peroxides in brain tissue in acute neural trauma (Table 10.1), as well as neurodegenerative diseases (Table 10.2). High levels of these lipid mediators along with impaired ion homeostasis, a persistent increase in intracellular Ca^{2+}, and decrease in ATP production, may be responsible for neural cell injury and death in ischemia. This suggests that neural cell injury mediated by PLA$_2$ in acute neural trauma and neurodegenerative diseases is a coordinated multistep process that involves interplay among excitotoxicity, oxidative stress, and neuroinflammation. The effect of interplay on "postmitotic cells," such as neurons, can be cumulative. Terminally differentiated neurons may commit to death in response to abnormal signal transduction processes initiated by the upregulation.

In non-neural cells, cPLA$_2$ activity fluctuates during the M, G1, and S-phases of the cell cycle. Inhibition of the relatively high activity during the initial phases of the cell cycle results in a drastic reduction in S-phase entry (Boonstra and van Rossum, 2003). Furthermore, cell cycle progression is also regulated by the generation of ROS mediated by PLA$_2$. Thus, ROS levels and the duration of ROS exposure regulate cell cycle progression through the modulation of signal transduction cascades, protein ubiquitination, and degradation of cytoskeleton structures. Cyclin kinase inhibitor protein p21 plays a prominent role, leading to cell cycle arrest at higher but not directly lethal levels of ROS. Dependent upon the nature of p21 induction, the cell cycle arrest may be transient, coupled to repair processes, or permanent. Similarly AACOCF$_3$, a cPLA$_2$ inhibitor, not only reduces DNA synthesis but also arrests the cell cycle (van Rossum et al., 2002), once again indicating that cPLA$_2$ activity plays an important role in modulation of the cell cycle. Collectively, these studies indicate that high concentrations of ROS initiate brain damage through signal transduction processes associated with both apoptosis and necrosis (Boonstra and Post, 2004). Depending upon genetic, environmental, and nutritional factors, the neurodegenerative process sometimes occurs through aberrant and uncoordinated re-entry of neural cells into the cell cycle mediated by PLA$_2$ (van Rossum et al., 2001, 2002; Manguikian and Barbour, 2004).

In AD, the affected neurons in the nucleus basalis and hippocampal regions leave the Go state and are arrested at both the G$_1$/S and G$_2$/M phases resulting in neurodegeneration (Munch et al., 2003). Moreover, in AD the neurofibrillary tangles and amyloid plaques are modified by advanced glycation endproducts that activate both mitogenic and redox-sensitive pathways involved in cell cycle re-entry and arrest (Munch et al., 2003). An abnormality in the cell cycle mediated by PLA$_2$ may not be mandatory for the execution of neural cell death. PLA$_2$ stimulation may occur through other mechanisms, such as phosphorylation/dephosphorylation or activation of caspases (Edgar et al., 1982; Wissing et al., 1997; Atsumi et al., 1998, 2000).

Based on PLA$_2$ activities and levels of PLA$_2$-generated metabolites (Tables 10.1 and 10.2), oxidative stress, and the extent of neuroinflammation, it is obvious that there are many similarities among various metabolic parameters in acute neural trauma and neurodegenerative diseases. Alterations in neural membrane glycerophospholipid metabolism, generation of free fatty acids, and production of ROS (oxidative stress) are the earliest events that occur at the onset of acute neural trauma (Bazan, 1970) and Alzheimer disease (Pettegrew et al., 1995; Nunomura et al., 2001; Zhu et al., 2005) before any clinical manifestations. As stated above, the most important risk factors for neurodegenerative diseases are old age and a positive family history. Initially, the coordinated interplay among excitotoxicity, oxidative stress, and neuroinflammation in aged humans and animals may cause abnormalities in motor and cognitive performance. An enhanced rate (upregulation) of interplay among the above processes may be associated with the increased vulnerability of neurons in neurodegenerative diseases. This interplay may be a common mechanism of brain damage in acute neural trauma and neurodegenerative diseases (Farooqui and Horrocks, 1994). Diet (Kidd, 2005), genetic, and environmental factors may also play a prominent role in modulating the interplay among excitotoxicity, oxidative stress, and neuroinflammation that results in neuronal demise.

Another important factor in the neurodegenerative process is the energy status of neurons. In acute neural trauma, neurons die rapidly, a matter of hours to days, because of the sudden lack of oxygen, decrease in ATP level, sudden collapse of ion gradients, and the rapid upregulation of interplay among excitotoxicity, oxidative stress, and neuroinflammation. In contrast, in neurodegenerative diseases, oxygen, nutrients, and ATP continue to be available to the nerve cells, and ionic homeostasis is maintained to a limited extent. The interplay among excito-toxicity, oxidative stress, and neuroinflammation occurs at a slow rate, resulting in a neurodegenerative process that takes several years to develop.

References

Abe K., Kogure K., Yamamoto H., Imazawa M., and Miyamoto K. (1987). Mechanism of arachidonic acid liberation during ischemia in gerbil cerebral cortex. *J. Neurochem.* 48:503–509.

Adibhatla R. M. and Hatcher J. F. (2006). Phospholipase A$_2$, reactive oxygen species, and lipid peroxidation in cerebral ischemia. *Free Radic. Biol. Med.* 40:376–387.

Adler D. H., Phillips J. A. I., Cogan J. D., Morrow I. D., Boutaud O., and Oates J. A. (2006). First description: cytosolic phospholipase A$_2$-alpha deficiency. *J. Invest. Med.* 54:S257.

Ahn M. J., Sherwood E. R., Prough D. S., Lin C. Y., and DeWitt D. S. (2004). The effects of traumatic brain injury on cerebral blood flow and brain tissue nitric oxide levels and cytokine expression. *J. Neurotrauma* 21:1431–1442.

Akaishi T., Nakazawa K., Sato K., Ohno Y., and Ito Y. (2004). 4-Hydroxynonenal modulates the long-term potentiation induced by L-type Ca^{2+} channel activation in the rat dentate gyrus in vitro. *Neurosci. Lett.* 370:155–159.

Alexandrov P. N., Cui J. G., and Lukiw W. J. (2006). Hypoxia-sensitive domain in the human cytosolic phospholipase A$_2$ promoter. *NeuroReport* 17:303–307.

Andersen J. K. (2004). Oxidative stress in neurodegeneration: cause or consequence? *Nature Rev. Neurosci.* S18–S25.

Anderson D. K. and Means E. D. (1985). Iron-induced lipid peroxidation in spinal cord: protection with mannitol and methylprednisolne. *J. Free Radic. Biol. Med.* 1:59–64.

Anderson D. K., Saunders R. D., Demediuk P., Dugan L. L., Braughler J. M., Hall E. D., Means E. D., and Horrocks L. A. (1985). Lipid hydrolysis and peroxidation in injured spinal cord: partial protection with methylprednisolone or vitamin E and selenium. *Cent. Nerv. Syst. Trauma* 2:257–267.

Arlt S., Kontush A., Zerr I., Buhmann C., Jacobi C., Schröter A., Poser S., and Beisiegel U. (2002). Increased lipid peroxidation in cerebrospinal fluid and plasma from patients with Creutzfeldt-Jakob disease. *Neurobiol. Dis.* 10:150–156.

Atsumi G., Tajima M., Hadano A., Nakatani Y., Murakami M., and Kudo I. (1998). Fas-induced arachidonic acid release is mediated by Ca^{2+}-independent phospholipase A$_2$ but not cytosolic phospholipase A$_2$ which undergoes proteolytic inactivation. *J. Biol. Chem.* 273:13870–13877.

Atsumi G., Murakami M., Kojima K., Hadano A., Tajima M., and Kudo I. (2000). Distinct roles of two intracellular phospholipase A$_2$s in fatty acid release in the cell death pathway. Proteolytic fragment of type IVA cytosolic phospholipase A$_{2\alpha}$ inhibits stimulus-induced arachidonate release, whereas that of type VI Ca^{2+}-independent phospholipase A$_2$ augments spontaneous fatty acid release. *J. Biol. Chem.* 275:18248–18258.

Auger C. and Attwell D. (2000). Fast removal of synaptic glutamate by postsynaptic transporters. *Neuron* 28:547–558.

Barrera G., Pizzimenti S., and Dianzani M. U. (2004). 4-Hydroxynonenal and regulation of cell cycle: effects on the pRb/E2F pathway. *Free Radic. Biol. Med.* 37:597–606.

Bate C. and Williams A. (2004). Role of glycosylphosphatidylinositols in the activation of phospholipase A$_2$ and the neurotoxicity of prions. *J. Gen. Virol.* 85:3797–3804.

Bate C., Reid S., and Williams A. (2004). Phospholipase A$_2$ inhibitors or platelet-activating factor antagonists prevent prion replication. *J. Biol. Chem.* 279:36405–36411.

Bazan N. G. (1970). Effects of ischemia and electroconvulsive shock on free fatty acid pool in the brain. *Biochim. Biophys. Acta* 218:1–10.

Bazan N. G. (1989). Arachidonic acid in the modulation of excitable membrane function and at the onset of brain damage. In: *Annals of the New York Academy of Sciences, 559.* New York Academy of Sciences, New York, pp. 1–16.

Bazan N. G., Bazan H. E. P., Kennedy W. G., and Joel C. D. (1971). Regional distribution and rate of production of free fatty acids in rat brain. *J. Neurochem.* 18:1387–1393.

Bazan N. G., Birkle D. L., Tang W., and Reddy T. S. (1986). The accumulation of free arachidonic acid, diacylglycerol, prostaglandins, and lipoxygenase reaction products in the brain during experimental epilepsy. *Adv. Neurol.* 44:879–902.

Bazan N. G., Colangelo V., and Lukiw W. J. (2002). Prostaglandins and other lipid mediators in Alzheimer's disease. *Prostaglandins Other Lipid Mediat.* 68–69:197–210.

Beattie M. S., Farooqui A. A., and Bresnahan J. C. (2000). Review of current evidence for apoptosis after spinal cord injury. *J. Neurotrauma* 17:915–925.

Beer R., Franz G., Srinivasan A., Hayes R. L., Pike B. R., Newcomb J. K., Zhao X., Schmutzhard E., Poewe W., and Kampfl A. (2000). Temporal profile and cell subtype distribution of activated caspase-3 following experimental traumatic brain injury. *J. Neurochem.* 75:1264–1273.

Bernoud-Hubac N., Fay L. B., Armarnath V., Guichardant M., Bacot S., Davies S. S., Roberts L. J., II, and Lagarde M. (2004). Covalent binding of isoketals to ethanolamine phospholipids. *Free Radic. Biol. Med.* 37:1604–1611.

Bonventre J. V., Huang Z. H., Taheri M. R., O'Leary E., Li E., Moskowitz M. A., and Sapirstein A. (1997). Reduced fertility and postischaemic brain injury in mice deficient in cytosolic phospholipase A$_2$. *Nature* 390:622–625.

Boonstra J. and Post J. A. (2004). Molecular events associated with reactive oxygen species and cell cycle progression in mammalian cells. *Gene* 337:1–13.

Boonstra J. and van Rossum G. S. A. T. (2003). The role of cytosolic phospholipase A$_2$ in cell cycle progression. *Prog. Cell Cycle Res.* 5:181–190.

Bosetti F. and Weerasinghe G. R. (2003). The expression of brain cyclooxygenase-2 is down-regulated in the cytosolic phospholipase A$_2$ knockout mouse. *J. Neurochem.* 87:1471–1477.

Boutaud O., Andreasson K. I., Zagol-Ikapitte I., and Oates J. A. (2005). Cyclooxygenase-dependent lipid-modification of brain proteins. *Brain Pathol.* 15:139–142.

Bramlett H. M. and Dietrich W. D. (2004). Pathophysiology of cerebral ischemia and brain trauma: Similarities and differences. *J. Cereb. Blood Flow Metab.* 24:133–150.

Brown D. R. (2005). Neurodegeneration and oxidative stress: prion disease results from loss of antioxidant defence. *Folia Neuropathol.* 43:229–243.

Chabot C., Gagné J., Giguère C., Bernard J., Baudry M., and Massicotte G. (1998). Bidirectional modulation of AMPA receptor properties by exogenous phospholipase A$_2$ in the hippocampus. *Hippocampus* 8:299–309.

Choi D. W. (1988). Glutamate neurotoxicity and diseases of the nervous system. *Neuron* 1:628–634.

Clemens J. A., Stephenson D. T., Smalstig E. B., Roberts E. F., Johnstone E. M., Sharp J. D., Little S. P., and Kramer R. M. (1996). Reactive glia express cytosolic phospholipase A$_2$ after transient global forebrain ischemia in the rat. *Stroke* 27:527–535.

Cowan M. J., Yao X. L., Pawliczak R., Huang X. L., Logun C., Madara P., Alsaaty S., Wu T., and Shelhamer J. H. (2004). The role of TFIID, the initiator element and a novel 5′

TFIID binding site in the transcriptional control of the TATA-less human cytosolic phospholipase A$_2$-α promoter. *Biochim. Biophys. Acta Gene Struct. Expression* 1680:145–157.

Corey E. J., Shih C., and Cashman J. R. (1983). Docosahexaenoic acid is a strong inhibitor of prostaglandin but not leukotriene biosynthesis. *Proc. Natl Acad. Sci. USA* 80:3581–3584.

Dalfo E., Portero-Otin M., Ayala V., Martinez A., Pamplona R., and Ferrer I. (2005). Evidence of oxidative stress in the neocortex in incidental Lewy body disease. *J. Neuropathol. Exp. Neurol.* 64:816–830.

DeArmond S. J. and Prusiner S. B. (2003). Perspectives on prion biology, prion disease pathogenesis, and pharmacologic approaches to treatment. *Clin. Lab. Med.* 23:1–41.

DeMedio G. E., Goracci G., Horrocks L. A., Lazarewicz J., Mazzari S., Porcellati G., Strosznajder J., and Trovarelli G. (1980). The effect of transient ischemia on fatty acid and lipid metabolism in the gerbil brain. *Ital. J. Biochem.* 29:412–432.

Demediuk P., Anderson D. K., Horrocks L. A., and Means E. D. (1985a). Mechanical damage to murine neuronal-enriched cultures during harvesting: effects on free fatty acids, diglycerides, Na$^+$K$^+$-ATPase, and lipid peroxidation. *In Vitro Cell Develop. Biol.* 21:569–574.

Demediuk P., Saunders R. D., Anderson D. K., Means E. D., and Horrocks L. A. (1985b). Membrane lipid changes in laminectomized and traumatized cat spinal cord. *Proc. Natl Acad. Sci. USA* 82:7071–7075.

Demediuk P., Saunders R. D., Clendenon N. R., Means E. D., Anderson D. K., and Horrocks L. A. (1985c). Changes in lipid metabolism in traumatized spinal cord. *Prog. Brain Res.* 63:211–226.

Demediuk P., Saunders R. D., Anderson D. K., Means E. D., and Horrocks L. A. (1987). Early membrane lipid changes in laminectomized and traumatized cat spinal cord. *Neurochem. Pathol.* 7:79–89.

Demediuk P., Daly M. P., and Faden A. I. (1988). Free amino acid levels in laminectomized and traumatized rat spinal cord. *Trans. Am. Soc. Neurochem.* 19:176.

Denecker G., Vercammen D., Declercq W., and Vandenabeele P. (2001). Apoptotic and necrotic cell death induced by death domain receptors. *Cell Mol. Life Sci.* 58:356–370.

Dienel G. A. (1984). Regional accumulation of calcium in postischemic rat brain. *J. Neurochem.* 43:913–925.

Doh-ura K., Iwaki T., and Caughey B. (2000). Lysosomotropic agents and cysteine protease inhibitors inhibit scrapie-associated prion protein accumulation. *J. Virol.* 74:4894–4897.

Edgar A. D., Strosznajder J., and Horrocks L. A. (1982). Activation of ethanolamine phospholipase A$_2$ in brain during ischemia. *J. Neurochem.* 39:1111–1116.

Eikelenboom P., Bate C., Van Gool W. A., Hoozemans J. J., Rozemuller J. M., Veerhuis R., and Williams A. (2002). Neuroinflammation in Alzheimer's disease and prion disease. *Glia* 40:232–239.

Ellis E. F., Wright K. F., Wei E. P., and Kontos H. A. (1981). Cyclooxygenase products of arachidonic acid metabolism in cat cerebral cortex after experimental concussive brain injury. *J. Neurochem.* 37:892–896.

Fallbrook A., Turenne S. D., Mamalias N., Kish S. J., and Ross B. M. (1999). Phosphatidylcholine and phosphatidylethanolamine metabolites may regulate brain phospholipid catabolism via inhibition of lysophospholipase activity. *Brain Res.* 834:207–210.

Farooqui A. A. and Horrocks L. A. (1991). Excitatory amino acid receptors, neural membrane phospholipid metabolism and neurological disorders. *Brain Res. Rev.* 16:171–191.

Farooqui A. A. and Horrocks L. A. (1994). Excitotoxicity and neurological disorders: involvement of membrane phospholipids. *Int. Rev. Neurobiol.* 36:267–323.

Farooqui A. A. and Horrocks L. A. (1998). Lipid peroxides in the free radical pathophysiology of brain diseases. *Cell Mol. Neurobiol.* 18:599–608.

Farooqui A. A. and Horrocks L. A. (2006a). Glutamate and cytokine-mediated alterations of phospholipids in head injury and spinal cord trauma. In: Banik N. (ed.), *Brain and Spinal Cord Trauma. Handbook of Neurochemistry*, Vol. 18. Springer, New York (in press).

Farooqui A. A. and Horrocks L. A. (2006b). Phospholipase A_2-generated lipid mediators in brain: the good, the bad, and the ugly. *Neuroscientist* 12:245–260.

Farooqui A. A., Liss L., and Horrocks L. A. (1988). Stimulation of lipolytic enzymes in Alzheimer's disease. *Ann. Neurol.* 23:306–308.

Farooqui A. A., Liss L., and Horrocks L. A. (1990). Elevated activities of lipases and lysophospholipases in Alzheimer's disease. *Dementia* 1:208–214.

Farooqui A. A., Anderson D. K., and Horrocks L. A. (1993). Effect of glutamate and its analogs on diacylglycerol and monoacylglycerol lipase activities of neuron-enriched cultures. *Brain Res.* 604:180–184.

Farooqui A. A., Haun S. E., and Horrocks L. A. (1994). Ischemia and hypoxia. In: Siegel G. J., Agranoff B. W., Albers R. W., and Molinoff P. B. (eds.), *Basic Neurochemistry.* Raven Press, New York, pp. 867–883.

Farooqui A. A., Rapoport S. I., and Horrocks L. A. (1997a). Membrane phospholipid alterations in Alzheimer disease: deficiency of ethanolamine plasmalogens. *Neurochem. Res.* 22:523–527.

Farooqui A. A., Yang H.-C., and Horrocks L. A. (1997b). Involvement of phospholipase A_2 in neurodegeneration. *Neurochem. Int.* 30:517–522.

Farooqui A. A., Ong W. Y., Horrocks L. A., and Farooqui T. (2000). Brain cytosolic phospholipase A_2: localization, role, and involvement in neurological diseases. *Neuroscientist* 6:169–180.

Farooqui A. A., Ong W. Y., Lu X. R., Halliwell B., and Horrocks L. A. (2001). Neurochemical consequences of kainate-induced toxicity in brain: involvement of arachidonic acid release and prevention of toxicity by phospholipase A_2 inhibitors. *Brain Res. Rev.* 38:61–78.

Farooqui A. A., Ong W. Y., Lu X. R., and Horrocks L. A. (2002). Cytosolic phospholipase A_2 inhibitors as therapeutic agents for neural cell injury. *Curr. Med. Chem. — Anti-Inflammatory Anti-Allergy Agents* 1:193–204.

Farooqui A. A., Ong W. Y., and Horrocks L. A. (2003a). Plasmalogens, docosahexaenoic acid, and neurological disorders. In: Roels F., Baes M., and de Bies S. (eds.), *Peroxisomal Disorders and Regulation of Genes*. Kluwer Academic/Plenum Publishers, London, pp. 335–354.

Farooqui A. A., Ong W. Y., and Horrocks L. A. (2003b). Stimulation of lipases and phospholipases in Alzheimer disease. In: Szuhaj B. and van Nieuwenhuyzen W. (eds.), *Nutrition and Biochemistry of Phospholipids*. AOCS Press, Champaign, pp. 14–29.

Farooqui A. A., Ong W. Y., and Horrocks L. A. (2004a). Biochemical aspects of neurodegeneration in human brain: involvement of neural membrane phospholipids and phospholipases A_2. *Neurochem. Res.* 29:1961–1977.

Farooqui A. A., Ong W. Y., and Horrocks L. A. (2004b). Neuroprotection abilities of cytosolic phospholipase A_2 inhibitors in kainic acid-induced neurodegeneration. *Curr. Drug Targets Cardiovasc. Haematol. Disord.* 4:85–96.

Fiskum G., Murphy A. N., and Beal M. F. (1999). Mitochondria in neurodegeneration: acute ischemia and chronic neurodegenerative diseases. *J. Cereb. Blood Flow Metab.* 19:351–369.

Follette P. (2003). New perspectives for prion therapeutics meeting. Prion disease treatment's early promise unravels. *Science* 299:191–192.

Gabriel C., Justicia C., Camins A., and Planas A. M. (1999). Activation of nuclear factor-κB in the rat brain after transient focal ischemia. *Brain Res. Mol. Brain Res.* 65:61–69.

Gasparini L., Ongini E., and Wenk G. (2004). Non-steroidal anti-inflammatory drugs (NSAIDs) in Alzheimer's disease: old and new mechanisms of action. *J. Neurochem.* 91:521–536.

Gattaz W. F., Maras A., Cairns N. J., Levy R., and Förstl H. (1995). Decreased phospholipase A$_2$ activity in Alzheimer brains. *Biol. Psychiatry* 37:13–17.

Gattaz W. F., Forlenza O. V., Talib L. L., Barbosa N. R., and Bottino C. M. (2004). Platelet phospholipase A$_2$ activity in Alzheimer's disease and mild cognitive impairment. *J. Neural Transm.* 111:591–601.

Ginsberg L., Xuereb J. H., and Gershfeld N. L. (1998). Membrane instability, plasmalogen content, and Alzheimer's disease. *J. Neurochem.* 70:2533–2538.

Gorman A. M., McGowan A., O'Neill C., and Cotter T. (1996). Oxidative stress and apoptosis in neurodegeneration. *J. Neurol. Sci.* 139(Suppl.):45–52.

Graeber M. B. and Moran L. B. (2002). Mechanisms of cell death in neurodegenerative diseases: fashion, fiction, and facts. *Brain Pathol.* 12:385–390.

Graham S. H. and Chen J. (2001). Programmed cell death in cerebral ischemia. *J. Cereb. Blood Flow Metab.* 21:99–109.

Griffiths T., Evans M. C., and Meldrum B. S. (1983). Temporal lobe epilepsy, excitotoxins and the mechanism of selective neuronal loss. In: Fuxe K., Roberts P., and Schwarcz R. (eds.), *Excitotoxins*. Macmillan Publ. Co. Inc., New York, pp. 331–342.

Grossman A., Zeiler B., and Sapirstein V. (2003). Prion protein interactions with nucleic acid: possible models for prion disease and prion function. *Neurochem. Res.* 28:955–963.

Guan Z., Söderberg M., Sindelar P., Prusiner S. B., Kristensson K., and Dallner G. (1996). Lipid composition in scrapie-infected mouse brain: prion infection increases the levels of dolichyl phosphate and ubiquinone. *J. Neurochem.* 66:277–285.

Guan Z. Z., Wang Y. A., Cairns N. J., Lantos P. L., Dallner G., and Sindelar P. J. (1999). Decrease and structural modifications of phosphatidylethanolamine plasmalogen in the brain with Alzheimer disease. *J. Neuropathol. Exp. Neurol.* 58:740–747.

Hall E. D. (1996). Free radicals and lipid peroxidation in neurotrauma. In: Narayan R. K., Wilberger J. E., and Povlishock J. T. (eds.), *Neurotrauma*. McGraw Hill, New York, pp. 1405–1419.

Han X. L., Holtzman D. M., and McKeel D. W., Jr. (2001). Plasmalogen deficiency in early Alzheimer's disease subjects and in animal models: molecular characterization using electrospray ionization mass spectrometry. *J. Neurochem.* 77:1168–1180.

Han W. K., Sapirstein A., Hung C. C., Alessandrini A., and Bonventre J. V. (2003). Crosstalk between cytosolic phospholipase A$_2$α (cPLA$_{2\alpha}$) and secretory phospholipase A$_2$ (sPLA$_2$) in hydrogen peroxide-induced arachidonic acid release in murine mesangial cells — sPLA$_2$ regulates cPLA$_{2\alpha}$ activity that is responsible for arachidonic acid release. *J. Biol. Chem.* 278:24153–24163.

Hayes R. L., Jenkins L. W., and Lyeth B. G. (1992). Neurotransmitter-mediated mechanisms of traumatic brain injury: Acetylcholine and excitatory amino acids. *J. Neurotrauma* 9:S173–S187.

Hayes K. C., Hull T. C., Delaney G. A., Potter P. J., Sequeira K. A., Campbell K., and Popovich P. G. (2002). Elevated serum titers of proinflammatory cytokines and CNS autoantibodies in patients with chronic spinal cord injury. *J. Neurotrauma* 19:753–761.

Hernández M., Nieto M. L., and Sánchez Crespo M. (2000). Cytosolic phospholipase A_2 and the distinct transcriptional programs of astrocytoma cells. *Trends Neurosci.* 23:259–264.

Hirashima Y., Koshu K., Kamiyama K., Nishijima M., Endo S., and Takaku A. (1984). The activities of phospholipase A_1, A_2, lysophospholipase and acyl CoA: Lysophospholipid acyltransferase in ischemic dog brain. In: Go K. G. and Baethmann A. (eds.), *Recent Progress in the Study and Therapy of Brain Edema.* Plenum Pub.Corp., New York, pp. 213–221.

Horrocks L. A., Demediuk P., Saunders R. D., Dugan L., Clendenon N. R., Means E. D., and Anderson D. K. (1985). The degradation of phospholipids, formation of metabolites of arachidonic acid, and demyelination following experimental spinal cord injury. *Cent. Nerv. Syst. Trauma* 2:115–120.

Husted C. A., Matson G. B., Adams D. A., Goodin D. S., and Weiner M. W. (1994). In vivo detection of myelin phospholipids in multiple sclerosis with phosphorus magnetic resonance spectroscopic imaging. *Ann. Neurol.* 36:239–241.

Huterer S. J., Tourtellotte W. W., and Wherrett J. R. (1995). Alterations in the activity of phospholipases A_2 in post-mortem white matter from patients with multiple sclerosis. *Neurochem. Res.* 20:1335–1343.

Ichinose F., Ullrich R., Sapirstein A., Jones R. C., Bonventre J. V., Serhan C. N., Bloch K. D., and Zapol W. M. (2002). Cytosolic phospholipase A_2 in hypoxic pulmonary vaso-constriction. *J. Clin. Invest.* 109:1493–1500.

Ikeda M., Yoshida S., Busto R., Santiso M., and Ginsberg M. D. (1986). Polyphosphoinositides as a probable source of brain free fatty acids accumulated at the onset of ischemia. *J. Neurochem.* 47:123–132.

Jeffrey M., Goodsir C. M., Bruce M. E., McBride P. A., Scott J. R., and Halliday W. G. (1992). Infection specific prion protein (PrP) accumulates on neuronal plasmalemma in scrapie infected mice. *Neurosci. Lett.* 147:106–109.

Jin J. K., Kim N. H., Min D. S., Kim J. I., Choi J. K., Jeong B. H., Choi S. I., Choi E. K., Carp R. I., and Kim Y. S. (2005). Increased expression of phospholipase D1 in the brains of scrapie-infected mice. *J. Neurochem.* 92:452–461.

Juranek I. and Bezek S. (2005). Controversy of free radical hypothesis: Reactive oxygen species – cause or consequence of tissue injury? *Gen. Physiol. Biophys.* 24:263–278.

Kajiwara K., Nagawawa H., Shimizu-Nishikawa S., Ookuri T., Kimura M., and Sugaya E. (1996). Molecular characterization of seizure-related genes isolated by differential screening. *Biochem. Biophys. Res. Commun.* 219:795–799.

Kalyvas A. and David S. (2004). Cytosolic phospholipase A_2 plays a key role in the pathogenesis of multiple sclerosis-like disease. *Neuron* 41:323–335.

Kanfer J. N., Sorrentino G., and Sitar D. S. (1998). Phospholipases as mediators of amyloid β-peptide neurotoxicity: an early event contributing to neurodegeneration characteristic of Alzheimer's disease. *Neurosci. Lett.* 257:93–96.

Kidd P. M. (2005). Neurodegeneration from mitochondrial insufficiency: nutrients, stem cells, growth factors, and prospects for brain rebuilding using integrative management. *Altern. Med. Rev.* 10:268–293.

Kihara Y., Ishii S., Kita Y., Toda A., Shimada A., and Shimizu T. (2005). Dual phase regulation of experimental allergic encephalomyelitis by platelet-activating factor. *J. Exp. Med.* 202:853–863.

Kim D. K., Rordorf G., Nemenoff R. A., Koroshetz W. J., and Bonventre J. V. (1995). Glutamate stably enhances the activity of two cytosolic forms of phospholipase A_2 in brain cortical cultures. *Biochem. J.* 310:83–90.

Klivenyi P., Beal M. F., Ferrante R. J., Andreassen O. A., Wermer M., Chin M. R., and Bonventre J. V. (1998). Mice deficient in group IV cytosolic phospholipase A$_2$ are resistant to MPTP neurotoxicity. *J. Neurochem.* 71:2634–2637.

Klunk W. E., Xu C. J., McClure R. J., Panchalingam K., Stanley J. A., and Pettegrew J. W. (1997). Aggregation of β-amyloid peptide is promoted by membrane phospholipid metabolites elevated in Alzheimer's disease brain. *J. Neurochem.* 69:266–272.

Klussmann S. and Martin-Villalba A. (2005). Molecular targets in spinal cord injury. *J. Mol. Med.* 83:657–671.

Korth C., May B. C., Cohen F. E., and Prusiner S. B. (2001). Acridine and phenothiazine derivatives as pharmacotherapeutics for prion disease. *Proc. Natl Acad. Sci. USA* 98:9836–9841.

Kriem B., Sponne I., Fifre A., Malaplate-Armand C., Lozac'h-Pillot K., Koziel V., Yen-Potin F. T., Bihain B., Oster T., Olivier J. L., and Pillot T. (2004). Cytosolic phospholipase A$_2$ mediates neuronal apoptosis induced by soluble oligomers of the amyloid-beta peptide. *FASEB J.* 18:doi:10.1096/fj.04–1807fje.

Kristensson K., Feuerstein B., Taraboulos A., Hyun W. C., Prusiner S. B., and DeArmond S. J. (1993). Scrapie prions alter receptor-mediated calcium responses in cultured cells. *Neurology* 43:2335–2341.

Kristiansen M., Messenger M. J., Klohn P. C., Brandner S., Wadsworth J. D., Collinge J., and Tabrizi S. J. (2005). Disease-related prion protein forms aggresomes in neuronal cells leading to caspase activation and apoptosis. *J. Biol. Chem.* 280:38851–38861.

LeBlanc A. C. (2005). The role of apoptotic pathways in Alzheimer's disease neurodegeneration and cell death. Curr. *Alzheimer Res.* 2:389–402.

Lee H. G., Casadesus G., Zhu X. W., Takeda A., Perry G., and Smith M. A. (2004). Challenging the amyloid cascade hypothesis — Senile plaques and amyloid-beta as protective adaptations to Alzheimer disease. In: DeGrey A. D. N. (ed.), *Strategies for Engineered Negligible Senescence: Why Genuine Control of Aging May Be Foreseeable.* New York Acad Sciences, pp. 1–4.

Lehtonen J. Y. A., Holopainen J. M., and Kinnunen P. K. J. (1996). Activation of phospholipase A$_2$ by amyloid β-peptides in vitro. *Biochemistry* 35:9407–9414.

Leker R. R. and Shohami E. (2002). Cerebral ischemia and trauma – different etiologies yet similar mechanisms: neuroprotective opportunities. *Brain Res. Rev.* 39:55–73.

Lev N., Melamed E., and Offen D. (2003). Apoptosis and Parkinson's disease. *Prog. Neuropsychopharmacol. Biol. Psychiatry* 27:245–250.

Lin T. N., Wang Q., Simonyi A., Chen J. J., Cheung W. M., He Y. Y., Xu J., Sun A. Y., Hsu C. Y., and Sun G. Y. (2004). Induction of secretory phospholipase A$_2$ in reactive astrocytes in response to transient focal cerebral ischemia in the rat brain. *J. Neurochem.* 90:637–645.

Liu D. X., Li L. P., and Augustus L. (2001). Prostaglandin release by spinal cord injury mediates production of hydroxyl radical, malondialdehyde and cell death: a site of the neuroprotective action of methylprednisolone. *J. Neurochem.* 77:1036–1047.

Love R. (2001). Old drugs to treat new variant Creutzfeldt-Jakob disease. Lancet 358:563.

Lukácová N., Halát G., Chavko M., and Maršala J. (1996). Ischemia-reperfusion injury in the spinal cord of rabbits strongly enhances lipid peroxidation and modifies phospholipid profiles. *Neurochem. Res.* 21:869–873.

Lukiw W. J., Cui J. G., Marcheselli V. L., Bodker M., Botkjaer A., Gotlinger K., Serhan C. N., and Bazan N. G. (2005). A role for docosahexaenoic acid-derived neuroprotectin D1 in neural cell survival and Alzheimer disease. *J. Clin. Invest.* 115:2774–2783.

Maeba R. and Ueta N. (2003). Ethanolamine plasmalogens prevent the oxidation of cholesterol by reducing the oxidizability of cholesterol in phospholipid bilayers. *J. Lipid Res.* 44:164–171.

Manguikian A. D. and Barbour S. E. (2004). Cell cycle dependence of group VIA calcium-independent phospholipase A_2 activity. *J. Biol. Chem.* 279:52881–52892.

Marusic S., Leach M. W., Pelker J. W., Azoitei M. L., Uozumi N., Cui J. Q., Shen M. W. H., DeClercq C. M., Miyashiro J. S., Carito B. A., Thakker P., Simmons D. L., Leonard J. P., Shimizu T., and Clark J. D. (2005). Cytosolic phospholipase $A_{2\alpha}$-deficient mice are resistant to experimental autoimmune encephalomyelitis. *J. Exp. Med.* 202:841–851.

Matute C., Domercq M., and Sánchez-Gómez M. V. (2006). Glutamate-mediated glial injury: Mechanisms and clinical importance. *Glia* 53:212–224.

May B. C. H., Fafarman A. T., Hong S. B., Rogers M., Deady L. W., Prusiner S. B., and Cohen F. E. (2003). Potent inhibition of scrapie prion replication in cultured cells by bis-acridines. *Proc. Natl Acad. Sci. USA* 100:3416–3421.

McGeer E. G. and McGeer P. L. (1998). The importance of inflammatory mechanisms in Alzheimer disease. *Exp. Gerontol.* 33:371–378.

McIntosh T. K., Saatman K. E., Raghupathi R., Graham D. I., Smith D. H., Lee V. M., and Trojanowski J. Q. (1998). The molecular and cellular sequelae of experimental traumatic brain injury: pathogenetic mechanisms. *Neuropathol. Appl. Neurobiol.* 24:251–267.

McKracken E., Graham D. I., Nilsen M., Stewart J., Nicoll J. A., and Horsburgh K. (2001). 4-Hydroxynonenal immunoreactivity is increased in human hippocampus after global ischemia. *Brain Pathol.* 11:414–421.

Minghetti L., Greco A., Cardone F., Puopolo M., Ladogana A., Almonti S., Cunningham C., Perry V. H., Pocchiari M., and Levi G. (2000). Increased brain synthesis of prostaglandin E_2 and F_2-isoprostane in human and experimental transmissible spongiform encephalopathies. *J. Neuropathol. Exp. Neurol.* 59:866–871.

Montine T. J. and Morrow J. D. (2005). Fatty acid oxidation in the pathogenesis of Alzheimer's disease. *Am. J. Pathol.* 166:1283–1289.

Montine T. J., Sidell K. R., Crews B. C., Markesbery W. R., Marnett L. J., Roberts L. J., and Morrow J. D. (1999). Elevated CSF prostaglandin E_2 levels in patients with probable AD. *Neurology* 53:1495–1498.

Moreira P. I., Oliveira C. R., Santos M. S., Nunomura A., Honda K., Zhu X. W., Smith M. A., and Perry G. (2005a). A second look into the oxidant mechanisms in Alzheimer's disease. *Curr. Neurovasc. Res.* 2:179–184.

Moreira P. L., Smith M. A., Zhu X. W., Honda K., Lee H. G., Aliev G., and Perry G. (2005b). Oxidative damage and Alzheimer's disease: Are antioxidant therapies useful? *Drug News Perspect.* 18:13–19.

Muller W. E. G., Ushijima H., Schroder H. C., Forrest J. M. S., Schatton W. F. H., Rytik P. G., and Heffner-Lauc M. (1993). Cytoprotective effect of NMDA receptor antagonists on prion protein (PrionSc)-induced toxicity in rat cortical cell cultures. *Eur. J. Pharmacol.* 246:261–267.

Munch G., Gasic-Milenkovic J., and Arendt T. (2003). Effect of advanced glycation end-products on cell cycle and their relevance for Alzheimer's disease. In: Horowski R., Mizuno Y., Olanow C. W., Poewe W. H., Riederer P., Stoessl J. A., and Youdim M. B. H. (eds.), *Advances in Research on Neurodegeneration.* Springer-Verlag Wien, Vienna, pp. 63–71.

Murakami M., Nakatani Y., Atsumi G., Inoue K., and Kudo I. (1997). Regulatory functions of phospholipase A_2. *Crit. Rev. Immunol.* 17:225–283.

Nagatsu T. and Sawada M. (2005). Inflammatory process in Parkinson's disease: role for cytokines. *Curr. Pharm. Des.* 11:999–1016.

Neu I. S., Metzger G., Zschocke J., Zelezny R., and Mayatepek E. (2002). Leukotrienes in patients with clinically active multiple sclerosis. *Acta Neurol. Scand.* 105:63–66.

Newcombe J., Li H., and Cuzner M. L. (1994). Low density lipoprotein uptake by macrophages in multiple sclerosis plaques: implications for pathogenesis. *Neuropathol. Appl. Neurobiol.* 20:152–162.

Nourooz-Zadeh J., Liu E. H. C., Yhlen B., Änggård E. E., and Halliwell B. (1999). F$_4$-isoprostanes as specific marker of docosahexaenoic acid peroxidation in Alzheimer's disease. *J. Neurochem.* 72:734–740.

Numazawa S., Ishikawa M., Yoshida A., Tanaka S., and Yoshida T. (2003). Atypical protein kinase C mediates activation of NF-E2-related factor 2 in response to oxidative stress. *Am. J. Physiol. Cell Physiol.* 285:C334–C342.

Nunomura A., Perry G., Aliev G., Hirai K., Takeda A., Balraj E. K., Jones P. K., Ghanbari H., Wataya T., Shimohama S., Chiba S., Atwood C. S., Petersen R. B., and Smith M. A. (2001). Oxidative damage is the earliest event in Alzheimer disease. *J. Neuropathol. Exp. Neurol.* 60:759–767.

Oka A., Belliveau M. J., Rosenberg P. A., and Volpe J. J. (1993). Vulnerability of oligodendroglia to glutamate: pharmacology, mechanisms, and prevention. *J. Neurosci.* 13:1441–1453.

Olney J. W., Fuller T., and de Gubareff T. (1979). Acute dendrotoxic changes in the hippocampus of kainate treated rats. *Brain Res.* 176:91–100.

Ong W. Y., Lu X. R., Ong B. K. C., Horrocks L. A., Farooqui A. A., and Lim S. K. (2003). Quinacrine abolishes increases in cytoplasmic phospholipase A$_2$ mRNA levels in the rat hippocampus after kainate-induced neuronal injury. *Exp. Brain Res.* 148:521–524.

Owada Y., Tominaga T., Yoshimoto T., and Kondo H. (1994). Molecular cloning of rat cDNA for cytosolic phospholipase A$_2$ and the increased gene expression in the dentate gyrus following transient forebrain ischemia. *Mol. Brain Res.* 25:364–368.

Pamplona R., Dalfó E., Ayala V., Bellmunt M. J., Prat J., Ferrer I., and Portero-Otín M. (2005). Proteins in human brain cortex are modified by oxidation, glycoxidation, and lipoxidation. Effects of Alzheimer disease and identification of lipoxidation targets. *J. Biol. Chem.* 280:21522–21530.

Panter S. S., Yum S. W., and Faden A. I. (1990). Alteration in extracellular amino acids after traumatic spinal cord injury. *Ann. Neurol.* 27:96–99.

Pasinetti G. M. and Aisen P. S. (1998). Cyclooxygenase-2 expression is increased in frontal cortex of Alzheimer's disease brain. *Neuroscience* 87:319–324.

Perovic S., Pergande G., Ushijima H., Kelve M., Forrest J., and Muller W. E. G. (1995). Flupirtine partially prevents neuronal injury induced by prion protein fragment and lead acetate. *Neurodegeneration* 4:369–374.

Peterson C. and Goldman J. E. (1986). Alterations in calcium content and biochemical processes in cultured skin fibroblasts from aged and Alzheimer donors. *Proc. Natl Acad. Sci. USA* 83:2758–2762.

Peterson C., Gibson G. E., and Blass J. P. (1985). Altered calcium uptake in cultured skin fibroblasts from patients with Alzheimer's disease. *New Engl. J. Med.* 312:1063–1069.

Pettegrew J. W. (1989). Molecular insights into Alzheimer disease. *Ann. NY Acad. Sci.* 568:5–28.

Pettegrew J. W., Klunk W. E., Kanal E., Panchalingam K., and McClure R. J. (1995). Changes in brain membrane phospholipid and high-energy phosphate metabolism precede dementia. *Neurobiol. Aging* 16:973–975.

Pettegrew J. W., Panchalingam K., Hamilton R. L., and McClure R. J. (2001). Brain membrane phospholipid alterations in Alzheimer's disease. *Neurochem. Res.* 26:771–782.

Peyrin J. M., Lasmezas C. I., Haik S., Tagliavini F., Salmona M., Williams A., Richie D., Deslys J. P., and Dormont D. (1999). Microglial cells respond to amyloidogenic PrP peptide by the production of inflammatory cytokines. *NeuroReport* 10:723–729.

Phillis J. W. and O'Regan M. H. (2004). A potentially critical role of phospholipases in central nervous system ischemic, traumatic, and neurodegenerative disorders. *Brain Res. Rev.* 44:13–47.

Phillis J. W., Horrocks L. A., and Farooqui A. A. (2006). Cyclooxygenases, lipoxygenases, and epoxygenases in CNS: their role and involvement in neurological disorders. *Brain Res. Rev.* (in press).

Pinto F., Brenner T., Dan P., Krimsky M., and Yedgar S. (2003). Extracellular phospholipase A_2 inhibitors suppress central nervous system inflammation. *Glia* 44:275–282.

Prasad M. R., Lovell M. A., Yatin M., Dhillon H., and Markesbery W. R. (1998). Regional membrane phospholipid alterations in Alzheimer's disease. *Neurochem. Res.* 23:81–88.

Prusiner S. B. (2001). Shattuck lecture – neurodegenerative diseases and prions. *New Engl. J. Med.* 344:1516–1526.

Raghupathi R. (2004). Cell death mechanisms following traumatic brain. *Brain Pathol.* 14:215–222.

Ray P., Ray R., Broomfield C. A., and Berman J. D. (1994). Inhibition of bioenergetics alters intracellular calcium, membrane composition, and fluidity in a neuronal cell line. *Neurochem. Res.* 19:57–63.

Ray S. K., Hogan E. L., and Banik N. L. (2003). Calpain in the pathophysiology of spinal cord injury: neuroprotection with calpain inhibitors. *Brain Res. Rev.* 42:169–185.

Refsgaard H. H. F., Tsai L., and Stadtman E. R. (2000). Modifications of proteins by polyunsaturated fatty acid peroxidation products. *Proc. Natl Acad. Sci. USA* 97:611–616.

Rordorf G., Uemura Y., and Bonventre J. V. (1991). Characterization of phospholipase A_2 (PLA_2) activity in gerbil brain: enhanced activities of cytosolic, mitochondrial, and microsomal forms after ischemia and reperfusion. *J. Neurosci.* 11:1829–1836.

Rosales-Corral S., Tan D. X., Reiter R. J., Valdivia-Velázquez M., Acosta-Martínez J. P., and Ortiz G. G. (2004). Kinetics of the neuroinflammation-oxidative stress correlation in rat brain following the injection of fibrillar amyloid-β onto the hippocampus in vivo. *J. Neuroimmunol.* 150:20–28.

Rosenberger T. A., Villacreses N. E., Contreras M. A., Bonventre J. V., and Rapoport S. I. (2003). Brain lipid metabolism in the $cPLA_2$ knockout mouse. *J. Lipid Res.* 44:109–117.

Ross B. M. and Kish S. J. (1994). Characterization of lysophospholipid metabolizing enzymes in human brain. *J. Neurochem.* 63:1839–1848.

Ross B. M., Moszczynska A., Erlich J., and Kish S. J. (1998). Low activity of key phospholipid catabolic and anabolic enzymes in human substantia nigra: possible implications for Parkinson's disease. *Neuroscience* 83:791–798.

Ross B. M., Mamalias N., Moszczynska A., Rajput A. H., and Kish S. J. (2001). Elevated activity of phospholipid biosynthetic enzymes in substantia nigra of patients with Parkinson's disease. *Neuroscience* 102:899–904.

Rossi G., Salmona M., Forloni G., Bugiani O., and Tagliavini F. (2003). Therapeutic approaches to prion diseases. *Clin. Lab. Med.* 23:187–208.

Rothstein J. D., Dykes-Hoberg M., Pardo C. A., Bristol L. A., Jin L., Kuncl R. W., Kanai Y., Hediger M. A., Wang Y., Schielke J. P., and Welty D. F. (1996). Knockout of glutamate transporters reveals a major role for astroglial transport in excitotoxicity and clearance of glutamate. *Neuron* 16:675–686.

Sandhya T. L., Ong W. Y., Horrocks L. A., and Farooqui A. A. (1998). A light and electron microscopic study of cytoplasmic phospholipase A$_2$ and cyclooxygenase-2 in the hippocampus after kainate lesions. *Brain Res.* 788:223–231.

Sanfeliu C., Hunt A., and Patel A. J. (1990). Exposure to N-methyl-D-aspartate increases release of arachidonic acid in primary cultures of rat hippocampal neurons and not in astrocytes. *Brain Res.* 526:241–248.

Sapirstein A. and Bonventre J. V. (2000). Phospholipases A$_2$ in ischemic and toxic brain injury. *Neurochem. Res.* 25:745–753.

Saresella M., Marventano I., Speciale L., Ruzzante S., Trabattoni D., Della B. S., Filippi M., Fasano F., Cavarretta R., Caputo D., Clerici M., and Ferrante P. (2005). Programmed cell death of myelin basic protein-specific T lymphocytes is reduced in patients with acute multiple sclerosis. *J. Neuroimmunol.* 166:173–179.

Saunders R. and Horrocks L. A. (1987). Eicosanoids, plasma membranes, and molecular mechanisms of spinal cord injury. *Neurochem. Pathol.* 7:1–22.

Schapira A. H. V. (1996). Oxidative stress and mitochondrial dysfunction in neurodegeneration. *Curr. Opin. Neurol.* 9:260–264.

Schneider A., Martin-Villalba A., Weih F., Vogel J., Wirth T., and Schwaninger M. (1999). NF-kappaB is activated and promotes cell death in focal cerebral ischemia. *Nat. Med.* 5:554–559.

Schuhmann M. U., Mokhtarzadeh M., Stichtenoth D. O., Skardelly M., Klinge P. A., Gutzki F. M., Samii M., and Brinker T. (2003). Temporal profiles of cerebrospinal fluid leukotrienes, brain edema and inflammatory response following experimental brain injury. *Neurol. Res.* 25:481–491.

Selley M. L., Close D. R., and Stern S. E. (2002). The effect of increased concentrations of homocysteine on the concentration of (E)-4-hydroxy-2-nonenal in the plasma and cerebrospinal fluid of patients with Alzheimer's disease. *Neurobiol. Aging* 23:383–388.

Shohami E., Shapira Y., Sidi A., and Cotev S. (1987). Head injury induces increased prostaglandin synthesis in rat brain. *J. Cereb. Blood Flow Metab.* 7:58–63.

Shohami E., Shapira Y., Yadid G., Reisfeld N., and Yedgar S. (1989). Brain phospholipase A$_2$ is activated after experimental closed head injury in the rat. *J. Neurochem.* 53:1541–1546.

Siesjö B. K. (1978). Brain Energy Metabolism. John Wiley & Sons, New York.

Siesjö B. K. (1988a). Historical overview: calcium, ischemia, and death of brain cells. *Ann. NY Acad. Sci.* 522:638–661.

Siesjö B. K. (1988b). Mechanisms of ischemic brain damage. Crit. Care Med. 16:954–963.

Singer T. P., Castagnoli N., Jr., Ramsay R. R., and Trevor A. J. (1987). Biochemical events in the development of parkinsonism induced by 1-methyl-4-phenyl-1,2,3,6-tetrahydropyridine. *J. Neurochem.* 49:1–8.

Söderberg M., Edlund C., Kristensson K., and Dallner G. (1990). Lipid compositions of different regions of the human brain during aging. *J. Neurochem.* 54:415–423.

Söderberg M., Edlund C., Kristensson K., and Dallner G. (1991). Fatty acid composition of brain phospholipids in aging and in Alzheimer's disease. *Lipids* 26:421–425.

Springer J. E., Azbill R. D., Mark R. J., Begley J. G., Wäg G., and Mattson M. P. (1997). 4-hydroxynonenal, a lipid peroxidation product, rapidly accumulates following traumatic spinal cord injury and inhibits glutamate uptake. *J. Neurochem.* 68:2469–2476.

Springer J. E., Azbill R. D., and Knapp P. E. (1999). Activation of the caspase-3 apoptotic cascade in traumatic spinal cord injury. *Nat. Med.* 5:943–946.

Stephenson D. T., Lemere C. A., Selkoe D. J., and Clemens J. A. (1996). Cytosolic phospholipase A$_2$ (cPLA$_2$) immunoreactivity is elevated in Alzheimer's disease brain. *Neurobiol. Dis.* 3:51–63.

Stephenson D., Rash K., Smalstig B., Roberts E., Johnstone E., Sharp J., Panetta J., Little S., Kramer R., and Clemens J. (1999). Cytosolic phospholipase A_2 is induced in reactive glia following different forms of neurodegeneration. *Glia* 27:110–128.

Stewart L. R., White A. R., Jobling M. F., Needham B. E., Maher F., Thyer J., Beyreuther K., Masters C. L., Collins S. J., and Cappai R. (2001). Involvement of the 5-lipoxygenase pathway in the neurotoxicity of the prion peptide PrP106–126. *J. Neurosci. Res.* 65:565–572.

Stokes C. E. and Hawthorne J. N. (1987). Reduced phosphoinositide concentration in anterior temporal cortex of Alzheimer's diseased brains. *J. Neurochem.* 48:1018–1021.

Stokes B. T. and Somerson S. K. (1987). Spinal cord extracellular microenvironment. Can the changes resulting from trauma be graded? *Neurochem. Pathol.* 7:47–55.

Stokes B. T., Fox P., and Hollinden G. (1983). Extracellular calcium activity in the injured spinal cord. *Exp. Neurol.* 80:561–572.

Sugaya K., Uz T., Kumar V., and Manev H. (2000). New anti-inflammatory treatment strategy in Alzheimer's disease. *Jpn J. Pharmacol.* 82:85–94.

Sun G. Y. and Foudin L. L. (1984). On the status of lysolecithin in rat cerebral cortex during ischemia. *J. Neurochem.* 43:1081–1086.

Sun G. Y., Xu J. F., Jensen M. D., and Simonyi A. (2004). Phospholipase A_2 in the central nervous system: implications for neurodegenerative diseases. *J. Lipid Res.* 45:205–213.

Sundström E. and Mo L. L. (2002). Mechanisms of glutamate release in the rat spinal cord slices during metabolic inhibition. *J. Neurotrauma* 19:257–266.

Syburra C. and Passi S. (1999). Oxidative stress in patients with multiple sclerosis. *Ukr. Biokhim. Zh.* 71:112–115.

Tabuchi S., Uozumi N., Ishii S., Shimizu Y., Watanabe T., and Shimizu T. (2003). Mice deficient in cytosolic phospholipase A_2 are less susceptible to cerebral ischemia/reperfusion injury. In: Kuroiwa T., Baethmann A., Czernicki Z., Hoff J. T., Ito U., Katayama Y., Mararou A., Mendelow A. D., and Reulen H. J. (eds.), *Brain Edema XII*. Springer-Verlag Wien, Vienna, pp. 169–172.

Taylor W. A. (1988). Effects of impact injury of rat spinal cord on activities of some enzymes of lipid hydrolysis. Dissertation. The Ohio State University, Columbus, OH.

Teismann P., Vila M., Choi D. K., Tieu K., Wu D. C., Jackson-Lewis V., and Przedborski S. (2003). COX-2 and neurodegeneration in Parkinson's disease. *Ann. NY Acad. Sci.* 991:272–277.

Trigueros S. D. A., Kalyvas A., and David S. (2003). Phospholipase A_2 plays an important role in myelin breakdown and phagocytosis during Wallerian degeneration. *Mol. Cell. Neurosci.* 24:753–765.

Tsutsui S., Schnermann J., Noorbakhsh F., Henry S., Yong V. W., Winston B. W., Warren K., and Power C. (2004). A1 adenosine receptor upregulation and activation attenuates neuroinflammation and demyelination in a model of multiple sclerosis. *J. Neurosci.* 24:1521–1529.

Uozumi N. and Shimizu T. (2002). Roles for cytosolic phospholipase $A_2\alpha$ as revealed by gene-targeted mice. *Prostaglandins Other Lipid Mediat.* 68–69:59–69.

van Rossum G. S. A. T., Vlug A. S., van den Bosch H., Verkleij A. J., and Boonstra J. (2001). Cytosolic phospholipase A_2 activity during the ongoing cell cycle. *J. Cell. Physiol.* 188:321–328.

van Rossum G. S. A. T., Bijvelt J. J. M., van den Bosch H., Verkleij A. J., and Boonstra J. (2002). Cytosolic phospholipase A_2 and lipoxygenase are involved in cell cycle progression in neuroblastoma cells. *Cell. Mol. Life Sci.* 59:181–188.

Viani P., Zini I., Cervato G., Biagini G., Agnati L. F., and Cestaro B. (1995). Effect of endothelin-1 induced ischemia on peroxidative damage and membrane properties in rat striatum synaptosomes. *Neurochem. Res.* 20:689–695.

Visioli F., Rodriguez de Turco E. B., Kreisman N. R., and Bazan N. G. (1994). Membrane lipid degradation is related to interictal cortical activity in a series of seizures. *Metab. Brain Dis.* 9:161–170.

Walton M., Sirimanne E., Williams C., Gluckman P. D., Keelan J., Mitchell M. D., and Dragunow M. (1997). Prostaglandin H synthase-2 and cytosolic phospholipase A$_2$ in the hypoxic–ischemic brain: role in neuronal death or survival? *Mol. Brain Res.* 50:165–170.

Wang Q., Yu S., Simonyi A., Sun G. Y., and Sun A. Y. (2005). Kainic acid-mediated excitotoxicity as a model for neurodegeneration. *Mol. Neurobiol.* 31:3–16.

Wei E. P., Lamb R. G., and Kontos H. A. (1982). Increased phospholipase C activity after experimental brain injury. *J. Neurosurg.* 56:695–698.

Wells K., Farooqui A. A., Liss L., and Horrocks L. A. (1995). Neural membrane phospholipids in Alzheimer disease. *Neurochem. Res.* 20:1329–1333.

Wilson R. and Tocher D. R. (1991). Lipid and fatty acid composition is altered in plaque tissue from multiple sclerosis brain compared with normal brain white matter. *Lipids* 26:9–15.

Wissing D., Mouritzen H., Egeblad M., Poirier G. G., and Jäättelä M. (1997). Involvement of caspase-dependent activation of cytosolic phospholipase A$_2$ in tumor necrosis factor-induced apoptosis. *Proc. Natl Acad. Sci. USA* 94:5073–5077.

Xu J., Hsu C. Y., Liu T. H., Hogan E. L., Perot P. L., Jr., and Tai H.-H. (1990). Leukotriene B4 release and polymorphonuclear cell infiltration in spinal cord injury. *J. Neurochem.* 55:907–912.

Xu J. F., Yu S., Sun A. Y., and Sun G. Y. (2003). Oxidant-mediated AA release from astrocytes involves cPLA$_2$ and iPLA$_2$. *Free Radic. Biol. Med.* 34:1531–1543.

Yegin A., Akhas S. H., Ozben T., and Korgun D. K. (2002). Secretory phospholipase A$_2$ and phospholipids in neural membranes in an experimental epilepsy model. *Acta Neurol. Scand.* 106:258–262.

Yoshinaga N., Yasuda Y., Murayama T., and Nomura Y. (2000). Possible involvement of cytosolic phospholipase A$_2$ in cell death induced by 1-methyl-4-phenylpyridinium ion, a dopaminergic neurotoxin, in GH3 cells. *Brain Res.* 855:244–251.

Zarkovic K. (2003). 4-Hydroxynonenal and neurodegenerative diseases. *Mol. Aspects Med.* 24:293–303.

Zhang J. P. and Sun G. Y. (1995). Free fatty acids, neutral glycerides, and phosphoglycerides in transient focal cerebral ischemia. *J. Neurochem.* 64:1688–1695.

Zhang D. Q., Dhillon H. S., Mattson M. P., Yurek D. M., and Prasad R. M. (1999). Immunohistochemical detection of the lipid peroxidation product 4-hydroxynonenal after experimental brain injury in the rat. *Neurosci. Lett.* 272:57–61.

Zhu X. W., Lee H. G., Casadesus G., Avila J., Drew K., Perry G., and Smith M. A. (2005). Oxidative imbalance in Alzheimer's disease. *Mol. Neurobiol.* 31:205–217.

11
Inhibitors of Phospholipases A$_2$ and Their Use for the Treatment of Neurological Disorders

11.1 Introduction

The stimulation of PLA$_2$ isoforms, release of arachidonic acid and its metabolites (prostaglandins and leukotrienes), and generation of platelet-activating factor (PAF) are important events in the inflammation and oxidative stress associated with acute neural trauma and chronic neurological disorders (Farooqui and Horrocks, 1994; Phillis and O'Regan, 2004). Nonsteroidal anti-inflammatory drugs (NSAID) and the COX-2 inhibitors celecoxib (Celebrex™) and rofecoxib (Vioxx™) inhibit the cyclooxygenase-mediated pathway for the synthesis of prostaglandins, but do not block the lipoxygenase-mediated generation of leukotrienes and the acetyl transferase-mediated synthesis of PAF. A PLA$_2$ inhibitor can potentially block all three pathways simultaneously. Thus, there is an urgent need for the development of potent, specific, nontoxic PLA$_2$ inhibitors that can be used as anti-inflammatory and antioxidant drugs for the treatment of inflammation and oxidative stress in acute neural trauma and chronic neurological disorders.

Research scientists at pharmaceutical companies are actively working on the discovery of PLA$_2$ inhibitors for these indications, but also many other peripheral diseases such as rheumatoid arthritis, sepsis, and asthma. Merckle GmbH introduced a series of Lehr's compounds that inhibit cPLA$_2$ (Lehr, 2000; Lehr et al., 2001; Griessbach et al., 2003). Elan patented a group of cPLA$_2$ inhibitors comprised substituted pyrimidines (Varghese et al., 2003). Bristol-Myers Squibb synthesized BMS-181162 (Tramposch et al., 1992). Shionogi discovered several pyrrolidine-based inhibitors that block cPLA$_2$ activity potently (Seno et al., 2000, 2001; Ghomashchi et al., 2001; Ono et al., 2002). Lilly Research Laboratories has a sPLA$_2$ inhibitor, LY311727 (Schevitz et al., 1995). These studies indicate clearly that the drug industry throughout the world pursues actively the development of PLA$_2$ inhibitors.

The problem with the available inhibitors of PLA$_2$ isoforms is their specificity. Many PLA$_2$ inhibitors originally thought to be selective for a specific PLA$_2$ isoform are now known to inhibit other PLA$_2$ isoforms and also inhibit other enzymes that are not involved in the release of arachidonic acid (Farooqui et al., 1999; Cummings et al., 2000; Fuentes et al., 2003). For example, in non-neural cells arachidonoyl trifluoromethyl ketone inhibits not only cPLA$_2$ activity, but also inhibits cyclooxygenase and acyltransferase activities (Cummings et al., 2000; Fuentes et al., 2003). Methyl arachidonoyl fluorophosphonate, another inhibitor of brain cPLA$_2$, also inhibits bovine brain iPLA$_2$ as well as hydrolysis of arachidonoyl ethanolamide (anandamide) by fatty acid amide hydrolase. Bromoenol lactone, a specific inhibitor of iPLA$_2$, blocks phosphatidic acid phosphatase (Balsinde and Dennis, 1997) and diacylglycerol lipase (Moriyama et al., 1999) activities. Another variable in the research on isoforms of PLA$_2$ and their inhibitors has been the discovery of new paralogs and splice variants of PLA$_2$ in brain and other body tissues (Masuda et al., 2005; Ohto et al., 2005). These paralogs and splice variants have different properties and respond to known inhibitors of PLA$_2$ differently than the native paralogs of PLA$_2$.

The discovery of potent and specific inhibitors of PLA$_2$ isoforms is an important approach for establishing functional roles of newly discovered PLA$_2$ molecular species in a specific type of neural cell in brain tissue and also for treating oxidative stress and inflammation caused by neurodegenerative process. Studies on this important topic are emerging (Farooqui et al., 1999; Cummings et al., 2000; Miele, 2003; Scott et al., 2003; Clark and Tam, 2004). These studies are complicated by the lack of information on the commercially available specific inhibitors. In addition, information is lacking on the in vivo effects of PLA$_2$ inhibitors on the activity of PLA$_2$ isoforms with the many different molecular species of glycerophospholipids. Furthermore, the effect of inhibitors on the physical state of substrate aggregates in neural membranes remains unknown. In searching for good cPLA$_2$ inhibitors, kinetic analysis is not enough to evaluate whether an inhibitor can block PLA$_2$ activity by affecting the interfacial quality of phospholipids in the lipid bilayer, or by directly inhibiting the interaction between the glycerophospholipids and the active site of the enzyme. An ideal inhibitor should be able to cross the blood–brain barrier, have regional specificity, and be able to reach the site where cells are under oxidative stress and inflammatory and neurodegenerative processes are taking place.

To overcome PLA$_2$ specificity, three approaches have been adopted. One is the discovery of antisense oligonucleotides (Roshak et al., 2000; Hannon, 2002). Another is the overexpression of a specific PLA$_2$ isoform (Kambe et al., 1999). The third (Aguzzi et al., 1996) is the development of transgenic (Tietge et al., 2000, 2002) and knockout mice (Burton et al., 2002; Bonventre and Sapirstein, 2002). Furthermore, transgenic and knockout mice for each PLA$_2$ isoform may not be suitable for studying neurodegenerative diseases. Studies on systemic administration of LPS in wild-type mice and mice deficient in cPLA$_2$-$\alpha^{(-/-)}$ indicate that inhibition of cPLA$_2$-α is a novel anti-inflammatory strategy that modulates but does not completely prevent eicosanoid responses (Sapirstein et al., 2005). All these approaches have limitations and suffer from the lack of sequence identity among PLA$_2$ isoforms and also from the continuous discovery of splice variants of various PLA$_2$ classes and subclasses (Pickard et al., 1999; Tanaka et al., 2000, 2004; Meyer et al., 2005; Ohto et al., 2005; Yamashita et al., 2005).

Neurons are more susceptible to free radical-mediated neuroinflammation and oxidative stress than glial cells (Adibhatla et al., 2003; Ajmone-Cat et al., 2003).

In fact, activated glial cells including astroglia and microglia sustain inflamma-tory processes initiated by metabolites generated from arachidonic acid. This sug-gests that signals modulating the induction, expression, and stimulation of PLA$_2$ isoforms may play an important role in neurodegenerative diseases associated with neuroinflammation and oxidative stress (Farooqui and Horrocks, 1994; Farooqui et al., 2003, 2004). For the successful treatment of inflammatory and oxidative stress in neurological disorders, timely delivery is required of a well-tolerated, chronically active, and specific inhibitor of PLA$_2$ that can bypass or cross the blood–brain barrier without harm. Some nonspecific PLA$_2$ inhibitors (see below) have been used for the treatment of ischemia, spinal cord injury, and AD (Sano et al., 1997), but no compound with an excellent clinical potential has emerged.

11.2 Physiological and Pharmacological Effects of PLA$_2$ Inhibitors

11.2.1 Arachidonoyl Trifluoromethyl Ketone (AACOCF$_3$)

Arachidonoyl trifluoromethyl ketone (Fig. 11.1) is a potent inhibitor of cPLA$_2$. NMR studies show that the carbon chain of the AACOCF$_3$ binds in a hydrophobic pocket and the carbonyl group of the AACOCF$_3$ forms a covalent bond with ser-ine 228 in the active site generating a charged hemiketal oxoanion that interacts with a positively charged group of the enzyme (Street et al., 1993; Trimble et al., 1993; Bartoli et al., 1994). The binding of AACOCF$_3$ is similar to the binding of the endogenous glycerophospholipid substrate. Thus, AACOCF$_3$ competes with glycerophospholipid substrates for the catalytic site on the enzyme molecule. AACOCF$_3$ is a 500-fold more potent inhibitor of cPLA$_2$ than of sPLA$_2$ (Trimble et al., 1993), indicating that it is a much more selective inhibitor of cPLA$_2$ than sPLA$_2$. This inhibitor also blocks cyclooxygenase activity (Riendeau et al., 1994).

Because of its physicochemical properties, AACOCF$_3$ can readily penetrate into cell membranes. At 5 to 20 µM it essentially blocks all liberation of arachi-donic acid in thrombin-stimulated platelets, in Ca^{2+} ionophore-stimulated human monocytic cells, and in interleukin 1-stimulated mesangial cells (Gronich et al., 1994). AACOCF$_3$ inhibits bovine brain cPLA$_2$ and iPLA$_2$ in a dose-dependent manner with IC$_{50}$ of 1.5 and 6.0 µM, respectively.

The treatment of NG 108-15 cells with AACOCF$_3$ decreases initial neurite formation in a concentration-dependent manner (Smalheiser et al., 1996). The pharmacological blockade of cPLA$_2$ by a low concentration, 10 µM, of AACOCF$_3$ significantly inhibits neuronal death in the CA1 region of rat hippocampus. In primary neuronal cultures, this PLA$_2$ inhibitor prevents caspase-3 activation and neurodegeneration induced by β-amyloid peptide (Aβ) and human prion protein peptide (Bate et al., 2004), suggesting the role of PLA$_2$ isoforms in neurode-generative processes (Farooqui and Horrocks, 1994; Farooqui et al., 1997). In

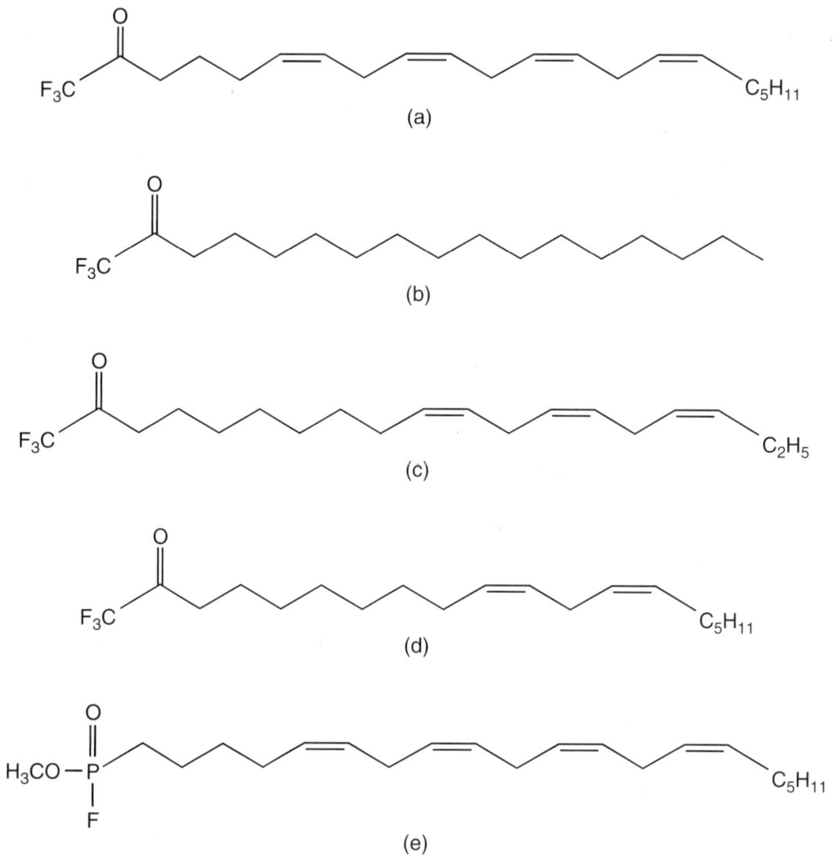

Fig. 11.1. Structures of fatty acid trifluoromethyl ketones and methyl arachidonoyl fluo-rophosphonate. Arachidonoyl trifluoromethyl ketone (a); palmitoyl trifluoromethyl ketone (b); α-linolenoyl trifluoromethyl ketone (c); linoleoyl trifluoromethyl ketone (d); and methyl arachidonoyl fluorophosphonate (e).

primary neuronal cultures, AACOCF$_3$ also abolishes the stimulation of cPLA$_2$ and arachidonic acid release mediated by methylmercury (MeHg^{2+}) (Shanker et al., 2004), suggesting that cPLA$_2$ plays an important role in MeHg^{2+}-induced neurotoxicity. Similarly, in astrocytes MeHg^{2+}-induced ROS generation is strongly inhibited by AACOCF$_3$ (Shanker and Aschner, 2003). In neural cell cultures, AACOCF$_3$ also shortens the association of protein kinase C gamma (PKC-γ) with the plasma membrane, indicating that this isoform of PKC may be involved in neuronal plasticity (Yagi et al., 2004). AACOCF$_3$ also blocks L-buthionine sulfoximine (BSO) toxicity in glutathione-depleted mesencephalic cultures (Kramer et al., 2004). Several analogs of AACOCF$_3$ have been synthe-sized and tested for their ability to inhibit cPLA$_2$ in assay systems in vitro (Ghomashchi et al., 2001). Very little information is available on their effects on brain tissue in intact animals (Schaeffer et al., 2005).

AACOCF$_3$ induces the dispersal of the Golgi stack and proteins resident in the *trans* Golgi network (Brown et al., 2003). This suggests that cPLA$_2$ isozymes play a crucial role in membrane trafficking and in maintenance of Golgi architecture. In non-neural cultured cells, AACOCF$_3$ inhibits the expression of interleukin-2 (IL-2) at both the mRNA and protein levels, indicating that cPLA$_2$ may have marked effects on T-cell function (Amandi-Burgermeister et al., 1997; Ouyang and Kaminski, 1999). This inhibitor inhibits DNA fragmentation during apoptosis in U937 cells, but failed to affect morphological changes that occur during apoptosis, suggesting that the use of AACOCF$_3$ may distinguish between cytoplasmic and nuclear events that occur during apoptotic cell death (Vanags et al., 1997; Wang et al., 2004). AACOCF$_3$ is described as a specific inhibitor of cPLA$_2$, but recent studies in non-neural cells indicate it may also inhibit cyclooxygenases and 5-lipoxygenase (Cummings et al., 2000; Fuentes et al., 2003). These observations strongly suggest that AACOCF$_3$ is not a specific inhibitor of cPLA$_2$.

Several other trifluoromethyl ketones have been synthesized for studies of their ability to inhibit cPLA$_2$ activity in non-neural tissues (Amandi-Burgermeister et al., 1997; Ghomashchi et al., 1999). Treatment of leukocytes with AACOCF$_3$ induces lipid body formation in them. In contrast, palmitoyl trifluoromethyl ketone (PACOCF$_3$) treatment has no effect on lipid body formation in leukocytes (Bozza and Weller, 2001). α-Linolenoyl trifluoromethyl ketone and linoleoyl trifluoromethyl ketone inhibit cPLA$_2$ activity to the same extent and in a dose-dependent manner with no measurable effect on sPLA$_2$ activity. All acyl trifluoromethyl ketones selectively suppress interleukin-1β synthesis, but have no effect on the synthesis of interleukin-6 and tumor necrosis factor-α (Amandi-Burgermeister et al., 1997). Based on pharmacological studies, the acyl trifluoromethyl ketones may interfere with either transcription or mRNA stability of interleukin-1β. These effects of acyl trifluoromethyl ketones are similar to those of arachidonic acid, which induces mRNA for the immediate-early genes egr-1 and c-fos (Danesch et al., 1994).

11.2.2 Methyl Arachidonoyl Fluorophosphonate (MAFP)

MAFP (Fig. 11.2) is an irreversible inhibitor of bovine brain cPLA$_2$ (IC50, 0.5 µM) and has no effect on sPLA$_2$. It inhibits enzymic activity by reacting with a serine residue at the active site. MAFP also inhibits bovine brain calcium-independent PLA$_2$ (iPLA$_2$) in a dose-dependent manner with an IC50 value of 0.75 µM. At 5.0 µM, MAFP completely inhibits bovine brain iPLA$_2$ activity. Also, MAFP inhibits Aβ-mediated stimulation of cPLA$_2$ activity in cortical neuronal cultures (Kriem et al., 2004). MAFP retards the cellular morphological alterations induced by hydrogen peroxide in H9o2 cells and protects them from hydrogen peroxide toxicity (Maoz et al., 2005).

MAFP induces irreversible inhibition of the enzymic hydrolysis of arachidonoyl ethanolamide (anandamide) by fatty acid amide hydrolase. Based on various pharmacological studies with cannabinoid CB$_1$ receptor and MAFP, MAFP may be an irreversible cannabinoid CB$_1$ receptor antagonist (Fernando and

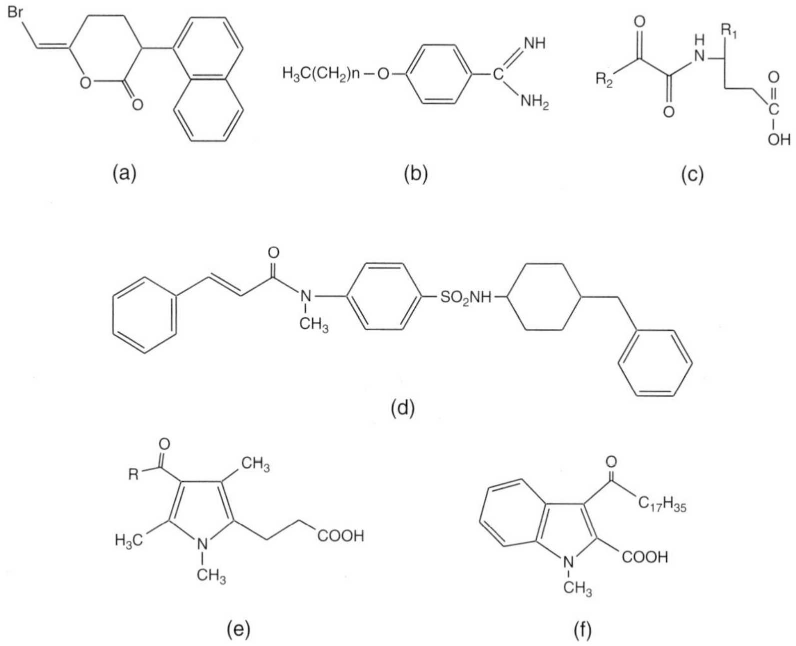

FIG. 11.2. Structures of some potent phospholipase A$_2$ inhibitors. Bromoenol lactone (a); 4-alkoxybenzamidine (b); long chain oxomide (c); benzenesulfonamide (d); 3-(4-acyl-1,3,5-dimethylpyrrol-2-yl) propionic acid (e); and 1-methyl-3-octadecanoylindole-2-carboxylic acid (f).

Pertwee, 1997). Since MAFP interacts with several PLA$_2$ isoforms (Ghomashchi et al., 1999) and with fatty amide hydrolase, it cannot be considered as a specific inhibitor of cPLA$_2$. MAFP also blocks BSO toxicity in glutathione-depleted mesencephalic cultures (Kramer et al., 2004). Intrathecal injections of MAFP in rats produce antinociceptive effects (Ates et al., 2003), suggesting that PLA$_2$ isoforms may play some role during pain states (see below).

11.2.3 Bromoenol Lactone (BEL)

BEL (Fig. 11.3) is a potent inhibitor of bovine brain iPLA$_2$ and PlsEtn-PLA$_2$ with IC50 values of 60 and 40 nM, respectively. BEL has a structural resemblance to plasmalogens. It inhibits brain cPLA$_2$ and sPLA$_2$ at a very high concentration (500 μM). Two forms of iPLA$_2$, namely iPLA$_2$γ and iPLA$_2$β, have been characterized and their activities have been implicated in glycerophospholipid homeostasis in membranes (Gross, 1998; Kinsey et al., 2005). Both iPLA$_2$ isoforms are inhibited by low concentrations of BEL. The racemic mixture of BEL can be separated into two enantiomers of BEL, namely (R)-BEL and (S)-BEL. These enantiomers inhibit iPLA$_2$γ and iPLA$_2$β with different inhibition potencies. (R)-BEL is 10-fold more selective for iPLA$_2$γ, whereas (S)-BEL is 10-fold more selective

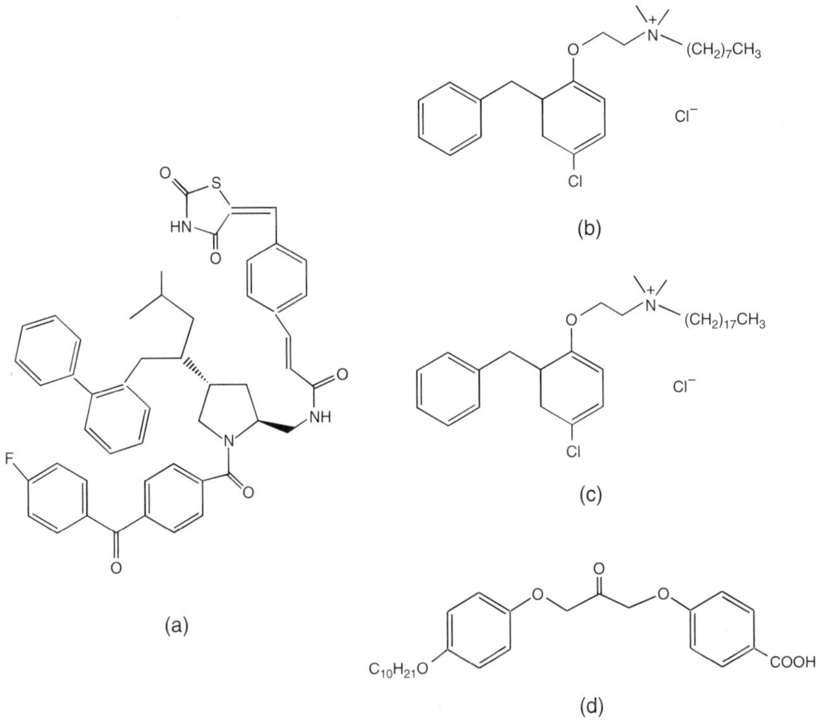

FIG. 11.3. Chemical structures of PLA$_2$ inhibitors. Pyrrolidine-1 (a); 2-(2-benzyl-4-chlorophenoxy)ethyldimethyl-n-octyl-ammonium chloride (b); 2-(2-benzyl-4-chlorophe-noxy)ethyldimethyl-n-octadecyl-ammonium chloride (c); and AR-C70484XX (d).

for iPLA$_2$β (Jenkins et al., 2002; Moran et al., 2005). Thus in non-neural A-10 cells arginine vasopressin-induced liberation of AA is selectively inhibited by (S)-BEL but not by (R)-BEL indicating that majority of AA release is mediated by iPLA$_2$β and not by iPLA$_2$β (Jenkins et al., 2002). Furthermore, pretreatment of A-10 cells with (S)-BEL has no effect on arginine vasopressin-induced MAPK phosphorylation or protein kinase C translocation. Most iPLA$_2$β Cys residues are alkylated at various BEL concentrations to form a thioester linkage to a BEL keto acid hydrolysis product (Song et al., 2006). The BEL concentration dependence of Cys (651) alkylation closely parallels to the loss of iPLA$_2$β activity. No amino acid residues other than Cys are modified during BEL treatment. These observations strongly indicate that Cys alkylation of iPLA$_2$β may be responsible for the loss of its activity (Song et al., 2006).

The injection of BEL (10 μM) into postsynaptic CA1 pyramidal neurons produces a robust increase in the amplitude of α-amino-3-hydroxy-5-methylisoxazole-4-propionate (AMPA) receptor-mediated excitatory postsynaptic currents (EPSCs), suggesting that iPLA$_2$ plays an important role in AMPA-mediated synaptic plasticity (St-Gelais et al., 2004). AACOCF$_3$ and palmitoyl trifluoromethyl ketone (PACOCF$_3$), which mainly interact with cPLA$_2$, have no effect on AMPA-mediated synaptic transmission. The inhibition of iPLA$_2$ by BEL and the enhancement of AMPA subunit immunoreactivity in brain homogenates and slices support the above electrophysiological studies. Taken together, these results support the hypothesis that BEL-mediated antagonism of AMPA receptors is involved in long-term potentiation and long-term depression during the regulation of synaptic plasticity. Based on the blockage of induction of hippocampal long-term potentiation, brain iPLA$_2$ may be involved in learning and memory (Wolf et al., 1995; Fujita et al., 2001). Intracerebroventricular injections of BEL, 3 nmol, markedly affect spatial performance in mice (Fujita et al., 2000), indicating that iPLA$_2$ is involved in spatial memory formation. BEL also modulates intracellular membrane trafficking (Kuroiwa et al., 2001; Brown et al., 2003) by inhibiting iPLA$_2$ activity in membrane tubule formation during reassembly of the Golgi complex. In addition, BEL treatment also interferes with membrane fusion events during endocytosis and exocytosis.

11.2.4 Benzenesulfonamides and Alkoxybenzamidines

Benzenesulfonamide (Fig. 11.3) and its piperidine derivative are the most potent inhibitors of membrane-bound heart PLA$_2$ activity with IC$_{50}$ values of 28.0 and 9.0 nM, respectively (Oinuma et al., 1991). Intravenous injections of these inhibitors protect rats against ischemic damage in acute myocardial infarction. These compounds are relatively metabolically stable in plasma with half lives of 1 to 2 h. These compounds also inhibit brain cPLA$_2$ activity in a dose-dependent manner with IC50 values of 23.0 and 10.0 nM, respectively. Nothing is known about their ability to cross the blood–brain barrier. Synthesis of 4-alkoxybenzamidines as PLA$_2$ inhibitors has also been described (Aitdafoun et al., 1996). These compounds competitively inhibit bovine pancreatic and rabbit platelet PLA$_2$ activities with IC$_{50}$ values of 3.0 and 5.0 μM, respectively. It is interesting to note that 4-tetradecyloxybenzamidine has an anti-inflammatory effect in vivo on carrageenan-mediated rat paw edema.

11.2.5 3-(Pyrrol)-2-propionic Acid

Lehr has synthesized many compounds (Fig. 11.3) that inhibit cPLA$_2$ activity in platelets with IC$_{50}$ values varying from 0.5 to 10 μM (Lehr, 1996, 1997a,b). Effects of these compounds on other isoforms of PLA$_2$ remain unknown. These inhibitors have not been used to block the activity of brain PLA$_2$ isoforms and have not been injected into intact animals or animal models of neurological disorders; therefore nothing is known about their tolerance, half lives, and toxicity. The ability of these inhibitors to cross the blood–brain barrier also remains unknown.

11.2.6 2-Oxoamide and 1,3-Disubstituted Propan-2-ones

Long-chain 2-oxoamides of γ-aminobutyric acid and γ-norleucine (AX006, AX007, and AX008) (Fig. 11.3) reversibly inhibit cPLA$_2$ activity in a dose- and time-dependent manner (Kokotos et al., 2004). These inhibitors block the

LPS-mediated release of arachidonic acid due to the stimulation of cPLA$_2$ in murine P388 D1 macrophages with IC50 values of 8.0, 7.6, and 4.6 µM, respectively. These IC50 values are lower than the IC50 value reported for MAFP (25 µM). This suggests that 2-oxoamides are more potent inhibitors than MAFP of cPLA$_2$. These inhibitors also block activities of cPLA$_2$ and iPLA$_2$ in inhibition assays using human recombinant enzyme (DeMar et al., 2006). The rank ordering of potency in blocking cPLA$_2$ is AX048, AX006, and AX057 > AX010 and for inhibiting iPLA$_2$ is AX048 and AX057 > AX006 and AX010. Oxoamide derivatives have no effect on recombinant cyclooxygenase activity. Carrageenan-induced edema in the rat paw was prevented with 2-oxoamides (Kokotos et al., 2004). Effects of these inhibitors on brain cPLA$_2$ remain unknown.

1,3-Disubstituted propan-2-ones (Fig. 11.4) were also recently synthesized (Connolly et al., 2002). These compounds inhibit cPLA$_2$ activity with an IC50 value of 0.03 µM in an in vitro assay. They are 10-fold more effective than 2-oxoamides and AACOCF$_3$ in inhibiting cPLA$_2$ activity. 1,3-Disubstituted propan-2-ones inhibit arachidonic acid production in HL60 cells with an IC50 value of 2.8 µM. These inhibitors have not been injected into intact animals or animal models of neurological disorders; therefore, nothing is known about their tolerance, half lives, and toxicity. The ability of these inhibitors to cross the blood–brain barrier also remains unknown.

11.2.7 Choline Derivatives with a Long Aliphatic Chain as PLA$_2$ Inhibitors

Recently, a new class of hydrophobic inhibitors that partition into the lipid bilayer and compete with monomers of the glycerophospholipid substrate was described

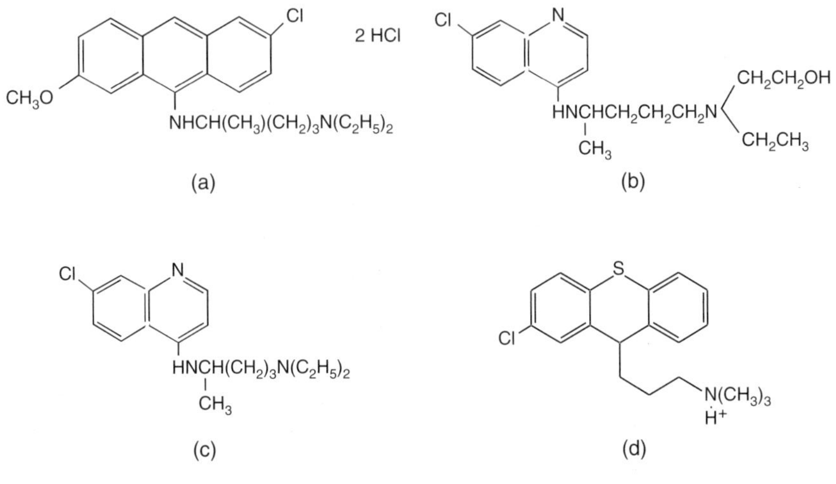

FIG. 11.4. Chemical structures of classical antimalarial drugs that inhibit isoforms of PLA$_2$ nonspecifically. Quinacrine (a); hydroxychloroquine (b); chloroquine (c); and chlorpromazine (d). These drugs have been used for the treatment of neurological disorders.

(Burke et al., 1999). These compounds include 2-(2-benzyl-4-cholorophenoxy) ethyldimethyl-n-octadecyl-ammonium chloride and 2-(2-benzyl-4-chlorophe-noxy)ethyldimethyl-n-octyl-ammonium bromide (Fig. 11.3). Both compounds inhibit cPLA$_2$ activity in a competitive manner with IC50 values of 5 and 13 µM, respectively. The length of the n-alkyl chain plays an important role in the degree of inhibition. Shortening of the n-alkyl chain considerably decreases the percentage of inhibitor partitioned into the glycerophospholipid bilayer and increases the value of IC50. This may be due to diminished hydrophobic interaction between the shorter alkyl chain and the fatty acid tails of the glycerophospholipids making up the bilayer. In contrast, lengthening of the n-alkyl chain increases the percentage of inhibitor partitioned into the lipid bilayer and decreases the IC50 value. The synthesis of these inhibitors represents an important step in the development of potent in vivo cPLA$_2$ inhibitors because these compounds inhibit the enzymic activity at the interface and provide a weak interaction with the glycerophospholipid bilayer (Burke et al., 1999). Based on kinetic studies, it is stated that the potential in vivo efficacy of these intracellular inhibitors can be more potent than other inhibitors such as AACOCF$_3$. These inhibitors have not been used for in vivo studies so nothing is known about their tolerance, toxicity, half life, and ability to cross the blood–brain barrier.

11.2.8 Pyrrolidine-Based Inhibitors of PLA$_2$

Pyrrolidine-containing compounds (Seno et al., 2000; Ghomashchi et al., 2001) markedly inhibit cPLA$_2$-α in vitro and block arachidonate release in Ca^{2+}-ionophore stimulated non-neural cells (Seno et al., 2000). The structure of the most potent inhibitor, pyrrolidine-1, is shown in Fig. 11.3. In a fluorometric assay, pyrrolidine-1 inhibits cPLA$_2$-α activity in a dose-dependent manner with an IC50 value of 1.8 nM. In a mixed-micelle assay system, this compound inhibits cPLA$_2$-α activity with an IC50 value of 1.8 µM. This difference in the IC50 values may be due to the differences in interface concentrations of pyrrolidine-1 in the different assay systems. The treatment of CHO cells with pyrrolidine-1 results in marked inhibition of A23187-induced arachidonic acid release with IC50 values of 0.2 to 0.5 µM. The degree of inhibition approaches 100% with 4 to 10 µM pyrrolidine-1 (Ghomashchi et al., 2001). Similarly, the treatment of MDCK cells with pyrrolidine-1 also results in marked inhibition of ATP-induced arachidonic acid release with an IC50 value of 0.8 µM. It must be stated here that pyrrolidine-1 also inhibits cPLA$_2$-γ and iPLA$_2$-β at a very high concentration but it does not inhibit sPLA$_2$.

Pyrrophenone, a triphenylmethylthioether derivative of pyrrolidine, is a 39-fold more potent inhibitor, Ki 4.2 nM, of cPLA$_2$ activity than pyrrolidine-1 (Ono et al., 2002). Pretreatment of rats with pyrrolidine dithiocarbamate, a powerful thiol antioxidant, protects against KA-mediated neurotoxicity (Shin et al., 2004). In vitro studies indicate that pyrrophenone may be a potential therapeutic agent for inflammatory diseases (Ono et al., 2002). Pyrrolidine-containing PLA$_2$ inhibitors have not been injected in animal models of neurological disorders so their half life and side effects remain unknown.

11.2.9 Antimalarial Drugs

Among antimalarial drugs, quinacrine, chloroquine, and hydroxychloroquine (Fig. 11.4) are very lipophilic compounds. All isoforms of brain PLA$_2$ (sPLA$_2$, cPLA$_2$, PlsEtn-PLA$_2$, and iPLA$_2$) are strongly inhibited by antimalarial drugs in a dose-dependent manner (Table 11.1) with rank order potency of chloroquine > quinacrine > hydroxychloroquine > quinine (Lu et al., 2001; Farooqui et al., 2005). Besides inhibiting activities of PLA$_2$ isoforms, antimalarial drugs also inhibit platelet aggregation in a dose-dependent manner with a similar pattern of inhibition. Metabolites of arachidonic acid metabolism may be involved in platelet aggregation (Chan et al., 1982; Nosal et al., 2000). Quinacrine increases lysosomal pH and blocks the activities of lysosomal enzymes (Di Cerbo et al., 1984; Nozawa et al., 1991). It inhibits cAMP accumulation through muscarinic receptors, and acetylcholine uptake by binding to nicotinic receptors (Table 11.2). At low concentrations, under 50 μM, these inhibitors have no effect on the growth of neuron-enriched cultures from rat brain cortex, but at high concentrations, above 1000 μM, these inhibitors are toxic.

Chloroquine, 7-chloro-4-(4′-diethylamino)-1-methylbutylamino-quinoline (Fig. 11.4c), is a small lipophilic base that diffuses into membranes in an unprotonated form and inhibits mitogen-activated protein kinase (Weber et al., 2002) in a dose-dependent manner. In neural cells, chloroquine induces the activation of nuclear factor-κB (NFκB) and expression of proinflammatory cytokines in

TABLE 11.1. Inhibitory effects of antimalarial drugs on partially purified preparations of PLA$_2$ isoforms from bovine brain.

Antimalarial Drug	IC50 sPLA$_2$	IC50 cPLA$_2$	IC50 PlsEtn-PLA$_2$	IC50 iPLA$_2$
Quinacrine	500 ± 60	200 ± 25	600 ± 70	800 ± 60
Chloroquine	250 ± 45	125 ± 20	175 ± 50	275 ± 55
Hydroxychloroquine	300 ± 80	185 ± 25	250 ± 40	350 ± 40
Quinine	400 ± 70	250 ± 45	550 ± 30	600 ± 80

IC50 values are expressed in μM. Modified from Lu et al. (2001).

TABLE 11.2. Neurochemical effects of antimalarial drugs.

Antimalarial drug	Target	Effect	Reference
Quinacrine	PLA$_2$ activity	Inhibition	Lu et al., 2001
	Muscarinic receptor	Inhibition	O'Donnell and Howlett, 1991
	Acetylcholine receptor	Inhibition	Holscher, 1995
Chloroquine	PLA$_2$ activity	Inhibition	Lu et al., 2001
	MAP-kinase	Inhibition	Weber et al., 2002
	Intracellular calcium release	Inhibition	Misra et al., 1997
	Tumor necrosis factor-α	Inhibition	Jeong and Jue, 1997
	NFκB	Activation	Park et al., 2003
	β-Amyloid deposition	Inhibition	Giulian, 1999

Modified from Farooqui et al. (2005).

human astroglia (Park et al., 2003). Chloroquine also inhibits platelet aggregation, lymphocyte responsiveness, and intracellular calcium release. Like chloroquine, hydroxychloroquine (Fig. 11.4b) penetrates the blood–brain barrier and is taken up by neural cells. It is an immunosuppressive agent. It suppresses acute-phase reactants, lymphocyte responsiveness, macrophage function, and cytokine release (Aisen and Davis, 1994), without affecting cerebral blood flow. This suggests that differences in the immunomodulatory effects of chloroquine on monocytes and astrocytes are determined at the level of NF-κB activation and the effects of this drug can be beneficial or detrimental depending upon the time and the type of cell involved. In vitro studies indicate that quinine, an antimalarial drug, enhances excitatory postsynaptic potentials and decreases fast and slow inhibitory postsynaptic potentials (Bikson et al., 2002). Quinine also possesses anticonvulsant properties in vivo during certain types of seizures (Wambebe et al., 1990).

Hydroxychloroquine is well tolerated by elderly people and the risk of neuropsychiatric side effects and retinopathy among patients receiving low doses of this drug is very low (Block, 1998). It was used for the treatment of inflammation in Alzheimer disease (Van Gool et al., 2001), but these double-blind randomized trials were not successful. The lack of benefit may be due to a short duration, 18 months, of therapy. Thus, more trials of longer duration are required to judge the efficacy of hydroxychloroquine for the treatment of inflammation in Alzheimer disease. The effect of antimalarial drugs depends not only on the dose but also on the stage of development of the neurodegenerative process.

Collectively these studies suggest that antimalarial drugs down-regulate the production of free radicals derived from oxygen and reduce cellular toxicity mediated by oxidative stress (Struhar et al., 1992; Alliangana, 1996). Chloroquine is specifically effective against β-amyloid protein-induced neurotoxicity (Giulian, 1999). Antimalarial drugs have anti-inflammatory, antioxidant, and immunomodulatory effects at low doses. They can cross the blood–brain barrier without harm and reach neural cells without producing toxic effects (Dubin et al., 1982; Estevez and Phillis, 1997; Van Gool et al., 2001).

11.2.10 Lithium and Carbamazepine

Lithium ion is a mood stabilizer. It has been used for the treatment of bipolar disorders for almost a half century (Corbella and Vieta, 2003). Recently its use was proposed for the treatment of ischemia and chronic neurodegenerative diseases (Stahelin et al., 2005). Lithium ion has a neuroprotective effect on brain tissue. Chronic lithium ion administration in rats results in a 50% reduction in mRNA and protein levels of cPLA$_2$ with no changes observed in iPLA$_2$ and sPLA$_2$ protein during these studies (Chang and Jones, 1998; Rintala et al., 1999). Lithium ion does not reduce the level of phosphorylated cPLA$_2$ protein. Thus, the decrease in brain cPLA$_2$ enzyme activity induced by chronic lithium ion is due to down-regulation of cPLA$_2$ transcription (Weerasinghe et al., 2004). This down-regulation of cPLA$_2$ transcription may be responsible for a selective reduction of arachidonic acid turnover compared to docosahexaenoic acid in rat brain glycerophospholipids (Basselin et al., 2003). The labeling of Purkinje cell dendrites with cPLA$_2$ and cyclooxygenase (COX-2) antibodies is inhibited by lithium ion indicating functional coupling at brain synapses between cPLA$_2$ and COX-2 enzymes (Weerasinghe et al., 2004). In bipolar disorders the mood-stabilizing effect of chronic lithium administration up-regulates cell survival molecules such as Bcl-2, cyclic AMP-responsive element binding protein, brain-derived neurotrophic factor, and heat shock protein HSP70. Lithium ion down-regulates proapoptotic activities such as excitotoxicity, activation of caspases, cytochrome c release, β-amyloid peptide synthesis, and tau hyperphosphorylation. The modulation of signaling processes and interplay among these processes results in prevention of neuronal cell death (Stahelin et al., 2005).

An anticonvulsant drug, carbamazepine (CBZ), has been used for the treatment of bipolar disorders for many years. Chronic administration of CBZ not only inhibits cPLA$_2$ activity, but also alters its protein and mRNA levels. In contrast, iPLA$_2$ and sPLA$_2$ activities and protein levels were not affected (Ghelardoni et al., 2004). These effects are accompanied by a decrease in COX-2 activity and prostaglandin E$_2$ levels in brain tissue, suggesting that CBZ blocks the cPLA$_2$-mediated release of arachidonic acid and its conversion via COX-2 to prostaglandin E$_2$ (Ghelardoni et al., 2004). The protein levels of other arachidonic acid metabolizing enzymes such as 5-lipoxygenase and cytochrome P450 and their reaction product leukotriene B$_4$ are not affected by CBZ. Thus, nonspecific PLA$_2$ inhibitors, like lithium ion and CBZ, may have beneficial effects, not only in neurological diseases (see below), but also in bipolar disorders and manic-depressive patients.

11.2.11 Vitamin E and Gangliosides

Vitamin E (α-tocopherol) (Fig. 11.5) is another nonspecific inhibitor of cPLA$_2$ activity (Douglas et al., 1986). It modulates the production of arachidonic acid and eicosanoids (Tran et al., 1996). It inhibits bovine brain cPLA$_2$ and iPLA$_2$ activities in a dose- and time-dependent manner with IC50 values of 500 and 750 μM, respectively. Vitamin E crosses the blood–brain barrier and with time accumulates in brain (Pentland et al., 1992). It reduces lipid peroxidation and stabilizes neuronal membranes. Several reports indicate that ischemia is accompanied by an increase in PLA$_2$ activity and a reduction in the levels of vitamin E and glutathione (Farooqui et al., 1994). A deficiency of vitamin E and selenium in rats leads to a biphasic increase in iPLA$_2$ activity in non-neural cells (Burgess and Kuo, 1996), once again supporting the view that PLA$_2$ activity is regulated by vitamin E. Vitamin E may modulate activities of PLA$_2$ isozymes by two mechanisms. First, by direct incorporation into substrate vesicles, and second, by stimulation of the activity of PLA$_2$ isoforms by up-regulating the rate of their synthesis at the transcriptional or translation level (Tran et al., 1996).

cPLA$_2$ and PlsEtn-PLA$_2$ activities are also inhibited by GM1 and GM3 gangliosides (Fig. 11.5) in a dose-dependent manner (Yang et al., 1994a,b). With

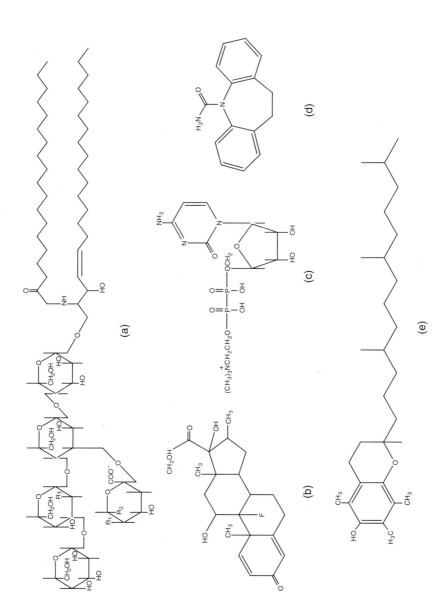

FIG. 11.5. Chemical structures of some nonspecific PLA₂ inhibitors used for the treatment of neurological disorders. GM1 ganglioside (a); dexamethasone (b); CDP-choline (c); carbamazepine (d); and vitamin E (e).

PlsEtn-PLA$_2$, the IC50 values for GM1 and GM3 gangliosides were 150 and 75 µg/ml, respectively. The IC50 values for brain cPLA$_2$ for GM1 and GM3 were 250 and 100 µg/ml, respectively. The mechanism of inhibition by gangliosides remains unknown. However, the orientation of N-acetylneuraminic acid residues in glycoconjugates is important for inhibitory activity (Yang et al., 1994b). Gangliosides not only stabilize neural membranes, but also regulate the influx of calcium ions and enzyme activities associated with signal transduction.

11.2.12 Cytidine 5-Diphosphoamines (CDP-amines)

CDP-amines (Fig. 11.5) are key intermediates in the biosynthesis of phosphatidylcholine and phosphatidylethanolamine. CDP-choline (citicoline) decreases cPLA$_2$ stimulation and hydroxyl radical generation after transient cerebral ischemia (Adibhatla and Hatcher, 2003, 2006). This process lowers the concentration of free fatty acids in a dose- and time-dependent manner. CDP-choline protects neural membranes, not only by accelerating the resynthesis of glycerophospholipids, but also by quenching free radicals generated by PLA$_2$ isozymes (Rao et al., 2001; Adibhatla and Hatcher, 2003, 2006). A mixture of CDP-ethanolamine and CDP-choline may be more effective than CDP-choline alone (Murphy and Horrocks, 1993).

11.2.13 Long-Chain Polyunsaturated Fatty Acids

Long-chain polyunsaturated fatty acids are normal constituents of neural membrane glycerophospholipids and are products of reactions catalyzed by PLA$_2$. They include arachidonic acid, belonging to the n-6 class, eicosapentaenoic acid (EPA), and docosahexaenoic acid (DHA), both belonging to the n-3 class. Arachidonic acid is released by the action of cPLA$_2$ and EPA and DHA are cleaved by the action of PlsEtn-PLA$_2$ on neural membrane glycerophospholipids. In vitro, the addition of these fatty acids to the reaction mixture inhibits the PLA$_2$-catalyzed reaction in a dose- and time-dependent manner. This inhibition can be reversed by the addition of bovine serum albumin. The in vivo effects of these fatty acids on brain metabolism are quite complex. Arachidonic acid is metabolized to prostaglandins, leukotrienes, and thromboxanes by cyclooxygenases and lipoxygenases. These metabolites can cause vasoconstriction and hence compromise blood flow and oxygen delivery to brain tissue. EPA competes with arachidonic acid at the cyclooxygenase level to produce the 3-series-prostaglandins (PGE$_3$, PGI$_3$, TXA$_3$) or the 5-series leukotrienes (LTB$_5$, LTC$_5$, LTD$_5$). These metabolites are less active than the corresponding arachidonic acid-derived compounds (Anderle et al., 2004). For example, TXA$_3$ is less active than TXA$_2$ in aggregating platelets and constricting blood vessels (James et al., 2000; Calder and Grimble, 2002).

DHA is not a substrate for cyclooxygenase, but it is an inhibitor. A 15-lipoxygenase-like enzyme metabolizes DHA to docosanoids. Docosanoids include 10,17S-docosatrienes and 17S-resolvins (Hong et al., 2003; Marcheselli et al., 2003; Serhan et al., 2004). They antagonize the effects of arachidonic acid-generated metabolites, and act potently on leukocyte trafficking as well as down-regulating the expression of cytokines in glial cells (Hong et al., 2003; Marcheselli et al., 2003; Mukherjee et al., 2004; Serhan et al., 2004). The specific receptors for these bioactive lipid metabolites occur in neural and non-neural tissues. These receptors include resolvin D receptors (ResoDR1), resolvin E receptors (resoER1), and neuroprotectin D receptors (NPDR). Characterization of these receptors in brain tissue is in progress. The generation of docosanoids may be an internal protective mechanism for preventing brain damage (Horrocks and Farooqui, 2004; Mukherjee et al., 2004; Serhan et al., 2004). Interference with the generation of docosanoids may explain part of the problems with COX-2 inhibitors.

11.2.14 PLA_2 Antisense Oligonucleotides and Interfering RNA (RNAi)

Antisense oligonucleotides have been synthesized to inhibit isoforms of PLA_2 (Locati et al., 1996; Yoo et al., 2001; Laktionova et al., 2004; Won et al., 2005). These antisense oligonucleotides efficiently inhibit the activity of various isoforms of PLA_2 and block their expression. They may be used for the treatment of inflammation and oxidative stress in neurological disorders. It must be emphasized here that the in vivo effects of antisense oligonucleotides may not be predictable from in vitro studies, partly because of the potential for the activation of the immune system by nucleotides. Furthermore, for neurological disorders there may be additional problems, including the efficient delivery of antisense oligonucleotides to a specific brain region in vivo and the high cost of manufacturing large quantities of antisense oligonucleotides.

An important development for inhibiting the enzymic activity of PLA_2 isoforms was the discovery of the RNA interference (RNAi) technique. This technology takes advantage of the evolutionary adaptation of neural cells to silence a gene whose corresponding double-stranded RNA molecule is present in the cell (Hannon, 2002). Introduction of a synthesized double-stranded RNA specific for a PLA_2 isoform gene may cause a rapid and prolonged reduction of mRNA and protein expression of that PLA_2 isoform in brain tissue. An RNAi was developed for $iPLA_2$ in non-neural cells (Shinzawa and Tsujimoto, 2003). It inhibits protein expression and $iPLA_2$ activity in a dose- and time-dependent manner. In vivo injections of RNAi have not been made in intact animals, so the therapeutic importance of RNAi remains unknown.

11.2.15 Diffusion Survival Evasion Peptide (DSEP)

DSEP is a peptide purified from the culture media of neural cell lines exposed to hydrogen peroxide (Cunningham et al., 1998). It promotes neuronal survival in vivo and in vitro by preventing differentiation in macrophages and microglia (Cunningham et al., 2000). The cDNA and the gene location for human DSEP are identified. Expression of the full human DSEP protein in either mouse or human neural cells results in resistance to a variety of toxic insults such as inflammatory and immune cell attacks. Based on structural studies, at least the N-terminal 30 amino acid sequence of the native protein may be responsible for the survival and immune evasion activities of DSEP.

CHEC-9 is a peptide having a similar sequence to DSEP (Cunningham et al., 2004). CHEC-9 inhibits serum sPLA$_2$ activity in a dose-dependent manner. This peptide increases the average Km of serum sPLA$_2$ by more than 3-fold. The inhibition of sPLA$_2$ by CHEC-9 is highly specific because inversion of a single pair of amino acids results in a complete loss of inhibitory effect (Cunningham et al., 2004).

11.2.16 sPLA$_2$ Inhibitors

LY311727, 3-(3-acetamide-1-benzyl-2-ethylindolyly-5-oxy) propane sulfonic acid (Fig. 11.6), is the best characterized potent specific inhibitor of sPLA$_2$ (Schevitz et al., 1995). At nanomolar concentrations, it binds to sPLA$_2$ group IIA from human platelets and synovial fluid as well as to group V sPLA$_2$ from P388D1 macrophages and inhibits their activities. Another LY311727 analog is [[3-(amino-oxoacetyl)-2-ethyl-1-(phenylmethyl)-1H-indol-4-yl] oxy]acetate, LY315920 (Snyder et al., 1999). It also selectively blocks sPLA$_2$ group IIA activity with an IC50 of 9 nM. Another group of selective sPLA$_2$ inhibitors includes oligomers of prostaglandin B1 (PGBx) (Rosenthal and Franson, 1989; Franson and Rosenthal, 1989). These inhibitors inhibit the release of arachidonic acid from human neutrophils. Later on a related compound, PX-52, was developed, but this compound also inhibits cPLA$_2$ (Franson and Rosenthal, 1997).

SB-203347 (Fig. 11.7) selectively inhibits human sPLA$_2$ group IIA at a relatively low concentration, IC50 value of 500 nM, but it also inhibits cPLA$_2$ and other PLA$_2$ isoforms. A series of sPLA$_2$ group IIA inhibitors were derived from

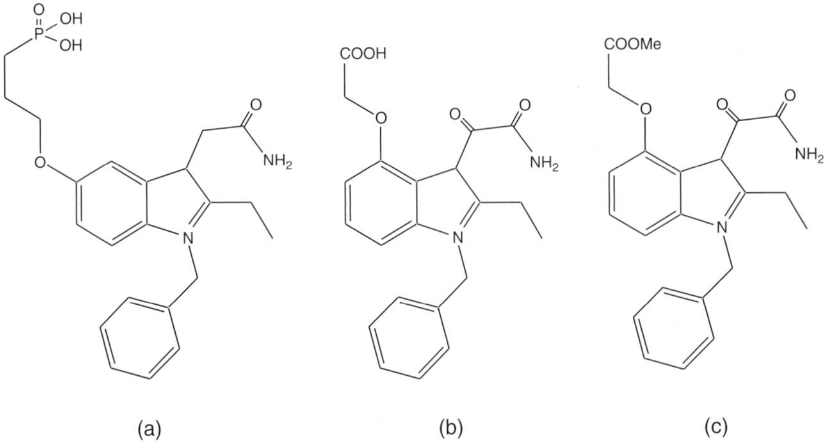

(a)   (b)   (c)

FIG. 11.6. Chemical structures of LY311727 and related compounds that inhibit sPLA$_2$ group IIA enzymes. LY311727 (a); LY333013 (b); and LY315920 (c).

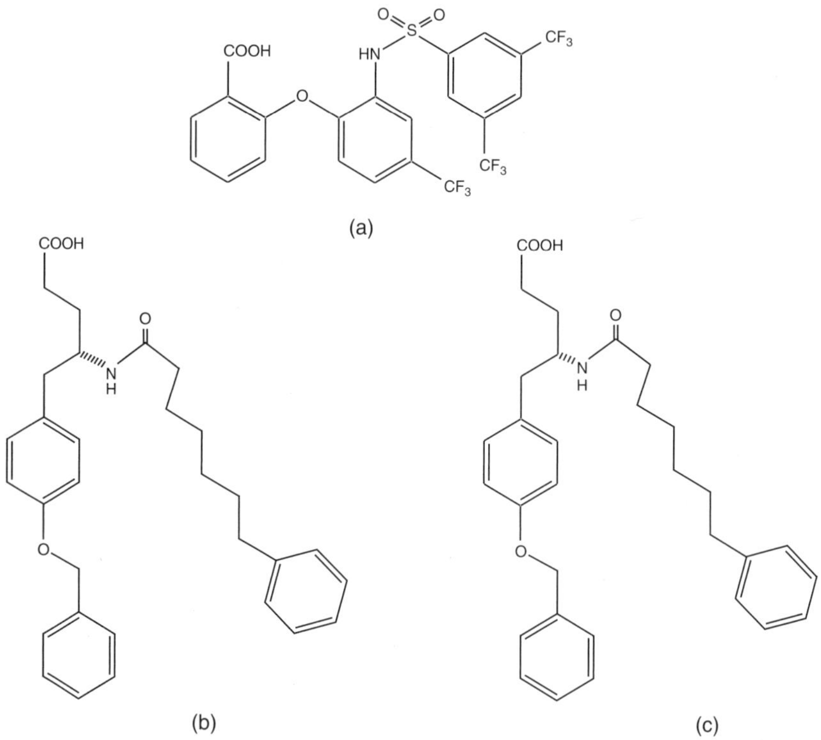

FIG. 11.7. Chemical structures of SB-203347, KH064, and KH067, the selective inhibitors of sPLA$_2$ group IIA enzymes. SB-203347 (a); KH064 (b); and KH067 (c).

D-tyrosine. They are KH064 and KH067 (Fig. 11.7). They inhibit sPLA$_2$ group IIA activity with IC50 values of 29 and 214 nM, respectively. These inhibitors were used in a rat model of intestinal ischemia (Hansford et al., 2003), but the results were not very encouraging. Pentapeptide inhibitors with amino acid sequences corresponding to residues 70 to 74 of the native sPLA$_2$ group IIA were described (Tseng et al., 1996; Church et al., 2001). Detailed investigations were performed with the peptide analog, FLSYK. Side-chain structural modifications of these pentapeptides markedly affect their inhibitory potency. Cyclization and the replacement of Phe and Tyr with larger aromatic side chains produce very potent inhibitors (Church et al., 2001) that can be used as potential therapeutic agents for inflammation.

BMS-181162 (Fig. 11.8) inhibits human platelet sPLA$_2$ group IIA with an IC50 value of 40 μM. It does not inhibit phospholipase A$_1$, phospholipase C, or phospholipase D in vitro. It prevents arachidonic acid release and synthesis of leukotriene B$_4$ and platelet-activating factor in human polymorphonuclear leukocytes (Tramposch et al., 1994). This compound has anti-inflammatory activity, but clinically failed to provide encouraging results in animal models and humans (Springer, 2001), so its development was discontinued.

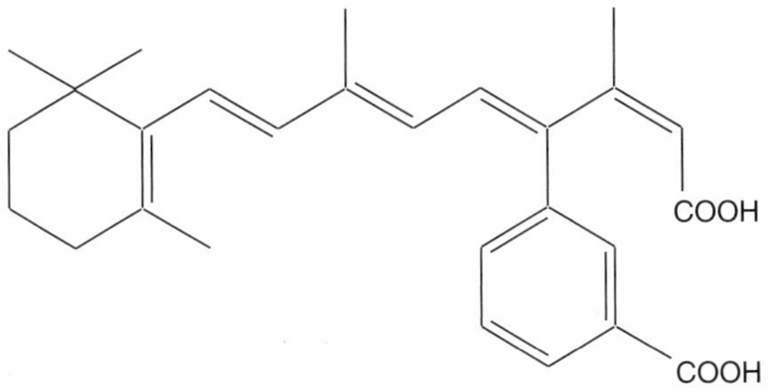

(a)

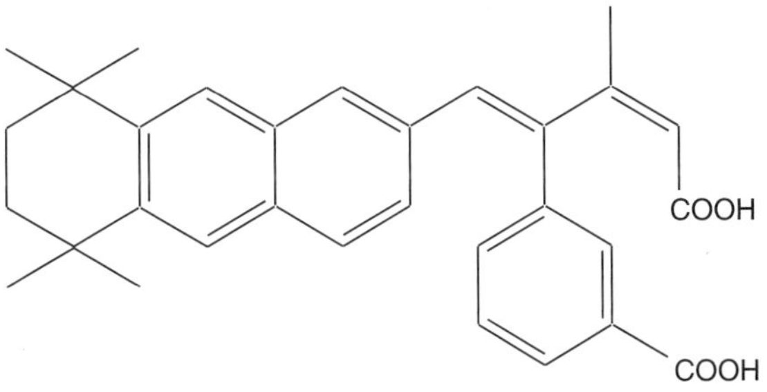

(b)

FIG. 11.8. Chemical structures of BMS-181162 and BMS-188184, the selective inhibitors of sPLA$_2$ group IIA enzymes. BMS-181162 (a); BMS-188184 (b).

11.2.17 Annexins (Lipocortins)

Annexins are a group of structurally related cytoplasmic proteins that interact with anionic phospholipids in a Ca^{2+}-dependent manner and inhibit activities of PLA$_2$ isoforms (Wahler et al., 1990; Wang and Robinson, 1997). To date, 12 unique members of this multigene family have been identified in a variety of mammalian tissues. A conserved 70-amino acid sequence is repeated either four or eight times in the sequences of annexin family members forming the core domain of the protein responsible for calcium and phospholipid binding (Gerke and Moss, 1997; Kamal et al., 2005). They display regulatory functions in diverse cellular processes, including inflammation, immune suppression, and membrane fusion (Kim et al., 2001b). Glucocorticoids induce the synthesis of annexin-1 with mol. mass 37 kDa. Annexins suppress inflammation through the inhibition of PLA$_2$ activity. All isoforms of PLA$_2$ are inhibited by annexins. Annexin-1 has received considerable attention as a mediator of glucocorticoid anti-inflammatory effects and as a substrate for protein kinases, as well as for calcium and phosphatidylserine-binding proteins in brain tissue. Immunocytochemical studies indicate that annexin-1 is located in neurons, astrocytes, and ramified microglia, and participates in inflammatory responses (McKanna and Zhang, 1997). The PLA$_2$ inhibitory activity of annexin-1 is regulated by phosphorylation (inactivation)/dephosphorylation (activation) mechanisms (Pepinsky et al., 1988; Gerke and Moss, 1997; Wang and Robinson, 1997).

Other proposed mechanisms of PLA$_2$ inhibition include substrate depletion and specific interaction with PLA$_2$. Annexin-1 deletion mutant data support the specific interaction mechanism of annexin-1 with PLA$_2$ (Kim et al., 2001b). However, inhibition of PLA$_2$ by specific interaction is not a general function of all annexins, and is rather a specific function of annexin-1 (Kim et al., 2001a). The tissues from mice lacking the annexin-1 gene exhibit an increased expression of several enzymes including cPLA$_2$ and COX-2 in experimental models of inflammation (Roviezzo et al., 2002). This suggests that mice lacking annexin-1 can provide useful information on the inflammatory mechanisms associated with cell signaling and proliferation. Amino acid sequencing studies indicate that a 9 amino acid sequence, with anti-inflammatory activity, is highly conserved in annexin-1 and annexin-V.

Synthetic peptides corresponding to the anti-inflammatory sequence are the antiflammins (Moreno, 2000). These peptides show anti-inflammatory activity on carrageenan-induced rat footpad edema. They are a potent inhibitor of PLA$_2$ activation both in vitro and in vivo. The mechanisms by which antiflammins protect against inflammation involve inhibition of PLA$_2$ and inducible nitric oxide synthase (iNOS). Antiflammins also inhibit neutrophil (PMN) adhesion to human leukocytes and coronary artery endothelial cells (HCAEC) by attenuating activation-induced up-regulation of CD11/CD18 expression on leukocytes. Thus, antiflammins may represent a novel therapeutic approach for blocking leukocyte trafficking in host defense and inflammation (Zouki et al., 2000).

11.3 Use of PLA$_2$ Inhibitors for the Treatment of Neurological Disorders

In organotypic hippocampal cultures, oxygen/glucose deprivation produces a 2-fold increase in PLA$_2$ activity with significant cell death. AACOCF$_3$ blocks this increase in PLA$_2$ activity in a dose- and time-dependent manner (Arai et al., 2001). sPLA$_2$ and iPLA$_2$ inhibitors were not effective in blocking cell death. In an attempt to evaluate the contribution of PLA$_2$ isoforms to the release of free fatty acids, rat cerebral cortex was superfused with inhibitors of PLA$_2$ activity. AACOCF$_3$ markedly inhibited the efflux of arachidonic, docosahexaenoic, linoleic, palmitic, and oleic acids from the ischemic/reperfused rat cerebral cortex (Phillis and O'Regan, 2004). Exposure to sPLA$_2$ and iPLA$_2$ inhibitors had a minimal effect on the efflux of free fatty acids. These observations strongly suggest that cPLA$_2$ plays an important role in ischemic injury and that PLA$_2$ inhibitors can be used for the treatment of ischemic injury (Table 11.3).

Pharmacokinetic studies indicate that all antimalarial drugs like quinacrine can be detected in monkey brain tissue 24 h after intravascular injection (Dubin et al., 1982). Incubation of guinea-pig brain slices with quinacrine results in localization of this antimalarial drug in cortical and basal ganglia neurons. Regional distribution studies indicate that cerebellum, cerebellar cortex, hippocampus, basal ganglion, and spinal cord contain quinacrine-positive neurons (Crowe and

TABLE 11.3. Therapeutic effect of quinacrine and other antimalarial drugs on neurological disorders.

Neurological disorder	Effect	Conc. of antimalarial drug (mg/kg)	Reference
Ischemia	Beneficial	5.0	Estevez and Phillis, 1997
Prion diseases	Beneficial	–	Korth et al., 2001; May et al., 2003
Alzheimer disease	Beneficial	100 to 150	Rogers et al., 1993
MPTP-induced Parkinsonism	Beneficial	60	Tariq et al., 2001
Kainic acid-induced neurodegeneration	Beneficial	5.0	Lu et al., 2001
Carrageenan-induced neurodegeneration	Beneficial	5.0	Ong et al., 2003

Modified from Farooqui et al. (2005).

Burnstock, 1984). These studies suggest that quinacrine is metabolically stable, crosses the blood–brain barrier, and localizes in neurons susceptible to ischemic injury. The administration of quinacrine results in a marked reduction in neurological deficits after 24 h of reperfusion. Importantly, the effects of quinacrine persist even after 7 days. These findings are supported by biochemical and histopathological analyses that indicate a significant decrease in infarct size in quinacrine-treated rats compared to saline-treated controls. Based on these studies (Estevez and Phillis, 1997), PLA$_2$ inhibitors may have cerebroprotective effects in focal as well as global models of cerebral ischemia. In brain, quinacrine (Fig. 11.4) protects gerbil CA1 hippocampal pyramidal cells during 5 min of forebrain ischemia (Estevez and Phillis, 1997).

In addition, quinacrine was proposed as a therapeutic agent for prion diseases (Korth et al., 2001). Quinacrine blocks prion protein peptide (PrP106–126)-mediated caspase-3 activation supporting the involvement of cPLA$_2$ in apoptotic cell death (Stewart et al., 2001). Quinacrine and a combination of quinacrine with chlorpromazine, a phenothiazine derivative, were used for the treatment of Creutzfeldt-Jakob disease (CJD) using compassionate use as a justification (Love, 2001; Follette, 2003; Kobayashi et al., 2003). During quinacrine treatment, the initial response of CJD patients have been positive, but within days of starting treatment, patients returned back to their previous states, indicating a transient recovery (Love, 2001; Follette, 2003; Kobayashi et al., 2003). The reason for the transient effect of quinacrine on CJD patients remains unknown, but may be due to the advanced stage of CJD. If quinacrine treatment could be started at the onset of CJD, patients would likely respond to this drug in a positive manner (Follette, 2003; Kobayashi et al., 2003). PLA$_2$ activities were not determined during these studies. Thus, no comments can be made about the levels of arachidonic acid and its metabolites, inflammatory reactions, and oxidative stress that occur in prion-mediated neurodegeneration in CJD. More studies are required on the involvement of PLA$_2$ isoforms and generation of proinflammatory mediators in the pathogenesis of prion diseases in animal and cell culture models.

The molecular mechanism involved in the inhibition of PrP^{sc} formation by quinacrine remains unknown. However, quinacrine may block channels formed by PrP (106–126) (Farrelly et al., 2003). NMR spectroscopic studies indicate that the PLA$_2$ inhibitor, quinacrine, binds to human prion protein at Tyr225, Tyr226, and Gln227 residues of helix α3 (Vogtherr et al., 2003). Similarly, other anti-malarial drugs, such as chloroquine and the phenothiazine derivatives acepromazine, chlorpromazine, and promazine, also bind to prion protein between residues 121 to 230. This suggests that Tyr225, Tyr226, and Gln227 residues are necessary for the binding of antimalarial drugs and phenothiazine derivatives (Vogtherr et al., 2003) to PrP^c. Quinacrine acts as an antioxidant and reduces the toxicity of PrP106–126 (Turnbull et al., 2003). This once again suggests that the release of arachidonic acid and the oxidative stress generated by altered arachidonic acid metabolism may play an important role in the pathogenesis of prion diseases (Guentchev et al., 2000; Milhavet et al., 2000).

Recent in vitro studies on prion-infected cell lines ScN2a, SMB, and ScGT1 also indicate that daily treatment of these cells with CDP, aristolochic acid, BEL, and AACOCF$_3$ causes a significant decrease in protease-resistant prion protein compared to untreated control cells. The treatment with PLA$_2$ inhibitors decreases protease-resistant prion protein but also reduces prostaglandin E$_2$ levels. This observation strongly suggests that PLA$_2$ activity may be closely related to the pathogenesis of prion diseases (Bate et al., 2004). Furthermore, corticosteroids that induce the formation of lipocortins (annexins), a family of PLA$_2$ inhibitory proteins (Kaetzel and Dedman, 1995), also reduce the content of protease-resistant prion protein in prion-infected cell lines. This once again supports an involvement of PLA$_2$ in prion diseases (Bate et al., 2004). However, the use of glucocorticoids in preventing prion diseases should be treated with caution because the chronic administration of glucocorticoids is known to produce neuronal atrophy (Abraham et al., 2001).

Platelet-activating factor (PAF) is generated by the acetylation of 1-alkyl-sn-glycero-3-phosphocholine, another product of PLA$_2$ catalyzed reactions. PAF increases the generation of protease-resistant prion protein and PAF antagonists block it. The mechanism by which PAF antagonists inhibit the formation of protease-resistant prion protein remains unknown. However, PAF antagonists and PLA$_2$ inhibitors may act by altering intracellular trafficking of cellular prion protein. These observations suggest the pivotal role of PLA$_2$ and PAF in modulating formation of protease-resistant prion protein, an agent that is suggested to be the main cause of prion diseases (Bate et al., 2004).

In lipopolysaccharide-induced injury, administration of methyl arachidonoyl fluorophosphonate reduces iNOS expression and NFκB activation in glial cells (Won et al., 2005), indicating the involvement of cPLA$_2$ in lipopolysaccharide-mediated brain injury.

Vitamin E protects from neuronal damage induced by cerebral ischemia by inhibiting apoptosis in hippocampal neurons (Tagami et al., 1999; Zhang et al., 2004). This suggests that vitamin E reacts with the free radicals and prevents neuronal apoptosis produced by cerebral ischemia and reperfusion. Vitamin E also protects neurons from a toxic concentration of sodium nitroprusside, a nitric oxide donor, in a dose-dependent manner, indicating that this vitamin protects brain tissue by inhibiting free radical generation and oxidative stress. Double-blind human trials of vitamin E either slow the progression of Alzheimer disease (Sano et al., 1997) or have only symptomatic effects with no alteration of the progression of AD (Table 11.4). Long-term combination therapy of donepezil and vitamin E has beneficial effects on AD patients (Klatte et al., 2003). High-doses of vitamin E are effective in modulating β-amyloid levels and deposition in Tg2576 mice only when administered at an early stage of its phenotype (Sung et al., 2004). In cat spinal cord, preloading with vitamin E and selenium promotes recovery following spinal cord injury (Anderson et al., 1985). Collective evidence suggests that vitamin E may be useful for the treatment of inflammation and oxidative stress in acute neural trauma and neurodegenerative diseases. Negative results in human trials are likely due to the lack of a range of redox inhibitors.

CDP-choline (citicoline) inhibits cPLA$_2$ activity and lowers the concentration of free fatty acids in a dose- and time-dependent manner (Adibhatla et al., 2002). This compound is an intermediate in PtdCho biosynthesis and was used for the treatment of ischemic and head injuries (Andersen et al., 1999; Dempsey and Rao, 2003). It not only restores the concentration of PtdCho following ischemic injury by increasing PtdCho synthesis from diacylglycerol but also blocks the activation of cPLA$_2$ activity (Adibhatla et al., 2002). The decrease in cPLA$_2$ activity may lead to a reduction in levels of arachidonic acid and reactive oxygen species, with stabilization of neural membranes.

TABLE 11.4. Beneficial effects of nonspecific PLA$_2$ inhibitors for the treatment of neurological disorders.

Neurological disorders	PLA$_2$ inhibitor	Therapeutic effect	Reference
Ischemia (stroke)	GM1 ganglioside	Beneficial	Hernandez et al., 1994
	Vitamin E	Beneficial	Farooqui et al., 1994
	CDP-choline	Beneficial	Wurtman et al., 1996
Spinal cord injury	GM1 ganglioside	Beneficial	Geisler et al., 1991
	Vitamin E	Beneficial	Hall et al., 1992
	CDP-choline	Not known	
Head injury	GM1 ganglioside	Not known	Chen et al., 2003
	Vitamin E	Not known	Ikeda et al., 2000
	CDP-choline	Beneficial	Maejima and Katayama, 2001; Adibhatla et al., 2002
Alzheimer disease	GM1 ganglioside	Beneficial	Svennerholm, 1994
	Vitamin E	Beneficial	Sano et al., 1997
	CDP-choline	Beneficial	Franco-Maside et al., 1994
Parkinson disease	GM1 ganglioside	Beneficial	Schneider, 1992
	Vitamin E	Beneficial	Dubin et al., 1982
	CDP-choline	Beneficial	Secades and Frontera, 1995

Beneficial refers to behavioral improvement in subjects treated with nonspecific inhibitors of PLA$_2$ inhibitors.

This drug can cross the blood–brain barrier and produces some improvement in the cognitive status of AD patients (Table 11.4). Long-term dietary CDP-choline supplementation can ameliorate hippocampal-dependent memory impairment caused by impoverished environmental conditions in the rat and suggest that its actions result, in part, from a long-term use that enhances membrane glycerophospholipid synthesis (Teather and Wurtman, 2005). CDP-choline also protects cerebellar granule neurons from glutamate-mediated neurotoxicity (Mir et al., 2003). CDP-choline was used in phase III clinical trials for stroke and is being evaluated for the treatment of AD and PD. It also improves the verbal memory of aged human subjects. The administration of CDP-choline in animal models of ischemia reduces neural membrane breakdown, leads to increased synthesis of PtdCho, and decreases levels of free fatty acids. From a behavioral viewpoint, CDP-choline improves neurologic signs, decreases neurologic deficits, restores animal learning performance, and improves neuronal survival (Adibhatla et al., 2002). Intravenous injections of CDP-choline increase blood pressure and reverse hypotension in hemorrhagic shock (Savci et al., 2003). This effect is mediated by activation of central nicotinic cholinergic receptors. These observations suggest that this cPLA$_2$ inhibitor can be used for treating acute neural trauma as well as neurodegenerative diseases (Table 11.4).

Neurotrophic effects of gangliosides have been demonstrated in AD, PD, spinal cord injury, and stroke (Geisler et al., 1991; Svennerholm, 1994). The mechanism underlying the ganglioside action is not fully understood. However, gangliosides are known to inhibit neurotransmitter release and activities of cPLA$_2$ and PlsEtn-PLA$_2$. Gangliosides also rescue neuronal cultures from death after neurotrophic factor deprivation (Ferrari et al., 1993). GM1 potentiates the effects of nerve growth factor on neural cells. This process may delay the neurodegenerative process in AD. NMR studies indicate that GM1 ganglioside binds tightly with β-amyloid peptide and inhibits the α-helix to β-sheet conformational change in β-amyloid peptide (Mandal and Pettegrew, 2004). This may be another mechanism, by which GM1 can preserve the integrity of degenerating neurons in cell culture and animal models of neurodegenerative diseases. Although attempts to treat AD with injections of GM1 have failed (Ala et al., 1990; Flicker et al., 1994), from a theoretical standpoint GM1 therapy still offers a valid way of delaying neuronal death in neurodegenerative diseases. In ischemic brain, gangliosides protect neural cells by scavenging free radicals generated during reperfusion (Fighera et al., 2004).

In the MPP$^+$-mediated cell culture model of PD (Yoshinaga et al., 2000), neurodegeneration is accompanied by the stimulation of PLA$_2$ and arachidonic acid release in GH3 cells. This release of arachidonic acid can be blocked by arachidonoyl trifluoromethyl ketone, a potent inhibitor of cPLA$_2$. This suggests the involvement of cPLA$_2$-mediated oxidative stress in MPP$^+$-mediated neurodegeneration. Similarly in the MPTP-induced model of Parkinsonism, quinacrine protects dopaminergic neurons from neurodegeneration (Tariq et al., 2001). In this system quinacrine may act not only as a PLA$_2$ inhibitor but also as a membrane stabilizer and antioxidant (Tariq et al., 2001; Turnbull et al., 2003). CDP-choline and vitamin E have also been used for the treatment of PD (Dubin et al., 1982; Schneider, 1992; Secades and Frontera, 1995).

Polyunsaturated fatty acids of the n-3 series have many beneficial effects in the central nervous system. These effects include generation of n-3 series prostaglandins and docosanoids, changes in membrane fluidity and lipid rafts, modulation of signal transduction, regulation of gene expression, and antigen presentation (Farooqui and Horrocks, 2004). Thus, EPA prevents LPS-mediated TNF-α expression by preventing NF-κB activation and protects rat hippocampus from LPS-mediated neurotoxicity (Zhao et al., 2004; Lonergan et al., 2004). In C6 glioma cells, EPA modulates myelin proteolipid gene expression (Salvati et al., 2004). This fatty acid is used for the treatment of schizophrenia (Peet and Ryles, 2001; Horrobin, 2003).

Chronic pre-administration of DHA prevents beta amyloid-induced impairment of an avoidance ability-related memory function in a rat model of AD (Hashimoto et al., 2002) and protects mice from synaptic loss and dendritic pathology in another model of AD (Calon et al., 2004). Thus, DHA is beneficial in preventing the learning deficiencies in these AD models (Hashimoto et al., 2005a,b). DHA suppresses increases in the levels of lipid peroxides and ROS in the cerebral cortex and hippocampus of Aβ-infused rats, indicating that DHA increases antioxidative defenses. DHA also affects amyloid precursor protein processing by inhibiting α- and β-secretase activities (de Wilde et al., 2003; Walsh and Selkoe, 2004). Supplements of DHA produce a neuroprotective effect on β-amyloid deposition without significant toxic effects (Hashimoto et al., 2005a). In contrast, in the Aβ-treated cortical cell culture model of AD, DHA does not act by blocking the oxidative stress induced by soluble Aβ peptides in neurons (Park et al., 2004). Instead, DHA protects neurons by preserving the microtubule organization of neurons. Furthermore, larger amounts of DHA induce a network of cells that contain more neurites with longer lengths compared with control neurons (Park et al., 2004). DHA reverses the age-related impairment in LTP and depolarization-induced glutamate release. It also inhibits the production of TNF-α, interleukin-1, and interleukin-6.

DHA protects the brain against ischemic and excitotoxic damage in rats (Gamoh et al., 1999; Terano et al., 1999). It also reduces the severity or delays the development of dyskinesias in a nonhuman primate model of PD (Samadi et al., 2006). DHA may act as an antioxidant (Hossain et al., 1998). DHA, a stimulant of peroxisomal enzymes, induces antioxidant defenses by enhancing cerebral activities of catalase, glutathione peroxidase, and levels of glutathione (Hossain et al., 1999). Thus, EPA and DHA exert their neuroprotective effects by modulating cytokines, inflammation, and oxidative stress. DHA has been used for the treatment of experimental epilepsy in rats (Yuen et al., 2005). Collectively these studies indicate that DHA and EPA not only regulate platelet aggregation, blood clotting, smooth muscle contraction, and leukocyte chemotaxis, but also modulate inflammatory cytokine production and immune function.

The treatment of Zellweger syndrome patients with purified DHA partially improves visual function, increases levels of plasmalogens, and reduces levels of saturated very long-chain fatty acids (Hossain et al., 1999). The level of DHA is also low in patients with multiple sclerosis. Fish oil supplements with vitamins improve the clinical outcome in MS patients (Nordvik et al., 2000). Collective evidence from many studies indicates that DHA supplementation restores signal transduction processes associated with behavioral deficits and learning activity in Alzheimer disease, schizophrenia, depression, hyperactivity, stroke, and peroxisomal disorders (Farooqui and Horrocks, 2004).

Injections of annexin-1 peptide (1–188) markedly inhibit the neuronal death, by up to 70%, and edema induced by focal cerebral ischemia in rats. Ischemic brain injury itself results in increased expression of lipocortin-1 (annexin-1) around the area of infarction. Furthermore, the intracerebroventricular administration of a lipocortin-1 fragment produces marked inhibition of infarct size and cerebral edema after cerebral ischemia in rats (Relton et al., 1991). Intracerebroventricular injections of neutralizing anti-lipocortin-1 fragment antiserum increased the size of the infarct and the development of edema. The anti-PLA$_2$ protein, annexin-1, is an endogenous inhibitor of cerebral ischemia. The annexin-1 fragment also blocks NMDA receptor stimulation, indicating that annexin-1 may have considerable therapeutic potential in vivo (Relton et al., 1991; Black et al., 1992). The expression of annexins is up-regulated in other pathologic conditions, such as kainic acid-lesioned cerebellum (Young et al., 1999), multiple sclerosis (Elderfield et al., 1992), EAE (Bolton et al., 1990; Elderfield et al., 1993), and spinal cord injury (Liu et al., 2004). Thus, increased annexin expression may be an inherent endogenous anti-inflammatory mechanism for protection of brain from damage. Annexin-1 also inhibits neutrophil and monocyte infiltration in experimental models of inflammation (Perretti et al., 1993; Harris et al., 1995). Annexins block the expression of proinflammatory cytokines such as TNF-α, and IL-1β (Harris et al., 1995), once again supporting the view that annexins are anti-inflammatory proteins. Annexins may also exert anti-inflammatory effects by binding to lipid inflammatory mediators. For example, annexin V binds with high affinity to phosphatidylserine in the presence of Ca^{2+} and thereby protects neural cells from apoptotic cell death (Reutelingsperger and van Heerde, 1997). Additional systematic studies on the pharmacology of annexins may aid in designing novel anti-inflammatory therapeutics based on this endogenous mediator.

All of the cPLA$_2$ inhibitors used in these studies are nonspecific. Thus, the design and synthesis of specific cPLA$_2$ inhibitors is urgently needed to make progress in this important area of research. The reaction catalyzed by cPLA$_2$ is a rate-limiting step for the generation of eicosanoids, lyso-glycerophospholipids, and platelet-activating factor. High levels of these metabolites are responsible for oxidative stress, inflammation, and neuronal death at the injury site. Potent PLA$_2$ inhibitors can effectively block the above events associated with neurodegenerative processes and rescue neural cells from cell death. It is hoped that a new generation of cPLA$_2$ inhibitors will have regional specificity. The inhibitors must be able to reach the injury site where neural cells are under oxidative stress and where neurodegenerative processes are taking place.

Many potent and selective inhibitors of human group IIA sPLA$_2$ are available for more than a decade and have provided compelling evidence for a causative role of group IIA sPLA$_2$ in numerous studies involving animal models of inflammatory diseases (Reid, 2005). These unrelated and structurally diverse groups of group IIA sPLA$_2$ inhibitors have been used for their biological activity in animal models with limited success.

LY315920NA/S-5920, a selective inhibitor of group IIA sPLA$_2$, is well tolerated by humans and shown to improve survival in a small group of patients who received this drug within 24 h of the first sepsis-induced organ failure. Confirmation of this study in a multicenter, double-blind, placebo-controlled manner on a larger patient population indicated that a continuous 7-day infusion of LY315920NA/S-5920 had no beneficial effect on severe sepsis patients. This study did not confirm earlier promising subgroup results with LY315920NA/S-5920, which provides a reminder that subgroup effects should be viewed cautiously, especially when primary effects are not significant (Zeiher et al., 2005). LY211727 has been used to block pain. Thus intrathecal administration of LY211727 in an experimental rat model of hyperalgesia blocks intraplantar carrageenan-induced thermal hyperalgesia and formalin-induced flinching (Svensson et al., 2005), indicating that this sPLA$_2$ inhibitor can be beneficial in spinal cord injury. Collectively these studies suggest that more studies are required on the therapeutic potentials of different PLA$_2$ inhibitors in human diseases.

11.4 Prevention of Pain by PLA$_2$ Inhibitors

Proinflammatory cytokines released at the site of neural trauma and nerve injury may be involved in sensitization of nociceptors leading to hyperalgesia (Walters, 1994). Injections of carrageenan into the paw or face have been widely used as a model to induce pain sensitization (Ng and Ong, 2001). We studied the effect of intracerebroventricular injections of a sPLA$_2$ inhibitor, 12-*epi*-scalaradial, a cPLA$_2$ inhibitor, AACOCF$_3$, and a iPLA$_2$ inhibitor, bromoenol lactone, on the development of allodynia after facial carrageenan injections in two strains of mice (Yeo et al., 2004). C57BL/6J (B6) mice show an increase in nociception from 8 h to 3 days after facial carrageenan injection. On the other hand, the BALB/c strain did not show an increase in allodynia at any of the time points. In both B6 and BALB/c mice, all PLA$_2$ inhibitors significantly reduced responses to von Frey hair stimulation at 8 h and 1 day. Only the sPLA$_2$ inhibitor had an effect at 3 days. Since BALB/c mice do not show increases in nociception after carrageenan injection, the reduction in responses seen with PLA$_2$ inhibitors actually means that these inhibitors produce a loss of normal sensitivity to von Frey hair stimulation.

The effects of PLA$_2$ inhibitors are unlikely to be due simply to inhibition of arachidonic acid generation, because intracerebroventricular injection of arachidonic acid also had an antinociceptive effect (Yeo et al., 2004). It is proposed that lysophosphatidylcholine mediates pain transmission in the central nervous system. The pronounced and long-lasting antinociceptive effect of 12-*epi*-scalaradial is consistent with our recent finding that sPLA$_2$ induces exocytosis and neurotransmitter release in neurons, and supports a key role of central nervous system sPLA$_2$ in synaptic and pain transmission. These results suggest that PLA$_2$ isoforms play an important role not only in pain transmission, but also in nonpainful, touch, or pressure sensation. Our studies on the antinociceptive effect of PLA$_2$ inhibitors are supported by recent studies on intrathecal injections of MAFP and AACOCF$_3$ in rats. MAFP has a significant antinociceptive effect in the rat formalin test (Ates et al., 2003). Similarly, in vivo systemic or intrathecal delivery of AX048, a potent cPLA$_2$ inhibitor prevents carrageenan hyperalgesia as well as spinally mediated hyperalgesia induced by intrathecal substance P. In contrast, patch-clamp technique studies indicate that melittin, an sPLA$_2$ activator, enhances spontaneous glutamatergic excitatory transmission in rat substantia gelatinosa (Yue et al., 2005). The spontaneous excitatory postsynaptic current frequency increase is reduced by 4-bromophenacyl bromide and is not affected by indomethacin, a cyclooxygenase inhibitor and nordihydroguaiaretic acid, a lipoxygenase inhibitor. It is proposed that melittin increases the spontaneous release of glutamate in substantia gelatinosa neurons by activating sPLA$_2$ and increasing Ca^{2+} influx through voltage-gated calcium channels and modulating glutamatergic neurotransmission (Yue et al., 2005). Collectively these studies (Kokotos et al., 2004; DeMar et al., 2006) suggest that cPLA$_2$ inhibitors mediate antinociceptive activity by blocking cPLA$_2$ activity and reducing lysophosphatidylcholine levels.

11.5 Perspective and Direction for Future Studies

PLA$_2$ isoforms along with cyclooxygenases have emerged as major players in modulating inflammation and oxidative stress in brain tissue. Elucidation of the mechanism of action of PLA$_2$ inhibitors in vivo is a critical area of research due to the potential pharmacologic benefits of these compounds as therapeutic agents for the treatment of inflammation and oxidative stress in neurotrauma and neurodegenerative diseases (Farooqui et al., 1999). Although several inhibitors of PLA$_2$ activity have been reported in the literature (Farooqui et al., 1999; Cummings et al., 2000; Miele, 2003), little information is available on the mechanism of their action. Different mechanisms of action are possible, e.g., an inhibitor can produce alterations in enzymic activity by perturbing the physicochemical properties of glycerophospholipid bilayers. A PLA$_2$ inhibitor can interact directly with the active site of an isoform, as AACOCF$_3$, MAFP, and BEL, or it can act on an allosteric site on the enzyme molecule to bring about changes in enzymic activity. An inhibitor may also possess a detergent-like structure that can induce nonspecific changes in membrane properties in vivo through the interaction of their amphiphilic groups with other membrane components to produce changes in enzymic activity.

Inhibitors of cPLA$_2$ modulate the expression of cytokines, growth factors, nuclear factor kappa B, and adhesion molecules, and thus can block endogenous inflammatory reactions. Some nonspecific inhibitors of PLA_2 have been used for the treatment of ischemia, spinal cord injury, and AD in animal models and in humans. It is clear from the above discussion that novel, potent, and specific inhibitors of PLA_2 are now emerging as potential therapeutic agents for neuroinflammation and oxidative stress in cell culture systems, but they have not yet been used in animal models of neurological disorders.

In brain, the PLA_2 occurs in multiple forms. Thus, specific PLA_2 inhibitors must be designed for individual PLA_2 isozymes to define their roles in brain metabolism. The design of PLA_2 inhibitors should be focused on our rapidly emerging understanding of the role of signal transduction pathways in neurological disorders. Since PLA_2-catalyzed reactions are the rate-limiting steps for the production of prostaglandins, leukotrienes, and thromboxanes, the identification of PLA_2-coupled receptors and their endogenous regulatory pathways that mediate proliferative, metabolic, and inflammatory signals can provide better targets for designing PLA_2 inhibitors. Specificity, selectivity, harmlessness, and the ability of a PLA_2 inhibitor to cross the blood–brain barrier are important qualities of a PLA_2 inhibitor as a potential therapeutic agent for neurological disorders.

At this time, it is quite difficult to predict the potential side effects of the chronic use of cell-permeable, specific, or nonspecific inhibitors of PLA_2. Hence, studies on the availability of specific, nontoxic potent inhibitors with greater blood–brain barrier permeability in animal models of neurodegenerative diseases are urgently needed. Surely, PLA_2 isoforms from different sources will have different inhibitor sensitivities and reactivity in vivo. Nevertheless, pharmacological studies in animal models of acute trauma and neurodegenerative diseases will provide directions that should be taken to develop better PLA_2 inhibitors for targeting isoforms of brain PLA_2 activities.

In recent years, a number of studies have utilized advanced molecular biology procedures to overcome some of the problems associated with the specificity of chemical inhibitors of PLA_2. For example, antisense oligonucleotides that inhibit specific $cPLA_2$ or $iPLA_2$ have been developed. Transgenic mice that are deficient in or overexpress $cPLA_2$ isoforms are now available (Bonventre et al., 1997). Overexpression of $cPLA_2$ allows one to study the effect of increased $cPLA_2$ activity, whereas a deficiency of $cPLA_2$ can be helpful in studying the consequences of reduced $cPLA_2$ activity on cellular metabolism in normal and diseased cells (Adler et al., 2006). Antisense for $cPLA_2$ has been developed and used for lowering lipopolysaccharide neurotoxicity in glial cell cultures (Won et al., 2005). RNAi for $iPLA_2$ has also been developed. Transfection studies with RNA interference (RNAi) of $iPLA_2$ indicate that the levels of $iPLA_2$ protein and $iPLA_2$ activity are decreased in a dose-dependent manner in transfected non-neural cells (Shinzawa and Tsujimoto, 2003). Such studies are needed in neuronal cell cultures and animal models to understand the neurophysiologic importance of the RNAi technique.

A comparison of activities of PLA_2 isoforms and intensity of signal transduction process between normal and genetically manipulated mice may provide further insight into the role of PLA_2 isoforms, their ligands, and their lipid mediators in neurodegenerative processes. Changes in mRNA expression of various PLA$_2$ isoforms and their second messengers in neural cells of a specific brain region may regulate activation of signaling pathways mediated by PLA$_2$ isoforms in response to external stimuli in normal and genetically manipulated mice. Network assembly of various signaling pathways that communicate information from neurons to glial cells to perform and complete physiological processes involved in cell survival or death may also regulate this activation. Therefore, recent advances in functional genomics, proteomics, and lipidomics in the presence and absence of PLA$_2$ inhibitors can provide a tremendous amount of information on signaling pathways associated with oxidative stress and inflammatory reactions during neurodegeneration in normal brain and brain tissue from neurological disorders.

In brain, the PLA$_2$ occurs in multiple forms. Thus, specific PLA$_2$ inhibitors must be designed for individual PLA$_2$ isozymes to define their roles in brain metabolism. The design of PLA$_2$ inhibitors should be focused on our rapidly emerging understanding of the role of signal transduction pathways in neurological disorders. Since PLA$_2$-catalyzed reactions are the rate-limiting steps for the production of prostaglandins, leukotrienes, and thromboxanes, the identification of PLA$_2$-coupled receptors and their endogenous regulatory pathways that mediate proliferative, metabolic, and inflammatory signals can provide better targets for designing PLA$_2$ inhibitors. Specificity, selectivity, harmlessness, and the ability of a PLA$_2$ inhibitor to cross the blood–brain barrier are important qualities of a PLA$_2$ inhibitor as a potential therapeutic agent for neurological disorders.

Thus, the development of specific inhibitors for different PLA$_2$ isoforms should be an important goal for future research on brain PLA$_2$ activities. The chemical approach, together with molecular biological procedures such as RNAi and alterations in signal transduction processes in knockout mice, may provide the important information needed to develop specific PLA$_2$ inhibitors that can be used to retard oxidative stress and inflammatory reactions during neurodegeneration in neurological disorders.

References

Abraham I. M., Harkany T., Horvath K. M., and Luiten P. G. (2001). Action of glucocorticoids on survival of nerve cells: promoting neurodegeneration or neuroprotection? *J. Neuroendocrinol.* 13:749–760.

Adibhatla R. M. and Hatcher J. F. (2003). Citicoline decreases phospholipase A2 stimulation and hydroxyl radical generation in transient cerebral ischemia. *J. Neurosci. Res.* 73:308–315.

Adibhatla R. M. and Hatcher J. F. (2006). Phospholipase A$_2$, reactive oxygen species, and lipid peroxidation in cerebral ischemia. *Free Radic. Biol. Med.* 40:376–387.

Adibhatla R. M., Hatcher J. F., and Dempsey R. J. (2002). Citicoline: neuroprotective mechanisms in cerebral ischemia. *J. Neurochem.* 80:12–23.

Adibhatla R. M., Hatcher J. F., and Dempsey R. J. (2003). Phospholipase A$_2$, hydroxyl radicals, and lipid peroxidation in transient cerebral ischemia. *Antioxid. Redox Signal.* 5:647–654.

Adler D. H., Phillips J. A. I., Cogan J. D., Morrow I. D., Boutaud O., and Oates J. A. (2006). First description: cytosolic phospholipase A$_2$-alpha deficiency. *J. Invest. Med.* 54:S257.

Aguzzi A., Brandner S., Marino S., and Steinbach J. P. (1996). Transgenic and knockout mice in the study of neurodegenerative diseases. *J. Mol. Med.* 74:111–126.

Aisen P. S. and Davis K. L. (1994). Inflammatory mechanisms in Alzheimer's disease: implications for therapy. *Am. J. Psychiatry* 151:1105–1113.

Aitdafoun M., Mounier C., Heymans F., Binisti C., Bon C., and Godfroid J. J. (1996). 4-Alkoxybenzamidines as new potent phospholipase A$_2$ inhibitors. *Biochem. Pharmacol.* 51:737–742.

Ajmone-Cat M. A., Nicolini A., and Minghetti L. (2003). Prolonged exposure of microglia to lipopolysaccharide modifies the intracellular signaling pathways and selectively promotes prostaglandin E-2 synthesis. *J. Neurochem.* 87:1193–1203.

Ala T., Romero S., Knight F., Feldt K., and Frey, W. H., II (1990). GM-1 treatment of Alzheimer's disease. A pilot study of safety and efficacy. *Arch. Neurol.* 47:1126–1130.

Alliangana D. M. (1996). Effects of beta-carotene, flavonoid quercitin and quinacrine on cell proliferation and lipid peroxidation breakdown products in BHK-21 cells. *East Afr. Med. J.* 73:752–757.

Amandi-Burgermeister E., Tibes U., Kaiser B. M., Friebe W. G., and Scheuer W. V. (1997). Suppression of cytokine synthesis, integrin expression and chronic inflammation by inhibitors of cytosolic phospholipase A$_2$. *Eur. J. Pharmacol.* 326:237–250.

Anderle P., Farmer P., Berger A., and Roberts M. A. (2004). Nutrigenomic approach to understanding the mechanisms by which dietary long-chain fatty acids induce gene signals and control mechanisms involved in carcinogenesis. *Nutrition* 20:103–108.

Andersen M., Overgaard K., Meden P., and Boysen G. (1999). Effects of citicoline combined with thrombolytic therapy in a rat embolic stroke model. *Stroke* 30:1464–1470.

Anderson D. K., Saunders R. D., Demediuk P., Dugan L. L., Braughler J. M., Hall E. D., Means E. D., and Horrocks L. A. (1985). Lipid hydrolysis and peroxidation in injured spinal cord: partial protection with methylprednisolone or vitamin E and selenium. *Cent. Nerv. Syst. Trauma* 2:257–267.

Arai K., Ikegaya Y., Nakatani Y., Kudo I., Nishiyama N., and Matsuki N. (2001). Phospholipase A$_2$ mediates ischemic injury in the hippocampus: a regional difference of neuronal vulnerability. *Eur. J. Neurosci.* 13:2319–2323.

Ates M., Hamza M., Seidel K., Kotalla C. E., Ledent C., and Guhring H. (2003). Intrathecally applied flurbiprofen produces an endocannabinoid-dependent antinociception in the rat formalin test. *Eur. J. Neurosci.* 17:597–604.

Balsinde J. and Dennis E. A. (1997). Function and inhibition of intracellular calcium-independent phospholipase A$_2$. *J. Biol. Chem.* 272:16069–16072.

Bartoli F., Lin H.-K., Ghomashchi F., Gelb M. H., Jain M. K., and Apitz-Castro R. (1994). Tight binding inhibitors of 85-kDa phospholipase A$_2$ but not 14-kDa phospholipase A$_2$ inhibit release of free arachidonate in thrombin-stimulated human platelets. *J. Biol. Chem.* 269:15625–15630.

Basselin M., Chang L., Seemann R., Bell J. M., and Rapoport S. I. (2003). Chronic lithium administration potentiates brain arachidonic acid signaling at rest and during cholinergic activation in awake rats. *J. Neurochem.* 85:1553–1562.

Bate C., Reid S., and Williams A. (2004). Phospholipase A$_2$ inhibitors or platelet-activating factor antagonists prevent prion replication. *J. Biol. Chem.* 279:36405–36411.

Bikson M., Id Bihi R., Vreugdenhil M., Kohling R., Fox J. E., and Jefferys J. G. (2002). Quinine suppresses extracellular potassium transients and ictal epileptiform activity without decreasing neuronal excitability in vitro. *Neuroscience* 115:251–261.

Black M. D., Carey F., Crossman A. R., Relton J. K., and Rothwell N. J. (1992). Lipocortin-1 inhibits NMDA receptor-mediated neuronal damage in the striatum of the rat. *Brain Res.* 585:135–140.

Block J. A. (1998). Hydroxychloroquine and retinal safety. *Lancet* 351:771.

Bolton C., Elderfield A. J., and Flower R. J. (1990). The detection of lipocortins 1, 2 and 5 in central nervous system tissues from Lewis rats with acute experimental allergic encephalomyelitis. *J. Neuroimmunol.* 29:173–181.

Bonventre J. V. and Sapirstein A. (2002). Group IV cytosolic phospholipase A_2 (PLA$_2$) function: insights from the knockout mouse. In: Honn K. V., Marnett L. J., Nigam S., Dennis E., and Serhan C. (eds.), *Eicosanoids and other Bioactive Lipids in Cancer, Inflammation, and Radiation Injury, 5.* Kluwer Academic/Plenum Publ, New York, pp. 25–31.

Bonventre J. V., Huang Z. H., Taheri M. R., O'Leary E., Li E., Moskowitz M. A., and Sapirstein A. (1997). Reduced fertility and postischaemic brain injury in mice deficient in cytosolic phospholipase A_2. *Nature* 390:622–625.

Bozza P. T. and Weller P. F. (2001). Arachidonyl trifluoromethyl ketone induces lipid body formation in leukocytes. *Prostaglandins Leukot. Essent. Fatty Acids* 64:227–230.

Brown W. J., Chambers K., and Doody A. (2003). Phospholipase A_2 (PLA$_2$) enzymes in membrane trafficking: mediators of membrane shape and function. *Traffic* 4:214–221.

Burgess J. R. and Kuo C. F. (1996). Increased calcium-independent phospholipase A_2 activity in vitamin E and selenium-deficient rat lung, liver, and spleen cytosol is time-dependent and reversible. *J. Nutr. Biochem.* 7:366–374.

Burke J. R., Witmer M. R., Zusi F. C., Gregor K. R., Davern L. B., Padmanabha R., Swann R. T., Smith D., Tredup J. A., Micanovic R., Manly S. P., Villafranca J. J., and Tramposch K. M. (1999). Competitive, reversible inhibition of cytosolic phospholipase A_2 at the lipid–water interface by choline derivatives that partially partition into the phospholipid bilayer. *J. Biol. Chem.* 274:18864–18871.

Burton C. A., Patel S., Mundt S., Hassing H., Zhang D., Hermanowski-Vosatka A., Wright S. D., Chao Y. S., Detmers P. A., and Sparrow C. P. (2002). Deficiency in sPLA$_2$ does not affect HDL levels or atherosclerosis in mice. *Biochem. Biophys. Res. Commun.* 294:88–94.

Calder P. C. and Grimble R. F. (2002). Polyunsaturated fatty acids, inflammation and immunity. *Eur. J. Clin. Nutr.* 56:S14-S19.

Calon F., Lim G. P., Yang F. S., Morihara T., Teter B., Ubeda O., Rostaing P., Triller A., Salem N. J., Ashe K. H., Frautschy S. A., and Cole G. M. (2004). Docosahexaenoic acid protects from dendritic pathology in an Alzheimer's disease mouse model. *Neuron* 43:633–645.

Chan A. C., Pritchard E. T., Gerrard J. M., Man R. Y., and Choy P. C. (1982). Biphasic modulation of platelet phospholipase A_2 activity and platelet aggregation by mepacrine (quinacrine). *Biochim. Biophys. Acta* 713:170–172.

Chang M. C. J. and Jones C. R. (1998). Chronic lithium treatment decreases brain phospholipase A_2 activity. *Neurochem. Res.* 23:887–892.

Chen Z. G., Lu Y. C., Zhu C., Zhang G. J., Ding X. H., and Jiang J. Y. (2003). Effects of ganglioside GM1 on reduction of brain edema and amelioration of cerebral metabolism after traumatic brain injury. *Chin. J. Traumatol.* 6:23–27.

Church W. B., Inglis A. S., Tseng A., Duell R., Lei P. W., Bryant K. J., and Scott K. F. (2001). A novel approach to the design of inhibitors of human secreted phospholipase A_2 based on native peptide inhibition. *J. Biol. Chem.* 276:33156–33164.

Clark J. D. and Tam S. (2004). Potential therapeutic uses of phospholipase A_2 inhibitors. *Expert Opin. Ther. Patents* 14:937–950.

Connolly S., Bennion C., Botterell S., Croshaw P. J., Hallam C., Hardy K., Hartopp P., Jackson C. G., King S. J., Lawrence L., Mete A., Murray D., Robinson D. H., Smith G. M., Stein L., Walters I., Wells E., and Withnall W. J. (2002). Design and synthesis of a novel and potent series of inhibitors of cytosolic phospholipase A_2 based on a 1,3-disubstituted propan-2-one skeleton. *J. Med. Chem.* 45:1348–1362.

Corbella B. and Vieta E. (2003). Molecular targets of lithium action. *Acta Neuropsychiatry* 15:316–340.

Crowe R. and Burnstock G. (1984). Quinacrine-positive neurones in some regions of the guinea-pig brain. *Brain Res. Bull.* 12:387–391.

Cummings B. S., McHowat J., and Schnellmann R. G. (2000). Phospholipase A_2s in cell injury and death. *J. Pharmacol. Exp. Ther.* 294:793–799.

Cunningham T. J., Hodge L., Speicher D., Reim D., Tyler-Polsz C., Levitt P., Eagleson K., Kennedy S., and Wang Y. (1998). Identification of a survival-promoting peptide in medium conditioned by oxidatively stressed cell lines of nervous system origin. *J. Neurosci.* 18:7047–7060.

Cunningham T. J., Jing H., Wang Y., and Hodge L. (2000). Calreticulin binding and other biological activities of survival peptide Y-P30 including effects of systemic treatment of rats. *Exp. Neurol.* 163:457–468.

Cunningham T. J., Souayah N., Jameson B., Mitchell J., and Yao L. H. (2004). Systemic treatment of cerebral cortex lesions in rats with a new secreted phospholipase A2 inhibitor. *J. Neurotrauma* 21:1683–1691.

Danesch U., Weber P. C., and Sellmayer A. (1994). Arachidonic acid increases c-*fos* and *Egr-1* mRNA in 3T3 fibroblasts by formation of prostaglandin E_2 and activation of protein kinase C. *J. Biol. Chem.* 269:27258–27263.

de Wilde M. C., Leenders I., Broersen L. M., Kuipers A. A. M., van der Beek E. M., and Kiliaan A. J. (2003). The omega-3 fatty acid docosahexaenoic acid (DHA) inhibits the formation of beta amyloid in CHO7PA2 cells. 2003 Abstract Viewer/Itinerary Planner, Program No. 730.11.

DeMar J. C. J., Ma K. Z., Bell J. M., Igarashi M., Greenstein D., and Rapoport S. I. (2006). One generation of n-3 polyunsaturated fatty acid deprivation increases depression and aggression test scores in rats. *J. Lipid Res.* 47:172–180.

Dempsey R. J. and Rao V. L. R. (2003). Cytidinediphosphocholine treatment to decrease traumatic brain injury-induced hippocampal neuronal death, cortical contusion volume, and neurological dysfunction in rats. *J. Neurosurg.* 98:867–873.

Di Cerbo A., Nandi P. K., and Edelhoch H. (1984). Interaction of basic compounds with coated vesicles. *Biochemistry* 23:6036–6040.

Douglas C. E., Chan A. C., and Choy P. C. (1986). Vitamin E inhibits platelet phospholipase A_2. *Biochim. Biophys. Acta* 876:639–645.

Dubin N. H., Blake D. A., DiBlasi M. C., Parmley T. H., and King T. M. (1982). Pharmacokinetic studies on quinacrine following intrauterine administration to cynomolgus monkeys. *Fert. Steril.* 38:735–740.

Elderfield A. J., Newcombe J., Bolton C., and Flower R. J. (1992). Lipocortins (annexins) 1, 2, 4 and 5 are increased in the central nervous system in multiple sclerosis. *J. Neuroimmunol.* 39:91–100.

Elderfield A. J., Bolton C., and Flower R. J. (1993). Lipocortin 1 (annexin 1) immunoreactivity in the cervical spinal cord of Lewis rats with acute experimental allergic encephalomyelitis. *J. Neurol. Sci.* 119:146–153.

Estevez A. Y. and Phillis J. W. (1997). The phospholipase A_2 inhibitor, quinacrine, reduces infarct size in rats after transient middle cerebral artery occlusion. *Brain Res.* 752:203–208.

Farooqui A. A. and Horrocks L. A. (1994). Excitotoxicity and neurological disorders: involvement of membrane phospholipids. *Int. Rev. Neurobiol.* 36:267–323.

Farooqui A. A. and Horrocks L. A. (2004). Beneficial effects of docosahexaenoic acid on health of the human brain. *Agro Food Ind. Hi-Tech* 15:52–53.

Farooqui A. A., Haun S. E., and Horrocks L. A. (1994). Ischemia and hypoxia. In: Siegel G. J., Agranoff B. W., Albers R. W., and Molinoff P. B. (eds.), *Basic Neurochemistry.* Raven Press, New York, pp. 867–883.

Farooqui A. A., Yang H. C., Rosenberger T. A., and Horrocks L. A. (1997). Phospholipase A$_2$ and its role in brain tissue. *J. Neurochem.* 69:889–901.

Farooqui A. A., Litsky M. L., Farooqui T., and Horrocks L. A. (1999). Inhibitors of intracellular phospholipase A$_2$ activity: their neurochemical effects and therapeutical importance for neurological disorders. *Brain Res. Bull.* 49:139–153.

Farooqui A. A., Ong W. Y., and Horrocks L. A. (2003). Stimulation of lipases and phospholipases in Alzheimer disease. In: Szuhaj B. and van Nieuwenhuyzen W. (eds.), *Nutrition and Biochemistry of Phospholipids.* AOCS Press, Champaign, pp. 14–29.

Farooqui A. A., Ong W. Y., and Horrocks L. A. (2004). Neuroprotection abilities of cytosolic phospholipase A$_2$ inhibitors in kainic acid-induced neurodegeneration. *Curr. Drug Targets Cardiovasc. Haematol. Disord.* 4:85–96.

Farooqui A. A., Ong W. Y., Go M. L., and Horrocks L. A. (2005). Inhibition of brain phospholipase A2 by antimalarial drugs: implications for neuroprotection in neurological disorders. *Med. Chem. Rev. Online* 2:379–392.

Farrelly P. V., Kenna B. L., Laohachai K. L., Bahadi R., Salmona M., Forloni G., and Kourie J. I. (2003). Quinacrine blocks PrP (106–126)-formed channels. *J. Neurosci. Res.* 74:934–941.

Fernando S. R. and Pertwee R. G. (1997). Evidence that methyl arachidonyl fluorophosphate is an irreversible cannabinoid receptor antagonist. *Br. J. Pharmacol.* 121:1716–1720.

Ferrari G., Batistatou A., and Greene L. A. (1993). Gangliosides rescue neuronal cells from death after trophic factor deprivation. *J. Neurosci.* 13:1879–1887.

Fighera M. R., Bonini J. S., Frussa R., Dutra C. S., Hagen M. E. K., Rubin M. A., and Mello C. F. (2004). Monosialoganglioside increases catalase activity in cerebral cortex of rats. *Free Radic. Res.* 38:495–500.

Flicker C., Ferris S. H., Kalkstein D., and Serby M. (1994). A double-blind, placebo-controlled crossover study of ganglioside GM$_1$ treatment for Alzheimer's disease. *Am. J. Psychiatry* 151:126–129.

Follette P. (2003). New perspectives for prion therapeutics meeting. Prion disease treatment's early promise unravels. *Science* 299:191–192.

Franco-Maside A., Caamaño J., Gómez M. J., and Cacabelos R. (1994). Brain mapping activity and mental performance after chronic treatment with CDP-choline in Alzheimer's disease. *Methods Find. Exp. Clin. Pharmacol.* 16:597–607.

Franson R. C. and Rosenthal M. D. (1989). Oligomers of prostaglandin B1 inhibit in vitro phospholipase A$_2$ activity. *Biochim. Biophys. Acta* 1006:272–277.

Franson R. C. and Rosenthal M. D. (1997). PX-52, a novel inhibitor of 14 kDa secretory and 85 kDa cytosolic phospholipases A2. *Adv. Exp. Med. Biol.* 400:365–373.

Fuentes L., Pérez R., Nieto M. L., Balsinde J., and Balboa M. A. (2003). Bromoenol lactone promotes cell death by a mechanism involving phosphatidate phosphohydrolase-1 rather than calcium-independent phospholipase A$_2$. *J. Biol. Chem.* 278:44683–44690.

Fujita S., Ikegaya Y., Nishiyama N., and Matsuki N. (2000). Ca^{2+}-independent phospholipase A$_2$ inhibitor impairs spatial memory of mice. *Jpn. J. Pharmacol.* 83:277–278.

Fujita S., Ikegaya Y., Nishikawa M., Nishiyama N., and Matsuki N. (2001). Docosahexaenoic acid improves long-term potentiation attenuated by phospholipase A$_2$ inhibitor in rat hippocampal slices. *Br. J. Pharmacol.* 132:1417–1422.

Gamoh S., Hashimoto M., Sugioka K., Hossain M. S., Hata N., Misawa Y., and Masumura S. (1999). Chronic administration of docosahexaenoic acid improves reference memory-related learning ability in young rats. *Neuroscience* 93:237–241.

Geisler F. H., Dorsey F. C., and Coleman W. P. (1991). Recovery of motor function after spinal-cord injury – a randomized, placebo-controlled trial with GM-1 ganglioside. *New Engl. J. Med.* 324:1829–1887.

Gerke V. and Moss S. E. (1997). Annexins and membrane dynamics. *Biochim. Biophys. Acta Mol. Cell Res.* 1357:129–154.

Ghelardoni S., Tomita Y. A., Bell J. M., Rapoport S. I., and Bosetti F. (2004). Chronic carbamazepine selectively downregulates cytosolic phospholipase A$_2$ expression and cyclooxygenase activity in rat brain. *Biol. Psychiatry* 56:248–254.

Ghomashchi F., Loo R., Balsinde J., Bartoli F., Apitz-Castro R., Clark J. D., Dennis E. A., and Gelb M. H. (1999). Trifluoromethyl ketones and methyl fluorophosphonates as inhibitors of group IV and VI phospholipases A$_2$: structure–function studies with vesicle, micelle, and membrane assays. *Biochim. Biophys. Acta* 1420:45–56.

Ghomashchi F., Stewart A., Hefner Y., Ramanadham S., Turk J., Leslie C. C., and Gelb M. H. (2001). A pyrrolidine-based specific inhibitor of cytosolic phospholipase A$_{2\alpha}$ blocks arachidonic acid release in a variety of mammalian cells. *Biochim. Biophys. Acta Biomembr.* 1513:160–166.

Giulian D. (1999). Microglia and the immune pathology of Alzheimer disease. *Am. J. Hum. Genet.* 65:13–18.

Griessbach K., Klimt M., Elfringhoff A. S., and Lehr M. (2003). Structure–activity relationship studies of 1-substituted 3-dodecanoylindole-2-carboxylic acids as inhibitors of cytosolic phospholipase A$_2$-mediated arachidonic acid release in intact platelets. *Arch. Pharm.* (Weinheim) 335:547–555.

Gronich J., Konieczkowski M., Gelb M. H., Nemenoff R. A., and Sedor J. R. (1994). Interleukin 1α causes rapid activation of cytosolic phospholipase A$_2$ by phosphorylation in rat mesangial cells. *J. Clin. Invest.* 93:1224–1233.

Gross R. W. (1998). Activation of calcium-independent phospholipase A$_2$ by depletion of internal calcium stores. *Biochem. Soc. Trans.* 26:345–349.

Guentchev M., Voigtlander T., Haberler C., Groschup M. H., and Budka H. (2000). Evidence for oxidative stress in experimental prion disease. *Neurobiol. Dis.* 7:270–273.

Hall E. D., Yonkers P. A., Andrus P. K., Cox J. W., and Anderson D. K. (1992). Biochemistry and pharmacology of lipid antioxidants in acute brain and spinal cord injury. *J. Neurotrauma* 9(Suppl. 2):S425–S442.

Hannon G. J. (2002). RNA interference. *Nature* 418:244–251.

Hansford K. A., Reid R. C., Clark C. I., Tyndall J. D., Whitehouse M. W., Guthrie T., McGeary R. P., Schafer K., Martin J. L., and Fairlie D. P. (2003). D-Tyrosine as a chiral precursor to potent inhibitors of human nonpancreatic secretory phospholipase A2 (IIa) with antiinflammatory activity. *Chembiochem* 4:181–185.

Harris J. G., Flower R. J., and Perretti M. (1995). Alteration of neutrophil trafficking by a lipocortin 1 N-terminus peptide. *Eur. J. Pharmacol.* 279:149–157.

Hashimoto M., Hossain S., Shimada T., Sugioka K., Yamasaki H., Fujii Y., Ishibashi Y., Oka J. I., and Shido O. (2002). Docosahexaenoic acid provides protection from impairment of learning ability in Alzheimer's disease model rats. *J. Neurochem.* 81:1084–1091.

Hashimoto M., Hossain S., Agdul H., and Shido O. (2005a). Docosahexaenoic acid-induced amelioration on impairment of memory learning in amyloid β-infused rats relates to the decreases of amyloid β and cholesterol levels in detergent-insoluble membrane fractions. *Biochim. Biophys. Acta Mol. Cell Biol. Lipids* 1738:91–98.

Hashimoto M., Tanabe Y., Fujii Y., Kikuta T., Shibata H., and Shido O. (2005b). Chronic administration of docosahexaenoic acid ameliorates the impairment of spatial cognition learning ability in amyloid β-infused rats. *J. Nutr.* 135:549–555.

Hernandez N. E., MacDonald J. S., Stier C. T., Belmonte A., Fernandez R., and Karpiak S. E. (1994). GM$_1$ ganglioside treatment of spontaneously hypertensive stroke prone rats. *Exp. Neurol.* 126:95–100.

Hirata M., Kohse K. P., Chang C. H., Ikebe T., and Murad F. (1990). Mechanism of cyclic GMP inhibition of inositol phosphate formation in rat aorta segments and cultured bovine aortic smooth muscle cells. *J. Biol. Chem.* 265:1268–1273.

Holscher C. (1995). Quinacrine acts like an acetylcholine receptor antagonist rather than like a phospholipase A$_2$ inhibitor in a passive avoidance task in the chick. *Neurobiol. Learn. Mem.* 63:206–208.

Hong S., Gronert K., Devchand P. R., Moussignac R. L., and Serhan C. N. (2003). Novel docosatrienes and 17S-resolvins generated from docosahexaenoic acid in murine brain, human blood, and glial cells — autacoids in anti-inflammation. *J. Biol. Chem.* 278:14677–14687.

Horrobin D. F. (2003). Eicosapentaenoic acid derivatives in the management of schizophrenia. In: Peet M., Glen L., and Horrobin D. F. (eds.), *Phospholipid Spectrum Disorders in Psychiatry and Neurology.* Marius Press, Carnforth, Lancashire, pp. 371–376.

Horrocks L. A. and Farooqui A. A. (2004). Docosahexaenoic acid in the diet: its importance in maintenance and restoration of neural membrane function. *Prostaglandins Leukot. Essent. Fatty Acids* 70:361–372.

Hossain M. S., Hashimoto M., Gamoh S., and Masumura S. (1999). Antioxidative effects of docosahexaenoic acid in the cerebrum versus cerebellum and brainstem of aged hypercholesterolemic rats. *J. Neurochem.* 72:1133–1138.

Hossain M. S., Hashimoto M., and Masumura S. (1998). Influence of docosahexaenoic acid on cerebral lipid peroxide level in aged rats with and without hypercholesterolemia. *Neurosci. Lett.* 244:157–160.

Ikeda Y., Mochizuki Y., Nakamura Y., Dohi K., Matsumoto H., Jimbo H., Hayashi M., Matsumoto K., Yoshikawa T., Murase H., and Sato K. (2000). Protective effect of a novel vitamin E derivative on experimental traumatic brain edema in rats — preliminary study. In: Mendelow A. D., Baethmann A., Czernick Z., Hoff J. T., Ito U., James H. E., Kuroiwa T., Marmarou A., Marshall L. F., and Reulen H. J. (eds.), *Brain Edema XI.* Springer-Verlag Wien, Vienna, pp. 343–345.

James M. J., Gibson R. A., and Cleland L. G. (2000). Dietary polyunsaturated fatty acids and inflammatory mediator production. *Am. J. Clin. Nutr.* 71:343S–348S.

Jenkins C. M., Han X. L., Mancuso D. J., and Gross R. W. (2002). Identification of calcium-independent phospholipase A$_2$ (iPLA$_2$β, and not iPLA$_2$γ, as the mediator of arginine vasopressin-induced arachidonic acid release in A-10 smooth muscle cells — enantioselective mechanism-based discrimination of mammalian iPLA$_2$s. *J. Biol. Chem.* 277:32807–32814.

Jeong J. Y. and Jue D. M. (1997). Chloroquine inhibits processing of tumor necrosis factor in lipopolysaccharide-stimulated RAW 264.7 macrophages. *J. Immunol.* 158:4901–4907.

Kaetzel M. A. and Dedman J. R. (1995). Annexins: novel Ca^{2+}-dependent regulators of membrane function. *News Physiol. Sci.* 10:171–176.

Kamal A. M., Flower R. J., and Perretti M. (2005). An overview of the effects of annexin 1 on cells involved in the inflammatory process. *Memorias do Instituto Oswaldo Cruz* 100:39–47.

Kambe T., Murakami M., and Kudo I. (1999). Polyunsaturated fatty acids potentiate inter-leukin-1-stimulated arachidonic acid release by cells overexpressing type IIA secretory phospholipase A_2. *FEBS Lett.* 453:81–84.

Kim S. W., Ko J., Kim J. H., Choi E. C., and Na D. S. (2001a). Differential effects of annexins I, II, III, and V on cytosolic phospholipase A_2 activity: specific interaction model. *FEBS Lett.* 489:243–248.

Kim S. W., Rhee H. J., Ko J. S., Kim Y. J., Kim H. G., Yang J. M., Choi E. C., and Na D. S. (2001b). Inhibition of cytosolic phospholipase A_2 by annexin I — specific interaction model and mapping of the interaction site. *J. Biol. Chem.* 276:15712–15719.

Kinsey G. R., Cummings B. S., Beckett C. S., Saavedra G., Zhang W. L., McHowat J., and Schnellmann R. G. (2005). Identification and distribution of endoplasmic reticulum $iPLA_2$. *Biochem. Biophys. Res. Commun.* 327:287–293.

Klatte E. T., Scharre D. W., Nagaraja H. N., Davis R. A., and Beversdorf D. Q. (2003). Combination therapy of donepezil and vitamin E in Alzheimer disease. *Alzheimer Dis. Assoc. Disord.* 17:113–116.

Kobayashi Y., Hirata K., Tanaka H., and Yamada T. (2003). [Quinacrine administration to a patient with Creutzfeldt-Jakob disease who received a cadaveric dura mater graft-an EEG evaluation]. *Rinsho Shinkeigaku* 43:403–408.

Kokotos G., Six D. A., Loukas V., Smith T., Constantinou-Kokotou., Hadjipavlou-Litina D., Kotsovolou S., Chiou A., Beltzner C. C., and Dennis E. A. (2004). Inhibition of group IVA cytosolic phospholipase A_2 by novel 2-oxoamides in vitro, in cells, and in vivo. *J. Med. Chem.* 47:3615–3628.

Korth C., May B. C., Cohen F. E., and Prusiner S. B. (2001). Acridine and phenothiazine derivatives as pharmacotherapeutics for prion disease. *Proc. Natl Acad. Sci. USA* 98:9836–9841.

Kramer B. C., Yabut J. A., Cheong J., Jnobaptiste R., Robakis T., Olanow C. W., and Mytilineou C. (2004). Toxicity of glutathione depletion in mesencephalic cultures: a role for arachidonic acid and its lipoxygenase metabolites. *Eur. J. Neurosci.* 19:280–286.

Kriem B., Sponne I., Fifre A., Malaplate-Armand C., Lozac'h-Pillot K., Koziel V., Yen-Potin F. T., Bihain B., Oster T., Olivier J. L., and Pillot T. (2004). Cytosolic phospholi-pase A_2 mediates neuronal apoptosis induced by soluble oligomers of the amyloid-beta peptide. *FASEB J.* 18:doi:10.1096/fj.04-1807fje.

Kuroiwa N., Nakamura M., Tagaya M., and Takatsuki A. (2001). Arachidonyltrifluoromethyl ketone, a phospholipase A_2 antagonist, induces dispersal of both Golgi stack- and trans Golgi network-resident proteins throughout the cytoplasm. *Biochem. Biophys. Res. Commun.* 281:582–588.

Laktionova P., Rykova E., Toni M., Spisni E., Griffoni C., Bryksin A., Volodko N., Vlassov V., and Tomasi V. (2004). Knock down of cytosolic phospholipase A2: an antisense oligonucleotide having a nuclear localization binds a C-terminal motif of glyc-eraldehyde-3-phosphate dehydrogenase. *Biochim. Biophys. Acta Mol. Cell Biol. Lipids* 1636:129–135.

Lehr M. (1996). 3-(3,5-dimethyl-4-octadecanoylpyrrol-2-yl)propionic acids as inhibitors of 85 kDa cytosolic phospholipase A_2. *Arch. Pharm.* (Weinheim) 329:483–488.

Lehr M. (1997a). Structure–activity relationship studies on (4-acylpyrrol-2-yl)alkanoic acids as inhibitors of the cytosolic phospholipase A2: Variation of the alkanoic acid substituent, the acyl chain and the position of the pyrrole nitrogen. *Eur. J. Med. Chem.* 32:805–814.

Lehr M. (1997b). Synthesis, biological evaluation, and structure–activity relationships of 3-acylindole-2-carboxylic acids as inhibitors of the cytosolic phospholipase A$_2$. *J. Med. Chem.* 40:2694–2705.

Lehr M. (2000). Cytosolic phospholipase A$_2$ as a target for drug design. *Drugs Future* 25:823–832.

Lehr M., Klimt M., and Elfringhoff A. S. (2001). Novel 3-dodecanoylindole-2-carboxylic acid inhibitors of cytosolic phospholipase A$_2$. *Bioorg. Med. Chem. Lett.* 11:2569–2572.

Liu N., Han S., Lu P. H., and Xu X. M. (2004). Upregulation of annexins I, II, and V after traumatic spinal cord injury in adult rats. *J. Neurosci. Res.* 77:391–401.

Locati M., Lamorte G., Luini W., Introna M., Bernasconi S., Mantovani A., and Sozzani S. (1996). Inhibition of monocyte chemotaxis to C–C chemokines by antisense oligonucleotide for cytosolic phospholipase A$_2$. *J. Biol. Chem.* 271:6010–6016.

Lonergan P. E., Martin D. S. D., Horrobin D. F., and Lynch M. A. (2004). Neuroprotective actions of eicosapentaenoic acid on lipopolysaccharide-induced dysfunction in rat hippocampus. *J. Neurochem.* 91:20–29.

Love R. (2001). Old drugs to treat new variant Creutzfeldt-Jakob disease. *Lancet* 358:563.

Lu X. R., Ong W. Y., Halliwell B., Horrocks L. A., and Farooqui A. A. (2001). Differential effects of calcium-dependent and calcium-independent phospholipase A$_2$ inhibitors on kainate-induced neuronal injury in rat hippocampal slices. *Free Radic. Biol. Med.* 30:1263–1273.

Maejima S. and Katayama Y. (2001). Neurosurgical trauma in Japan. *World J. Surg.* 25:1205–1209.

Mandal P. K. and Pettegrew J. W. (2004). Alzheimer's disease: NMR studies of asialo (GM1) and trisialo (GT1b) ganglioside interactions with A beta(1–40) peptide in a membrane mimic environment. *Neurochem. Res.* 29:447–453.

Maoz D., Lee H. J., Deutsch J., Rapoport S. I., and Bazinet R. P. (2005). Immediate no-flow ischemia decreases rat heart nonesterified fatty acid and increases acyl-CoA species concentrations. *Lipids* 40:1149–1154.

Marcheselli V. L., Hong S., Lukiw W. J., Tian X. H., Gronert K., Musto A., Hardy M., Gimenez J. M., Chiang N., Serhan C. N., and Bazan N. G. (2003). Novel docosanoids inhibit brain ischemia-reperfusion-mediated leukocyte infiltration and pro-inflammatory gene expression. *J. Biol. Chem.* 278:43807–43817.

Masuda S., Murakami M., Takanezawa Y., Aoki J., Arai H., Ishikawa Y., Ishii T., Arioka M., and Kudo I. (2005). Neuronal expression and neuritogenic action of group X secreted phospholipase A$_2$. *J. Biol. Chem.* 280:23203–23214.

May B. C. H., Fafarman A. T., Hong S. B., Rogers M., Deady L. W., Prusiner S. B., and Cohen F. E. (2003). Potent inhibition of scrapie prion replication in cultured cells by bis-acridines. *Proc. Natl Acad. Sci. USA* 100:3416–3421.

McKanna J. A. and Zhang M. Z. (1997). Immunohistochemical localization of lipocortin 1 in rat brain is sensitive to pH, freezing, and dehydration. *J. Histochem. Cytochem.* 45:527–538.

Meyer M. C., Rastogi P., Beckett C. S., and McHowat J. (2005). Phospholipase A$_2$ inhibitors as potential anti-inflammatory agents. *Curr. Pharm. Des.* 11:1301–1312.

Miele L. (2003). New weapons against inflammation: dual inhibitors of phospholipase A$_2$ and transglutaminase. *J. Clin. Invest.* 111:19–21.

Milhavet O., McMahon H. E., Rachidi W., Nishida N., Katamine S., Mange A., Arlotto M., Casanova D., Riondel J., Favier A., and Lehmann S. (2000). Prion infection impairs the cellular response to oxidative stress. *Proc. Natl Acad. Sci. USA* 97:13937–13942.

Mir C., Clotet J., Aledo R., Durany N., Argemi J., Lozano R., Cervos-Navarro J., and Casals N. (2003). CDP-choline prevents glutamate-mediated cell death in cerebellar granule neurons. *J. Mol. Neurosci.* 20:53–59.

Misra U. K., Gawdi G., and Pizzo S. V. (1997). Chloroquine, quinine and quinidine inhibit calcium release from macrophage intracellular stores by blocking inositol 1,4,5-trisphosphate binding to its receptor. *J. Cell. Biochem.* 64:225–232.

Moran J. M., Buller R. M. L., McHowat J., Turk J., Wohltmann M., Gross R. W., and Corbett J. A. (2005). Genetic and pharmacologic evidence that calcium-independent phospholipase $A_2\beta$ regulates virus-induced inducible nitric-oxide synthase expression by macrophages. *J. Biol. Chem.* 280:28162–28168.

Moreno J. J. (2000). Antiflammin peptides in the regulation of inflammatory response. In: Mukherjee A. B. and Chilton B. S. (eds.), *Uteroglobin/Clara Cell Protein Family*. New York Acad Sciences, New York, pp. 147–153.

Moriyama T., Urade R., and Kito M. (1999). Purification and characterization of diacylglycerol lipase from human platelets. *J. Biochem.* (Tokyo) 125:1077–1085.

Mukherjee P. K., Marcheselli V. L., Serhan C. N., and Bazan N. G. (2004). Neuroprotectin D1: a docosahexaenoic acid-derived docosatriene protects human retinal pigment epithelial cells from oxidative stress. *Proc. Natl Acad. Sci. USA* 101:8491–8496.

Murphy E. J. and Horrocks L. A. (1993). CDPcholine, CDPethanolamine, lipid metabolism and disorders of the central nervous system. In: Massarelli R., Horrocks L., Kanfer J. N., and Löffelholz K. (eds.), *Phospholipids and Signal Transmission*. Springer-Verlag GmbH, Heidelberg, pp. 353–372.

Ng C. H. and Ong W. Y. (2001). Increased expression of γ-aminobutyric acid transporters GAT-1 and GAT-3 in the spinal trigeminal nucleus after facial carrageenan injections. *Pain* 92:29–40.

Nordvik I., Myhr K. M., Nyland H., and Bjerve K. S. (2000). Effect of dietary advice and n-3 supplementation in newly diagnosed MS patients. *Acta Neurol. Scand.* 102:143–149.

Nosal R., Jancinova V., and Danihelova E. (2000). Chloroquine: a multipotent inhibitor of human platelets in vitro. *Thromb. Res.* 98:411–421.

Nozawa Y., Nakashima S., and Nagata K. (1991). Phospholipid-mediated signaling in receptor activation of human platelets. *Biochim. Biophys. Acta Lipids Lipid Metab.* 1082:219–238.

O'Donnell K. A. and Howlett A. C. (1991). Muscarinic receptor binding is inhibited by quinacrine. *Neurosci. Lett.* 127:46–48.

Ohto T., Uozumi N., Hirabayashi T., and Shimizu T. (2005). Identification of novel cytosolic phospholipase A_2s, murine cPLA$_2$δ, ε, and ζ, which form a gene cluster with cPLA$_2\beta$. *J. Biol. Chem.* 280:24576–24583.

Oinuma H., Takamura T., Hasegawa T., Nomoto K. I., Naitoh T., Daiku Y., Hamano S., Kakisawa H., and Minami N. (1991). Synthesis and biological evaluation of substituted benzenesulfonamides as novel potent membrane-bound phospholipase A_2 inhibitors. *J. Med. Chem.* 34:2260–2267.

Ong W. Y., Lu X. R., Horrocks L. A., Farooqui A. A., and Garey L. J. (2003). Induction of astrocytic cytoplasmic phospholipase A_2 and neuronal death after intracerebroventricular carrageenan injection, and neuroprotective effects of quinacrine. *Exp. Neurol.* 183:449–457.

Ono T., Yamada K., Chikazawa Y., Ueno M., Nakamoto S., Okuno T., and Seno K. (2002). Characterization of a novel inhibitor of cytosolic phospholipase A$_2\alpha$, pyrrophenone. *Biochem. J.* 363:727–735.

Ouyang Y. and Kaminski N. E. (1999). Phospholipase A$_2$ inhibitors *p*-bromophenacyl bromide and arachidonyl trifluoromethyl ketone suppressed interleukin-2 (IL-2) expression in murine primary splenocytes. *Arch. Toxicol.* 73:1–6.

Park E., Velumian A. A., and Fehlings M. G. (2004). The role of excitotoxicity in secondary mechanisms of spinal cord injury: a review with an emphasis on the implications for white matter degeneration. *J. Neurotrauma* 21:754–774.

Park J., Kwon D., Choi C., Oh J. W., and Benveniste E. N. (2003). Chloroquine induces activation of nuclear factor-κB and subsequent expression of pro-inflammatory cytokines by human astroglial cells. *J. Neurochem.* 84:1266–1274.

Peet M. and Ryles S. (2001). Eicosapentaenoic acid — a potential new treatment for schizophrenia? In: Mostofsky D. I., Yehuda S., and Salem N. (eds.), *Fatty Acids: Physiological and Behavioral Functions.* Humana Press Inc., Totowa, pp. 345–356.

Pentland A. P., Morrison A. R., Jacobs S. C., Hruza L. L., Hebert J. S., and Packer L. (1992). Tocopherol analogs suppress arachidonic acid metabolism via phospholipase inhibition. *J. Biol. Chem.* 267:15578–15584.

Pepinsky R. B., Tizard R., Mattaliano R. J., Sinclair L. K., Miller G. T., Browning J. L., Chow E. P., Burne C., Huang K.-S., Pratt D., Wachter L., Hession C., Frey A. Z., and Wallner B. P. (1988). Five distinct calcium and phospholipid binding proteins share homology with lipocortin I. *J. Biol. Chem.* 263:10799–10811.

Perretti M., Ahluwalia A., Harris J. G., Goulding N. J., and Flower R. J. (1993). Lipocortin-1 fragments inhibit neutrophil accumulation and neutrophil-dependent edema in the mouse: a qualitative comparison with an anti-CD11b monoclonal antibody. *J. Immunol.* 151:4306–4314.

Phillis J. W. and O'Regan M. H. (2004). A potentially critical role of phospholipases in central nervous system ischemic, traumatic, and neurodegenerative disorders. *Brain Res. Rev.* 44:13–47.

Pickard R. T., Strifler B. A., Kramer R. M., and Sharp J. D. (1999). Molecular cloning of two new human paralogs of 85-kDa cytosolic phospholipase A$_2$. *J. Biol. Chem.* 274:8823–8831.

Rao A. M., Hatcher J. F., and Dempsey R. J. (2001). Does CDP-choline modulate phospholipase activities after transient forebrain ischemia? *Brain Res.* 893:268–272.

Reid R. C. (2005). Inhibitors of secretory phospholipase A2 group IIA. *Curr. Med. Chem.* 12:3011–3026.

Relton J. K., Strijbos P. J. L. M., O'Shaughnessy C. T., Carey F., Forder R. A., Tilders F. J. H., and Rothwell N. J. (1991). Lipocortin-1 is an endogenous inhibitor of ischemic damage in the rat brain. *J. Exp. Med.* 174:305–310.

Reutelingsperger C. P. M. and van Heerde W. L. (1997). Annexin V, the regulator of phosphatidylserine-catalyzed inflammation and coagulation during apoptosis. *Cell Mol. Life Sci.* 53:527–532.

Riendeau D., Guay J., Weech P. K., Laliberté F., Yergey J., Li C., Desmarais S., Perrier H., Liu S., Nicoll-Griffith D., and Street I. P. (1994). Arachidonyl trifluoromethyl ketone, a potent inhibitor of 85-kDa phospholipase A$_2$, blocks production of arachidonate and 12-hydroxyeicosatetraenoic acid by calcium ionophore-challenged platelets. *J. Biochem.* 269:15619–15624.

Rintala J., Seemann R., Chandrasekaran K., Rosenberger T. A., Chang L., Contreras M. A., Rapoport S. I., and Chang M. C. J. (1999). 85 kDa cytosolic phospholipase A$_2$ is a target for chronic lithium in rat brain. *NeuroReport* 10:3887–3890.

Rogers J., Kirby L. C., Hempelman S. R., Berry D. L., McGeer P. L., Kaszniak A. W., Zalinski J., Cofield M., Mansukhani L., Willson P., et al. (1993). Clinical trial of indomethacin in Alzheimer's disease. *Neurology* 43:1609–1611.

Rosenthal M. D. and Franson R. C. (1989). Oligomers of prostaglandin B1 inhibit arachidonic acid mobilization in human neutrophils and endothelial cells. *Biochim. Biophys. Acta* 1006:278–286.

Roshak A. K., Capper E. A., Stevenson C., Eichman C., and Marshall L. A. (2000). Human calcium-independent phospholipase A_2 mediates lymphocyte proliferation. *J. Biol. Chem.* 275:35692–35698.

Roviezzo F., Getting S. J., Paul-Clark M. J., Yona S., Gavins F. N. E., Perretti M., Hannon R., Croxtall J. D., Buckingham J. C., and Flower R. J. (2002). The annexin-1 knockout mouse: what it tells us about the inflammatory response. *J. Physiol. Pharmacol.* 53:541–553.

Salvati S., Natali F., Attorri L., Raggi C., Di Biase A., and Sanchez M. (2004). Stimulation of myelin proteolipid protein gene expression by eicosapentaenoic acid in C6 glioma cells. *Neurochem. Int.* 44:331–338.

Samadi P., Gregoire L., Rouillard C., Bedard P. J., Di Paolo T., and Levesque D. (2006). Docosahexaenoic acid reduces levodopa-induced dyskinesias in 1-methyl-4-phenyl-1,2,3,6-tetrahydropyridine monkeys. *Ann. Neurol.* 59:282–288.

Sano M., Ernesto C., Thomas R. G., Klauber M. R., Schafer K., Grundman M., Woodbury P., Growdon J., Cotman D. W., Pfeiffer E., Schneider L. S., and Thal L. J. (1997). A controlled trial of selegiline, alpha-tocopherol, or both as treatment for Alzheimer's disease. *New Engl. J. Med.* 336:1216–1222.

Sapirstein A., Saito H., Texel S. J., Samad T. A., O'Leary E., and Bonventre J. V. (2005). Cytosolic phospholipase $A_2\alpha$ regulates induction of brain cyclooxygenase-2 in a mouse model of inflammation. *Am. J. Physiol. Regul. Integr. Comp. Physiol.* 288:R1774–R1782.

Savci V., Goktalay G., Cansev M., Cavun S., Yilmaz M. S., and Ulus I. H. (2003). Intravenously injected CDP-choline increases blood pressure and reverses hypotension in haemorrhagic shock: effect is mediated by central cholinergic activation. *Eur. J. Pharmacol.* 468:129–139.

Schaeffer E. L., Bassi F. J., and Gattaz W. F. (2005). Inhibition of phospholipase A_2 activity reduces membrane fluidity in rat hippocampus. *J. Neural Transm.* 112:641–647.

Schevitz R. W., Bach N. J., Carlson D. G., Chirgadze N. Y., Clawson D. K., Dillard R. D., Draheim S. E., Hartley L. W., Jones N. D., Mihelich E. D., Olkowski J. L., Snyder D. W., Sommers C., and Wery J.-P. (1995). Structure-based design of the first potent and selective inhibitor of human non-pancreatic secretory phospholipase A_2. *Nat. Struct. Biol.* 2:458–465.

Schneider J. S. (1992). MPTP-induced Parkinsonism: Acceleration of biochemical and behavioral recovery by GM_1 ganglioside treatment. *J. Neurosci. Res.* 31:112–119.

Scott K. F., Graham G. G., and Bryant K. J. (2003). Secreted phospholipase A_2 enzymes as therapeutic targets. *Expert Opin. Ther. Targets* 7:427–440.

Secades J. J. and Frontera G. (1995). CDP-choline: pharmacological and clinical review. *Methods Find. Exp. Clin. Pharmacol.* 17(Suppl. B):1–54.

Seno K., Okuno T., Nishi K., Murakami Y., Watanabe F., Matsuura T., Wada M., Fujii Y., Yamada M., Ogawa T., Okada T., Hashizume H., Kii M., Hara S., Hagishita S., Nakamoto S., Yamada K., Chikazawa Y., Ueno M., Teshirogi I., Ono T., and Ohtani M. (2000). Pyrrolidine inhibitors of human cytosolic phospholipase A_2. *J. Med. Chem.* 43:1041–1044.

Seno K., Okuno T., Nishi K., Murakami Y., Yamada K., Nakamoto S., and Ono T. (2001). Pyrrolidine inhibitors of human cytosolic phospholipase A_2. Part 2: Synthesis of potent and crystallized 4-triphenylmethylthio derivative 'pyrrophenone'. *Bioorg. Med. Chem. Lett.* 11:587–590.

Serhan C. N., Gotlinger K., Hong S., and Arita M. (2004). Resolvins, docosatrienes, and neuroprotectins, novel omega-3-derived mediators, and their aspirin-triggered endogenous epimers: an overview of their protective roles in catabasis. *Prostaglandins Other Lipid Mediat.* 73:155–172.

Shanker G. and Aschner M. (2003). Methylmercury-induced reactive oxygen species formation in neonatal cerebral astrocytic cultures is attenuated by antioxidants. *Mol. Brain Res.* 110:85–91.

Shanker G., Hampson R. E., and Aschner M. (2004). Methylmercury stimulates arachidonic acid release and cytosolic phospholipase A$_2$ expression in primary neuronal cultures. *Neurotoxicology* 25:399–406.

Shin E. J., Jhoo J. H., Kim W. K., Jhoo W. K., Lee C., Jung B. D., and Kim H. C. (2004). Protection against kainate neurotoxicity by pyrrolidine dithiocarbamate. *Clin. Exp. Pharmacol. Physiol* 31:320–326.

Shinzawa K. and Tsujimoto Y. (2003). PLA$_2$ activity is required for nuclear shrinkage in caspase-independent cell death. *J. Cell Biol.* 163:1219–1230.

Smalheiser N. R., Dissanayake S., and Kapil A. (1996). Rapid regulation of neurite outgrowth and retraction by phospholipase A$_2$-derived arachidonic acid and its metabolites. *Brain Res.* 721:39–48.

Snyder D. W., Bach N. J., Dillard R. D., Draheim S. E., Carlson D. G., Fox N., Roehm N. W., Armstrong C. T., Chang C. H., Hartley L. W., Johnson L. M., Roman C. R., Smith A. C., Song M., and Fleisch J. H. (1999). Pharmacology of LY315920/S-5920, [[3-(aminooxoacetyl)-2-ethyl-1-(phenylmethyl)-1H-indol-4-yl]oxy] acetate, a potent and selective secretory phospholipase A2 inhibitor: a new class of anti-inflammatory drugs, SPI. *J. Pharmacol. Exp. Ther.* 288:1117–1124.

Song H. W., Ramanadham S., Bao S. Z., Hsu F. F., and Turk J. (2006). A bromoenol lactone suicide substrate inactivates group VIA phospholipase A$_2$ by generating a diffusible bromomethyl keto acid that alkylates cysteine thiols. *Biochemistry* 45:1061–1073.

Springer D. M. (2001). An update on inhibitors of human 14 kDa Type II s-PLA$_2$ in development. *Curr. Pharm. Des.* 7:181–198.

St-Gelais F., Ménard C., Congar P., Trudeau L. E., and Massicotte G. (2004). Postsynaptic injection of calcium-independent phospholipase A2 inhibitors selectively increases AMPA receptor-mediated synaptic transmission. *Hippocampus* 14:319–325.

Stahelin R. V., Hwang J. H., Kim J. H., Park Z. Y., Johnson K. R., Obeid L. M., and Cho W. H. (2005). The mechanism of membrane targeting of human sphingosine kinase 1. *J. Biol. Chem.* 280:43030–43038.

Stewart L. R., White A. R., Jobling M. F., Needham B. E., Maher F., Thyer J., Beyreuther K., Masters C. L., Collins S. J., and Cappai R. (2001). Involvement of the 5-lipoxygenase pathway in the neurotoxicity of the prion peptide PrP106–126. *J. Neurosci. Res.* 65:565–572.

Street I. P., Lin H. K., Laliberté F., Ghomashchi F., Wang Z., Perrier H., Tremblay N. M., Huang Z., Weech P. K., and Gelb M. H. (1993). Slow- and tight-binding inhibitors of the 85-kDa human phospholipase A$_2$. *Biochemistry* 32:5935–5940.

Struhar D., Kivity S., and Topilsky M. (1992). Quinacrine inhibits oxygen radicals release from human alveolar macrophages. *Int. J. Immunopharmacol.* 14:275–277.

Sung S., Yao Y., Uryu K., Yang H., Lee V. M., Trojanowski J. Q., and Pratico D. (2004). Early vitamin E supplementation in young but not aged mice reduces Aβ levels and amyloid deposition in a transgenic model of Alzheimer's disease. *FASEB J.* 18:323–325.

Svennerholm L. (1994). Gangliosides — a new therapeutic agent against stroke and Alzheimer's disease. *Life Sci.* 55:2125–2134.

Svensson C. I., Lucas K. K., Hua X. Y., Powell H. C., Dennis E. A., and Yaksh T. L. (2005). Spinal phospholipase A$_2$ in inflammatory hyperalgesia: role of the small, secretory phospholipase A$_2$. *Neuroscience* 133:543–553.

Tagami M., Ikeda K., Yamagata K., Nara Y., Fujino H., Kubota A., Numano F., and Yamori Y. (1999). Vitamin E prevents apoptosis in hippocampal neurons caused by cerebral ischemia and reperfusion in stroke-prone spontaneously hypertensive rats. *Lab. Invest.* 79:609–615.

Tanaka H., Takeya R., and Sumimoto H. (2000). A novel intracellular membrane-bound calcium-independent phospholipase A$_2$. *Biochem. Biophys. Res. Commun.* 272:320–326.

Tanaka H., Minakami R., Kanaya H., and Sumimoto H. (2004). Catalytic residues of group VIB calcium-independent phospholipase A$_2$ (iPLA$_2$γ). *Biochem. Biophys. Res. Commun.* 320:1284–1290.

Tariq M., Khan H. A., Al Moutaery K., and Al Deeb S. (2001). Protective effect of quinacrine on striatal dopamine levels in 6-OHDA and MPTP models of Parkinsonism in rodents. *Brain Res. Bull.* 54:77–82.

Teather L. A. and Wurtman R. J. (2005). Dietary CDP-choline supplementation prevents memory impairment caused by impoverished environmental conditions in rats. *Learn. Memory* 12:39–43.

Terano T., Fujishiro S., Ban T., Yamamoto K., Tanaka T., Noguchi Y., Tamura Y., Yazawa K., and Hirayama T. (1999). Docosahexaenoic acid supplementation improves the moderately severe dementia from thrombotic cerebrovascular diseases. *Lipids* 34(Suppl.):S345–S346.

Tietge U. J. F., Maugeais C., Cain W., Grass D., Glick J. M., de Beer F. C., and Rader D. J. (2000). Overexpression of secretory phospholipase A$_2$ causes rapid catabolism and altered tissue uptake of high density lipoprotein cholesteryl ester and apolipoprotein A-I. *J. Biol. Chem.* 275:10077–10084.

Tietge U. J. F., Maugeais C., Lund-Katz S., Grass D., deBeer F. C., and Rader D. J. (2002). Human secretory phospholipase A$_2$ mediates decreased plasma levels of HDL cholesterol and apoA-I in response to inflammation in human apoA-I transgenic mice. *Arterioscler. Thromb. Vasc. Biol.* 22:1213–1218.

Tramposch K. M., Steiner S. A., Stanley P. L., Nettleton D. O., Franson R. C., Lewin A. H., and Carroll F. I. (1992). Novel inhibitor of phospholipase A$_2$ with topical anti-inflammatory activity. *Biochem. Biophys. Res. Commun.* 189:272–279.

Tramposch K. M., Chilton F. H., Stanley P. L., Franson R. C., Havens M. B., Nettleton D. O., Davern L. B., Darling I. M., and Bonney R. J. (1994). Inhibitor of phospholipase A$_2$ blocks eicosanoid and platelet activating factor biosynthesis and has topical anti-inflammatory activity. *J. Pharmacol. Exp. Ther.* 271:852–859.

Tran K., Wong J. T., Lee E., Chan A. C., and Choy P. C. (1996). Vitamin E potentiates arachidonate release and phospholipase A$_2$ activity in rat heart myoblastic cells. *Biochem. J.* 319:385–391.

Trimble L. A., Street I. P., Perrier H., Tremblay N. M., Weech P. K., and Bernstein M. A. (1993). NMR structural studies of the tight complex between a trifluoromethyl ketone inhibitor and the 85-kDa human phospholipase A$_2$. *Biochemistry* 32:12560–12565.

Tseng A., Inglis A. S., and Scott K. F. (1996). Native peptide inhibition. Specific inhibition of type II phospholipases A$_2$ by synthetic peptides derived from the primary sequence. *J. Biol. Chem.* 271:23992–23998.

Turnbull S., Tabner B. J., Brown D. R., and Allsop D. (2003). Quinacrine acts as an antioxidant and reduces the toxicity of the prion peptide PrP106–126. *NeuroReport* 14:1743–1745.

Van Gool W. A., Weinstein H. C., Scheltens P., Walstra G. J., and Scheltens P. K. (2001). Effect of hydroxychloroquine on progression of dementia in early Alzheimer's disease: an 18-month randomised, double-blind, placebo-controlled study. *Lancet* 358:455–460.

Vanags D. M., Larsson P., Feltenmark S., Jakobsson P. J., Orrenius S., Claesson H. E., and Aguilar-Santelises M. (1997). Inhibitors of arachidonic acid metabolism reduce DNA and nuclear fragmentation induced by TNF plus cycloheximide in U937 cells. *Cell Death Differ.* 4:479–486.

Varghese, J., Rydel, R. E., Dappen, M. S., and Thorsett, E. D. (2003). Substituted pyrimidine compositions and methods of use. U.S. Patent 6,518,424. *Elan* Pharmaceuticals, Inc.

Vogtherr M., Grimme S., Elshorst B., Jacobs D. M., Fiebig K., Griesinger C., and Zahn R. (2003). Antimalarial drug quinacrine binds to C-terminal helix of cellular prion protein. *J. Med. Chem.* 46:3563–3564.

Wahler G. M., Rusch N. J., and Sperelakis N. (1990). 8-Bromo-cyclic GMP inhibits the calcium channel current in embryonic chick ventricular myocytes. *Can. J. Physiol. Pharmacol.* 68:531–534.

Walsh D. M. and Selkoe D. J. (2004). Deciphering the molecular basis of memory failure in Alzheimer's disease. *Neuron* 44:181–193.

Walters E. T. (1994). Injury-related behavior and neuronal plasticity: an evolutionary perspective on sensitization, hyperalgesia, and analgesia. *Int. Rev. Neurobiol.* 36:325–427.

Wambebe C., Sokomba E., and Amabeoku G. (1990). Effect of quinine on electroshock and pentylenetetrazol-induced seizures in mice. *Prog. Neuropsychopharmacol. Biol. Psychiatry* 14:121–127.

Wang X. and Robinson P. J. (1997). Cyclic GMP-dependent protein kinase and cellular signaling in the nervous system. *J. Neurochem.* 68:443–456.

Wang Y., Zhou X., Wang B. H., Chen L. D., Zhang J., and Cao J. X. (2004). Cytosolic phospholipase A_2 mediates MM-LDL-induced apoptosis in human umbilical vein endothelial cells. *Prog. Biochem. Biophys.* 31:350–355.

Weber S. M., Chen J. M., and Levitz S. M. (2002). Inhibition of mitogen-activated protein kinase signaling by chloroquine. *J. Immunol.* 168:5303–5309.

Weerasinghe G. R., Rapoport S. I., and Bosetti F. (2004). The effect of chronic lithium on arachidonic acid release and metabolism in rat brain does not involve secretory phospholipase A_2 or lipoxygenase/cytochrome P450 pathways. *Brain Res. Bull.* 63:485–489.

Wolf M. J., Izumi Y., Zorumski C. F., and Gross R. W. (1995). Long-term potentiation requires activation of calcium-independent phospholipase A_2. *FEBS Lett.* 377:358–362.

Won J. S., Im Y. B., Khan M., Singh A. K., and Singh I. (2005). Involvement of phospholipase A_2 and lipoxygenase in lipopolysaccharide-induced inducible nitric oxide synthase expression in glial cells. *Glia* 51:13–21.

Wurtman R. J., Sandage B. W., Jr., and Warach S. (1996). Advances in understanding cholinergic brain neurons: implications in the use of citicoline (CDP-choline) to treat stroke. In: Becker R. and Giacobini E. (eds.), *Alzheimer Disease: from Molecular Biology to Therapy.* Birkhauser, Boston, pp. 179–185.

Yagi K., Shirai Y., Hirai M., Sakai N., and Saito N. (2004). Phospholipase A2 products retain a neuron specific γ isoform of PKC on the plasma membrane through the C1 domain – a molecular mechanism for sustained enzyme activity. *Neurochem. Int.* 45:39–47.

Yamashita A., Kamata R., Kawagishi N., Nakanishi H., Suzuki H., Sugiura T., and Waku K. (2005). Roles of C-terminal processing, and involvement in transacylation reaction of human group IVC phospholipase A_2 (cPLA$_2\gamma$). *J. Biochem.* 137:557–567.

Yang H.-C., Farooqui A. A., and Horrocks L. A. (1994a). Effects of glycosaminoglycans and glycosphingolipids on cytosolic phospholipases A$_2$ from bovine brain. *Biochem. J.* 299:91–95.

Yang H.-C., Farooqui A. A., and Horrocks L. A. (1994b). Effects of sialic acid and sialo-glycoconjugates on cytosolic phospholipases A$_2$ from bovine brain. *Biochem. Biophys. Res. Commun.* 199:1158–1166.

Yeo J. F., Ong W. Y., Ling S. F., and Farooqui A. A. (2004). Intracerebroventricular injection of phospholipases A$_2$ inhibitors modulates allodynia after facial carrageenan injection in mice. *Pain* 112:148–155.

Yoo M. H., Woo C. H., You H. J., Cho S. H., Kim B. C., Choi J. E., Chun J. S., Jhun B. H., Kim T. S., and Kim J. H. (2001). Role of the cytosolic phospholipase A$_2$-linked cascade in signaling by an oncogenic, constitutively active Ha-Ras isoform. *J. Biol. Chem.* 276:24645–24653.

Yoshinaga N., Yasuda Y., Murayama T., and Nomura Y. (2000). Possible involvement of cytosolic phospholipase A$_2$ in cell death induced by 1-methyl-4-phenylpyridinium ion, a dopaminergic neurotoxin, in GH3 cells. *Brain Res.* 855:244–251.

Young K. A., Hirst W. D., Solito E., and Wilkin G. P. (1999). De novo expression of lipocortin-1 in reactive microglia and astrocytes in kainic acid lesioned rat cerebellum. *Glia* 26:333–343.

Yue H. Y., Fujita T., and Kumamoto E. (2005). Phospholipase A$_2$ activation by melittin enhances spontaneous glutamatergic excitatory transmission in rat substantia gelatinosa neurons. *Neuroscience* 135:485–495.

Yuen A. W. C., Sander J. W., Fluegel D., Patsalos P. N., Bell G. S., Johnson T., and Koepp M. J. (2005). Omega-3 fatty acid supplementation in patients with chronic epilepsy: A randomized trial. *Epilepsy Behav.* 7:253–258.

Zeiher B. G., Steingrub J., Laterre P. F., Dmitrienko A., Fukiishi Y., and Abraham E. (2005). LY315920NA/S-5920, a selective inhibitor of group IIA secretory phospholipase A$_2$, fails to improve clinical outcome for patients with severe sepsis. *Crit. Care Med.* 33:1741–1748.

Zhang B., Tanaka J., Yang L., Yang L., Sakanaka M., Hata R., Maeda N., and Mitsuda N. (2004). Protective effect of vitamin E against focal brain ischemia and neuronal death through induction of target genes of hypoxia-inducible factor-1. *Neuroscience* 126:433–440.

Zhao Y., Joshi-Barve S., Barve S., and Chen L. H. (2004). Eicosapentaenoic acid prevents LPS-induced TNF-α expression by preventing NF-κB activation. *J. Am. Coll. Nutr.* 23:71–78.

Zouki C., Ouellet S., and Filep J. G. (2000). The anti-inflammatory peptides, antiflammins, regulate the expression of adhesion molecules on human leukocytes and prevent neutrophil adhesion to endothelial cells. *FASEB J.* 14:572–580.

12
Assay Methods for Phospholipase A$_2$ Activities in Brain

12.1 Assay Methods

Two major problems complicate studies on the isolation and characterization of brain PLA$_2$. First, the activities of these enzymes in the brain tissue are quite low when compared with other hydrolytic enzymes. Second, assays for PLA$_2$ activities are complex, laborious, and time consuming. Furthermore, progress on the development of rapid and sensitive assay procedures for these enzymes has been quite slow. The development of rapid and sensitive PLA$_2$ assay procedures requires the selection of a glycerophospholipid substrate with appropriate interfacial properties (physical form) in aqueous solution, an appropriate procedure for the separation of substrate from products, and finally the quantitation of the product generated by PLA$_2$ (Reynolds et al., 1991).

Several methods for the assay of PLA$_2$ activity have been described (Table 12.1) (Aarsman and van den Bosch, 1979; Cox and Horrocks, 1981; Farooqui et al., 1984; Hendrickson, 1994). These methods include titrimetric, radiochemical, spectrophotometric, fluorometric, and immunological procedures (Farooqui and Horrocks, 1988). Radiochemical procedures are sensitive, but suffer from the disadvantage of being discontinuous, requiring separation of the radiochemical substrate from the labeled products. They are also time-consuming and expensive. Furthermore, handling radioactive compounds is undesirable, due to safety issues and the high cost of radioactive materials, and because of high disposal costs for long-lived radioactive material.

Although continuous and discontinuous spectrophotometric and fluorometric assay procedures are less sensitive than radiochemical procedures, they are preferred because of their rapidity, reliability, reproducibility, and availability of their substrates in large quantities at a low cost. However, these assays require the use of nonphysiological substrates. These substrates include thioester analogs of glycerophospholipid substrates (Aarsman and van den Bosch, 1979; Farooqui et al., 1984; Farooqui and Horrocks, 1988; Reynolds et al., 1994; Fuji et al., 1997) and analogs of glycerophospholipid substrates with a fluorescent label (Hendrickson, 1994). With the discovery of various PLA$_2$ isoforms, many assay procedures with different fluorophores and coupling procedures for the detection

TABLE 12.1. Assay procedures used for the determination of PLA$_2$ isoforms and their kinetic properties.

PLA$_2$ isoform	Method	Substrate	pH optimum	Km value (μM)	V$_{max}$ (nmol/ min/mg)	Reference
cPLA$_2$ (human)	Spectrophotometric	1	7.4	830	0.28	Reynolds et al., 1994
sPLA$_2$ (hog)	Spectrophotometric	2	8.5	4.5	1,800	Jiménez et al., 2003
PlsEtn-PLA$_2$ (*Naja naja*)	Spectrophotometric	3	7.2	–	0.040	Hirashima et al., 1989b
sPLA$_2$ (*Naja naja*)	Spectrophotometric	4	8.5	1890	99,600	Yu et al., 1998
sPLA$_2$ (human)	Fluorometric	5	9.0	13	77	Blanchard et al., 1998
cPLA$_2$ (human)	Fluorometric	6	8.0	–	117	Huang et al., 1994
cPLA$_2$ (bovine brain)	Fluorometric	7	7.4	29	13	Hirashima et al., 1992
PlsEtn-PLA$_2$ (bovine brain)	Fluorometric	8	8.0	70	36	Hirashima et al., 1992
Lyso- plasmalogenase (rat liver)	Fluorometric	9	7.4	15	121	Hirashima et al., 1989a

Substrates: 2-*S*-arachidonoyl-1-*O*-hexadecyl-*sn*-2-thioglycero-3-*O*-phosphocholine (1); [dilinoleoyl] phosphatidylcholine (2); 1-alkenyl-2-acyl-Gro*P*Cho (3); 1-decanoyl-2-octylcarbonothioyl-*sn*-glycero-3-phosphocholine (4); 1-acyl-2-(*N*-4-nitrobenzo-2-oxo-1,3-diazole)aminododecanoyl-*sn*-Gro*P*Cho (5); 7-hydroxycoumarinyl γ-linolenate (6); 1,2-diacyl-*sn*-Gro*P*Etn(Pyr) (7); 1-alk-1-enyl-2-acyl-*sn*-Gro*P*Etn(Pyr) (8); and 1-alk-1-enyl-*sn*-Gro*P*Cho (9).

of products generated by PLA$_2$ exist. Continuous spectrophotometric and fluorometric assay procedures are available for sPLA$_2$, cPLA$_2$, PlsEtn-PLA$_2$, iPLA$_2$, and lysoplasmalogenase (Hirashima et al., 1989a, 1990; Reynolds et al., 1994; Hendrickson, 1994; Farooqui et al., 1999). PLA$_2$ assay procedures were designed with specific inhibitors to distinguish various isoforms in biological samples (Yang et al., 1999; Lucas and Dennis, 2005).

12.2 Titrimetric Procedures

In this method, the released fatty acid is continuously titrated at constant pH and the activity of PLA$_2$ is calculated from the recorded alkali consumption. This method can be used with a pH stat for determining initial velocities of reactions catalyzed by PLA$_2$ (De Haas et al., 1971; Wells, 1972). It is restricted to neural or alkaline pH values because of the pKa value of the released fatty acid. Thus, at pH 6.0 and 5.0, the titration efficiencies are about 90% and 50%, respectively. This assay cannot be performed at acidic pH values, because at the acidic pH value the released fatty acid is not sufficiently ionized. Even at neutral and alkaline pH values, this procedure is not very sensitive. The lower limit of detection is about 50 to 100 nmol/min. Thus, it cannot be applied to tissue homogenates, cultured cells, and subcellular fractions that usually display activities in the order of 1 to 5 nmol/min/mg protein. This procedure can be used for the determination of extracellular PLA$_2$ activity, such as that present in pancreatic juice and snake venom. In this procedure the released fatty acids are detected by either observing the amount of base consumed or through the conversion of fatty acid to Cu-soaps, which are measured in a spectrophotometer after reaction with diethyl dithiocarbamate (Duncombe, 1963). Collectively, these studies suggest that titrimetric assay methods are continuous, straightforward, and use natural substrates, but suffer from low sensitivity and limitation of the pH range.

12.3 Radiochemical Procedures

Radiochemical procedures are the most sensitive methods for the determination of activities of PLA$_2$ isoforms in brain homogenates, cell culture preparations, and subcellular fractions. These procedures require the use of radiolabeled glycerophospholipids, which can be either synthesized (Farooqui and Horrocks, 1988) or obtained commercially. The sensitivity of radiochemical procedures depends on the specific radioactivity of the labeled glycerophospholipids. Commercially available ^{3}H- or ^{14}C-labeled glycerophospholipids have specific activities of 50 to 100 mCi/mmol (DuPont NEN, Boston and Amersham Life Science, Arlington Heights, IL), which correspond to detection limits of about 1 fmol and 1 pmol, respectively. Radiochemical procedures are discontinuous, laborious, and time consuming. These procedures require separation of the radioactive substrate from the radioactive products. Briefly, labeled glycerophospholipids and their hydrolysis products, lyso glycerophospholipids and labeled fatty acids, are extracted (Bligh and Dyer, 1959) using chloroform, methanol, and acetic acid followed by TLC. Spots are visualized, identified using standards, scraped into scintillation fluid, and counted. Radiolabeled substrates and fatty acids can also be separated by the Dole extraction procedure (Dole, 1956) using 2-propanol, heptane, and sulfuric acid. This separation procedure is not as efficient as the TLC procedure. Although the majority of glycerophospholipids and lyso glycerophospholipids generated by PLA$_2$ remain in the aqueous phase, small portions are always extracted into the heptane phase and interfere with the measurement of radioactivity in fatty acids. Furthermore, interference problems can be encountered in studies requiring the use of PLA$_2$ inhibitors. Many PLA$_2$ inhibitors are amphiphilic and therefore can interfere with the Dole extraction procedure and give false values.

The use of radioiodinatable 1-fatty acyl-2-(12-(3-(4-hydroxyphenyl)propionyl) amino dodecanoyl)-GroPCho (BHC12-PtdCho) (Fig. 12.1) as a substrate was

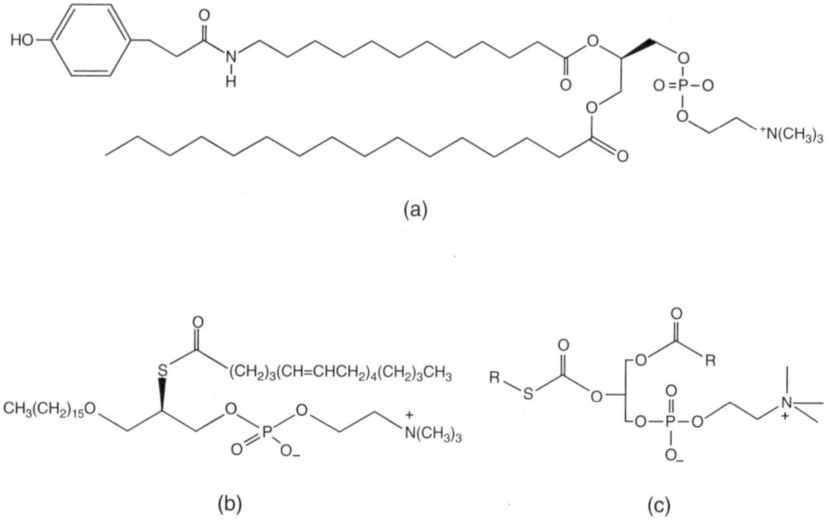

FIG. 12.1. Chemical structures of 1-fatty acyl-2-(12-(3-(4-hydroxyphenyl)propionyl) aminododecanoyl)-sn-GroPCho (BHC12-PtdCho) (a); 2-S-arachidonyl-1-O-hexadecyl-sn-2-thio-GroPCho (b); and a carbonothioate glycerophospholipid analog (c).

recently proposed (Caramelo and Delfino, 2004). Attachment of a 4-hydroxy-phenyl group at the end of fatty acyl chain located at the sn-2-position of PtdCho enables its radioiodination with Na[^{135}I] in the presence of chloramine T. The radioiodinated BHC12-PtdCho resembles natural PtdCho in its interfacial and other physical properties (Caramelo and Delfino, 2004). *Naja naja naja* PLA$_2$ hydrolyzes it in a dose and time-dependent manner in the presence of Triton-X-100. The progress of the reaction can be monitored either by TLC or by an alternative method based on the selective adsorption of BHC12-PtdCho to silica gel. An additional advantage of this procedure is that the cost of ^{135}I-labeled BHC12-PtdCho is significantly lower than that of ^{3}H, ^{14}C, or ^{32}P-labeled PtdCho.

12.4 Spectrophotometric Procedures

12.4.1 Use of Thioester Substrate Analogs

Spectrophotometric methods are less sensitive than radiochemical procedures, but they have an advantage over radiochemical procedures in that the spec-trophotometric substrate can be synthesized in large quantities at a lower cost than the radioactive counterpart. Continuous spectrophotometric methods permit the easy calculation of initial velocity from recorder tracings. Spectrophotometric procedures require chemical modification of the native glycerophospholipid sub-strates, because the action of PLA$_2$ on the native glycerophospholipid generates reaction products, i.e., lyso glycerophospholipids and fatty acids that are not detectable spectrophotometrically. Aarsman and van den Bosch (1977) developed a continuous spectrophotometric assay procedure for PLA$_2$ using thioester substrate analogs. Initially, they synthesized a glycol analog of PtdCho with a thioester linkage in place of an oxyester linkage. Hydrolysis of this substrate by PLA$_2$ produces a thiol group, which is detected continuously by the increase in absorption using thiol reagents. The yellow chromophore produced during this reaction can be monitored continuously at 412 nm (Fig. 12.2). Two thiol reagents, 5,5-dithiobis(2-nitrobenzoic acid) (DTNB) and 4,4-dithiobispyridine (DTP), are commonly used to detect free thiol groups. The selection of the thiol reagent for the assay procedure depends on several factors, including solubility in water, extinction coefficient, and effect on the enzymic activity.

The thioester substrate analog procedure has several advantages over titrimetric and radiochemical procedures. Assays with thioester substrates are convenient, fast, continuous, and inexpensive. This assay procedure can be used for the determination of activities of PLA$_2$ isoforms in a large number of samples. Thioester substrate analogs for PtdCho can be either synthesized (Farooqui and Horrocks, 1988; Reynolds et al., 1994) or obtained commercially. The hydrolysis of thioester substrate analogs by PLA$_2$ follows simple Michaelis–Menten kinetics and can be used for the assay of sPLA$_2$ as well as cPLA$_2$ activities in neural and nonneural tissues (Farooqui et al., 1984; Yu and Dennis, 1991; Reynolds et al., 1994). The procedures are simple, rapid, and convenient and all reagents including substrate are available commercially at a low cost.

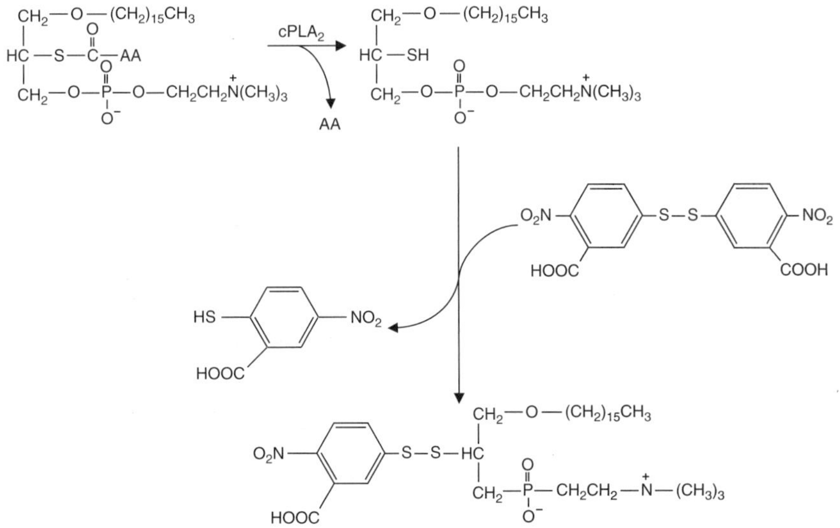

FIG. 12.2. Hydrolysis of 2-S-arachidonoyl-1-O-hexadecyl-sn-2-thio-GroPCho by cPLA$_2$ and reaction of DTNB with the thiol group of a lysoglycerophospholipid product.

An excellent use of thioester substrates for cPLA₂ assays was made with a microtiter plate assay procedure using 1-hexadecyl-2-arachidonoyl-thio-2-deoxy-sn-glycero-3-phosphocholine (Reynolds et al., 1994). This procedure utilizes 30% glycerol, 4 mM Triton-X-100, 10 mM calcium chloride, and 1 mg/ml bovine serum albumin to solubilize, stabilize, and optimize the hydrolysis of the thio substrate. This assay of cPLA₂ follows normal Michaelis–Menten kinetics. This procedure can be used for the determination of cPLA₂ activity in a large number of samples in a short time at a very low cost. It is also useful for routine screening of cPLA₂ activities in biological samples and column eluates during the purification of cPLA₂ (Farooqui and Horrocks, 1988; Reynolds et al., 1994).

The most serious drawback of the thioester substrate assay is the necessity for reagents to capture the liberated thiols. These reagents may inhibit those PLA₂ isoforms that require sulfhydryl groups for their activity. Although cPLA₂ has a hidden thiol group that participates in the reaction catalyzed by cPLA₂, blocking with thiol reagents or iodoacetate requires preincubation of enzyme with thiol reagents. In assay procedures using microtiter plates that do not require preincubation with thiol reagents, there is no interference. Mercaptoethanol or dithiothreitol cannot be included during enzyme purification.

Carbonothioate glycerophospholipids have been used for assays of cobra venom PLA₂ activity (Yu et al., 1998). The hydrolysis of carbonothioate glycerophospholipids by PLA₂ generates an alkyl mercaptan. As in thioester substrate procedures, the formation of an alkyl mercaptan can be monitored continuously by following the release of free thiol using DTNB (Figs. 12.1 and 12.2). Carbonothioate glycerophospholipids, similar to natural glycerophospholipids, exhibit an interfacial activation phenomenon. Their hydrolysis follows simple Michaelis–Menten kinetics (Yu et al., 1998). Although this assay is simple, reproducible, and convenient, it requires a higher concentration of enzyme than that used in the thioester assay.

12.4.2 Use of Coupled Enzyme Assays

Coupled enzyme assays have been developed for PLA₂ hydrolyzing PtdCho (Jiménez et al., 2003). In this coupling assay procedure, dilinoleoyl-GroPCho is the PLA₂ substrate, hog pancreatic PLA₂ is the enzyme source (500 U/mg), and soybean lipoxygenase (1,000,000 U/mg) is the coupling enzyme. Lipoxygenase oxidizes the linoleic acid released by PLA₂. PLA₂ activity is followed spectrophotometrically by measuring the increase in absorbance at 234 nm due to the formation of the corresponding hydroperoxide from the linoleic acid (Jiménez et al., 2003). This method provides a continuous record of glycerophospholipid hydrolysis. It is specific because the record shows no activity in the absence of PLA₂. This procedure is reproducible and requires a short analysis time with a straightforward measurement technique. All reagents are available commercially and are inexpensive. Due to the high value for the extinction coefficient of the hydroperoxide at 234 nm ($\varepsilon_{234} = 25{,}000\ \mathrm{M^{-1}\ cm^{-1}}$), the limit of sensitivity is about 0.4 nmol/ml of the product (Jiménez et al., 2003).

The coupling assay for plasmalogen selective-PLA$_2$ (Hirashima et al., 1989b; Jurkowitz-Alexander et al., 1991) is a continuous spectrophotometric procedure that requires rat liver lysoplasmalogenase and horse liver alcohol dehydrogenase as coupling enzymes (Fig. 12.3). *Naja naja* venom PLA$_2$ was used as a source of PLA$_2$ activity (Jurkowitz-Alexander and Horrocks, 1990; Hirashima et al., 1990). PLA$_2$ hydrolyzes choline plasmalogens yielding lyso plasmalogens, which lysoplasmalogenase cleaves into glycerophosphocholine and free aldehyde. Alcohol dehydrogenase quantitatively converts the free aldehyde to an alcohol with the concomitant oxidation of NADH. The disappearance of NADH is measured continuously with a spectrophotometer at 340 nm. The assay is rapid, convenient, and sensitive to about 0.2 nmol aldehyde/ml/min. All reagents can be purchased commercially except choline plasmalogen and lysoplasmalogenase, which can be prepared by adequately described, well-established procedures (Hirashima et al., 1990; Jurkowitz-Alexander et al., 1991).

The coupling assay for lysoplasmalogenase requires choline lysoplasmalogen as substrate and alcohol dehydrogenase as a coupling enzyme. Rat liver lysoplasmalogenase was the PLA$_2$ source. In this assay, formation of the fatty aldehyde is measured directly by coupling with alcohol dehydrogenase. The rate of fatty aldehyde formation is directly proportional to the loss of NADH that is monitored by the decrease in absorbance at 340 nm. In this assay, the amount of alcohol dehydrogenase is chosen to ensure that it is not rate-limiting. This procedure is simple, rapid, convenient, and reproducible. All reagents are available commercially except the lysoplasmalogenase that is assayed (Jurkowitz-Alexander and Horrocks, 1990).

A continuous spectrofluorometric assay for the determination of lysoplasmalogenase using horse liver alcohol dehydrogenase as a coupling enzyme was also developed (Hirashima et al., 1989a). During this assay, lysoplasmalogenase hydrolyzes lysoPlsCho to GroPCho and free aldehyde. Alcohol dehydrogenase quantitatively converts the free aldehyde to an alcohol with oxidation of the NADH. NADH is fluorescent, whereas NAD$^+$ is not; hence the disappearance of NADH is measured spectrofluorometrically at 340 nm (excitation) and 460 nm

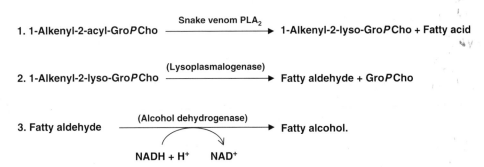

FIG. 12.3. This scheme shows the coupling between a PLA$_2$ and the fatty aldehyde generated by lysoplasmalogenase and alcohol dehydrogenase.

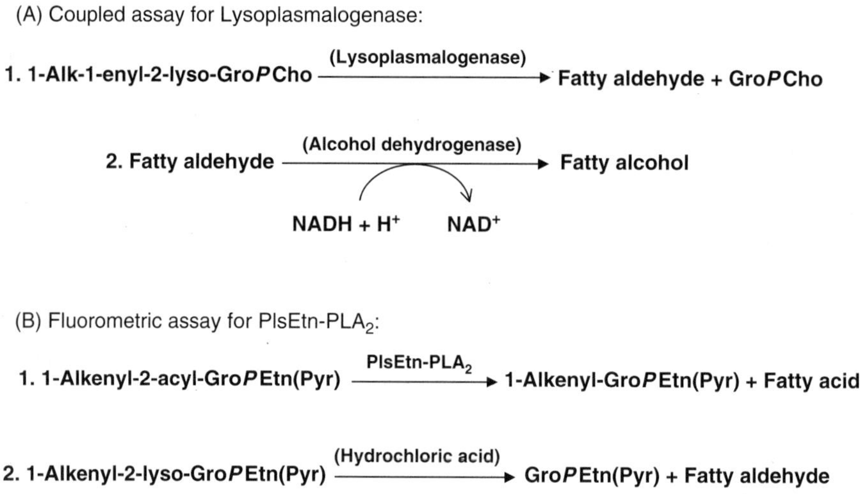

(A) Coupled assay for Lysoplasmalogenase:

(Lysoplasmalogenase)

1. 1-Alk-1-enyl-2-lyso-Gro$P$Cho ⎯⎯⎯⎯⎯⎯⎯⎯⎯⎯→ **Fatty aldehyde + Gro$P$Cho**

(Alcohol dehydrogenase)

2. Fatty aldehyde ⎯⎯⎯⎯⎯⎯⎯⎯⎯⎯→ **Fatty alcohol**

NADH + H$^+$ **NAD$^+$**

(B) Fluorometric assay for PlsEtn-PLA$_2$:

PlsEtn-PLA$_2$

1. 1-Alkenyl-2-acyl-Gro$P$Etn(Pyr) ⎯⎯⎯⎯⎯⎯⎯⎯→ **1-Alkenyl-Gro$P$Etn(Pyr) + Fatty acid**

(Hydrochloric acid)

2. 1-Alkenyl-2-lyso-Gro$P$Etn(Pyr) ⎯⎯⎯⎯⎯⎯⎯⎯→ **Gro$P$Etn(Pyr) + Fatty aldehyde**

Fɪɢ. 12.4. The principle behind fluorometric assays of lysoplasmalogenase and plasmalo-gen-selective PLA$_2$. This scheme shows the reactions involved in the fluorometric assay of lysoplasmalogenase (A) and the action of plasmalogen-selective-PLA$_2$ on pyrene-labeled 1-alkenyl-2-acyl-*sn*-Gro$P$Etn and subsequent generation of fatty aldehyde by hydrochloric acid vapors (B).

(emission) (Fig. 12.4A). This assay procedure is 10-fold more sensitive than a spectrophotometric procedure (Hirashima et al., 1989a). The lower limit of detection is 20 pmol/min/ml.

12.5 Fluorometric Procedures

Both continuous and discontinuous fluorometric procedures have been described for the determination of sPLA$_2$, cPLA$_2$, plasmalogen-selective PLA$_2$, and lyso-plasmalogenase activities in the brain tissue (Hirashima et al., 1989a,b, 1990; Hendrickson, 1994; Farooqui et al., 1999). In the continuous assay, the hydroly-sis of fluorophore-labeled glycerophospholipid substrate by PLA$_2$ is monitored by measuring changes in the fluorescence properties of the fluorophore (Hendrickson and Rauk, 1981). Fluorophore-labeled glycerophospholipid can be synthesized (Sunamoto et al., 1980), or can be bought commercially from Molecular Probes, Eugene, OR. Several factors should be considered for the flu-orometric determination of PLA$_2$. These factors include the interfacial properties of the fluorophore-labeled glycerophospholipids, perturbing effects of the fluo-rophore, and intrinsic substrate specificity of the PLA$_2$ isoforms. Assays of enzymic activity by continuous fluorescence assay procedures depend on a change in the fluorescence properties of the probe as PLA$_2$ isoforms hydrolyze the substrate. Several probes including dansyl; pyrene; 4,4-difluoro-4-bora-3α, 4α-diaza-S-indacene (BODIPY); 7-hydroxycoumarin; 7-nitrobenzo-2-oxa-1, 3-diazol-4-yl (NBD); and naphthyl groups have been used for the synthesis of PLA_2 substrates (Fig. 12.5). The sensitivity of substrate probe substrates in a nonpolar environment is different from that in the polar environment of the probe in the product (Hendrickson, 1994). This property facilitates the rapid detection of fluorescent product. Pyrene is the most frequently used fluorophore for PLA_2 assays. Its most characteristic features are a long excised state lifetime and concentration-dependent formation of excimers (Somerharju, 2002). Pyrene is hydrophobic and its attachment does not significantly distort the conformation of the labeled glycerophospholipid molecule. Its monomer emits at 382 and 400 nm, but as an excited dimer its emission shifts from 400 to 480 nm. Thus, the assay of PLA_2 activity utilizes excimer emitting pyrene-labeled glycerophospholipid (1,2-bis[4-(1-pyreno) butanoyl]-sn-glycero-3-phosphocholine), which on hydrolysis gives monomer fluorescence that is measured at 382 nm (Hendrickson, 1991, 1994). Although detergents may affect the fluorescent properties of fluorophore

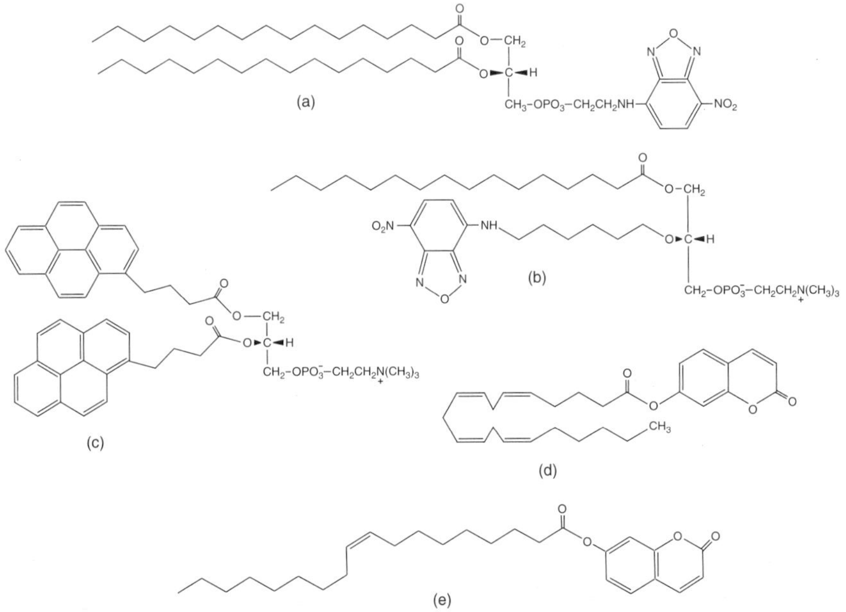

FIG. 12.5. Chemical structures of dansyl-PtdEtn (a); 2-(6-(7-nitro-benz-2-oxa-1,3-diazol-4-yl)amino-hexanoyl-1-hexadecanoyl-sn-GroPCho (NBD-PtdCho) (b); [bis-pyrenebutanoyl]phosphatidylcholine ([DPyb]PtdCho) (c); umbelliferone-arachidonate (UMB-arachidonate) (d); and umbelliferone-oleate (UMB-oleate) (e).

in the substrate and products, their use is required to produce a substrate interface suitable for the catalytic action of PLA$_2$.

12.5.1. Continuous Fluorometric Procedures

Several continuous fluorescence procedures have been described for the assay of sPLA$_2$ activity found in pancreatic juice and snake venom. A continuous fluorescent procedure involves the displacement of the highly fluorescence fatty acid probe 11-(dansylamino)undecanoic acid (DAUDA) from rat fatty acid-binding protein (FABP) by long-chain fatty acids generated by the action of PLA$_2$ on glycerophospholipids (Wilton, 1990). Displacement of DAUDA by long-chain fatty acids produces a decrease in the fluorescence signal. The initial rate of decrease in fluorescence is linearly related to the PLA$_2$ activity over a 100-fold range of enzyme concentration (Wilton, 1990). In the absence of PLA$_2$, or in the presence of excess of EDTA to remove Ca^{2+}, the initial fluorescence reading is very stable with no detectable fall after 30 min. Some variability in the overall shape of the time course is observed, but this is similar to other PLA$_2$ assay procedures and the initial rate of displacement of DAUDA is not affected (Wilton, 1990). This procedure is simple, convenient, versatile, sensitive, and initial rates are reproducible. Furthermore, no lag phase is observed before the fall in fluorescence. The lower limit of detection is 20 pmol/min/ml. There are some disadvantages to this procedure. They include the requirement for liver FABP, interference by detergents, and reduction of sensitivity at higher glycerophospholipid concentration. A modification of this displacement assay procedure using albumin and a medium-chain fatty acid glycerophospholipid substrate has also been described (Kinkaid and Wilton, 1993).

Another continuous fluorescence-based procedure for assay of cPLA$_2$ was developed using fatty acid esters of 7-hydroxycoumarin. These esters of 7-hydroxycoumarin are not fluorescent, but hydrolysis by cPLA$_2$ results in the generation of highly fluorescent 7-hydroxycoumarin at 460 nm (excitation 360 nm at pH 8 or 335 nm at pH 7.2) (Huang et al., 1994). This procedure is sensitive and rapid, but can be used only for the purified PLA$_2$ isoforms because other esterases and lipases in the crude homogenate can also hydrolyze 7-hydroxycoumarin.

Two bromoacyl analogs of PtdCho, 1-ω-bromoundecanoyl-2-[4-(pyren-1-yl) butyroyl]-sn-glycero-3-phosphocholine (B-PtdCho) and 1-(9,10-dibromostearoyl-2-[4-(pyren-1-yl)butyroyl]-sn-glycero-3-phosphocholine (DB-PtdCho) (Fig. 12.6), with intramolecular fluorescence quenching have been synthesized for continuous monitoring of PLA$_2$ activity (Babitskaya et al., 2004). The pyrenylbutyric acid residue in these substrates does not disturb the balance of hydrophobicity and hydrophilicity in the glycerophospholipid molecule. Bromine-containing fatty acids are good intramolecular quenchers of fluorescence in this procedure (Babitskaya et al., 2004). When pancreatic PLA$_2$ hydrolyzes these substrates, the enzymic reaction can be followed continuously by monitoring the intensity of fluorescence emission and the amount of the pyrenylbutyric acid can be determined from the calibration curve. This procedure

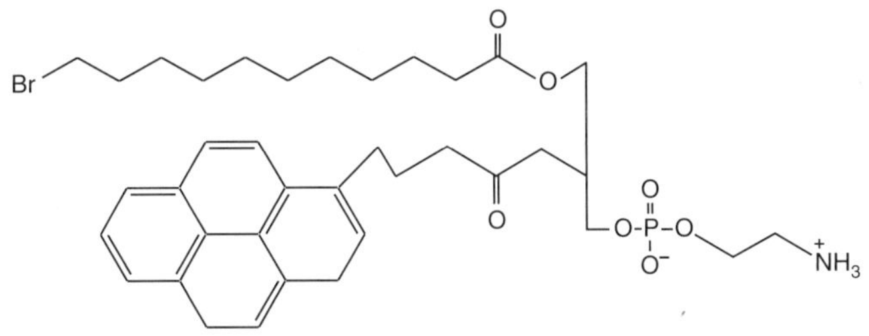

(a)

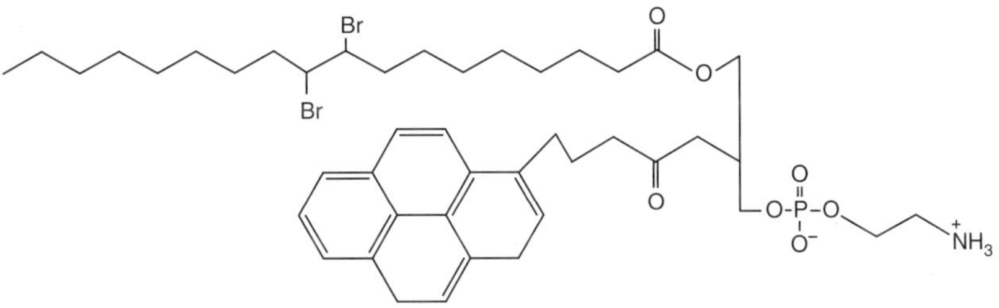

(b)

FIG. 12.6. Chemical structures of 1-ω-bromoundecanoyl-2-[4-(pyren-1-yl)butyroyl]-*sn*-Gro*P*Cho (B-PtdCho) (a); and 1-(9,10-dibromo)stearoyl-2-[4-(pyren-1-yl)butyroyl]-*sn*-Gro*P*Cho (DB-PtdCho) (b).

is sensitive and rapid. Its lower limit of the detection is 10 pmol/min. This value is similar to the range of other fluorometric substrates.

In addition, other continuous fluorometric assay procedures were also described using hexadecanoyl-2-(1-pyrenedecanol)-*sn*-glycero-3-phosphocholine (Radvanyi et al., 1989; Bayburt et al., 1995; Yarger et al., 2000). These procedures are simple, rapid, and reproducible. All reagents are commercially available. These procedures do not work well with crude tissue homogenates and membrane suspensions. They can be used for determining PLA$_2$ activities in clear purified enzyme and cytosolic preparations.

Fluorescence-labeled PtdEtn is also used as a substrate for determining type II sPLA$_2$ activity. This enzyme follows simple Michaelis–Menten kinetics and hydrolyzes 1-acyl-2-(*N*-4-nitrobenzo-2-oxo-1,3-diazole)aminododecanoyl-*sn*-Gro*P*Etn (NBD-C$_{12}$-PtdEtn). This can be followed continuously with a linear increase in fluorescence intensity. Excitation and emission are monitored at 485 and 535 nm, respectively (Blanchard et al., 1994). NBD-C$_{12}$-PtdEtn suspensions are prepared without detergent. They exhibit a low fluorescence due to self-quenching. Substrate hydrolysis results in a release of quenching. The fluorescence signal, therefore, comes from changes in the local environment of the fluorophore and not from intrinsic changes in the quantum yields of substrate and products. This method is simple, convenient, and economical and was used for determination of sPLA$_2$ IIA in human synovial fluid (Blanchard et al., 1994).

12.5.2. Discontinuous Fluorometric Procedures

Discontinuous fluorometric procedures fall into two groups, i.e., those that require separation of substrate from its hydrolyzed products (separation-dependent) by HPLC or TLC, and those that do not require separation of substrate from its products (separation-independent). In the first group of assay procedures, 1-O-[12-(2-naphthyl)-dodec-11-enyl]-2-decanoyl-sn-glycero-3-phosphocholine, rac 1-O-(N-dansyl-11-amino-1-undecyl)-2-O-decanoyl-sn-glycero-3-phospho-choline (dansyl-PtdCho), and 1-acyl-2-{6-[(7-nitrobenzo-2-oxa-1,3-diazol-4-yl)amino]-caproyl}-sn-glycero-3-phosphocholine (NBD-PtdCho) are often used as PLA$_2$ substrates (Fig. 12.7). Following the enzymic reaction, either HPLC or TLC separates substrate and product. The ratio of substrate to product can be determined by using a fluorescence detector or quantitative TLC analysis. These procedures are very convenient, sensitive, economical, and activities as low as 10 pmol/min in 100 μl are measured easily (Hendrickson et al., 1990).

For procedures that do not require the separation of substrate from products, novel analogs of glycerophospholipid substrates were synthesized. They contain both a fluorescent BODIPY-FL-C$_5$ (4,4-difluoro-5,7-dimethyl-4-bora-3a, 4a-diaza-S-indacene-3-pentanoic acid) group at the sn-1 position and a quench-ing 2,4-dinitrophenyl (DPN) at the sn-2 position of the glycerol moiety. Bis-BODIPY-C$_{11}$-PtdCho and BC$_{11}$-DHPC$_s$-PtdCho, and BC$_{11}$-DNPC$_8$-PtdCho show very little fluorescence because of intramolecular quenching by the DPN group at the sn-2 position, but BODIPY-PtdCho becomes fluorescent after hydrolysis by PLA$_2$ (Hendrickson et al., 1999). These substrate analogs can be used for the determination of sPLA$_2$, cPLA$_2$, and platelet-activating factor acetylhydrolase activities (PAF-AH). BC$_{11}$-DHPC$_s$-PtdCho is a poor substrate for sPLA$_2$, but a good substrate for cPLA$_2$ and plasma PAF-AH. Cytosolic PAF-AH, which requires an acetyl group at the sn-2 position of the glycerol moiety, does not hydrolyze it. N-((6-(2,4-dinitrophenyl)amino)hexanoyl)-1-palmitoyl-2-BODIPY-FL-pentanoyl-sn-glycero-3-phosphoethanolamine (PBPEC$_6$DNP) was injected into living zebra fish embryos at cell stages one to four. Embryos were allowed to develop until early somitogenesis. At early somitogenesis, a marked increase in PLA$_2$ activity was observed, indicating the generation of second messengers by PLA$_2$ for the survival of the developing embryo (Hendrickson et al., 1999).

Pyrenesulfonyl-labeled plasmalogen, 1-alk-1-enyl-2-acyl-sn-GroPEtn(Pyr), is synthesized and used for the determination of PlsEtn-PLA$_2$ activity, not only in brain homogenate and homogenates from cultured cells of neuronal and glial origin (Hirashima et al., 1990) but also for following the purification of PlsEtn-PLA$_2$ from bovine brain (Hirashima et al., 1992). This procedure is as sensitive as radiolabeled substrate and is specific for plasmalogen. In this method, the liberated 1-alk-1-enyl-sn-GroPEtn(Pyr) is converted to GroPEtn(Pyr) by expo-sure to HCl vapors (Fig. 12.4B) on a TLC plate, and then separated from the

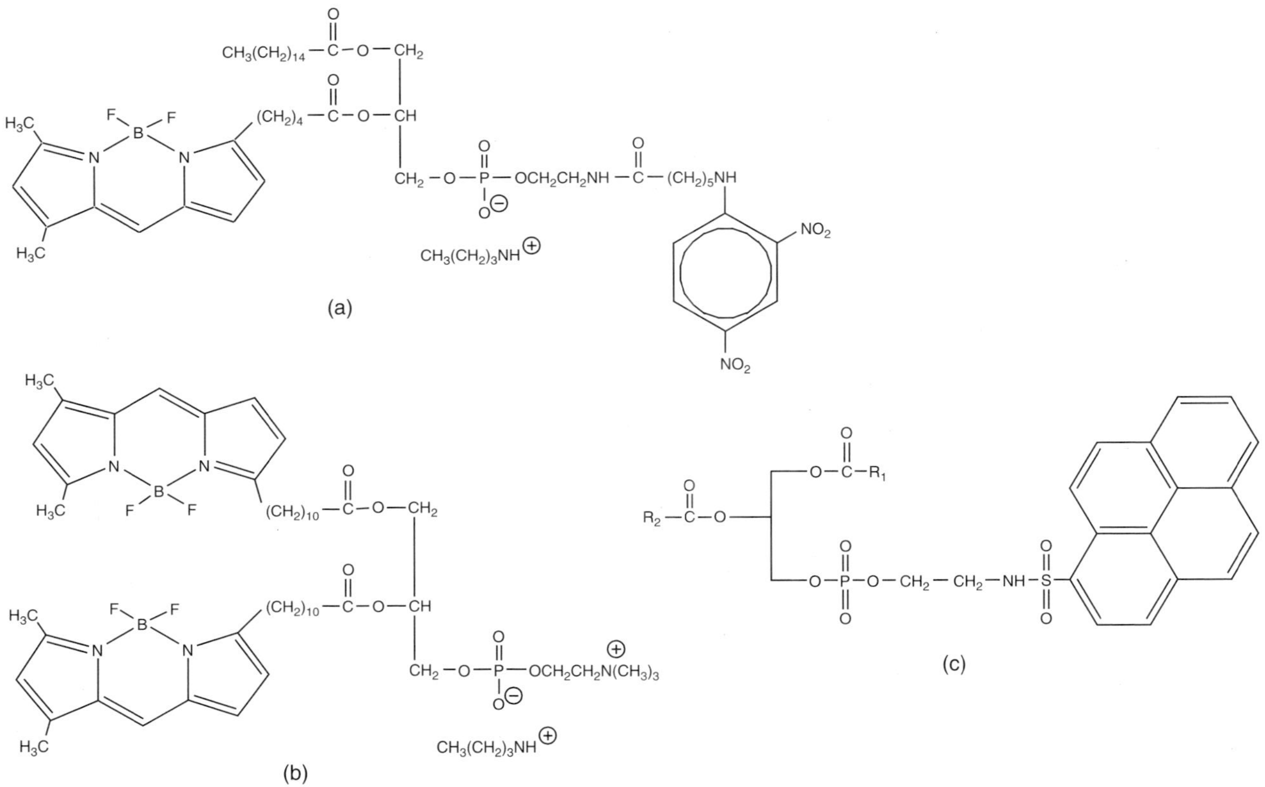

FIG. 12.7. Chemical structures of N-((6-(2,4-dinitrophenyl)aminohexyl)-2(4,4-difluoro-5,7-dimethyl-4-bora-3a,4a-diaza-S-indacene-3-pentanoyl)-1-hexadecanoyl-sn-GroPEtn (a); 1,2-bis(4,4-difluoro-5,7-dimethyl-4-bora-3a,4a-diaza-S-indacene-3-undecanoyl)-sn-GroPCho (BODIPY-C11-PtdCho); (b); and pyrene-GroPEtn (c).

remaining lysoPtdEtn(Pyr) using a solvent system composed of choloroform/methanol/NH$_4$OH (65:25:4 v/v). The spots of GroPEtn(Pyr) are scraped and extracted with 2 ml of methanol. The fluorescence of GroPEtn(Pyr) is measured using excitation and emission wavelengths 340 and 378 nm, respectively. PlsEtn-PLA$_2$ activity can be calculated from the fluorescence of GroPEtn(Pyr) after subtracting appropriate control values (Hirashima et al., 1990; Farooqui et al., 1999). This method is simple, convenient, and sensitive. It can be used for the purification and characterization of PlsEtn-PLA$_2$ (Hirashima et al., 1992).

12.6. Assay of Multiple Forms of PLA$_2$ in Biological Samples

Studies on PLA$_2$ isoforms in the brain are complicated not only by the occurrence of multiple forms and their paralogs but also by the lack of information on the effect of various exogenous and endogenous activators and inhibitors. The addition of activators or inhibitors can affect the physical state of the glycerophospholipid substrate making it more or less susceptible to hydrolysis by PLA$_2$ isoforms. These effects can be minimized by using high substrate concentrations or by using more potent activators or inhibitors whose concentration in the assay system is much less than that of the substrate (Reynolds et al., 1991). Utilizing specific properties of partially purified and purified cPLA$_2$, iPLA$_2$, and sPLA$_2$, attempts have been made to develop assay procedures to distinguish among them (Yang et al., 1999; Lucas and Dennis, 2005; Markova et al., 2005). These properties include substrate preference, use of activators and inhibitors, calcium ion dependence, and susceptibility of disulfide bonds to DTT. Activators include phosphatidylinositol 4,5-bisphosphate (PIP$_2$) and calcium ion. Inhibitors include MAFP, BEL, LY311727, and DTT. PIP$_2$ and Ca^{2+} activate cPLA$_2$, whereas MAFP inhibits both cPLA$_2$ as well as iPLA$_2$. BEL inhibits iPLA$_2$. LY31127 and DTT inhibit sPLA$_2$ activity. Use of these activators and inhibitors at the appropriate concentration in the presence of optimal Ca^{2+} inhibits one form and allows the assay of the other PLA$_2$ isoform (Lucas and Dennis, 2005; Markova et al., 2005).

An assay system for cPLA$_2$ uses 1-palmitoyl-2-arachidonoyl-sn-GroPCho and PIP$_2$ as a cPLA$_2$ activator. It can detect 0.1 ng of cPLA$_2$ and has 30-fold selectivity for cPLA$_2$ over iPLA$_2$ and more than a 10,000-fold selectivity over the group IIA and V sPLA$_2$. Similarly, an iPLA$_2$ assay system uses 1,2-dipalmitoyl-sn-glycero-3-GroPCho as a substrate. It can detect 0.3 ng of iPLA$_2$ and has a 5,000-fold selectivity for iPLA$_2$ over cPLA$_2$ and more than a 50,000-fold selectivity over group IIA and V sPLA$_2$ (Lucas and Dennis, 2005). The group V sPLA$_2$ assay system uses 1-palmitoyl-2-oleoyl-sn-GroPSer and has a 10,000-, 5,000-, and 30-fold selectivity for group V sPLA$_2$ over cPLA$_2$, iPLA$_2$, and group IIA sPLA$_2$, respectively. This is the best set of assay procedures for the isoforms of PLA$_2$ in tissue homogenates and biological samples (Akbar et al., 2005). It is simple, economical, convenient, and sensitive. One drawback of all PLA$_2$ assay procedures, including this one, is the nature and stability of the interfacial form of the glycerophospholipid substrates in detergent. The nature and stability of glycerophospholipid substrates in detergent varies from one day to another, resulting in 2- to 3-fold differences in the specific activity of a PLA$_2$ preparation from one day to the next. Thus, it is very important to prepare PLA$_2$ substrates by a rigidly established procedure and to perform PLA$_2$ assays on the same day using the same substrate preparation (Lucas and Dennis, 2005). Another important issue is the handling and storage of glycerophospholipids. Glycerophospholipids should be stored carefully under nitrogen in the dark because they are prone to oxidation, especially those glycerophospholipids that contain polyunsaturated fatty acids such as arachidonic or docosahexaenoic acids.

12.6.1. Immunological Procedures

Western blot analysis has been used to detect cPLA$_2$ levels (Nakamura et al., 1992; Bolognese et al., 1995), but these procedures require substantial amounts of protein, and are time consuming and laborious. ELISA for sPLA$_2$ (Roshak et al., 1994; Rosenthal et al., 1995; Bolognese et al., 1995) and cPLA$_2$ (Zhu et al., 1996) were developed. The antibodies used in ELISA sandwich assays do not crossreact with other PLA$_2$ isoforms and other proteins present in the tissue and thus provide an accurate measure of PLA$_2$ content. ELISA for sPLA$_2$ and cPLA$_2$ are simple, precise, reliable, specific, and sensitive, namely linear within the range of 0.10 to 30 ng/ml.

Time-resolved fluoroimmunoassays for pancreatic sPLA$_2$ have also been developed (Santavuori et al., 1991). In this assay, the labeled antibody in combination with the time-resolved fluorometric detection of the europium label essentially eliminates all background fluorescence. This results in high sensitivity and a wide linear range. The sensitivity of this method is 10 ng/ml of pancreatic sPLA$_2$ in the preparation. Another advantage of this procedure is that the presence of an endogenous inhibitor(s) of pancreatic sPLA$_2$ activity does not affect measurements. Time-resolved fluoroimmunoassays for multiple forms of sPLA$_2$ in human serum were developed (Nevalainen et al., 2005). These are simple, specific, and more sensitive than radioimmunoassays and obviate the use of radioactive material (Nevalainen et al., 2005). The lower limit of detection varies from 15 ng to 20 μg in serum and other body fluids.

The assay procedures for PLA$_2$ described above are based on the detection of release of fatty acid and lysoglycerophospholipid from exogenously added substrate (radiolabeled, fluorescent-labeled, or thioester glycerophospholipid analogs). Using the above strategy to determine PLA$_2$ activity, the rate of glycerophospholipid hydrolysis depends not only on the choice of substrate employed during the assay, i.e., PtdCho, PtdEtn, or PlsCho, etc., but also on the physical state of the phospholipids (Vesterqvist et al., 1994). Synthetic short-chain glycerophospholipids below their critical micellar concentration (CMC) exist as monomers, or above their CMC aggregate into micelles. In contrast, native glycerophospholipids with long-chain fatty acid chains form mixed micelles in the presence of detergent. In most of the assay procedures described above, the exogenously added glycerophospholipids exist in a mixture of different aggregated forms such as mixed micelles and vesicles. PLA$_2$ activities with these aggregated glycerophospholipids can be many-fold higher than that observed with soluble glycerophospholipid substrates because interactions of these aggregates with PLA$_2$ at the lipid–water interface induce a conformational change in the enzyme leading to increased catalytic efficiency (Reynolds et al., 1991). The exogenously added glycerophospholipid substrate cannot resemble the complex natural state of the same glycerophospholipid found in membranes. Intact membranes with their endogenous glycerophospholipid substrates, such as radiolabeled *E. coli* glycerophospholipids or lyophilized rabbit myocardial membranes, have been used as substrates for assays of PLA$_2$ activity (Elsbach and Weiss, 1991; Vesterqvist et al., 1994). Since these endogenous glycerophospholipids have a more complex composition than the exogenously added glycerophospholipids, it is quite difficult to calculate the exact substrate concentration in the membranes during these assays. The situation would be more complex for brain membranes than for other visceral membranes, because the brain has several types of cells, neurons, astrocytes, oligodendrocytes, and microglia, with different glycerophospholipid compositions. Thus, these assay procedures may have limited value for brain tissue. Additional novel assay procedures are needed for the determination of PLA$_2$ activity.

Another important issue is the use of these procedures for assaying activities of PLA$_2$ isoforms in neural and nonneural tissues and biological fluids from neuropsychiatric and neurological disorders. Limited studies have been performed with inconsistent and controversial results (Gattaz et al., 1987; Albers et al., 1993; Ross et al., 1997; Katila et al., 1997; Farooqui et al., 2003a,b). A fluorometric assay was used for PLA$_2$ activity in EDTA-plasma and serum (Gattaz et al., 1987), a radiochemical assay was used for PLA$_2$ in serum (Schulze et al., 1988), and radiochemical and photometric assays were done with several body fluids (Marki et al., 1990). Based on recent studies, separation of fluorogenic substrates from hydrolytic products prior to quantitation by video imaging may be mandatory. Therefore, it is recommended for clinical use (Lasch et al., 2003).

References

Aarsman A. J. and van den Bosch H. (1977). A continuous spectrophotometric assay for membrane-bound lysophospholipases using a thioester substrate analog. *FEBS Lett.* 79:317–320.

Aarsman A. J. and van den Bosch H. (1979). A comparison of acyl-oxyester and acyl-thioester substrates for some lipolytic enzymes. *Biochim. Biophys. Acta* 572:519–530.

Akbar M., Calderon F., Wen Z. M., and Kim H. Y. (2005). Docosahexaenoic acid: a positive modulator of Akt signaling in neuronal survival. *Proc. Natl Acad. Sci. USA* 102:10858, 12997.

Albers M., Meurer H., Marki F., and Klotz J. (1993). Phospholipase A$_2$ activity in serum of neuroleptic-naive psychiatric inpatients. *Pharmacopsychiatry* 26:94–98.

Babitskaya S. V., Kisel M. A., and Kisselev P. A. (2004). Bromoacyl analogues of phosphatidylcholine with intramolecular fluorescence quenching and their use as substrates for continuous monitoring of phospholipase A_2 activity. *Appl. Biochem. Microbiol.* 40:351–356.

Bayburt T., Yu B. Z., Street I., Ghomashchi F., Laliberte F., Perrier H., Wang Z., Homan R., Jain M. K., and Gelb M. H. (1995). Continuous, vesicle-based fluorimetric assays of 14- and 85-kDa phospholipases A_2. *Anal. Biochem.* 232:7–23.

Blanchard S. G., Harris C. O., and Parks D. J. (1994). A fluorescence-based assay for human type II phospholipase A_2. *Anal. Biochem.* 222:435–440.

Blanchard S. G., Andrews R. C., Brown P. J., Gan L. S., Lee F. W., Sinhababu A. K., and Wheeler T. N. (1998). Discovery of bioavailable inhibitors of secretory phospholipase A_2. *Pharm. Biotechnol.* 11:445–463.

Bligh E. G. and Dyer W. J. (1959). A rapid method of total lipid extraction and purification. *Can. J. Biochem. Physiol.* 37:911–917.

Bolognese B., McCord M., and Marshall L. A. (1995). Differential regulation of elicited-peritoneal macrophage 14 kDa and 85 kDa phospholipase A_2(s) by transforming growth factor-beta. *Biochim. Biophys. Acta* 1256:201–209.

Caramelo J. J. and Delfino J. M. (2004). A subnanogram assay for phospholipase activity based on a long-chain radioiodinatable phosphatidylcholine. *Anal. Biochem.* 333:289–295.

Cox J. W. and Horrocks L. A. (1981). Preparation of thioester substrates and development of continuous spectrophotometric assays for phospholipase A_1 and monoacylglycerol lipase. *J. Lipid Res.* 22:496–505.

De Haas G. H., Bonsen P. P. M., Pieterson W. A., and van Deenen L. L. M. (1971). Studies on phospholipase A and its zymogen from porcine pancreas. 3. Action of the enzyme on short-chain lecithins. *Biochim. Biophys. Acta* 239:252–266.

Dole V. P. (1956). A relation between non-esterified fatty acids in plasma and the metabolism of glucose. *J. Clin. Invest.* 35:150–154.

Duncombe W. G. (1963). The colorimetric micro-determination of long-chain fatty acids. *Biochem. J.* 88:7–12.

Elsbach P. and Weiss J. (1991). Utilization of labeled *Escherichia coli* as phospholipase substrate. *Methods Enzymol.* 197:24–31.

Farooqui A. A. and Horrocks L. A. (1988). Methods for the determination of phospholipases, lipases and lysophospholipases. In: Boulton A. A., Baker G. B., and Horrocks L. A. (eds.), *Neuromethods, Vol. 7, Lipids and Related Compounds*. Humana Press, New Jersey, pp. 179–209.

Farooqui A. A., Taylor W. A., Pendley C. E. [**]2., Cox J. W., and Horrocks L. A. (1984). Spectrophotometric determination of lipases, lysophospholipases, and phospholipases. *J. Lipid Res.* 25:1555–1562.

Farooqui A. A., Yang H.-C., Hirashima Y., and Horrocks L. A. (1999). Determination of plasmalogen-selective phospholipase A_2 activity by radiochemical and fluorometric assay procedures. In: Doolittle M. H. and Reue K. (eds.), *Mammalian Lipases and Phospholipases*. Humana Press, Totowa, NJ, pp. 39–47.

Farooqui A. A., Ong W. Y., and Horrocks L. A. (2003a). Plasmalogens, docosahexaenoic acid, and neurological disorders. In: Roels F., Baes M., and de Bies S. (eds.), *Peroxisomal Disorders and Regulation of Genes*. Kluwer Academic/Plenum Publishers, London, pp. 335–354.

Farooqui A. A., Ong W. Y., and Horrocks L. A. (2003b). Stimulation of lipases and phospholipases in Alzheimer disease. In: Szuhaj B. and van Nieuwenhuyzen W. (eds.), *Nutrition and Biochemistry of Phospholipids*. AOCS Press, Champaign, pp. 14–29.

Fuji M., Watanabe F., Fujii Y., Hashizume H., Okuno T., Shirahase K., Teshirogi I., and Ohtani M. (1997). A stereoselective and highly practical synthesis of cytosolic phospholipase A2 substrate, 2-S-arachidonoyl-1-O-hexadecyl-sn-2-thioglycero-3-O-phosphocholine. *J. Org. Chem.* 62:6804–6809.

Gattaz W. F., Kollisch M., Thuren T., Virtanen J. A., and Kinnunen P. K. (1987). Increased plasma phospholipase A$_2$ activity in schizophrenic patients: reduction after neuroleptic therapy. *Biol. Psychiatry* 22:421–426.

Hendrickson H. S. (1991). Phospholipase A$_2$ assays with fluorophore-labeled lipid substrates. *Methods Enzymol.* 197:90–94.

Hendrickson H. S. (1994). Fluorescence-based assays of lipases, phospholipases, and other lipolytic enzymes. *Anal. Biochem.* 219:1–8.

Hendrickson H. S. and Rauk P. N. (1981). Continuous fluorometric assay of phospholipase A$_2$ with pyrene-labeled lecithin as a substrate. *Anal. Biochem.* 116:553–558.

Hendrickson H. S., Kotz K. J., and Hendrickson E. K. (1990). Evaluation of fluorescent and colored phosphatidylcholine analogs as substrates for the assay of phospholipase A$_2$. *Anal. Biochem.* 185:80–83.

Hendrickson H. S., Hendrickson E. K., Johnson I. D., and Farber S. A. (1999). Intramolecularly quenched BODIPY-labeled phospholipid analogs in phospholipase A$_2$ and platelet-activating factor acetylhydrolase assays and *in vivo* fluorescence imaging. *Anal. Biochem.* 276:27–35.

Hirashima Y., Farooqui A. A., and Horrocks L. A. (1989a). Fluorimetric coupled enzyme assay for lysoplasmalogenase activity in liver. *Biochem. J.* 260:605–608.

Hirashima Y., Jurkowitz-Alexander M. S., Farooqui A. A., and Horrocks L. A. (1989b). Continuous spectrophotometric assay of phospholipase A$_2$ activity hydrolyzing plasmalogens using coupling enzymes. *Anal. Biochem.* 176:180–184.

Hirashima Y., Mills J. S., Yates A. J., and Horrocks L. A. (1990). Phospholipase A$_2$ activities with a plasmalogen substrate in brain and in neural tumor cells: a sensitive and specific assay using pyrenesulfonyl-labeled plasmenylethanolamine. *Biochim. Biophys. Acta* 1074:35–40.

Hirashima Y., Farooqui A. A., Mills J. S., and Horrocks L. A. (1992). Identification and purification of calcium-independent phospholipase A$_2$ from bovine brain cytosol. *J. Neurochem.* 59:708–714.

Huang Z., Laliberté F., Tremblay N. M., Weech P. K., and Street I. P. (1994). A continuous fluorescence-based assay for the human high-molecular-weight cytosolic phospholipase A$_2$. *Anal. Biochem.* 222:110–115.

Jiménez M., Cabanes J., Gandía-Herrero F., Escribano J., García-Carmona F., and Pérez-Gilabert M. (2003). A continuous spectrophotometric assay for phospholipase A$_2$ activity. *Anal. Biochem.* 319:131–137.

Jurkowitz-Alexander M. S. and Horrocks L. A. (1990). Lysoplasmalogenase: solubilization and partial purification from liver microsomes. *Methods Enzymol.* 197:483–490.

Jurkowitz-Alexander M. S., Hirashima Y., and Horrocks L. A. (1991). Coupled enzyme assays for phospholipase activities with plasmalogen substrates. *Methods Enzymol.* 197:79–89.

Katila H., Appelberg B., and Rimon R. (1997). No differences in phospholipase-A$_2$ activity between acute psychiatric patients and controls. *Schizophr. Res.* 26:103–105.

Kinkaid A. R. and Wilton D. C. (1993). A continuous fluorescence displacement assay for phospholipase A$_2$ using albumin and medium chain phospholipid substrates. *Anal. Biochem.* 212:65–70.

Lasch J., Willhardt I., Kinder D., Sauer H., and Smesny S. (2003). Fluorometric assays of phospholipase A$_2$ activity with three different substrates in biological samples of patients with schizophrenia. *Clin. Chem. Lab. Med.* 41:908–914.

Lucas K. K. and Dennis E. A. (2005). Distinguishing phospholipase A_2 types in biological samples by employing group-specific assays in the presence of inhibitors. *Prostaglandins Other Lipid Mediat.* 77:235–248.

Marki F., Pignat W., Steinbruckner B., and Hoffmann G. E. (1990). Determination of human serum phospholipase A_2. Comparison of two methods. *J. Clin. Chem. Clin. Biochem.* 28:543–544.

Markova M., Koratkar R. A., Silverman K. A., Sollars V. E., MacPhee-Pellini M., Walters R., Palazzo J. P., Buchberg A. M., Siracusa L. D., and Farber S. A. (2005). Diversity in secreted PLA_2-IIA activity among inbred mouse strains that are resistant or susceptible to $Apc^{Min/+}$ tumorigenesis. *Oncogene* 24:6450–6458.

Nakamura T., Lin L. L., Kharbanda S., Knopf J., and Kufe D. (1992). Macrophage colony stimulating factor activates phosphatidylcholine hydrolysis by cytoplasmic phospholipase A2. *EMBO J.* 11:4917–4922.

Nevalainen T. J., Eerola L. I., Rintala E., Jukka V., Laine O., Lambeau G., and Timo J. N. A. (2005). Time-resolved fluoroimmunoassays of the complete set of secreted phospholipases A_2 in human serum. *Biochim. Biophys. Acta Mol. Cell Biol. Lipids* 1733:210–223.

Radvanyi F., Jordan L., Russo-Marie F., and Bon C. (1989). A sensitive and continuous fluorometric assay for phospholipase A_2 using pyrene-labeled phospholipids in the presence of serum albumin. *Anal. Biochem.* 177:103–109.

Reynolds L. J., Washburn W. N., Deems R. A., and Dennis E. A. (1991). Assay strategies and methods for phospholipases. *Methods Enzymol.* 197:3–23.

Reynolds L. J., Hughes L. L., Yu L., and Dennis E. A. (1994). 1-Hexadecyl-2-arachidonoylthio-2-deoxy-*sn*-glycero-3-phosphorylcholine as a substrate for the microtiterplate assay of human cytosolic phospholipase A_2. *Anal. Biochem.* 217:25–32.

Rosenthal M. D., Gordon M. N., Buescher E. S., Slusser J. H., Harris L. K., and Franson R. C. (1995). Human neutrophils store type II 14-kDa phospholipase A_2 in granules and secrete active enzyme in response to soluble stimuli. *Biochem. Biophys. Res. Commun.* 208:650–656.

Roshak A., Sathe G., and Marshall L. A. (1994). Suppression of monocyte 85-kDa phospholipase A_2 by antisense and effects on endotoxin-induced prostaglandin biosynthesis. *J. Biol. Chem.* 269:25999–26005.

Ross B. M., Hudson C., Erlich J., Warsh J. J., and Kish S. J. (1997). Increased phospholipid breakdown in schizophrenia — evidence for the involvement of a calcium-independent phospholipase A_2. *Arch. Gen. Psychiatry* 54:487–494.

Santavuori S. A., Kortesuo P. T., Eskola J. U., and Nevalainen T. J. (1991). Application of a new monoclonal antibody for time-resolved fluoroimmunoassay of human pancreatic phospholipase A_2. *Eur. J. Clin. Chem. Clin. Biochem.* 29:819–826.

Schulze R. M., Muller W. E., and Gattaz W. F. (1988). A radioenzymatic assay for the determination of phospholipase A_2 in serum suitable for psychiatric and non-psychiatric patients. *Pharmacopsychiatry* 21:348–349.

Somerharju P. (2002). Pyrene-labeled lipids as tools in membrane biophysics and cell biology. *Chem. Phys. Lipids* 116:57–74.

Sunamoto J., Kondo H., Nomura T., and Okamoto M. (1980). Liposomal membranes. 2. Synthesis of a novel pyrene-labeled lecithin and structural studies on liposomal bilayers. *J. Am. Chem. Soc.* 102:1146–1152.

Vesterqvist O., Sargent C. A., Grover G. J., Warrack B. M., DiDonato G. C., and Ogletree M. L. (1994). Characterization of rabbit myocardial phospholipase A_2 activity using endogenous phospholipid substrates. *Anal. Biochem.* 217:210–219.

Wells M. A. (1972). A kinetic study of the phospholipase A2 (*Crotalus adamanteus*) catalyzed hydrolysis of 1,2-dibutyryl-*sn*-glycero-3-phosphorylcholine. *Biochemistry* 11:1030–1041.

Wilton D. C. (1990). A continuous fluorescence displacement assay for the measurement of phospholipase A$_2$ and other lipases that release long-chain fatty acids. *Biochem. J.* 266:435–439.

Yang H. C., Mosior M., Johnson C. A., Chen Y. J., and Dennis E. A. (1999). Group-specific assays that distinguish between the four major types of mammalian phospholipase A$_2$. *Anal. Biochem.* 269:278–288.

Yarger D. E., Patrick C. B., Rapoport S. I., and Murphy E. J. (2000). A continuous fluorometric assay for phospholipase A$_2$ activity in brain cytosol. *J. Neurosci. Methods* 100:127–133.

Yu L. and Dennis E. A. (1991). Thio-based phospholipase assay. *Methods Enzymol.* 197:65–75.

Yu L., Ternansky R. J., Crisologo J. F., Chang J., Baker B. L., and Coutts S. M. (1998). Carbonothioate phospholipids as substrate for a spectrophotometric assay of phospholipase A$_2$. *Anal. Biochem.* 265:35–41.

Zhu X., Munoz N. M., Rubio N., Herrnreiter A., Mayer D., Douglas I., and Leff A. R. (1996). Quantitation of the cytosolic phospholipase A$_2$ (type IV) in isolated human peripheral blood eosinophils by sandwich-ELISA. *J. Immunol. Methods* 199:119–126.

13
Glycerophospholipids and Phospholipases A$_2$ in Neuropsychiatric Disorders

13.1 Introduction

Neuropsychiatric disorders include both neurodevelopmental disorders and neurodegenerative diseases. Alterations in glycerophospholipids and PLA$_2$ activities in neurodegenerative disorders are discussed in Chapter 10. Neurodevelopmental disorders include schizophrenia, some forms of bipolar affective disorders, autism, mood disorders, and certain forms of manic depression. Epidemiology studies indicate that genetic factors have a major role in the risk for schizophrenia, bipolar affective disorder, and dyslexia, although vulnerability genes have not yet been identified in unequivocal form (Harrison and Owen, 2003). One of the most important characteristics of neuropsychiatric disorders, in general, and in schizophrenia in particular, is the impairment of cognitive processing. Cognitive processing refers to signal transduction-mediated processes associated with every day problem-solving behavior. This includes the ability to learn and store the memory, to retrieve stored memory for further use, and to apply the stored memory to efficiently solve problems (Gallagher, 2004). The impairment of cognitive processes may be caused by over-expression or under-expression of certain genes or other unknown factors that result in behavioral symptoms such as thoughts or actions, delusions, and hallucinations that are the hallmarks of schizophrenia and bipolar disorders.

Like neurodegenerative diseases, neurodevelopmental disorders are also characterized by neuronal death (Margolis et al., 1994). It is well known that as many as 50% of all originally formed neurons die during the formation and maturation of the central nervous system (Oppenheim, 1991). This cell death occurs through apoptosis and is caused by the activation of intrinsic pathways associated with signal transduction and second messenger-mediated neural cell remodeling and pruning in the developing brain. Apoptosis, along with genetic and environmental factors, modulates the ways in which surviving neurons are laid down and differentiated into mature neurons through second messenger-mediated expansion and retraction of dendrites and synaptic connections (Margolis et al., 1994). Apoptotic cell death can occur at the synapse as well as at the cell body (Mattson et al., 1998). Apoptosis is accompanied by caspase-3 activation and DNA fragmentation (Sastry and Rao, 2000). There is much less DNA fragmentation in individuals with schizophrenia than in healthy controls and bipolar subjects suggesting reduced neuronal apoptosis in schizophrenic patients. Furthermore, levels of the antiapoptotic Bcl-2 protein are also low in the temporal cortex of schizophrenic patients. Bcl-2 interacts with the proapoptotic Bax protein at an upstream checkpoint to regulate the activation of apoptosis by caspase-3 and other proteolytic caspases. A high Bax/Bcl-2 ratio is associated with greater vulnerability to apoptosis, while a high caspase-3 level is often associated with apoptotic activity. The Bax/Bcl-2 ratio, but not caspase-3, may be high in the temporal cortex of patients with chronic schizophrenia (Jarskog et al., 2004). Reduced apoptotic cell death may contribute to the pathophysiology of schizophrenia (Benes et al., 2003).

In neuropsychiatric disorders the survival of neurons in the brain is modulated not only by genes in utero but also by certain events during pregnancy including stress and starvation and by obstetric complications and viral infections around birth. The neurochemical and neurophysiological effects of these events are fully expressed in early adulthood, around puberty, and even at an older age (Horrobin, 1998). These effects may involve changes in neural membrane glycerophospholipids because they are crucial for synaptic remodeling in the developing brain and are also involved in learning and memory processes as the developing brain matures into the adult brain. Thus abnormalities in genes that code and modulate enzymes of glycerophospholipid metabolism may contribute to risk factors and physiopathological mechanisms underlying neuropsychiatric disorders (Horrobin, 1998).

13.2 Schizophrenia

Schizophrenia is a complex neuropsychiatric disorder with a prevalence of nearly 1% of the world population. Clinically, schizophrenia is characterized by chronic psychotic symptoms and psychosocial impairment. At least two core syndromes of schizophrenia, the positive and the negative, are recognized (Liddle, 1987). Those in whom positive symptoms predominate have hallucinations, delusions, and paranoid ideation and those who have negative symptoms show apathy and anledonia. Beside impairment in the cognitive domain, individuals with schizophrenia show a deficit in emotion processing, as indicated by a markedly reduced ability to perceive, process, and express facial emotions (Aleman et al., 1999). Not all, but many of these individuals have low levels of arachidonic acid and docosahexaenoic acid in membrane glycerophospholipids and also fail the niacin flush test (Glen et al., 1994).

Marked elevations are found in iPLA$_2$ activity in the brain tissue of some schizophrenic patients (Table 13.1) (Hudson et al., 1996a; Ross et al., 1997, 1999; Ross, 2003). This results in accelerated glycerophospholipid metabolism and oxidative stress in schizophrenia. Levels of PtdCho and EtnGpl are decreased while the levels of lyso-PtdCho are increased in the brain, erythrocytes, platelets, and skin fibroblasts of patients with schizophrenia (Yao et al., 2000; Ross, 2003).

TABLE 13.1. Status of glycerophospholipid metabolism and activities of PLA$_2$ in neuropsychiatric disorders.

Disorder	Glycerophospholipids/ FAA Metabolism	PLA$_2$ Isoform	References
Schizophrenia	Abnormal	iPLA$_2$ ($\uparrow$)	Ross et al., 1997, 1999; Yao et al., 2000; Ross, 2003
Schizophrenia	Abnormal	cPLA$_2$ ($\uparrow$)($\downarrow$)	Ross et al., 1997; Albers et al., 1993; Katila et al., 1997; Pae et al., 2004b
Cocaine user	Unknown	cPLA$_2$ ($\downarrow$)	Ross and Turenne, 2002
Bipolar disorders	Abnormal	Unknown	Pae et al., 2004a; Yildiz et al., 2001; Kato et al., 1993
Dyslexia	Abnormal	cPLA$_2$ ($\uparrow$)	Taylor et al., 2000; Richardson et al., 1997; MacDonell et al., 2000
Autism	Abnormal	cPLA$_2$ ($\uparrow$)	Bell et al., 2004
ADHD	Abnormal	–	Young et al., 2004

Downward and upward arrows in parentheses indicate increase ($\uparrow$) or decrease ($\downarrow$). FAA is free arachidonic acid.

Elevated levels of lyso-PtdCho and lyso-PtdEtn in schizophrenic patients are significantly reduced after three weeks of pharmacotherapy with haloperidol (Schmitt et al., 2001). This effect of haloperidol is caused by a dopamine-mediated decrease in PLA$_2$ activity. Other neuroleptic drugs also decrease iPLA$_2$ activity in the blood of patients with schizophrenia (Gattaz et al., 1987). These studies are supported by recent studies on rats. Haloperidol exerts its effect by downregulating D$_2$-mediated PLA$_2$ signaling associated with AA release in basal ganglia–frontal cortex circuitry (Myers et al., 2001). In general, reduced PLA$_2$ activity through the action of antipsychotic drugs may result either from the binding of the drug to the interface enzyme–substrate complex or from a downregulation of protein-coupled PLA$_2$ signaling.

Increased iPLA$_2$ activity in schizophrenic subjects can change the membrane glycerophospholipid composition, disrupt membrane fluidity, and therefore, the activity of membrane-dependent proteins such as Na$^+$-K$^+$-ATPase, β2- and α2-adrenergic receptors, and MAO, and uptake of norepinephrine and serotonin. Disturbances in other membrane-dependent proteins, tyrosine and tryptophan hydroxylase, may also occur and this may explain the dopamine hypothesis. The mechanisms of action of tricyclic antidepressants, lithium, electroconvulsive shock, and some novel antimanic agents can be explained in terms of alterations of iPLA$_2$ activity (Horrobin, 1998).

^{31}P-Magnetic resonance spectroscopic (^{31}P-MRS) studies of frontal lobe metabolism of living schizophrenic patients show a reduction in resonances of phosphomonoesters (PME) and/or increase in phosphodiesters (PDE) and ATP in the dorsolateral prefrontal cortex of drug-naïve schizophrenic patients, once again indicating an accelerated glycerophospholipid metabolism (Pettegrew et al., 1991; Stanley et al., 1994; Richardson et al., 2001; Yacubian et al., 2002). Changes in neural membrane glycerophospholipids may be related to molecular changes that precede the onset of clinical symptoms and structural changes in the brain in schizophrenia, whereas changes in high-energy phosphate metabolism may be state-dependent. Furthermore, the decline in PtdCho and EtnGpl levels in schizophrenic patients is also accompanied by the depletion of arachidonic and docosahexaenoic acid levels (Yao et al., 2000; Horrobin et al., 1991). This suggests that increased PLA$_2$ activity may be responsible for the low arachidonic acid and docosahexaenoic acid levels in schizophrenic patients.

Arachidonic acid is a second messenger that regulates glutamatergic neurotransmission (Barbour et al., 1989). Activation of NMDA receptors by glutamate activates the PLA$_2$-mediated release of arachidonic acid and in turn facilitates long-term potentiation at the glutamate synapse in hippocampus by blocking glutamate uptake. Reduced levels of arachidonic acid in neural membranes of schizophrenic patients would therefore impair glutamatergic neurotransmission (Peet et al., 1994), and these events may be closely associated with the pathophysiology of schizophrenia (Horrobin, 1998). Glycerophospholipids are not only precursors for a number of signaling molecules such as platelet-activating factor, lysophosphatidic acid, and eicosanoids but also provide a suitable lipid environment for neurotransmitter-mediated signal transduction processes. Collectively these studies suggest that the rate of membrane turnover is accelerated in schizophrenia. This accelerated glycerophospholipid metabolism may have significant effects on neuronal development and communication resulting in behavioral abnormalities in schizophrenic individuals.

The cause of the increased iPLA$_2$ activity is not known. However, it may be due to several mechanisms that are altered in schizophrenia. These mechanisms include (a) the upregulation of retinoic acid receptor-α (RAR-α) expression (Rioux and Arnold, 2005). Increased expression of RAR-α may be involved in the pathophysiology of schizophrenia (Goodman, 1995; LaMantia, 1999) and also with the stimulation of iPLA$_2$ in the nucleus (Antony et al., 2003; Farooqui et al., 2004). Polyunsaturated fatty acids generated through the activation of iPLA$_2$ can bind to RXR-α and cause excessive stimulation (Lengqvist et al., 2004) resulting in abnormalities in memory formation and consolidation (Das, 2003). (b) RAR-α receptors also upregulate the expression of dopamine D$_2$ receptors (Samad et al., 1997), suggesting that RAR-α-mediated expression of dopamine D$_2$ receptors may contribute to the symptoms of schizophrenia. (c) Also, increased levels of cytokines in schizophrenia may contribute to the stimulation of iPLA$_2$ in these subjects (Buka et al., 2001; Farooqui and Horrocks, 2006). Collectively these studies suggest that elevated dopamine and retinoid metabolism along with upregulation of cytokines and the stimulation of iPLA$_2$ activity are closely associated with the etiology of schizophrenia (Goodman, 1998; Smesny, 2004; Yao and Van Kammen, 2004; Laruelle et al., 1999; Farooqui et al., 2004). An understanding of the molecular basis of RAR-α-mediated upregulation of iPLA$_2$ and how it affects downstream molecular pathways for generation of prostaglandins involved in hippocampal plasticity may provide clues to the mechanism responsible for the generation of abnormal brain connectivity in schizophrenia (Rioux and Arnold, 2005).

In contrast, studies on cPLA$_2$ activity in schizophrenic patients have been controversial (Ross et al., 1997; Hudson et al., 1999). Some investigators found elevated $cPLA_2$ activity (Table 13.1), while others report markedly lower $cPLA_2$ activity in the brain and peripheral tissues including blood from schizophrenic subjects (Ross, 2003; Albers et al., 1993). A lower $cPLA_2$ activity in schizophrenic patients emerges only after the subjects are differentiated with regard to their niacin sensitivity (Hudson et al., 1999). Collectively, these studies indicate multiple etiologies for schizophrenia.

Studies on the genetic basis of altered PLA_2 activity in schizophrenia have also been controversial. Some studies indicate differences in allele frequencies of a polymorphism close to the promoter region of the $cPLA_2$ gene. A dimorphic site within the first intron of $cPLA_2$ was also linked to schizophrenia (Peet et al., 1998b; Rybakowski et al., 2003). It is speculated that the gene function can be influenced by allele length in schizophrenic subjects (Hudson et al., 1996a,b; Rybakowski et al., 2003). Others failed to observe abnormalities in the promoter region of the gene encoding $cPLA_2$ (Doris et al., 1998). Thus more studies are needed on a larger population to understand the involvement of PLA_2 polymorphism and glycerophospholipid alterations in the pathophysiology of schizophrenia (Junqueira et al., 2004). Genes for other PLA_2 subtypes ($sPLA_2$ and platelet-activating factor acetylhydrolase) show no linkage with schizophrenia (Bell et al., 1997; Frieboes et al., 2001). In contrast, genes encoding $iPLA_2$ show significant associations with schizophrenic population (Junqueira et al., 2004).

13.3 Cocaine Addiction

Cocaine is a strong central nervous system stimulant. The primary mechanism of cocaine-induced actions is a blockade of the monoamine transporters, resulting in elevated extracellular monoamine (dopamine, serotonin, and epinephrine) concentrations. An increase in dopamine levels at the nerve terminal causes continuous stimulation of "receiving" neurons. This is associated with the euphoria that is known to occur in cocaine abusers. Targets for cocaine also include norepinephrine and serotonin transporters as well as at dopamine transporters, blocking reuptake of these monoamines and increasing their synaptic levels. Detailed investigations on the glycerophospholipid composition of a cocaine user's brain have not been performed, but these individuals show reduced $cPLA_2$ activity in their striatum (Table 13.1) (Ross and Turenne, 2002). Since PLA_2 receptors are coupled to serotonin and dopamine receptors (Kolko et al., 1996; Ross, 2003; Qu et al., 2003) on neural membranes, it is proposed that serotonergic and dopaminergic hyperactivity in cocaine users may be responsible for the decreased $cPLA_2$ activity (Ross and Turenne, 2002).

Assays of enzymic activities in the striatum of rats exposed to cocaine also show a decrease in PLA_2 activity that can be reversed by haloperidol, a dopamine receptor antagonist (Ross and Turenne, 2002). This confirms results obtained with human subjects (Ross and Turenne, 2002). To establish whether the decrease in $cPLA_2$ is specific for cocaine users or a general feature of all abused drugs that enhance dopaminergic neurotransmission, enzymes of glycerophospholipid metabolism have been assayed in dopamine-rich (putamen) and dopamine-poor brain areas of chronic users of cocaine and of methamphetamine (Ross et al., 2002b). In cocaine and methamphetamine users, cPLA$_2$ and phosphocholine cytidylyltransferase activities in dopamine-rich areas are decreased when compared to control subjects. A decrease in striatal cPLA$_2$ and/or PCCT activities in cocaine users might also help in explaining why CDP-choline, which enhances glycerophospholipid synthesis, reduces craving in some users of cocaine (Ross et al., 2002a). At present it is not known whether the decrease in PLA$_2$ activity is due to the stimulant-sensitization effects of cocaine and methamphetamine or is caused by some other unknown mechanism. However, PLA$_2$ is associated with stimulant-induced behavioral sensitization in rats (Reid et al., 1996). PLA$_2$ activity in mesolimbic dopamine neurons, at the level of the cell bodies and perhaps the nerve terminals, may be involved in the biochemical mechanisms mediating stimulant sensitization effects.

13.4 Depression and Bipolar Disorders

Bipolar disorders are common and often disabling mood disorders from which individuals suffer from episodes of mania and depression. Depression is characterized by feelings of unhappiness, loss of energy and interest, fatigue, poor concentration, altered appetite, sleep disturbance, diminished cognitive function, weight gain or loss, anxiety, agitation or irritability, and chronic indecisiveness. The symptoms of mania include irritable mood, inflated self-esteem, increased talkativeness, distractibility, increased goal-directed activity, and excessive involvement in pleasurable activities with a high potential for painful consequences (NIMH Genetic Workshop, 1999). The biological cause of depression and bipolar disorders is unknown. Both may be due partially to an imbalance in some brain neurotransmitters. Some studies indicate that a low activity of monoamine neurotransmitter systems results in depression (Charney et al., 1990). Depression and bipolar disorders are commonly treated with a variety of antidepressant drugs such as the selective serotonin-reuptake inhibitors.

Mitochondrial dysfunction and abnormalities in glycerophospholipid metabolism are also implicated in the pathophysiology of depression and bipolar disorders (Kato et al., 1993). Cytokines play a pivotal role in the communication between the immune system and the CNS. In rodents, cytokines produce symptoms commonly referred to as "sickness behavior." Some of these, including reduced feeding and decreased social and exploratory behavior, are reminiscent of those seen in depressed patients. Some studies in humans indicate that major depression is also accompanied by an immune response with an increased production of proinflammatory cytokines, such as interleukin 1(IL-1), IL-6, TNF-α, and interferon gamma (IFN-γ) (Maes et al., 1997; Tuglu et al., 2003). These cytokines may bind to their receptors on astrocytes and induce the enhancement of glycerophospholipid metabolism through the activation of PLA$_2$. Significantly high calcium levels (Dubovsky et al., 1989) in bipolar disorders may also facilitate

PLA_2 stimulation. However, PLA_2 activities have not been determined in bipolar disorders. Collectively these studies suggest that cytokine-mediated neurochemical changes in brain may have a pronounced effect on glycerophospholipid metabolism in individuals with bipolar disorders.

^{31}P-MRS studies provide important information on membrane glycerophospholipid abnormalities in depression and bipolar disorders. Depressed bipolar patients have significantly greater PME levels, especially PEtn, than control human subjects (Yildiz et al., 2001; Kato et al., 1993), indicating an accelerated glycerophospholipid metabolism in these individuals. Although PLA_2 activities have not been assayed in the brain or peripheral tissue from depressed bipolar patients, an association between major depressive disorders and a polymorphism within $sPLA_2$ has been reported in some patients (Papadimitriou et al., 2003). Furthermore, a relationship between Ban1 bimorphism and the $cPLA_2$ gene has been reported in Korean patients having major depressive disorder and schizophrenia (Pae et al., 2004a,b). Ban1 polymorphism of the $cPLA_2$ gene may be related to the pathogenesis of major depressive disorder and schizophrenia (Pae et al., 2004a,b). These studies support the notion that activities of PLA_2 isoforms may be altered in certain forms of depression (Table 13.1) and detailed studies are required on a larger human population with depressed bipolar patients.

[3]H-MRS studies on glycerophospholipid metabolites demonstrate alterations in resonance intensities of choline in both depressed and bipolar patients (Charles et al., 1994; Ende et al., 2000). The choline is primarily derived from phosphocholine and is used for the synthesis of acetylcholine in the brain. Determinations of the rate of oxygen consumption of freshly prepared mitochondria in the presence and absence of various glycerophospholipid degradation products indicate that phosphoethanolamine and ethanolamine inhibit mitochondrial respiration in a dose-dependent manner, whereas choline, glycerophosphoethanolamine, and glycerophosphocholine have no effect. This suggests a specific inhibition by ethanolamine and phosphoethanolamine. Although the concentrations of phosphoethanolamine and ethanolamine used in this study are quite high and nonphysiological, it is likely that during episodes of depression high concentrations of these metabolites occur in the brain tissue (Kato et al., 1993). The mechanism of inhibition of mitochondrial respiration by these metabolites remains unknown (Modica-Napolitano and Renshaw, 2004); hence, more studies on this important topic are required.

The use of lithium for the treatment of bipolar disorders is based on the inhibition of the PtdIns cycle and the upregulation of adenylate cyclase by this mood-stabilizer (Horrobin and Bennett, 1999). However, several studies indicate that chronic lithium administration in rats results in a 50% reduction in mRNA and protein levels of $cPLA_2$ with no changes in $iPLA_2$ and $sPLA_2$ proteins (Chang and Jones, 1998; Rintala et al., 1999). Detailed investigations on the mechanism of lithium inhibition indicate that the reduction of $cPLA_2$ activity is caused by the downregulation of $cPLA_2$ transcription (Weerasinghe et al., 2004). It is interesting to note that the effect of lithium on $cPLA_2$ occurs at lower concentrations than for the PtdIns cycle (Chang and Jones, 1998), indicating that lithium is a powerful cPLA$_2$ inhibitor. Collectively these studies suggest that lithium acts on cPLA$_2$ and the PLC–PtdIns cycle and produces its therapeutic effect through synergistic effects on glycerophospholipid metabolism in bipolar disorders.

13.5 Dyslexia

Dyslexia is a complex syndrome whose exact cause remains unknown. In general, dyslexic signs and symptoms include the auditory-linguistic and spoken language difficulties traditionally associated with the disorder, as well as visual problems, both with reading and more generally, and motor problems. It is proposed that a problem with fatty acid and membrane glycerophospholipid metabolism together with an increase in cPLA$_2$ activity may play a role in the pathophysiology of dyslexia (Taylor and Richardson, 2000; MacDonell et al., 2000). ^{31}P-MSR studies on PME and PDE composition in dyslexic patients indicate that the PME peak area is significantly elevated in the dyslexic group, as evidenced by higher ratios of PME/total phosphorus, PME/beta NTP, and PME/PDE (Richardson et al., 1997). No other spectral measurements related to other glycerophospholipid metabolites differ significantly between dyslexic and nondyslexic adults. The PME peak has several components, but predominantly consists of phosphoethanolamine (PEtn) and phosphocholine (PCho), which are precursors of membrane glycerophospholipids. The PME increase in dyslexia may be due to reduced incorporation of glycerophospholipids into cell membranes. These findings are consistent with the hypothesis that membrane glycerophospholipid metabolism is abnormal in dyslexia.

Another hypothesis related to the pathogenesis of dyslexia is the involvement of n-3 fatty acids in this disorder. Mothers whose diet during pregnancy has lower levels of n-3 fatty acids developed a dark adaptation defect and gave birth to children who developed dyslexia. In contrast, mothers whose diet was enriched with n-3 fatty acids did not develop the dark adaptation defect and had normal children. Four weeks of a high intake of n-3 fatty acids in the first group normalized the dark adaptation defect (Stordy, 1995). This suggests that the pathophysiology of dyslexia involves a defect in the incorporation of n-3 fatty acids into membrane glycerophospholipids (Taylor et al., 2000).

13.6 Autism

Autism is a complex neurodevelopmental disorder of unknown etiology. It is characterized by deficits in social and language development and communicative abnormalities as well as repetitive and stereotyped behaviors (American Psychiatric Association, 1994). Genetic and environmental factors are closely involved in the etiology of autism (Acosta and Pearl, 2003). At present there is no biochemical test to assist in the behavioral diagnosis of autism. Levels of phosphatidylethanolamine are decreased while levels of phosphatidylserine are increased in the erythrocyte membranes of children with autism as compared to their nonautistic developmentally normal siblings (Chauhan et al., 2004). Highly unsaturated fatty acids in red blood cell glycerophospholipids are decreased in autistic subjects (Bell et al., 2000), suggesting an abnormality in unsaturated fatty acid-mediated signal transduction that may be associated with the pathophysiology of autism. Similarly a marked decrease in n-3 fatty acids has been reported in the plasma of autistic subjects (Vancassel et al., 2001). No changes were observed in levels of n-6 fatty acids and consequently a significant increase in the (n-6)/(n-3) ratio was reported in autistic subjects. The decrease in levels of n-3 fatty acids is accompanied by higher levels of erythrocyte lipid peroxides and urinary isoprostanes indicating oxidative stress in autism (McGinnis, 2004).

13.7 Status of n-3 and n-6 Fatty Acids in Neuropsychiatric Disorders

13.7.1 Introduction

As described in Chapter 6, the oxidation of arachidonic acid by the cyclooxygenase enzyme system produces the "2" series of prostaglandins such as PGE_2, $PGF_{2\alpha}$, and so on, so called because of the loss of two unsaturated bonds, leaving two unsaturated bonds. Lipoxygenase converts arachidonic acid to the "4" series of leukotrienes, such as LTB_4. In contrast, n-3 fatty acids, particularly eicosapentaenoic acid, are not good substrates for the cyclooxygenase enzyme system and in fact competitively inhibit the oxidation of n-6 fatty acids (Fig. 13.1). The action of cyclooxygenase on eicosapentaenoic acid produces PGE_3, which is less potent than PGE_2 in producing biological effects related to inflammation. Eicosapentaenoic acid is a good substrate for lipoxygenase and produces LTB_5, which is less active as an activator of neutrophils than LTB_4 (Phillis et al., 2006). These metabolites are collectively called eicosanoids. In contrast, docosahexaenoic acid is not metabolized by a cyclooxygenase. It inhibits cyclooxygenase activity. The action of 15-lipoxygenase on docosahexaenoic acid produces docosanoids (Fig. 13.1) (Serhan, 2005; Marcheselli et al., 2003).

Besides being essential components of neural cell membranes, n-6 and n-3 fatty acids are precursors for eicosanoids and docosanoids, respectively (Phillis et al., 2006). These metabolites have antagonistic activity against each other in the brain tissue. Eicosanoids are proinflammatory, whereas docosanoids are anti-inflammatory (Phillis et al., 2006). In normal brain tissue these n-6 and n-3 fatty acids and their oxygenated products modulate glutamatergic, dopaminergic, and serotonergic neurotransmission (Horrocks and Farooqui, 2004; Ross et al., 2002a; Evans et al., 2001) and are involved in long-term potentiation, sleep, pain, and locomotion (Ross and Glen, 2004).

13.7.2 Depression and Bipolar Disorder

Major depression is accompanied by an increased secretion of eicosanoids and excessive production of proinflammatory cytokines such as interleukin-1β, IL-6,

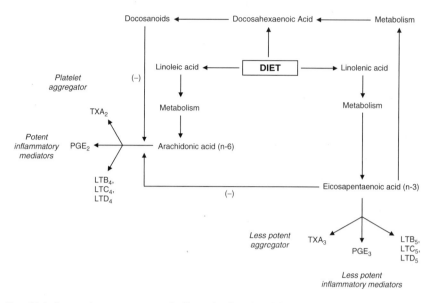

F$_{IG}$. 13.1. Interactions among metabolites of n-3 and n-6 fatty acid metabolites. Note that arachidonic acid is metabolized by cyclooxygenases and lipoxygenases to generate potent inflammatory lipid mediators, eicosanoids. The action of cyclooxygenase on eicosapentaenoic acid produces less active inflammatory lipid mediators. Cyclooxygenase does not act on docosahexaenoic acid. The action of a 15-lipoxygenase-like enzyme on this fatty acid produces docosanoids. (–) indicates inhibition.

IL-2, and interferon-γ (Maes et al., 1997). Increases in cytokines can induce an imbalance in the n-6 to n-3 fatty acid ratio through the activation of PLA$_2$ activity. Thus changes in the levels of eicosanoids and cytokines and the n-6 to n-3 fatty acid ratio in depressed individuals may interfere with serotonin receptor function and can cause depression. In Finland, a low frequency of fish consumption was significantly associated with depression in women, but not in men (Timonen et al., 2004). The n-3 fatty acids from fish are lower in persons with major depression than in controls (van West and Maes, 2003).

Levels of n-3 but not n-6 fatty acids are decreased in peripheral cells of bipolar depressed patients (Edwards et al., 1998; Peet et al., 1998a). In contrast, studies on the fatty acid composition of peripheral cells in schizophrenia have been controversial. Both n-3 and n-6 fatty acids are frequently decreased in schizophrenia (Yao et al., 1994; Peet et al., 2004; Reddy et al., 2004), whereas others found a decrease in n-3 or n-6 fatty acids (Vaddadi et al., 1996; Evans et al., 2003). Collectively these studies suggest that there is no evidence for a specific decrease in n-3 fatty acids in schizophrenia, whereas in bipolar disorders a specific n-3 deficiency exists in their peripheral cells such as red blood cells (Table 13.2) (Peet et al., 1998a). Cross-national comparisons of seafood consumption and rates of psychiatric disorders show a robust correlation between higher seafood consumption and a lower prevalence of bipolar disorders, but not of schizophrenia

TABLE 13.2. Status of n-3 fatty acids and their supplementation in neuropsychiatric disorders.

Disorders	Fatty acid status	Fatty acid supplementation	References
Schizophrenia	n-3 fatty acids ($\downarrow$) n-6 fatty acids ($\downarrow$)	Beneficial	Das, 2004
Bipolar disorders	n-3 fatty acids ($\downarrow$)	Beneficial	Marangell et al., 2003
Dyslexia	n-3 fatty acid ($\downarrow$)	Unknown	Taylor and Richardson, 2000; Taylor et al., 2000
Autism	n-3 fatty acids ($\downarrow$)	Beneficial	Vancassel et al., 2001; Bell et al., 2004
ADHD	n-3 fatty acids ($\downarrow$)	Beneficial	Young et al., 2004; Stevens et al., 2003

A downward arrow in parentheses indicates a decrease.

(Noaghiul and Hibbeln, 2003). The same correlation, but including a lower prevalence of suicide, was found in Finland (Tanskanen et al., 2001a,b).

13.7.3 Aggressive Disorders and Cocaine Addiction

Low levels of n-3 fatty acids may play a role in aggressive disorders. Low levels of plasma DHA are associated with increased fear and anxiety, components of defensive and violent behaviors (Hibbeln et al., 2004a). High dietary intake of DHA is related to a lower likelihood of hostility in young adults (Iribarren et al., 2004). Among cocaine addicts, aggressive persons had lower levels of n-3 fatty acids, including DHA (Buydens-Branch et al., 2003a). Treated cocaine addicts who relapsed after three months had lower baseline levels of AA and n-3 fatty acids (Buydens-Branch et al., 2003b). Higher consumption of linoleic acid, the n-6 precursor of AA, correlates with higher rates of homicide mortality across countries and time (Hibbeln et al., 2004b).

13.7.4 Attention-Deficit Hyperactivity Disorder

Attention-deficit hyperactivity disorder (ADHD) is a debilitating childhood psychiatric disorder characterized by severe and persistent impulsiveness, inattention, and hyperactivity resulting in long-term educational and social disadvantages (American Psychiatric Association, 1994). Pharmacological, neuroimaging, and animal-model studies indicate an associated imbalance in monoaminergic neurotransmission in ADHD. The abnormalities in monoaminergic neurotransmission (Spencer et al., 2005) in ADHD are coupled to alterations in activities of enzymes associated with glycerophospholipid metabolism, specifically a $\Delta6$-desaturase deficit (Ward, 2000). Adult ADHD patients have significantly lower levels of total polyunsaturated fatty acids, total n-3 fatty acids, and docosahexaenoic acid, and significantly higher levels of total saturated fatty acids in erythrocyte membrane glycerophospholipids. The proportion of docosahexaenoic acid in serum and erythrocyte membrane glycerophospholipids is not related to symptom severity in these ADHD subjects (Young et al., 2004). The exact cause of the fatty acid alterations is unknown, but a zinc deficiency may be related (Arnold and DiSilvestro, 2005). However, since the diet is not deficient in n-3 fatty acids, genetic and environmental factors together with abnormalities in fatty acid metabolism may be involved in the pathophysiology of ADHA.

Boys with ADHD are inattentive, impulsive, and hyperactive. The disorder appears to be multifactorial. Their content of plasma arachidonic acid, EPA, and DHA is significantly lower than in the control boys (Stevens et al., 1995). They also had some signs of essential fatty acid deficiency, but did have an elevation of n-9 eicosatrienoic acid, an indicator of that deficiency. The lower level of the essential fatty acids was not caused by diet; therefore, it could be due to impaired conversion of essential fatty acids to AA, EPA, and DHA. The boys with lower plasma phospholipid total n-3 fatty acids had more behavior, learning, and health problems than boys with higher levels (Stevens et al., 1996; Burgess and Stevens, 2003). Delta-6 desaturase deficiency may be one cause of ADHD (Arnold et al., 1994). Preliminary results suggest that some children with ADHD have higher rates of oxidative breakdown of n-3 fatty acids (Ross et al., 2003). This would account for the low levels of n-3 fatty acids found in these children. Adults with ADHD also have lower DHA levels in plasma and erythrocytes, but without correlation to ADHD symptom severity (Young et al., 2004).

13.8 Effects of n-3 Fatty Acid Supplementation in Neuropsychiatric Disorders

13.8.1 Depression and Bipolar Disorder

Reduced dietary intake of n-3 fatty acids may result in neuropsychiatric problems in humans. However, studies on this topic have been inconsistent and controversial. Some studies report no correlation between dietary intake of fish (a food rich in n-3 fatty acid) and depression in women (Jacka et al., 2005), whereas other studies indicate that feeding fish oil to bipolar disorder patients can improve bipolar disorder symptoms (Stoll et al., 1999). Furthermore, a lower n-3 fatty acid content in mother's milk and lower seafood consumption by the mother are associated with higher rates of postpartum depression in women (Hibbeln, 2002). Many studies in this area report no statistically different result and claim no effect of dietary differences on depression. A prime example is a study of the correlation of postpartum depression and fish consumption during pregnancy in relatively small groups of women (Browne et al., 2006). Also, in that study, no differentiation was made between oily fish with high DHA and whitefish with low DHA content. None of the women consumed oily fish regularly, thus the study was useless. A much better study confirmed that lowered serum n-3 fatty acid levels are present in major depression and postpartum depression (De Vriese et al., 2003).

Similarly, in awake rats, a dietary deficiency of n-3 fatty acids decreases the rate of release and turnover of n-3 from neural membrane glycerophospholipids (Contreras et al., 2001), but it remains to be seen whether dietary supplementation with n-3 fatty acid can restore normal turnover or have an ameliorative biological effect on neural membrane glycerophospholipids. A potential synergism of uridine and omega-3 fatty acids for production of antidepressant effects was found in rats (Carlezon et al., 2005). Uridine stimulates synthesis of cytidine 5′-diphosphocholine, which increases glycerophospholipid biosynthesis.

13.8.2 Treatment with High-Dose EPA

Supplementation of n-3 fatty acids in the diet also improves symptoms of schizophrenia, bipolar disorder, dyslexia, autism, and ADHD (Peet et al., 2004; Das, 2004; Bell et al., 2004; Stevens et al., 2003; Young et al., 2004; Yao et al., 2004). High doses of EPA given to schizophrenics markedly enhanced the responsivity to 5-hydroxytryptamine (serotonin). This correlates inversely with severity of the psychosis (Yao et al., 2004). Collectively these studies suggest that n-3 fatty acids are well tolerated by humans and have beneficial effects when supplemented in persons with neuropsychiatric disorders. Larger human trials are needed to confirm the above studies. The n-3 fatty acids are particularly useful in the management of bipolar disorders and major depression (Sarmiento et al., 2003; Severus et al., 2001). At the same time, the n-3 fatty acids reduce the risk of cardiovascular mortality in these patients (Severus et al., 2001).

A group associated with the late David Horrobin used high-dose EPA in several conditions (Horrobin, 2002), including schizophrenia (Horrobin, 2003) and depression (Murck et al., 2004). It rapidly improved severe anorexia nervosa (Ayton et al., 2004). No clinically important changes were found after 12 weeks of treatment of Alzheimer patients in a pilot study (Boston et al., 2004).

13.8.3 ADHD

Children with ADHD were supplemented with various polyunsaturated fatty acids including DHA or EPA (Stevens et al., 2003). This pilot study found some positive effects with those n-3 long-chain fatty acids. The greatest improvement was in oppositional defiant behavior. Another study with children with specific learning difficulties, particularly dyslexia, combined with ADHD showed significant improvement and reduction in ADHD symptoms after 12 weeks of treatment with polyunsaturated fatty acids (Richardson and Puri, 2002; Richardson et al., 2003; Richardson, 2003a,b, 2004a). Although both n-6 and n-3 fatty acids are necessary for brain development, n-3 fatty acids appear most promising for the treatment of childhood developmental and psychiatric disorders (Richardson, 2004b; Richardson and Montgomery, 2005). Alternative treatments for adults with ADHD were described, but most apply to a specific subgroup or have not been tested rigorously (Arnold, 2001). Supplementation with zinc ion or with long-chain n-3 fatty acids is most promising. Relatively high doses of fish oil will be needed for adults with ADHD (Young et al., 2005).

13.8.4 Mechanism of Action of n-3 Fatty Acids

The molecular mechanism of action of n-3 fatty acids in neuropsychiatric disorders remains unknown. However, n-3 fatty acids may have a direct action on one or more neurotransmitter systems such as glutamatergic, dopaminergic, and serotonergic neurotransmission (Evans et al., 2001; Ross et al., 2002a; Horrocks and Farooqui, 2004), and may also act through their immunosuppression effect (Murck et al., 2004). This effect is characterized by the impairment of antigen presentation and of T helper cell type-1 responses. n-3 Fatty acids also decrease the production of inflammatory cytokines and eicosanoids. These mediators are closely associated with the pathogenesis of neuropsychiatric disorders. Supplementation with n-3 fatty acids increases membrane fluidity (Hirashima et al., 2004). This may account for effects on neurotransmission. A high dose of EPA did not benefit patients with Huntington disease, but control patients showed improved motor function (Puri et al., 2005).

Serotonergic neurotransmission plays an important role in bipolar depression and is the site of action of several antidepressants (Delgado, 2004). It is interesting to note that n-3 fatty acid supplementation increases the concentration of serotonin in pig frontal cortex (De la Presa-Owens and Innis, 1999), whereas n-3 fatty acid depletion reduces the ability of fenfluramine, an appetite suppressant, to stimulate serotonin release in rat hippocampus (Kodas et al., 2004). The neurochemical changes in serotonin levels are reversed by a supply of balanced diet provided at birth or during the first 2 weeks of life through maternal milk. However, alterations in serotonin levels persist if the balanced diet is provided from weaning (at 3 weeks of age). This suggests that the provision of essential fatty acids is durably able to affect brain function and is related to the developmental stage during which the deficiency occurs (Kodas et al., 2004). Furthermore, depletion of n-3 fatty acids in rats results in the modification of glycerophospholipid composition and neurochemical function of specific cerebral areas such as striatum and frontal cortex. Thus rats given an n-3 fatty acid deficient diet have an increased serotonin 2_A receptor density in the frontal cortex and decreased D_2 receptors (Delion et al., 1997). Similar results have been reported in the frontal cortex of suicide victims (Maggioni et al., 1990).

A diet deficient in n-3 fatty acids also produces a decrease in the dopamine concentration in rat frontal cortex (Delion et al., 1996). Inversely, a diet enriched in n-3 fatty acids produces a 40% increase in the dopamine concentration in rat frontal cortex (Chalon et al., 1998). Thus the modulation of brain dopamine levels by dietary n-3 fatty acids may have an effect on dopamine-mediated behavior in individuals with neuropsychiatric disorders.

n-3 fatty acid deficiency produces a decrease in NMDA receptor subunits NR2A and NR2B in the cortex of transgenic mice overexpressing the human Alzheimer disease gene APPswe (Calon et al., 2005). Dietary supplementation with n-3 fatty acids partly protects these mice from NMDA receptor subunit loss, indicating that dietary n-3 fatty acids can influence cognitive processes in Alzheimer disease and other disorders. These fatty acids also increase the resistance of forebrain cholinergic neurons against NMDA-mediated neurotoxicity (Hogyes et al., 2003), indicating that n-3 fatty acid supplementation increases neural cell resistance against the excitotoxic damage by being incorporated into neural membrane glycerophospholipids. A decrease in n-3 fatty acids in the diet affects the aging process by decreasing longevity and learning ability in rats (Yamamoto et al., 1987). n-3 Fatty acids modulate responses to γ-aminobutyric acid (GABA) and shift the inactivation curve to a more hyperpolarized potential in both Na^+ and Ca^{2+} currents in primary neuronal cultures (Hamano et al., 1996).

Collective evidence suggests that depletion of n-3 fatty acids can increase the risk of developing neuropsychiatric disorders. The neurochemical mechanism underlying this effect is the deficiency of docosanoids. As stated earlier these metabolites are antiinflammatory and they antagonize the effects of eicosanoids. They decrease the transcription activation gene for adhesion molecules, chemoattractant, and inflammatory cytokines involved in endothelial activation in response to inflammatory stimuli. Furthermore, n-3 fatty acids also modulate gene expression (Horrocks and Farooqui, 2004). Thus microarray studies indicate that a diet enriched in fish oil modulates the overexpression of 55 genes and the suppression of 47 genes in the brain. These genes include genes controlling synaptic plasticity, cytoskeleton, and membrane association, signal transduction, ion channels, energy metabolism, and regulatory proteins (Farkas et al., 2000; Kitajka et al., 2002; Puskás et al., 2003). DHA stimulates the expression of peroxisomal enzymes needed for the synthesis of plasmalogens (Farooqui and Horrocks, 2001; Martinez, 2001; Brites et al., 2004; André et al., 2005, 2006).

13.8.5 Genetic Involvement

Recent DNA microarray studies indicate that genes involved in synaptic neurotransmission, signal transduction, and glutamate/GABA regulation are differentially regulated in the brains of subjects with schizophrenia and bipolar disorders (Fatemi et al., 2006; Ogden et al., 2004). Thus 177 putative schizophrenia risk genes have been identified in the brain, 28 of which map to linked chromosomal loci (Glatt et al., 2005). These genes include MAG, CNP, SOX10, CLDN11, and PMP22 (Dracheva et al., 2006; Wan et al., 2005). Furthermore, 123 putative biomarkers for schizophrenia have been described in blood, 6 of which (BTG1, GSK3A, HLA-DRB1, HNRPA3, SELENBP1, and SFRS1) have corresponding differential expression in the brain (Glatt et al., 2005). Similarly genes for DARPP-32, PENK (preproenkephalin), and TAC1 (tachykinin 1, substance P) have been identified in bipolar subjects (Ogden et al., 2004). These studies suggest that molecular mechanisms involved in pleasure and pain may have been recruited by evolution to play a role in higher mental functions such as mood. The analysis also revealed other high-probability candidate genes (neurogenesis, neurotrophic, neurotransmitter, signal transduction, circadian, synaptic, and myelin related), pathways, and mechanisms of likely importance in the pathophysiology of bipolar disorders. The continued application of this approach in larger populations should facilitate the discovery of highly reliable and reproducible candidate risk genes and biomarkers that can be used for the identification of neuropsychiatric disorder patients in a human population (Konradi, 2005). This information may be useful for early diagnosis and for monitoring the effects of therapeutic drugs for the treatment of neuropsychiatric disorders.

References

Acosta M. T. and Pearl P. L. (2003). The neurobiology of autism: new pieces of the puzzle. *Curr. Neurol. Neurosci. Rep.* 3:149–156.

Albers M., Meurer H., Marki F., and Klotz J. (1993). Phospholipase A$_2$ activity in serum of neuroleptic-naive psychiatric inpatients. *Pharmacopsychiatry* 26:94–98.

Aleman A., Hijman R., de Haan E. H., and Kahn R. S. (1999). Memory impairment in schizophrenia: a meta-analysis. *Am. J. Psychiatry* 156:1358–1366.

American Psychiatric Association (1994). Diagnostic and Statistical Manual of Mental Disorders.

André A., Juanéda P., Sébédio J. L., and Chardigny J. M. (2005). Effects of aging and dietary n-3 fatty acids on rat brain phospholipids: focus on plasmalogens. *Lipids* 40:799–806.

André A., Juanéda P., Sébédio J. L., and Chardigny J. M. (2006). Plasmalogen metabolism-related enzymes in rat brain during aging: influence of n-3 fatty acid intake. *Biochimie* 88:103–111.

Antony P., Freysz L., Horrocks L. A., and Farooqui A. A. (2003). Ca^{2+}-independent phospholipases A$_2$ and production of arachidonic acid in nuclei of LA-N-1 cell cultures: a specific receptor activation mediated with retinoic acid. *Mol. Brain Res.* 115:187–195.

Arnold L. E. (2001). Alternative treatments for adults with attention-deficit hyperactivity disorder (ADHD). In: Wasserstein J., Wolf L. E., and LeFever F. F. (eds.), *Adult Attention Deficit Disorder*. New York Academy of Sciences, New York, pp. 310–341.

Arnold L. E. and DiSilvestro R. A. (2005). Zinc in attention-deficit/hyperactivity disorder. *J. Child Adolesc. Psychopharmacol.* 15:619–627.

Arnold L. E., Kleykamp D., Votolato N. A., Gibson R. A., and Horrocks L. (1994). Potential link between dietary intake of fatty acids and behavior: pilot exploration of serum lipids in attention-deficit hyperactivity disorder. *J. Child Adolesc. Psychopharmacol.* 4:171–182.

Ayton A. K., Azaz A., and Horrobin D. F. (2004). Rapid improvement of severe anorexia nervosa during treatment with ethyl-eicosapentaenoate and micronutrients. *Eur. Psychiatry* 19:317–319.

Barbour B., Szatkowski M., Ingledew N., and Attwell D. (1989). Arachidonic acid induces a prolonged inhibition of glutamate uptake into glial cells. *Nature* 342:918–920.

Bell R., Collier D. A., Rice S. Q., Roberts G. W., Macphee C. H., Kerwin R. W., Price J., and Gloger I. S. (1997). Systematic screening of the LDL-PLA$_2$ gene for polymorphic variants and case-control analysis in schizophrenia. *Biochem. Biophys. Res. Commun.* 241:630–635.

Bell J. G., Sargent J. R., Tocher D. R., and Dick J. R. (2000). Red blood cell fatty acid compositions in a patient with autistic spectrum disorder: a characteristic abnormality in neurodevelopmental disorders? *Prostaglandins Leukot. Essent. Fatty Acids* 63:21–25.

Bell J. G., MacKinlay E. E., Dick J. R., Macdonald D. J., Boyle R. M., and Glen A. C. A. (2004). Essential fatty acids and phospholipase A$_2$ in autistic spectrum disorders. *Prostaglandins Leukot. Essent. Fatty Acids* 71:201–204.

Benes F. M., Walsh J., Bhattacharyya S., Sheth A., and Berretta S. (2003). DNA fragmentation decreased in schizophrenia but not bipolar disorder. *Arch. Gen. Psychiatry* 60:359–364.

Boston P. F., Bennett A., Horrobin D. F., and Bennett C. N. (2004). Ethyl-EPA in Alzheimer's disease – a pilot study. *Prostaglandins Leukot. Essent. Fatty Acids* 71:341–346.

Brites P., Waterham H. R., and Wanders R. J. A. (2004). Functions and biosynthesis of plasmalogens in health and disease. *Biochim. Biophys. Acta Mol. Cell Biol. Lipids* 1636:219–231.

Browne J. C., Scott K. M., and Silvers K. M. (2006). Fish consumption in pregnancy and omega-3 status after birth are not associated with postnatal depression. *J. Affect. Disord.* 90:131–139.

Buka S. L., Tsuang M. T., Torrey E. F., Klebanoff M. A., Wagner R. L., and Yolken R. H. (2001). Maternal cytokine levels during pregnancy and adult psychosis. *Brain Behav. Immun.* 15:411–420.

Burgess J. R. and Stevens L. (2003). Essential fatty acids in relation to attention-deficit/hyperactivity disorder: an update. In: Peet M., Glen L., and Horrobin D. F. (eds.), *Phospholipid Spectrum Disorders in Psychiatry and Neurology*. Marius Press, Carnforth, Lancashire, pp. 511–519.

Buydens-Branch, Branchey M., McMakin D. L., and Hibbeln J. R. (2003a). Polyunsaturated fatty acid status and aggression in cocaine addicts. *Drug Alcohol Depend.* 71:319–323.

Buydens-Branch, Branchey M., McMakin D. L., and Hibbeln J. R. (2003b). Polyunsaturated fatty acid status and relapse vulnerability in cocaine addicts. *Psychiatry Res.* 120:29–35.

Calon F., Lim G. P., Morihara T., Yang F. S., Ubeda O., Salem N. J., Frautschy S. A., and Cole G. M. (2005). Dietary n-3 polyunsaturated fatty acid depletion activates caspases and decreases NMDA receptors in the brain of a transgenic mouse model of Alzheimer's disease. *Eur. J. Neurosci.* 22:617–626.

Carlezon W. A. J., Mague S. D., Parow A. M., Stoll A. L., Cohen B. M., and Renshaw P. F. (2005). Antidepressant-like effects of uridine and omega-3 fatty acids are potentiated by combined treatment in rats. *Biol. Psychiatry.* 57:343–350.

Chalon S., Delion-Vancassel S., Belzung C., Guilloteau D., Leguisquet A. M., Besnard J. C., and Durand G. (1998). Dietary fish oil affects monoaminergic neurotransmission and behavior in rats. *J. Nutr.* 128:2512–2519.

Chang M. C. J. and Jones C. R. (1998). Chronic lithium treatment decreases brain phospholipase A_2 activity. *Neurochem. Res.* 23:887–892.

Charles H. C., Lazeyras F., Krishnan K. R., Boyko O. B., Payne M., and Moore D. (1994). Brain choline in depression: in vivo detection of potential pharmacodynamic effects of antidepressant therapy using hydrogen localized spectroscopy. *Prog. Neuropsychopharmacol. Biol. Psychiatry* 18:1121–1127.

Charney D. S., Southwick S. M., Delgado P. L., and Krystal J. H. (1990). Current status of the receptor sensitivity hypothesis of antidepressant action. In: Amsterdam J. D. (ed.), *Psychopharmacology of Depression*. Marcel Dekker, New York, pp. 13–34.

Chauhan V., Chauhan A., Cohen I. L., Brown W. T., and Sheikh A. (2004). Alteration in amino-glycerophospholipids levels in the plasma of children with autism: a potential biochemical diagnostic marker. *Life Sci.* 74:1635–1643.

Contreras M. A., Chang M. C. J., Rosenberger T. A., Greiner R. S., Myers C. S., Salem N. J., and Rapoport S. I. (2001). Chronic nutritional deprivation of n-3 α-linolenic acid does not affect n-6 arachidonic acid recycling within brain phospholipids of awake rats. *J. Neurochem.* 79:1090–1099.

Das U. N. (2003). Long-chain polyunsaturated fatty acids in memory formation and consolidation: Further evidence and discussion. *Nutrition* 19:988–993.

Das U. N. (2004). Can perinatal supplementation of long-chain polyunsaturated fatty acids prevents schizophrenia in adult life? Med. Sci. *Monitor* 10:HY33–HY37.

De la Presa-Owens S. and Innis S. M. (1999). Docosahexaenoic and arachidonic acid prevent a decrease in dopaminergic and serotoninergic neurotransmitters in frontal cortex caused by a linoleic and α-linolenic acid deficient diet in formula-fed piglets. *J. Nutr.* 129:2088–2093.

Delgado P. L. (2004). Common pathways of depression and pain. *J. Clin. Psychiatry* 65(Suppl. 12):16–19.

Delion S., Chalon S., Guilloteau D., Besnard J. C., and Durand G. (1996). α-Linolenic acid dietary deficiency alters age-related changes of dopaminergic and serotoninergic neurotransmission in the rat frontal cortex. *J. Neurochem.* 66:1582–1591.

Delion S., Chalon S., Guilloteau D., Lejeune B., Besnard J. C., and Durand G. (1997). Age-related changes in phospholipid fatty acid composition and monoaminergic neurotransmission in the hippocampus of rats fed a balanced or an n-3 polyunsaturated fatty acid-deficient diet. *J. Lipid Res.* 38:680–689.

De Vriese S. R., Christophe A. B., and Maes M. (2003). Lowered serum n-3 polyunsaturated fatty acid (PUFA) levels predict the occurrence of postpartum depression: further evidence that lowered n-PUFAs are related to major depression. *Life Sci.* 73:3181–3187.

Doris A. B., Wahle K., MacDonald A., Morris S., Coffey I., Muir W., and Blackwood D. (1998). Red cell membrane fatty acids, cytosolic phospholipase-A$_2$ and schizophrenia. *Schizophr. Res.* 31:185–196.

Dracheva S., Davis K. L., Chin B., Woo D. A., Schmeidler J., and Haroutunian V. (2006). Myelin-associated mRNA and protein expression deficits in the anterior cingulate cortex and hippocampus in elderly schizophrenia patients. *Neurobiol. Dis.* 21:531–540.

Dubovsky S. L., Christiano J., Daniell L. C., Franks R. D., Murphy J., Adler L., Baker N., and Harris R. A. (1989). Increased platelet intracellular calcium concentration in patients with bipolar affective disorders. *Arch. Gen. Psychiatry* 46:632–638.

Edwards R., Peet M., Shay J., and Horrobin D. (1998). Omega-3 polyunsaturated fatty acid levels in the diet and in red blood cell membranes of depressed patients. *J. Affect. Disord.* 48:149–155.

Ende G., Braus D. F., Walter S., Weber-Fahr W., and Henn F. A. (2000). The hippocampus in patients treated with electroconvulsive therapy: a proton magnetic resonance spectroscopic imaging study. *Arch. Gen. Psychiatry* 57:937–943.

Evans K. L., Cropper J. D., Berg K. A., and Clarke W. P. (2001). Mechanisms of regulation of agonist efficacy at the 5-HT$_{1A}$ receptor by phospholipid-derived signaling components. *J. Pharmacol. Exp. Ther.* 297:1025–1035.

Evans D. R., Parikh V. V., Khan M. M., Coussons C., Buckley P. F., and Mahadik S. P. (2003). Red blood cell membrane essential fatty acid metabolism in early psychotic patients following antipsychotic drug treatment. *Prostaglandins Leukot. Essent. Fatty Acids* 69:393–399.

Farkas T., Kitajka K., Fodor E., Csengeri I., Lahdes E., Yeo Y. K., Krasznai Z., and Halver J. E. (2000). Docosahexaenoic acid-containing phospholipid molecular species in brains of vertebrates. *Proc. Natl Acad. Sci. USA* 97:6362–6366.

Farooqui A. A. and Horrocks L. A. (2001). Plasmalogens, phospholipase A$_2$, and docosahexaenoic acid turnover in brain tissue. *J. Mol. Neurosci.* 16:263–272.

Farooqui A. A. and Horrocks L. A. (2006). Phospholipase A$_2$-generated lipid mediators in brain: the good, the bad, and the ugly. *Neuroscientist* 12:245.

Farooqui A. A., Antony P., Ong W. Y., Horrocks L. A., and Freysz L. (2004). Retinoic acid-mediated phospholipase A$_2$ signaling in the nucleus. *Brain Res. Rev.* 45:179–195.

Fatemi S. H., Reutiman T. J., Folsom T. D., Bell C., Nos L., Fried P., Pearce D. A., Singh S., Siderovski D. P., Willard F. S., and Fukuda M. (2006). Chronic olanzapine treatment causes differential expression of genes in frontal cortex of rats as revealed by DNA microarray technique. *Neuropsychopharmacology* doi:10.1038/sj.npp.1301002.

Frieboes R. M., Moises H. W., Gattaz W. F., Yang L., Li T., Liu X. H., Vetter P., Macciardi F., Hwu H. G., and Henn F. (2001). Lack of association between schizophrenia and the phospholipase-A_2 genes cPLA$_2$ and sPLA$_2$. *Am. J. Med. Genet.* 105:246–249.

Gallagher S. (2004). Neurocognitive models of schizophrenia: a neurophenomenological critique. *Psychopathology* 37:8–19.

Gattaz W. F., Kollisch M., Thuren T., Virtanen J. A., and Kinnunen P. K. (1987). Increased plasma phospholipase A$_2$ activity in schizophrenic patients: reduction after neuroleptic therapy. *Biol. Psychiatry* 22:421–426.

Glatt S. J., Everall I. P., Kremen W. S., Corbeil J., Sasik R., Khanlou N., Han M., Liew C. C., and Tsuang M. T. (2005). Comparative gene expression analysis of blood and brain provides concurrent validation of SELENBP1 up-regulation in schizophrenia. *Proc. Natl Acad. Sci. USA* 102:15533–15538.

Glen A. I. M., Glen E. M. T., Horrobin D. F., Vaddadi K. S., Spellman M., Morse-Fisher N., Ellis K., and Skinner F. S. (1994). A red cell membrane abnormality in a subgroup of schizophrenic patients: evidence for two diseases. *Schizophr. Res.* 12:53–61.

Goodman A. B. (1995). Chromosomal locations and modes of action of genes of the retinoid (vitamin A) system support their involvement in the etiology of schizophrenia. *Am. J. Med. Genet.* 60:335–348.

Goodman A. B. (1998). Three independent lines of evidence suggest retinoids as causal to schizophrenia. *Proc. Natl Acad. Sci. USA* 95:7240–7244.

Hamano H., Nabekura J., Nishikawa M., and Ogawa T. (1996). Docosahexaenoic acid reduces GABA response in substantia nigra neuron of rat. J. Neurophysiol. 75:1264–1270.

Harrison P. J. and Owen M. J. (2003). Genes for schizophrenia? Recent findings and their pathophysiological implications. *Lancet* 361:417–419.

Hibbeln J. R. (2002). Seafood consumption, the DHA content of mothers' milk and prevalence rates of postpartum depression: a cross-national, ecological analysis. *J. Affect. Disord.* 69:15–29.

Hibbeln J. R., Bissette G., Umhau J. C., and George D. T. (2004a). Omega-3 status and cerebrospinal fluid corticotrophin releasing hormone in perpetrators of domestic violence. *Biol. Psychiatry* 56:895–897.

Hibbeln J. R., Nieminen L. R. G., and Lands W. E. M. (2004b). Increasing homicide rates and linoleic acid consumption among five western countries, 1961–2000. *Lipids* 39:1207–1213.

Hirashima F., Parow A. M., Stoll A. L., Demopulos C. M., Damico K. E., Rohan M. L., Eskesen J. G., Zuo C. S., Cohen B. M., and Renshaw P. F. (2004). Omega-3 fatty acid treatment and T-2 whole brain relaxation times in bipolar disorder. *Am. J. Psychiatry* 161:1922–1924.

Hogyes E., Nyakas C., Kiliaan A., Farkas T., Penke B., and Luiten P. G. (2003). Neuroprotective effect of developmental docosahexaenoic acid supplement against excitotoxic brain damage in infant rats. *Neuroscience* 119:999–1012.

Horrobin D. F. (1998). The membrane phospholipid hypothesis as a biochemical basis for the neurodevelopmental concept of schizophrenia. *Schizophr. Res.* 30:193–208.

Horrobin D. F. (2002). A new category of psychotropic drugs: neuroactive lipids as exemplified by ethyl eicosapentaenoate (E-E). In: Jucker E. (ed.), *Progress in Drug Research, Vol 59*. Birkhauser Verlag AG, Basel, pp. 171–199.

Horrobin D. F. (2003). Omega-3 fatty acid for schizophrenia. *Am. J. Psychiatry* 160:188–189.

Horrobin D. F. and Bennett C. N. (1999). New gene targets related to schizophrenia and other psychiatric disorders: enzymes, binding proteins and transport proteins involved in phospholipid and fatty acid metabolism. *Prostaglandins Leukot. Essent. Fatty Acids* 60:141–167.

Horrobin D. F., Manku M. S., Hillman H., Iain A., and Glen M. (1991). Fatty acid levels in the brains of schizophrenics and normal controls. *Biol. Psychiatry* 30:795–805.

Horrocks L. A. and Farooqui A. A. (2004). Docosahaenoic acid in the diet: its importance in maintenance and restoration of neural membrane function. *Prostaglandins Leukot. Essent. Fatty Acids* 70:361–372.

Hudson C. J., Kennedy J. L., Gotowiec A., Lin A., King N., Gojtan K., Macciardi F., Skorecki K., Meltzer H. Y., Warsh J. J., and Horrobin D. F. (1996a). Genetic variant near cytosolic phospholipase A$_2$ associated with schizophrenia. *Schizophr. Res.* 21:111–116.

Hudson C. J., Lin A., and Horrobin D. F. (1996b). Phospholipases: in search of a genetic base of schizophrenia. *Prostaglandins Leukot. Essent. Fatty Acids* 55:119–122.

Hudson C., Gotowiec A., Seeman M., Warsh J., and Ross B. M. (1999). Clinical subtyping reveals significant differences in calcium-dependent phospholipase A$_2$ activity in schizophrenia. *Biol. Psychiatry* 46:401–405.

Iribarren C., Markovitz J. H., Jacobs D. R. J., Schreiner P. J., Daviglus M., and Hibbeln J. R. (2004). Dietary intake of n-3, n-6 fatty acids and fish: relationship with hostility in young adults – the CARDIA study. *Eur. J. Clin. Nutr.* 58:24–31.

Jacka F. N., Pasco J. A., Henry M. J., Kotowicz M. A., Dodd S., Nicholson G. C., and Berk M. (2005). Depression and bone mineral density in a community sample of perimenopausal women: Geelong Osteoporosis Study. *Menopause* 12:88–91.

Jarskog L. F., Selinger E. S., Lieberman J. A., and Gilmore J. H. (2004). Apoptotic proteins in the temporal cortex in schizophrenia: high Bax/Bcl-2 ratio without caspase-3 activation. *Am. J. Psychiatry* 161:109–115.

Junqueira R., Cordeiro Q., Meira-Lima I., Gattaz W. F., and Vallada H. (2004). Allelic association analysis of phospholipase A2 genes with schizophrenia. *Psychiatr. Genet.* 14:157–160.

Katila H., Appelberg B., and Rimon R. (1997). No differences in phospholipase-A$_2$ activity between acute psychiatric patients and controls. *Schizophr. Res.* 26:103–105.

Kato T., Takahashi S., Shioiri T., and Inubushi T. (1993). Alterations in brain phosphorous metabolism in bipolar disorder detected by in vivo ^{31}P and ^{7}Li magnetic resonance spectroscopy. *J. Affect. Disord.* 27:53–59.

Kitajka K., Puskás L. G., Zvara A., Hackler L. J., Barceló-Coblijn G., Yeo Y. K., and Farkas T. (2002). The role of n-3 polyunsaturated fatty acids in brain: Modulation of rat brain gene expression by dietary n-3 fatty acids. *Proc. Natl Acad. Sci. USA* 99:2619–2624.

Kodas E., Galineau L., Bodard S., Vancassel S., Guilloteau D., Besnard J. C., and Chalon S. (2004). Serotoninergic neurotransmission is affected by n-3 polyunsaturated fatty acids in the rat. *J. Neurochem.* 89:695–702.

Kolko M., DeCoster M. A., Rodriguez de Turco E. B., and Bazan N. G. (1996). Synergy by secretory phospholipase A$_2$ and glutamate on inducing cell death and sustained arachidonic acid metabolic changes in primary cortical neuronal cultures. *J. Biol. Chem.* 271:32722–32728.

Konradi C. (2005). Gene expression microarray studies in polygenic psychiatric disorders: applications and data analysis. *Brain Res. Brain Res. Rev.* 50:142–155.

LaMantia A. S. (1999). Forebrain induction, retinoic acid, and vulnerability to schizophrenia: insights from molecular and genetic analysis in developing mice. *Biol. Psychiatry* 46:19–30.

Laruelle M., Abi-Dargham A., Gil R., Kegeles L., and Innis R. (1999). Increased dopamine transmission in schizophrenia: relationship to illness phases. *Biol. Psychiatry* 46:56–72.

Lengqvist J., Mata de Urquiza A., Bergman A. C., Willson T. M., Sjövall J., Perlmann T., and Griffiths W. J. (2004). Polyunsaturated fatty acids including docosahexaenoic and arachidonic acid bind to the retinoid X receptor α ligand-binding domain. *Mol. Cell. Proteomics* 3:692–703.

Liddle P. F. (1987). The symptoms of chronic schizophrenia. A re-examination of the positive–negative dichotomy. *Br. J. Psychiatry* 151:145–151.

MacDonell L. E., Skinner F. K., Ward P. E., Glen A. I., Glen A. C., Macdonald D. J., Boyle R. M., and Horrobin D. F. (2000). Increased levels of cytosolic phospholipase A2 in dyslexics. *Prostaglandins Leukot. Essent. Fatty Acids* 63:37–39.

Maes M., Bosmans E., de Jongh R., Kenis G., Vandoolaeghe E., and Neels H. (1997). Increased serum IL-6 and IL-1 receptor antagonist concentrations in major depression and treatment resistant depression. *Cytokine* 9:853–858.

Maggioni M., Picotti G. B., Bondiolotti G. P., Panerai A., Cenacchi T., Nobile P., and Brambilla F. (1990). Effects of phosphatidylserine therapy in geriatric patients with depressive disorders. *Acta Psychiatr. Scand.* 81:265–270.

Marangell L. B., Martinez J. M., Zboyan H. A., Kertz B., Kim H. F. S., and Puryear L. J. (2003). A double-blind, placebo-controlled study of the omega-3 fatty acid docosahexaenoic acid in the treatment of major depression. *Am. J. Psychiatry* 160:996–998.

Marcheselli V. L., Hong S., Lukiw W. J., Tian X. H., Gronert K., Musto A., Hardy M., Gimenez J. M., Chiang N., Serhan C. N., and Bazan N. G. (2003). Novel docosanoids inhibit brain ischemia-reperfusion-mediated leukocyte infiltration and pro-inflammatory gene expression. *J. Biol. Chem.* 278:43807–43817.

Margolis R. L., Chuang D. M., and Post R. M. (1994). Programmed cell death: implications for neuropsychiatric disorders. *Biol. Psychiatry* 35:946–956.

Martinez M. (2001). Restoring the DHA levels in the brains of Zellweger patients. *J. Mol. Neurosci.* 16:309–316.

Mattson M. P., Keller J. N., and Begley J. G. (1998). Evidence for synaptic apoptosis. *Exp. Neurol.* 153:35–48.

McGinnis W. R. (2004). Oxidative stress in autism. *Altern. Ther. Health Med.* 10:22–36.

Modica-Napolitano J. S. and Renshaw P. F. (2004). Ethanolamine and phosphoethanolamine inhibit mitochondrial function in vitro: implications for mitochondrial dysfunction hypothesis in depression and bipolar disorder. *Biol. Psychiatry* 55:273–277.

Murck H., Song C., Horrobin D. F., and Uhr M. (2004). Ethyl-eicosapentaenoate and dexamethasone resistance in therapy-refractory depression. *Int. J. Neuropsychopharmacol.* 7:341–349.

Myers C. S., Contreras M. A., Chang M. C. J., Rapoport S. I., and Appel N. M. (2001). Haloperidol downregulates phospholipase A_2 signaling in rat basal ganglia circuits. *Brain Res.* 896:96–101.

NIMH Genetic Workshop (1999). Genetics and mental disorders. *Biol. Psychiatry* 45:559–602.

Noaghiul S. and Hibbeln J. R. (2003). Cross-national comparisons of seafood consumption and rates of bipolar disorders. *Am. J. Psychiatry* 160:2222–2227.

Ogden C. A., Rich M. E., Schork N. J., Paulus M. P., Geyer M. A., Lohr J. B., Kuczenski R., and Niculescu A. B. (2004). Candidate genes, pathways and mechanisms for bipolar (manic-depressive) and related disorders: an expanded convergent functional genomics approach. *Mol. Psychiatry* 9:1007–1029.

Oppenheim R. W. (1991). Cell death during development of the nervous system. *Annu. Rev. Neurosci.* 14:453–501.

Pae C. U., Yu H. S., Kim J. J., Lee C. U., Lee S. J., Lee K. U., Jun T. Y., Paik I. H., Serretti A., and Lee C. (2004a). BanI polymorphism of the cytosolic phospholipase A$_2$ gene and mood disorders in the Korean population. *Neuropsychobiology* 49:185–188.

Pae C. U., Yu H. S., Lee K. U., Kim J. J., Lee C. U., Lee J. S., Jun T. Y., Lee C., and Paik I. H. (2004b). BanI polymorphism of the cytosolic phospholipase A2 gene may confer susceptibility to the development of schizophrenia. *Prog. Neuro-Psychopharmacol. Biol. Psychiat.* 28:739–741.

Papadimitriou G. N., Dikeos D. G., Souery D., Del Favero J., Massat I., Avramopoulos D., Blairy S., Cichon S., Ivezic S., Kaneva R., Karadima G., Lilli R., Milanova V., Nothen M., Oruc L., Rietschel M., Serretti A., Van Broeckhoven C., Stefanis C. N., and Mendlewicz J. (2003). Genetic association between the phospholipase A$_2$ gene and unipolar affective disorder: a multicentre case-control study. *Psychiatr. Genet.* 13:211–220.

Peet M., Laugharne J. D., Horrobin D. F., and Reynolds G. P. (1994). Arachidonic acid: a common link in the biology of schizophrenia? [letter]. *Arch. Gen. Psychiatry* 51:665–666.

Peet M., Murphy B., Shay J., and Horrobin D. (1998a). Depletion of omega-3 fatty acid levels in red blood cell membranes of depressive patients. *Biol. Psychiatry* 43:315–319.

Peet M., Ramchand C. N., Lee J., Telang S. D., Vankar G. K., Shah S., and Wei J. (1998b). Association of the Ban I dimorphic site at the human cytosolic phospholipase A$_2$ gene with schizophrenia. *Psychiatr. Genet.* 8:191–192.

Peet M., Shah S., Selvam K., and Ramchand C. N. (2004). Polyunsaturated fatty acid levels in red cell membranes of unmedicated schizophrenic patients. *World J. Biol. Psychiatry* 5:92–99.

Pettegrew J. W., Keshavan M. S., Panchalingam K., Strychor S., Kaplan D. B., Tretta M. G., and Allen M. (1991). Alterations in brain high-energy phosphate and membrane phospholipid metabolism in first-episode, drug-naive schizophrenics: a pilot study of the dorsal prefrontal cortex by in vivo phosphorus 31 nuclear magnetic resonance spectroscopy. *Arch. Gen. Psychiatry* 48:563–568.

Phillis J. W., Horrocks L. A., and Farooqui A. A. (2006). Cyclooxygenases, lipoxygenases, and epoxygenases in CNS: their role and involvement in neurological disorders. *Brain Res. Rev.* (in press).

Puri B. K., Leavitt B. R., Hayden M. R., Ross C. A., Rosenblatt A., Greenamyre J. T., Hersch S., Vaddadi K. S., Sword A., Horrobin D. F., Manku M., and Murck H. (2005). Ethyl-EPA in Huntington disease – a double-blind, randomized, placebo-controlled trial. *Neurology* 65:286–292.

Puskás L. G., Kitajka K., Nyakas C., Barcelo-Coblijn G., and Farkas T. (2003). Short-term administration of omega 3 fatty acids from fish oil results in increased transthyretin transcription in old rat hippocampus. *Proc. Natl Acad. Sci. USA* 100:1580–1585.

Qu Y., Chang L., Klaff J., Seeman R., Balbo A., and Rapoport S. I. (2003). Imaging of brain serotonergic neurotransmission involving phospholipase A$_2$ activation and arachidonic acid release in unanesthetized rats. *Brain Res. Protocols* 12:16–25.

Reddy R. D., Keshavan M. S., and Yao J. K. (2004). Reduced red blood cell membrane essential polyunsaturated fatty acids in first episode schizophrenia at neuroleptic-naive baseline. *Schizophr. Bull.* 30:901–911.

Reid M. S., Hsu K., Tolliver B. K., Crawford C. A., and Berger S. P. (1996). Evidence for the involvement of phospholipase A$_2$ mechanisms in the development of stimulant sensitization. *J. Pharmacol. Exp. Ther.* 276:1244–1256.

Richardson A. J. (2003a). Clinical trials of fatty acid supplementation in ADHD. In: Peet M., Glen L., and Horrobin D. F. (eds.), *Phospholipid Spectrum Disorders in Psychiatry and Neurology*. Marius Press, Carnforth, Lancashire, pp. 529–541.

Richardson A. J. (2003b). Clinical trials of fatty acid supplementation in dyslexia and dyspraxia. In: Peet M., Glen L., and Horrobin D. F. (eds.), *Phospholipid Spectrum Disorders in Psychiatry and Neurology*. Marius Press, Carnforth, Lancashire, pp. 491–500.

Richardson A. J. (2004a). Clinical trials of fatty acid treatment in ADHD, dyslexia, dyspraxia and the autistic spectrum. *Prostaglandins Leukot. Essent. Fatty Acids* 70:383–390.

Richardson A. J. (2004b). Long-chain polyunsaturated fatty acids in childhood developmental and psychiatric disorders. *Lipids* 39:1215–1222.

Richardson A. J. and Montgomery P. (2005). The Oxford-Durham study: A randomized, controlled trial of dietary supplementation with fatty acids in children with developmental coordination disorder. *Pediatrics* 115:1360–1366.

Richardson A. J. and Puri B. K. (2002). A randomized double-blind, placebo-controlled study of the effects of supplementation with highly unsaturated fatty acids on ADHD-related symptoms in children with specific learning difficulties. *Prog. Neuropsychopharmacol. Biol. Psychiatry* 26:233–239.

Richardson A. J., Cox I. J., Sargentoni J., and Puri B. K. (1997). Abnormal cerebral phospholipid metabolism in dyslexia indicated by phosphorus-31 magnetic resonance spectroscopy. *NMR Biomed.* 10:309–314.

Richardson A. J., Allen S. J., Hajnal J. V., Cox I. J., Easton T., and Puri B. K. (2001). Associations between central and peripheral measures of phospholipid breakdown revealed by cerebral 31-phosphorus magnetic resonance spectroscopy and fatty acid composition of erythrocyte membranes. *Prog. NeuroPsychopharmacol. Biol. Psychiatry* 25:1513–1521.

Richardson A. J., Cyhlarova E., and Puri B. K. (2003). Clinical and biochemical fatty acid abnormalities in dyslexia, dyspraxia and schizotypy: an overview. In: Peet M., Glen L., and Horrobin D. F. (eds.), *Phospholipid Spectrum Disorders in Psychiatry and Neurology*. Marius Press, Carnforth, Lancashire, pp. 477–490.

Rintala J., Seemann R., Chandrasekaran K., Rosenberger T. A., Chang L., Contreras M. A., Rapoport S. I., and Chang M. C. J. (1999). 85 kDa cytosolic phospholipase A_2 is a target for chronic lithium in rat brain. *NeuroReport* 10:3887–3890.

Rioux L. and Arnold S. E. (2005). The expression of retinoic acid receptor alpha is increased in the granule cells of the dentate gyrus in schizophrenia. *Psychiatry Res.* 133:13–21.

Ross B. M. (2003). Phospholipase A2-associated processes in the human brain and their role in neuropathology and psychopathology. In: Peet M., Glen L., and Horrobin D. F. (eds.), *Phospholipid Spectrum Disorders in Psychiatry and Neurology*. Marius Press, Carnforth, Lancashire, pp. 163–182.

Ross B. M. and Glen I. (2004). Prostaglandins and eicosanoids in the CNS. In: Curtis-Prior P. B. (ed.), *The Eicosanoids*. Wiley, London, pp. 434–441.

Ross B. M. and Turenne S. D. (2002). Chronic cocaine administration reduces phospholipase A_2 activity in rat brain striatum. *Prostaglandins Leukot. Essent. Fatty Acids* 66:479–483.

Ross B. M., Hudson C., Erlich J., Warsh J. J., and Kish S. J. (1997). Increased phospholipid breakdown in schizophrenia — evidence for the involvement of a calcium-independent phospholipase A_2. *Arch. Gen. Psychiatry* 54:487–494.

Ross B. M., Turenne S., Moszczynska A., Warsh J. J., and Kish S. J. (1999). Differential alteration of phospholipase A_2 activities in brain of patients with schizophrenia. *Brain Res.* 821:407–413.

Ross B. M., Brooks R. J., Lee M., Kalasinsky K. S., Vorce S. P., Seeman M., Fletcher P. J., and Turenne S. D. (2002a). Cyclooxygenase inhibitor modulation of dopamine-related behaviours. *Eur. J. Pharmacol.* 450:141–151.

Ross B. M., Moszczynska A., Peretti F. J., Adams V., Schmunk G. A., Kalasinsky K. S., Ang L., Mamalias N., Turenne S. D., and Kish S. J. (2002b). Decreased activity of brain phospholipid metabolic enzymes in human users of cocaine and methamphetamine. *Drug Alcohol Depend.* 67:73–79.

Ross B. M., McKenzie I., Glen I., and Bennett C. P. W. (2003). Increased levels of ethane, a non-invasive marker of n-3 fatty acid oxidation, in breath of children with attention deficit hyperactivity disorder. *Nutr. Neurosci.* 6:277–281.

Rybakowski J. K., Borkowska A., Czerski P. M., Dmitrzak-Weglarz M., and Hauser J. (2003). The study of cytosolic phospholipase A$_2$ gene polymorphism in schizophrenia using eye movement disturbances as an endophenotypic marker. *Neuropsychobiology* 47:115–119.

Samad T. A., Krezel W., Chambon P., and Borrelli E. (1997). Regulation of dopaminergic pathways by retinoids: activation of the D2 receptor promoter by members of the retinoic acid receptor-retinoid X receptor family. *Proc. Natl Acad. Sci. USA* 94:14349–14354.

Sarmiento I. A., Stoll A. L., and Cohen B. M. (2003). The role of essential lipids in the management of bipolar disorder. In: Peet M., Glen L., and Horrobin D. F. (eds.), *Phospholipid Spectrum Disorders in Psychiatry and Neurology.* Marius Press, Carnforth, Lancashire, pp. 457–462.

Sastry P. S. and Rao K. S. (2000). Apoptosis and the nervous system. *J. Neurochem.* 74:1–20.

Schmitt A., Maras A., Braus D. F., Petroianu G., Jatzko A., and Gattaz W. F. (2001). Antipsychotics and phospholipid metabolism in schizophrenia. *Fortschr. Neurol. Psychiatry* 69:503–509.

Serhan C. N. (2005). Novel eicosanoid and docosanoid mediators: resolvins, docosatrienes, and neuroprotectins. *Curr. Opin. Clin. Nutr. Metab. Care* 8:115–121.

Severus W. E., Littman A. B., and Stoll A. L. (2001). Omega-3 fatty acids, homocysteine, and the increased risk of cardiovascular mortality in major depressive disorder. *Harvard Rev. Psychiatry* 9:280–293.

Smesny S. (2004). Prostaglandin-mediated signaling in schizophrenia. In: Smythies J. (ed.), *Disorders of Synaptic Plasticity and Schizophrenia.* Academic Press Inc., San Diego, pp. 255–271.

Spencer T. J., Biederman J., Madras B. K., Faraone S. V., Dougherty D. D., Bonab A. A., and Fischman A. J. (2005). In vivo neuroreceptor imaging in attention-deficit/hyperactivity disorder: a focus on the dopamine transporter. *Biol. Psychiatry* 57:1293–1300.

Stanley J. A., Williamson P. C., Drost D. J., Carr T. J., Rylett R. J., Morrison-Stewart S., and Thompson R. T. (1994). Membrane phospholipid metabolism and schizophrenia: an in vivo 31P-MR spectroscopy study. *Schizophr. Res.* 13:209–215.

Stevens L. J., Zentall S. S., Deck J. L., Abate M. L., Watkins B. A., Lipp S. R., and Burgess J. R. (1995). Essential fatty acid metabolism in boys with attention-deficit hyperactivity disorder. *Am. J. Clin. Nutr.* 62:761–768.

Stevens L. J., Zentall S. S., Abate M. L., Kuczek T., and Burgess J. R. (1996). Omega-3 fatty acids in boys with behavior, learning, and health problems. *Physiol. Behav.* 59:915–920.

Stevens L., Zhang W., Peck L., Kuczek T., Grevstad N., Mahon A., Zentall S. S., Arnold L. E., and Burgess J. R. (2003). EFA supplementation in children with inattention, hyperactivity, and other disruptive behaviors. *Lipids* 38:1007–1021.

Stoll A. L., Severus W. E., Freeman M. P., Rueter S., Zboyan H. A., Diamond E., Cress K. K., and Marangell L. B. (1999). Omega 3 fatty acids in bipolar disorder: a preliminary double-blind, placebo-controlled trial. *Arch. Gen. Psychiatry* 56:407–412.

Stordy B. J. (1995). Benefit of docosahexaenoic acid supplements to dark adaptation in dyslexics. *Lancet* 346:385.

Tanskanen A., Hibbeln J. R., Hintikka J., Haatainen K., Honkalampi K., and Viinamaki H. (2001a). Fish consumption, depression, and suicidality in a general population. *Arch. Gen. Psychiatry* 58:512–513.

Tanskanen A., Hibbeln J. R., Tuomilehto J., Uutela A., Haukkala A., Viinamaki H., Lehtonen J., and Vartiainen E. (2001b). Fish consumption and depressive symptoms in the general population in Finland. *Psychiatr. Services* 52:529–531.

Taylor K. E. and Richardson A. J. (2000). Visual function, fatty acids and dyslexia. *Prostaglandins Leukot. Essent. Fatty Acids* 63:89–93.

Taylor K. E., Higgins C. J., Calvin C. M., Hall J. A., Easton T., McDaid A. M., and Richardson A. J. (2000). Dyslexia in adults is associated with clinical signs of fatty acid deficiency. *Prostaglandins Leukot. Essent. Fatty Acids* 63:75–78.

Timonen M., Horrobin D., Jokelainen J., Laitinen J., Herva A., and Rasanen P. (2004). Fish consumption and depression: the Northern Finland 1966 birth cohort study. *J. Affect. Disord.* 82:447–452.

Tuglu C., Kara S. H., Caliyurt O., Vardar E., and Abay E. (2003). Increased serum tumor necrosis factor-alpha levels and treatment response in major depressive disorder. *Psychopharmacology* (Berl.) 170:429–433.

Vaddadi K. S., Gilleard C. J., Soosai E., Polonowita A. K., Gibson R. A., and Burrows G. D. (1996). Schizophrenia, tardive dyskinesia and essential fatty acids. *Schizophr. Res.* 20:287–294.

Vancassel S., Durand G., Barthelemy C., Lejeune B., Martineau J., Guilloteau D., Andres C., and Chalon S. (2001). Plasma fatty acid levels in autistic children. Prostaglandins *Leukot. Essent. Fatty Acids* 65:1–7.

van West D. and Maes M. (2003). Fatty acid composition in major depression. In: Peet M., Glen L., and Horrobin D. F. (eds.), *Phospholipid Spectrum Disorders in Psychiatry and Neurology*. Marius Press, Carnforth, Lancashire, pp. 423–429.

Wan C., Yang Y., Feng G., Gu N., Liu H., Zhu S., He L., and Wang L. (2005). Polymorphisms of myelin-associated glycoprotein gene are associated with schizophrenia in the Chinese Han population. *Neurosci. Lett.* 388:126–131.

Ward P. E. (2000). Potential diagnostic aids for abnormal fatty acid metabolism in a range of neurodevelopmental disorders. *Prostaglandins Leukot. Essent. Fatty Acids* 63:65–68.

Weerasinghe G. R., Rapoport S. I., and Bosetti F. (2004). The effect of chronic lithium on arachidonic acid release and metabolism in rat brain does not involve secretory phospholipase A_2 or lipoxygenase/cytochrome P450 pathways. *Brain Res. Bull.* 63:485–489.

Yacubian J., de Castro C. C., Ometto M., Barbosa E., de Camargo C. P., Tavares H. J., Cerri G. G., and Gattaz W. F. (2002). P-31-spectroscopy of frontal lobe in schizophrenia: alterations in phospholipid and high-energy phosphate metabolism. *Schizophr. Res.* 58:117–122.

Yamamoto N., Saitoh M., Moriuchi A., Nomura M., and Okuyama H. (1987). Effect of dietary alpha-linolenic/linoleate balance on brain lipid compositions and learning ability of rats. *J. Lipid Res.* 28:144–151.

Yao J. K. and Van Kammen D. P. (2004). Membrane phospholipids and cytokine interaction in schizophrenia. In: Smythies J. (ed.), *Disorders of Synaptic Plasticity and Schizophrenia*. Academic Press Inc., San Diego, pp. 297–326.

Yao J. K., Van Kammen D. P., and Welker J. A. (1994). Red blood cell membrane dynamics in schizophrenia. II. Fatty acid composition. *Schizophr. Res.* 13:217–226.

Yao J. K., Leonard S., and Reddy R. D. (2000). Membrane phospholipid abnormalities in postmortem brains from schizophrenic patients. *Schizophr. Res.* 42:7–17.

Yao J. K., Magan S., Sonel A. F., Gurklis J. A., Sanders R., and Reddy R. D. (2004). Effects of omega-3 fatty acid on platelet serotonin responsivity in patients with schizophrenia. *Prostaglandins Leukot. Essent. Fatty Acids* 71:171–176.

Yildiz A., Sachs G. S., Dorer D. J., and Renshaw P. F. (2001). [31]P Nuclear magnetic resonance spectroscopy findings in bipolar illness: a meta-analysis. *Psychiatry Res.* 106:181–191.

Young G. S., Maharaj N. J., and Conquer J. A. (2004). Blood phospholipid fatty acid analysis of adults with and without Attention Deficit/Hyperactivity Disorder. *Lipids* 39:117–123.

Young G. S., Conquer J. A., and Thomas R. (2005). Effect of randomized supplementation with high dose olive, flax or fish oil on serum phospholipid fatty acid levels in adults with attention deficit hyperactivity disorder. *Reprod. Nutr. Dev.* 45:549–558.

14
Future Perspectives: Metabolic and Functional Aspects of Neural Membrane Glycerophospholipids

Glycerophospholipids are an integral component of neural membranes in which they exist in a dynamic flux, with continuous biosynthesis countered by continuous degradation. The turnover of acyl groups is much more rapid than thought previously. The consumption of ATP for glycerophospholipid metabolism in brain accounts for up to 20% of net brain ATP consumption (Purdon et al., 2002). Glycerophospholipid homeostasis is based on a balance between catabolism and re-synthesis in the reacylation/deacylation cycle and pathways for de novo synthesis (Farooqui et al., 2000a,b). The differential packing of phospholipids, glycolipids, cholesterol, and proteins leads to the formation of microdomains (lipid rafts), which diffuse laterally. These microdomains serve as mobile platforms for signal transduction, clustering and organizing bilayer constituents including receptors, enzymes, and ion-channels. This provides neural membranes with structural and functional integrity that facilitates the appropriate interactions with integral membrane proteins, which modulate their regular function and control adaptive responses (Ivanova et al., 2004). In general, the function of the signal transduction network is to convey extracellular signals from the cell surface to the nucleus to induce a biological response at the gene level.

Lipid mediators convey the messages and modulate the intensity of signal transduction processes associated with intracellular metabolism of glycerophospholipids and gene expression. Membranes sense temperature changes and control a regulatory loop with chaperone proteins. This loop seems to need the existence of specific membrane microdomains and also includes the association of chaperone (heat stress) proteins with the membrane (Vigh et al., 2005). Alterations in microdomains may be associated with various human pathologies such as cardiovascular disease, cancer, and neurodegenerative diseases (Vigh et al., 2005). Collectively, these studies suggest that neural membranes are not simply an inert physical barrier, but complex, well organized, and highly specialized structures involved in receiving, processing, transporting, and transmitting information, not only from the plasma membrane to the nucleus, but also from one cell to another.

Two fundamental questions related to glycerophospholipid metabolism in neural membranes remain unresolved. First, what mechanisms regulate the composition and total content of glycerophospholipids in membranes of neurons, astrocytes, oligodendrocytes, and microglia? To respond to this question, one must have complete knowledge of the biosynthesis of each molecular species of glycerophospholipids in various pools of brain tissue. Second, how do glycerophospholipids move between membranes of different subcellular organelles in neurons, astrocytes, and oligodendrocytes? For example, the synthesis of glycerophospholipids mainly occurs in the endoplasmic reticulum (ER). Membranes of other subcellular organelles are not capable of synthesizing their own glycerophospholipids. Therefore, the intracellular transport and sorting of glycerophospholipids from the site of synthesis (ER) to their final destination is an essential event in glycerophospholipid metabolism. Several mechanisms have been proposed for glycerophospholipid transport and sorting including carrier proteins, transport vesicles, and contact zones between donor and acceptor membranes (Vallée et al., 1999; Voelker, 2003; Oram et al., 2003), but the specificity and modulation of mechanisms associated with the transport process and its regulation by specific genes remains unknown (Van Meer and Sprong, 2004).

The development of mutant neural cell lines with defective glycerophospholipid trafficking and sorting would help in the identification of genes associated with glycerophospholipid trafficking and sorting, and would also provide information on the molecular mechanisms involved in modulation of glycerophospholipid trafficking and sorting (Voelker, 2004). For example, genetic analysis studies of the amino glycerophospholipid transport process are now providing important new information about specific proteins and lipid components that are involved (Voelker, 2003).

Decarboxylation of PtdSer to PtdEtn is a biochemical indicator of transport from the ER to mitochondria. The transport of PtdSer to the locus of PtdSer decarboxylase-2 in mitochondria requires phosphatidylinositol-4-kinase, phosphatidylinositol-binding protein, and the C2 domain of the PtdSer decarboxylase-2. PtdSer transport to mitochondria is modulated by ubiquitination via the action of the ubiquitin ligase subunit Met30p (Voelker, 2005). Mutant strains with lesions in the MET30 gene are defective in PtdSer transport and exhibit altered ubiquitination of specific target proteins. Collectively these studies support a model in which specific proteins and lipids are required for PtdSer transport.

In contrast, studies on PtdCho transport demonstrate the involvement of the prevacuolar compartment and a requirement for multiple genes associated with the regulation of protein sorting for transport of the phospholipids to the vacuole (Voelker, 2004). Thus, detailed investigations are required not only on transport machinery of other glycerophospholipids but also on segregation of membrane glycerophospholipids for microdomain formation and mechanism of sorting at various stages of the secretory and endocytic pathways in developing adult brains (Voelker, 2003, 2004).

Lipidomics has emerged as an important technology for the identification and full characterization of glycerophospholipid molecular species found in developing, adult, and aging brain (Piomelli, 2005; Lee et al., 2005). Synaptic function and signal transduction processes depend on the temporal and spatially coordinated interactions between lipid mediators with their receptors and on their inter-relationships with the organization of lipid mediator network. Recent advances in shotgun lipidomics and multidimensional mass spectrometry will provide new insights into the roles of phospholipid molecular species in neuronal function (Gross et al., 2005). With the development of proteomics technology and DNA microarray analysis one can not only identify specific genes involved in regulation of biosynthesis of individual molecular species of glycerophospholipid, but also identify genes related to its sorting and transport (Voelker, 2003; Forrester et al., 2004; Lee et al., 2005).

Another technique that can provide useful information on rates of glycerophospholipid metabolic pathways is quantitative autoradiography or positron emission tomography (PET) (Rapoport, 1999, 2005). This procedure utilizes incorporation of fatty acids labeled with a radioactive or heavy isotope followed by determination of its distribution in brain regions and their lipid compartments as a function of time. From measurements, fluxes, turnover rates, half-lives, and ATP consumption rates, fatty acid metabolism in vivo can be determined and its incorporation can be imaged. This technique has provided information on metabolism in vivo of palmitic acid, arachidonic acid, and docosahexaenoic acid metabolism in rat brain (Rapoport, 1999, 2005). Based on the in vivo metabolism of these fatty acids, PET is used to image brain signaling and neuroplasticity in humans in health and diseases. Initial experiments on animal models of Alzheimer and Parkinson disease with chronic unilateral lesions of nucleus basalis or substantia nigra indicate that PET and [^{11}C]arachidonic acid can be used with drug activation to image signal transduction. Detailed investigations are required on the use of MRI along with PET imaging to judge the severity and progression of dementia during the course of various neurodegenerative diseases in patients and normal human subjects (Rapoport, 2001; Hampel et al., 2002).

Only a few enzymes of glycerophospholipid metabolism have been purified and characterized from brain tissue (Hirashima et al., 1992; Negre-Aminou et al., 1996; Pete et al., 1994; Pete and Exton, 1996; Yang et al., 1999). Proteomics and molecular biological approaches such as cloning the cDNA for enzymes synthesizing and degrading glycerophospholipids and functionally expressing them in neurons, astrocytes, oligodendrocytes, and microglia will advance the understanding of glycerophospholipid metabolism at cellular and subcellular levels in brain tissue. The use of proteomics and genomics will lead to the identification and expression profile of genes involved in the modulation of enzymes associated with the synthesis and degradation of glycerophospholipids in neurons and glial cells (Hovland et al., 2001) and also in monitoring alterations in gene expression profiles in neurodegenerative diseases (Colangelo et al., 2002; Thomas et al., 2006).

Furthermore, the development of mice deficient in specific enzyme(s) of glycerophospholipids will provide animal models for diseases involving defective glycerophospholipid metabolism, which will also result in better understanding of roles of glycerophospholipid species in neural membranes (Uozumi and Shimizu, 2002; Bonventre and Sapirstein, 2002). Although considerable information is available on cPLA$_2$-α gene deletion in the mouse (Bonventre et al., 1997; Klivenyi et al., 1998; Uozumi and Shimizu, 2002; Rosenberger et al., 2003), only one case of an inherited cPLA$_2$-α deficiency in a 45-year-old male with chronic gastrointestinal blood loss and recurrent small intestinal ulcers has been reported (Adler et al., 2006). It is not known whether the mechanism by which a deficiency of cPLA$_2$-α exerts its effect on brain and other tissues in mice and humans is similar or not. Thus, detailed comparative studies using lipidomics and proteomics can provide information on the mechanisms involved. This information would be useful in developing drugs that target cPLA$_2$-α (see below). Similarly, mice over-expressing enzymes associated with glycerophospholipid metabolism and neural cells transfected with genes overexpressing glycerophospholipid metabolizing enzymes can provide model system analogous to neurological disorders.

Although transcripts, activities, and immunoreactive proteins for enzymes synthesizing and degrading glycerophospholipids are widely expressed throughout the brain (Zanassi et al., 1998; Molloy et al., 1998; Kishimoto et al., 1999; Balboa et al., 2002; Phillis and O'Regan, 2004), very little is known about their interactions with each other at cellular and subcellular levels in neurons and glial cells. Proteomics-related procedures are available for the purification and characterization of these enzymes. The genes that encode them can be identified and mapped to chromosomes by genomics and genetic analysis procedures. Identification of substrates (molecular species) for PLA$_2$, PLC, and PLD in brain tissue can provide information about turnover in vivo and phospholipid homeostasis in neural membranes of neurons and glial cells. The occurrence of isoforms of enzymes degrading glycerophospholipids, such as PLA$_2$, PLC, PLD, and their downstream enzymes, cyclooxygenases, lipoxygenases, and epoxygenases, in cytoplasm, and plasma and nuclear membranes complicates the analysis of their function at cellular and subcellular levels. Future studies on this multiplicity using lipidomics and proteomics will provide information on the diversity of their function and selectivity of molecular species as substrates and on the way neural cells utilize arachidonic acid and docosahexaenoic acid for the production of eicosanoids and docosanoids in response to a wide range of extracellular signals (Serhan, 2005a,b; Bazan, 2005a,b). An important question that must be addressed in future studies is what factors determine the specificity of neural cell responses at subcellular and microdomain levels and how much of this specificity is dictated by the interplay among second messengers generated by PLA$_2$, PLC, and PLD. Thus, more studies are required to understand the metabolic significance of the interplay among PLA$_2$, PLC, and PLD at nuclear and non-nuclear levels in cultured cells of neuronal and glial origin and in nuclear and non-nuclear preparations of neural cells in developing, adult, and aging brains.

Many enzymes related to glycerophospholipid metabolism have C2 domains. These enzymes include protein kinases, phospholipases A$_2$, lipoxygenases, GTPases and proteins involved in membrane trafficking (Davletov et al., 1998; Cafiso, 2005). These domains facilitate the docking of enzymes to their glycerophospholipid substrate on the surface in the presence of Ca^{2+}. Some enzymes dock on membrane surfaces through ionic interactions with PtdSer, whilst others, such as PLA$_2$ and 5-lipoxygenase, employ a hydrophobic mechanism using neutral phospholipids like PtdCho (Perisic et al., 1999). Currently, the structure of the interface formed between the enzyme and glycerophospholipid bilayer is not accessible to high-resolution structure determination. However, a combination of high-resolution structural investigations and NMR and EPR studies and fluorescence quenching by spin-labeled glycerophospholipids can provide information on the nature and mechanism of docking of enzymes containing a C2 domain on bilayer phospholipids (Malmberg et al., 2003; Cafiso, 2005).

The interactions among metabolites generated by PLA_2, PLC, or PLD at plasma membrane, cytoplasmic and nuclear membrane levels (Fig. 14.1) may provide neural cells and brain tissue with great versatility in ensuring that arachidonic acid and docosahexaenoic acid are efficiently utilized in brain tissue (Farooqui and Horrocks, 2005, 2006). It is tempting to speculate that coordinated cross-talk, not only among PLA_2, PLC, and PLD and downstream cyclooxygenase and lipoxygenase isozymes (Farooqui and Horrocks, 2005; Phillis et al., 2006), but also with upstream acyltransferases and cytidylyltransferases (Karim et al., 2003), is essential for maintaining normal neuronal and glial cell growth. In the nuclear membrane and nucleus, signaling mediated by PLA_2, PLC, and PLD has the advantage over plasma membrane signaling in that second messengers generated by these enzymes during differentiation may directly interact with nuclear factors producing physiological responses and morphological changes (Farooqui et al., 2000b). In brain tissue, activities of isoforms of enzymes synthesizing and degrading phospholipids depend on not only the structural, physicochemical, and dynamic properties of neural membranes, but also on the type and metabolic state of neural cells. The activation of PLA_2, PLC, and PLD isoforms at the subcellular level is the rate-limiting step for the generation of lipid mediators such as eicosanoids, docosanoids, platelet-activating factor, diacylglycerols, and lysophosphatidic acid (Fukami, 2002; Banno, 2002; Farooqui and Horrocks, 2004). Therefore, tight regulation of PLA_2, PLC, PLD and their downstream cyclooxygenases, lipoxygenases, and epoxygenases and upstream acyltransferases and cytidylyltransferases at subcellular and microdomain levels is very important for normal brain function (Farooqui et al., 2004).

The complexity of signal transduction processes associated with multiple forms of PLA_2, PLC, PLD, and enzymes metabolizing arachidonic acid becomes obvious when one considers the coupling mechanisms of various isoforms with different receptors at cellular and subcellular levels and tries to relate them to neuronal and glial cell functions. To understand the contribution of isoforms of PLA_2, PLC, and PLD in physiological and disease processes, a systematic approach is necessary to identify the phospholipid substrates (molecular species) and the second messengers and signaling pathways by which each isoform couples to its receptor in neuronal and glial cells at various subcellular levels. Some isoforms of the above enzymes are constitutively expressed whereas others are inducible in response to cytokines and growth factors (Farooqui and Horrocks, 2005). These isoforms may not function interchangeably but act in parallel to transducer signals. It is likely that various isoforms of PLA_2, PLC, PLD, cyclooxygenases, lipoxygenases, and epoxygenases act on different cellular pools of arachidonic and docosahexaenoic acids located in different subcellular

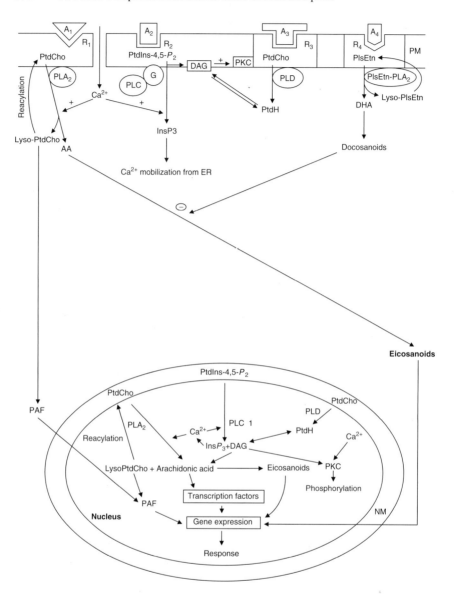

FIG. 14.1. A hypothetical diagram showing the existence of independent glycerophospholipid metabolism in plasma membrane (PM) and nucleus (NM). Plasma membrane (PM); agonists (A$_1$, A$_2$, A$_3$, and A$_4$); receptors (R$_1$, R$_2$, R$_3$, and R$_4$); phosphatidylcholine (PtdCho); phosphatidylinositol 4,5-bisphosphate (PtdIns (4,5)P$_2$); diacylglycerol (DAG); ethanolamine plasmalogen (PlsEtn); phospholipase A$_2$ (PLA$_2$); phospholipase C (PLC), phospholipase D (PLD); plasmalogen-selective phospholipase A$_2$ (PlsEtn-PLA$_2$); lysophosphatidylcholine (lyso-PtdCho); inositol 1,4,5-trisphosphate (InsP$_3$); phosphatidic acid (PtdH); ethanolamine lysoplasmalogen (lyso-PlsEtn); arachidonic acid (AA), docosahexaenoic acid (DHA); protein kinase C (PKC), and endoplasmic reticulum (ER). Nuclear membrane (NM); platelet activating factor (PAF); and all other abbreviations are same as plasma membrane.

organelles of various types of neural cells. Different coupling mechanisms may regulate these isoforms, generating common second messengers. Intracellular signaling cascades involving multiple forms of PLA_2, PLC, and PLD can no longer be viewed as a linear pathway that relays information from the outer cell surface to intracellular organelles. Neural cells use these enzymes to regulate multiple functions. Coordination and integration of second messengers produced by PLA_2, PLC, and PLD isozymes in various subcellular compartments is necessary for optimal functioning of signal transduction processes.

Elevated activities of PLA_2, PLC, and PLD are important in the inflammation and oxidative stress associated with numerous acute and chronic neurological disorders (Farooqui et al., 2000c, 2006; Phillis and O'Regan, 2004; Kim et al., 2004; Jin et al., 2005; Farooqui and Horrocks, 2006). For their treatment, the development of specific inhibitors of PLA_2, C, and D that can cross the blood-brain barrier without harm would be important. The approach for designing inhibitors of enzymes of glycerophospholipid metabolism should be based on our rapidly emerging concept of signal transduction pathways in neurological disorders. Better drug delivery systems that target brain need to be developed to protect PLA_2, PLC, and PLD inhibitors from in vivo degradation or detoxification. Drugs delivered through these drug delivery systems must reach the site where inflammatory processes are taking place (Yoshikawa et al., 1999; Andresen and Jorgensen, 2005). This would enhance their efficacy. The effects of these drugs on genes can be monitored by microarray procedures (Colangelo et al., 2002; Bosetti et al., 2005). These studies can lead to better therapeutic agents for the treatment of neurological disorders involving glycerophospholipid alterations. The next 25 years should witness the understanding of the role of glycerophospholipid molecular species in metabolic processes in brain tissue (Farooqui et al., 2002), and the development of concepts based on signal transduction for the molecular mechanisms utilized in intracellular glycerophospholipid trafficking, sorting, and metabolic regulation at cellular and subcellular levels in normal as well as diseased neural cells.

References

Adler D. H., Phillips J. A. I., Cogan J. D., Morrow I. D., Boutaud O., and Oates J. A. (2006). First description: cytosolic phospholipase A_2-alpha deficiency. *J. Invest. Med.* 54:S257.

Andresen T. L. and Jorgensen K. (2005). Synthesis and membrane behavior of a new class of unnatural phospholipid analogs useful as phospholipase A2 degradable liposomal drug carriers. *Biochim. Biophys. Acta Biomembr.* 1669:1–7.

Balboa M. A., Varela-Nieto I., Lucas K. K., and Dennis E. A. (2002). Expression and function of phospholipase A_2 in brain. *FEBS Lett.* 531:12–17.

Banno Y. (2002). Regulation and possible role of mammalian phospholipase D in cellular functions. *J. Biochem. (Tokyo)* 131:301–306.

Bazan N. G. (2005a). Lipid signaling in neural plasticity, brain repair, and neuroprotection. *Mol. Neurobiol.* 32:89–103.

Bazan N. G. (2005b). Neuroprotectin D1 (NPD1): a DHA-derived mediator that protects brain and retina against cell injury-induced oxidative stress. *Brain Pathol.* 15:159–166.

Bonventre J. V. and Sapirstein A. (2002). Group IV cytosolic phospholipase A_2 (PLA_2) function: Insights from the knockout mouse. In: Honn K. V., Marnett L. J., Nigam S., Dennis E., and Serhan C. (eds.), *Eicosanoids and Other Bioactive Lipids in Cancer, Inflammation, and Radiation Injury, 5.* Kluwer Academic/Plenum Publ., New York, pp. 25–31.

Bonventre J. V., Huang Z. H., Taheri M. R., O'Leary E., Li E., Moskowitz M. A., and Sapirstein A. (1997). Reduced fertility and postischaemic brain injury in mice deficient in cytosolic phospholipase A_2. *Nature* 390:622–625.

Bosetti F., Bell J. M., and Manickam P. (2005). Microarray analysis of rat brain gene expression after chronic administration of sodium valproate. *Brain Res. Bull.* 65:331–338.

Cafiso D. S. (2005). Structure and interactions of C2 domains at membrane surfaces. In: Tamm L. K. (ed.), *Membrane Domains to Cellular Networks.* Wiley-VCH Verlag GmbH, Weinheim, pp. 403–422.

Colangelo V., Schurr J., Ball M. J., Pelaez R. P., Bazan N. G., and Lukiw W. J. (2002). Gene expression profiling of 12633 genes in Alzheimer hippocampal CA1: transcription and neurotrophic factor down-regulation and up-regulation of apoptotic and pro-inflammatory signaling. *J. Neurosci. Res.* 70:462–473.

Davletov B., Perisic O., and Williams R. L. (1998). Calcium-dependent membrane penetration is a hallmark of the C2 domain of cytosolic phospholipase A_2 whereas the C2A domain of synaptotagmin binds membranes electrostatically. *J. Biol. Chem.* 273:19093–19096.

Farooqui A. A. and Horrocks L. A. (2004). Brain phospholipases A_2: a perspective on the history. *Prostaglandins Leukot. Essent. Fatty Acids* 71:161–169.

Farooqui A. A. and Horrocks L. A. (2005). Signaling and interplay mediated by phospholipases A_2, C, and D in LA-N-1 cell nuclei. *Reprod. Nutr. Dev.* 45:613–631.

Farooqui A. A. and Horrocks L. A. (2006). Phospholipase A_2-generated lipid mediators in brain: the good, the bad, and the ugly. *Neuroscientist* 12:245.

Farooqui A. A., Horrocks L. A., and Farooqui T. (2000a). Deacylation and reacylation of neural membrane glycerophospholipids. *J. Mol. Neurosci.* 14:123–135.

Farooqui A. A., Horrocks L. A., and Farooqui T. (2000b). Glycerophospholipids in brain: their metabolism, incorporation into membranes, functions, and involvement in neurological disorders. *Chem. Phys. Lipids* 106:1–29.

Farooqui A. A., Ong W. Y., Horrocks L. A., and Farooqui T. (2000c). Brain cytosolic phospholipase A_2: localization, role, and involvement in neurological diseases. *Neuroscientist* 6:169–180.

Farooqui A. A., Farooqui T., and Horrocks L. A. (2002). Molecular species of phospholipids during brain development. Their occurrence, separation and roles. In: Skinner E. R. (ed.), *Brain Lipids and Disorders in Biological Psychiatry.* Elsevier Science B.V., Amsterdam, pp. 147–158.

Farooqui A. A., Antony P., Ong W. Y., Horrocks L. A., and Freysz L. (2004). Retinoic acid-mediated phospholipase A_2 signaling in the nucleus. *Brain Res. Rev.* 45:179–195.

Farooqui A. A., Ong W. Y., and Horrocks L. A. (2006). Inhibitors of brain phospholipase A_2 activity: their neuropharmacologic effects and therapeutic importance for the treatment of neurologic disorders. *Pharm. Rev.* (in press).

Forrester J. S., Milne S. B., Ivanova P. T., and Brown H. A. (2004). Computational lipidomics: a multiplexed analysis of dynamic changes in membrane lipid composition during signal transduction. *Mol. Pharmacol.* 65:813–821.

Fukami K. (2002). Structure, regulation, and function of phospholipase C isozymes. *J. Biochem. (Tokyo)* 131:293–299.

Gross R. W., Jenkins C. M., Yang J. Y., Mancuso D. J., and Han X. L. (2005). Functional lipidomics: the roles of specialized lipids and lipid–protein interactions in modulating neuronal function. *Prostaglandins Other Lipid Mediat.* 77:52–64.

Hampel H., Teipel S. J., Alexander G. E., Pogarell O., Rapoport S. I., and Moller H. J. (2002). In vivo imaging of region and cell type specific neocortical neurodegeneration in Alzheimer's disease — perspectives of MRI derived corpus callosum measurement for mapping disease progression and effects of therapy. Evidence from studies with MRI, EEG and PET. *J. Neural Transm.* 109:837–855.

Hirashima Y., Farooqui A. A., Mills J. S., and Horrocks L. A. (1992). Identification and purification of calcium-independent phospholipase A_2 from bovine brain cytosol. *J. Neurochem.* 59:708–714.

Hovland A. R., Nahreini P., Andreatta C. P., Edwards-Prasad J., and Prasad K. N. (2001). Identifying genes involved in regulating differentiation of neuroblastoma cells. *J. Neurosci. Res.* 64:302–310.

Ivanova P. T., Milne S. B., Forrester J. S., and Brown H. A. (2004). Lipid arrays: new tools in the understanding of membrane dynamics and lipid signaling. *Mol. Interv.* 4:86–96.

Jin J. K., Kim N. H., Min D. S., Kim J. I., Choi J. K., Jeong B. H., Choi S. I., Choi E. K., Carp R. I., and Kim Y. S. (2005). Increased expression of phospholipase D1 in the brains of scrapie-infected mice. *J. Neurochem.* 92:452–461.

Karim M., Jackson P., and Jackowski S. (2003). Gene structure, expression and identification of a new CTP:phosphocholine cytidylyltransferase isoform. *Biochim. Biophys. Acta Mol. Cell Biol. Lipids* 1633:1–12.

Kim M. D., Min D. S., Sim K. B., Cho H. J., and Shin T. (2004). Expression and potential role of phospholipase D1 in cryoinjured cerebral cortex of rats. *Histol. Histopathol.* 19:1015–1019.

Kishimoto K., Matsumura K., Kataoka Y., Morii H., and Watanabe Y. (1999). Localization of cytosolic phospholipase A_2 messenger RNA mainly in neurons in the rat brain. *Neuroscience* 92:1061–1077.

Klivenyi P., Beal M. F., Ferrante R. J., Andreassen O. A., Wermer M., Chin M. R., and Bonventre J. V. (1998). Mice deficient in group IV cytosolic phospholipase A_2 are resistant to MPTP neurotoxicity. *J. Neurochem.* 71:2634–2637.

Lee S. H., Williams M. V., and Blair I. A. (2005). Targeted chiral lipidomics analysis. *Prostaglandins Other Lipid Mediat.* 77:141–157.

Malmberg N. J., Van Buskirk D. R., and Falke J. J. (2003). Membrane-docking loops of the cPLA2 C2 domain: detailed structural analysis of the protein–membrane interface via site-directed spin-labeling. *Biochemistry* 42:13227–13240.

Molloy G. Y., Rattray M., and Williams R. J. (1998). Genes encoding multiple forms of phospholipase A_2 are expressed in rat brain. *Neurosci. Lett.* 258:139–142.

Negre-Aminou P., Nemenoff R. A., Wood M. R., de la Houssaye B. A., and Pfenninger K. H. (1996). Characterization of phospholipase A_2 activity enriched in the nerve growth cone. *J. Neurochem.* 67:2599–2608.

Oram J. F., Wolfbauer G., Vaughan A. M., Tang C. R., and Albers J. J. (2003). Phospholipid transfer protein interacts with and stabilizes ATP-binding cassette transporter A1 and enhances cholesterol efflux from cells. *J. Biol. Chem.* 278:52379–52385.

Perisic O., Paterson H. F., Mosedale G., Lara-González S., and Williams R. L. (1999). Mapping the phospholipid-binding surface and translocation determinants of the C2 domain from cytosolic phospholipase A_2. *J. Biol. Chem.* 274:14979–14987.

Pete M. J. and Exton J. H. (1996). Purification of a lysophospholipase from bovine brain that selectively deacylates arachidonoyl-substituted lysophosphatidylcholine. *J. Biol. Chem.* 271:18114–18121.

Pete M. J., Ross A. H., and Exton J. H. (1994). Purification and properties of phospholipase A₁ from bovine brain. *J. Biol. Chem.* 269:19494–19500.

Phillis J. W. and O'Regan M. H. (2004). A potentially critical role of phospholipases in central nervous system ischemic, traumatic, and neurodegeneretive disorders. *Brain Res. Rev.* 44:13–47.

Phillis J. W., Horrocks L. A., and Farooqui A. A. (2006). Cyclooxygenases, lipoxygenases, and epoxygenases in CNS: their role and involvement in neurological disorders. *Brain Res. Rev.* (in press).

Piomelli D. (2005). The challenge of brain lipidomics. *Prostaglandins Other Lipid Mediat.* 77:23–34.

Purdon A. D., Rosenberger T. A., Shetty H. U., and Rapoport S. I. (2002). Energy consumption by phospholipid metabolism in mammalian brain. *Neurochem. Res.* 27:1641–1647.

Rapoport S. I. (1999). In vivo fatty acid incorporation into brain phospholipids in relation to signal transduction and membrane remodeling. *Neurochem. Res.* 24:1403–1415.

Rapoport S. I. (2001). In vivo fatty acid incorporation into brain phospholipids in relation to plasma availability, signal transduction and membrane remodeling. *J. Mol. Neurosci.* 16:243–261.

Rapoport S. I. (2005). In vivo approaches and rationale for quantifying kinetics and imaging brain lipid metabolic pathways. *Prostaglandins Other Lipid Mediat.* 77:185–196.

Rosenberger T. A., Villacreses N. E., Contreras M. A., Bonventre J. V., and Rapoport S. I. (2003). Brain lipid metabolism in the cPLA₂ knockout mouse. *J. Lipid Res.* 44:109–117.

Serhan C. N. (2005a). Novel eicosanoid and docosanoid mediators: resolvins, docosatrienes, and neuroprotectins. *Curr. Opin. Clin. Nutr. Metab. Care* 8:115–121.

Serhan C. N. (2005b). Novel ω-3-derived local mediators in anti-inflammation and resolution. *Pharmacol. Ther.* 105:7–21.

Thomas D. M., Francescutti-Verbeem D. M., and Kuhn D. M. (2006). Gene expression profile of activated microglia under conditions associated with dopamine neuronal damage. *FASEB J.* 20:515–517.

Uozumi N. and Shimizu T. (2002). Roles for cytosolic phospholipase A₂α as revealed by gene-targeted mice. *Prostaglandins Other Lipid Mediat.* 68–69:59–69.

Vallée B., Teyssier C., Maget-Dana R., Ramstein J., Bureaud N., and Schoentgen F. (1999). Stability and physicochemical properties of the bovine brain phosphatidylethanolamine-binding protein. *Eur. J. Biochem.* 266:40–52.

Van Meer G. and Sprong H. (2004). Membrane lipids and vesicular traffic. *Curr. Opin. Cell Biol.* 16:373–378.

Vigh L., Escriba P. V., Sonnleitner A., Sonnleitner M., Piotto S., Maresca B., Horvath I., and Harwood J. L. (2005). The significance of lipid composition for membrane activity: new concepts and ways of assessing function. *Prog. Lipid Res.* 44:303–344.

Voelker D. R. (2003). New perspectives on the regulation of intermembrane glycerophospholipid traffic. *J. Lipid Res.* 44:441–449.

Voelker D. R. (2004). Genetic analysis of intracellular aminoglycerophospholipid traffic. *Biochem. Cell Biol.* 82:156–169.

Voelker D. R. (2005). Protein and lipid motifs regulate phosphatidylserine traffic in yeast. *Biochem. Soc. Trans.* 33:1141–1145.

Yang H. C., Mosior M., Ni B., and Dennis E. A. (1999). Regional distribution, ontogeny, purification, and characterization of the Ca²⁺-independent phospholipase A₂ from rat brain. *J. Neurochem.* 73:1278–1287.

Yoshikawa T., Sakaeda T., Sugawara T., Hirano K., and Stella V. J. (1999). A novel chemical delivery system for brain targeting. *Adv. Drug Deliv. Rev.* 36:255–275.

Zanassi P., Paolillo M., and Schinelli S. (1998). Coexpression of phospholipase A₂ isoforms in rat striatal astrocytes. *Neurosci. Lett.* 247:83–86.

Index

Page numbers followed by f and t indicate figures and tables, respectively

Printed in the United States of America